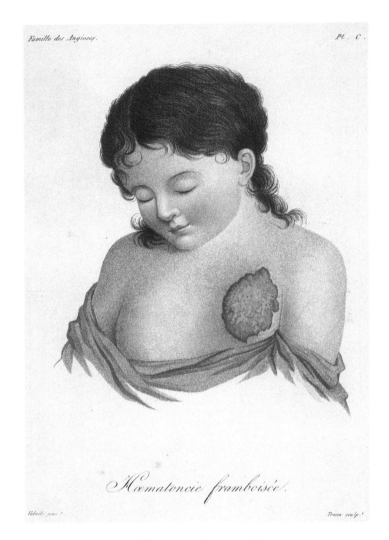

Famille des Angioses.   Pl. C.

Hœmatoncie framboisée.

Valois pinx.t   Troxcn sculp.t

From Alibert's *Nosologie Naturelle*, 1817

VASCULAR BIRTHMARKS

Hemangiomas and Malformations

John B. Mulliken
M.D., F.A.C.S.

Associate Professor of Surgery
Harvard Medical School

Children's Hospital and
Brigham and Women's Hospital
Boston, Massachusetts

Anthony E. Young
M.A., M. Chir., F.R.C.S.

Consultant Surgeon
St. Thomas' Hospital
London, England

1988

W. B. SAUNDERS COMPANY
Harcourt Brace Jovanovich, Inc.

Philadelphia   London   Toronto   Montreal   Sydney   Tokyo

W. B. SAUNDERS COMPANY
Harcourt Brace Jovanovich, Inc.

The Curtis Center
Independence Square West
Philadelphia, PA 19106-3399

Library of Congress Cataloging-in-Publication Data

Mulliken, John B.

Vascular birthmarks.

Includes index.

1. Birthmarks.   2. Hemangioma.   3. Blood-vessels—
   Abnormalities.   I. Young, Anthony E.   II. Title.
   [DNLM: 1. Arteriovenous Malformations.
   2. Hemangioma. WG 500 M959v]

RL793.M84 1988   616.1'48   88–3143

ISBN 0–7216–6601–9

Editor: Lisa McAllister
Designer: W. B. Saunders Staff
Production Manager: Peter Faber
Manuscript Editor: Tom Stringer
Illustration Coordinator: Peg Shaw
Indexer: Ellen Murray

Vascular Birthmarks: Hemangiomas and Malformations   ISBN 0–7216–6601–9

Last digit is the print number: 9   8   7   6   5   4   3   2   1

Contributors

Michael J. Aminoff, M.D., F.R.C.P.

Professor of Neurology, University of California; Attending Physician and Director, Clinical Neurophysiology Laboratories, University of California Medical Center, San Francisco, California.

Vascular Malformations of the Central Nervous System

Alexandra M. Harrison, M.D.

Clinical Instructor in Psychiatry, Harvard Medical School, Boston, Massachusetts; Faculty, Cambridge Hospital Child Psychiatry Training Program, Cambridge, Massachusetts.

The Emotional Impact of a Vascular Birthmark

Jean-Jacques Merland, M.D.

Professor, University of Paris VII; Chief of the Department of Neuroradiology, Hôpital Lariboisière, University of Paris VII, Paris, France.

Embolization of Vascular Malformations

John B. Mulliken, M.D., F.A.C.S.

Associate Professor of Surgery, Harvard Medical School; Director of Craniofacial Centre, Division of Plastic Surgery, Children's Hospital and Brigham and Women's Hospital, Boston, Massachusetts.

Vascular Birthmarks in Folklore, History, Art, and Literature; Classification of Vascular Birthmarks; Diagnosis and Natural History of Hemangiomas; Pathogenesis of Hemangiomas; Treatment of Hemangiomas; Capillary (Port-Wine) and Other Telangiectatic Stains; Vascular Malformations of the Head and Neck

Joel M. Noe, M.D., F.A.C.S.

Clinical Assistant Professor of Surgery (Plastic Surgery), Harvard Medical School; Associate Surgeon, Beth Israel Hospital, Boston, Massachusetts.

Laser Therapy of Port-Wine Stains

Marie-Claire Riché, M.D.

Chef de Clinique, Neuroradiology and Therapeutic Angiography, Hôpital Lariboisière, University of Paris VII, Paris, France.

Embolization of Vascular Malformations

M. Lea Thomas, M.A., Ph.D. (Cantab.), F.R.C.P. (Lond.), F.R.C.R., D.M.R.D.

Lecturer, United Medical and Dental Schools of Guy's and St. Thomas' Hospitals; Clinical Teacher, Faculty of Medicine, University of London; Senior Physician in Radiology, St. Thomas' Hospital, London, England.

Radiological Assessment of Vascular Malformations

Joseph Upton, III, M.D., F.A.C.S.

Assistant Professor of Surgery, Harvard Medical School; Associate in Surgery, Division of Plastic Surgery, Children's Hospital and Brigham and Women's Hospital, Boston, Massachusetts.

Vascular Malformations of the Upper Limb

Anthony E. Young, M.A., M. Chir., F.R.C.S.

Consultant Surgeon, St. Thomas' Hospital, London, England.

Vascular Birthmarks in Folklore, History, Art, and Literature; Pathogenesis of Vascular Malformations; Clinical Assessment of Vascular Malformations; Investigation of Vascular Malformations; Venous and Arterial Malformations; Lymphatic Malformations; Arteriovenous Malformations; Combined Vascular Malformations; Intra-abdominal and Pelvic Malformations; Vascular Malformations of the Lower Limb

Preface

Of every three children born, one will have a vascular birthmark, a red, blue, or purple blemish. The great majority of these stains will fade or remain small and inconsequential. One child in a hundred will have a vascular birthmark that requires an opinion from a doctor or referral to a specialist. Fortunately, gross and disfiguring lesions are rare; however, many of these patients will become, in a sense, medical nomads, searching for someone who understands their problems. The primary practitioner, whether he be a family physician, pediatrician, or surgeon, will usually have had little or no experience with diagnosis and management of the uncommon vascular birthmarks. It is to these doctors, together with those familiar and fascinated, that this book is directed.

Parents with blemished or malformed children put enormous pressures on medical advisors. The burden of perinatal anxiety is such that early and accurate diagnosis and prognosis are essential. At the earliest opportunity, parents should be given some indication of what the future may hold, including what kind of treatment may be feasible or necessary. Our experience has been that both the referring physician and the referral clinic may lack the expertise to give this advice, and that months or even years can elapse before the patient reaches someone familiar with these conditions. By this time, the family may be discouraged after needless investigation and searching for a knowledgeable physician, or after unnecessary or even counterproductive procedures may have been performed.

This book is both medical and surgical. It is intended as a reference for both primary and secondary care physicians and surgeons. Wherever possible, biological and physiological data are given. Our purpose is that this text will help in the diagnosis and differential diagnosis, and allow rational investigation, correct prognosis, and proper treatment. The journals are largely unhelpful for this task, as papers tend to be single case reports or discuss small series. The general textbooks may be disappointingly brief or inaccurate. Of the two specialist volumes, one is out of print and the other is not written in English.

A confusing nomenclature has been largely responsible for illogical thinking on the subject of vascular birthmarks. Edward Sapir, the American anthropologist and linguist, believed that "language structures thought." Mindful of this concept, we have made a concerted effort to free our subject from its old terminological chamber of horrors. Based on clinical and cellular studies, vascular birthmarks are divided into two major categories: *hemangiomas* and *malformations*. The chapters are organized under these headings. We have used a consistent terminology throughout this book and have provided a glossary to relate our nosological system to terms found elsewhere in the literature. This field is also replete with syndromic designations, usually prefixed with personal names. All too often, eponymy lulls us into a false sense of knowledge. Hence, we have tried whenever possible to define these syndromes in anatomical words. We hope that by presenting vascular birthmarks in clear and understandable terminology, our book will not only assist in improved patient care but will also stimulate studies of pathogenesis.

The expression "vascular birthmark," used in the title, is necessarily broad, and the intention was to signal that in this book we hope to encompass the common hemangiomas of infancy as well as the developmental aberrations of the vascular system—arterial, venous, capillary, and lymphatic—that show themselves on the skin. We have, in addition, included chapters on vascular abnormalities affecting the central nervous system and abdominal viscera, as these may be associated with cutaneous marks. We have not touched on anomalies of the heart, great vessels, the eye, or the lung, as these are amply discussed elsewhere.

This book was written by two surgeons, one from Old England and one from New England, who share a fascination with vascular birthmarks. In a desire for textual uniformity, the authors have taken great pains to edit one another's chapters as well as those of their contributing specialists. The stimulus to write this book has been our biennial meeting of the International Workshop for the Study of Vascular Anomalies, beginning in Boston (1976, 1978) and later in London (1980), Paris (1982), Milan (1984), and again in Boston (1986). It is a pleasure to acknowledge that many of the views voiced in this work are consensus opinions derived from the meetings of this group and the individual participants.

JOHN B. MULLIKEN
ANTHONY E. YOUNG

Acknowledgments

The authors recognize the important contributions of Dr. Michael J. Aminoff, Dr. Alexandra M. Harrison, Dr. Jean Jacques Merland, Dr. Joel M. Noe, Dr. Marie-Claire Riché, Dr. M. Lea Thomas, and Dr. Joseph Upton. Their chapters, dealing with individual specialties, make this text comprehensive. In addition, we are grateful for the assistance of the following: Jennifer Ackroyd, Paul Baskerville, Asha Senapati, Michael Smith, and Gordon Stewart, all of St. Thomas' Hospital. We express our gratitude to our teachers, Dr. Joseph E. Murray, Professor of Surgery, Harvard Medical School; and the late John B. Kinmonth, Professor of Surgery at St. Thomas' Hospital.

Many others gladly helped in the preparation of the manuscripts. In particular, for their scientific contributions, we are indebted to Julie Glowacki, Ph.D.; Judah Folkman, M.D.; Kenneth E. Fellows, M.D.; Diana Beardsley, M.D., Ph.D.; Lawrence N. Rappaport, M.D.; Christine M. Rodgers, M.D.; and James K. Wallman, M.D. The historical background was amplified with the help of the indefatigably resourceful Mr. Richard J. Wolfe, Curator of Rare Books and Manuscripts at the Francis A. Countway Library of Medicine. For their willingness to fossick in dusty books, we thank the research staff at the Boston Public Library, National Library of Medicine, Wellcome Library of History of Medicine, The Library of The Royal Society of Medicine, and St. Thomas' Hospital Medical School. The manuscripts were constructively criticized by Dr. Julie Glowacki and Ms. Claire Henneberry, and by Prof. Norman Browse and Kevin Burnand, F.R.C.S. Sandy M. Dethlefsen, M.A., deserves credit for the light and electron photomicrographs; as does Jean Kanski for her artistic renderings and Harry P.W. Kozakewich, M.D., for his histopathological assistance. Miss Karen Golden and Miss Kate McDowell were tireless in applying their typing skills. Mr. Paul Gramer entered the text into a word processor and earned the authors' gratitude with each revision thereafter.

To Lisa McAllister and her staff at W. B. Saunders Company, we express our sincere appreciation for their skillful production and generous allotment of color reproductions.

Finally, we owe a special debt to all of our patients and their parents who have taught us about vascular birthmarks and made this book possible.

JOHN B. MULLIKEN
ANTHONY E. YOUNG

Contents

PART ONE

Background

CHAPTER ONE

Vascular Birthmarks in Folklore, History, Art, and Literature

John B. Mulliken and Anthony E. Young

Folklore

Fortis imaginatio generat casum.
Axiom. Scholast. (Montaigne)

INTRODUCTION

The human mind cannot easily accept random mischance as a cause for an event. Something or somebody, divine or human, must have induced it, probably for some purpose. Thus, when a child is born less than perfect, it is impossible to regard the imperfection as mere misadventure. In European cultures, extensive folklore surrounds different birth defects; it was believed that children so affected were born of some improper behavior either at the time of conception or during pregnancy.

MATERNAL IMPRESSIONS: FOLKLORE TO DOCTRINE

Birthmark

The very word *birthmark* infers a causal relationship between the mother's experience and her child's blemish. Mother is reproached by Latin medical terms, such as *naevus maternus* or *stigma metrocelis*. She is held responsible because of her longing, craving, or aversion to those things that indelibly marked her unborn child. The French call a birthmark *envie*, a desire; the Italians, *vòglia*, a wish or craving; and if the mother is overly fond of strawberries, her child may have a *vòglia di fragola*. In German, the word is *muttermal*, mother's mark; in Spanish, *estigma*. This same linguistic indictment of the mother is shared by all Indo-European languages.

These words, used to describe vascular birthmarks, derive from the concept known as *maternal impressions*—that an influence on a mother's emotions can affect her child's phenotype. This belief can be traced to antiquity, originating independently among peoples of widely separated cultures. From its beginnings, this psychic imprinting of the child was not only a teratogenic theory; it was also used to explain how human and animal offspring came to be of special colors, especially if the tint differed from that of the parents. The force of maternal impression was once an accepted breeding technique, as told in the Biblical story of Jacob (Genesis XXX, vs. 32–41). In order to upgrade the

3

plain colored sheep, Jacob placed peeled tree branches before the flocks when they mated at the watering trough. Those animals that saw the branches brought forth vigorous, hybrid speckled lambs. By these and other stratagems, Jacob became a prosperous stock-breeder and the putative father of experimental embryology. In ancient Greece, women were believed to give birth to infants who resembled the statues that the mothers had admired during the pregnancy. King Lycurgus, as part of his eugenics program, required Spartan wives to look upon statues of the strong and beautiful, such as the twins Castor and Pollux (Ballantyne, 1905). In a treatise, questionably attributed to Hippocrates, it is said that "when pregnant women long to eat coals and earth, the likeness of these things can appear on the head of the child" (Adams, 189?). The elder Pliny (A.D. 23–79), in his *Natural History*, noted that the Romans believed that both maternal and paternal sensations could affect the embryo at the time of conception (Plinius). Pliny also explained how man, because of his complex mind, is thus capable of impressing a great diversity of patterns in his children; whereas sluggish minded animals cannot produce such phenotypic variety in their offspring. Galen (A.D. 131–201) believed that even the sight of a picture was sufficient to alter the fetus into the appearance of the depicted likeness (Turner, 1731).

The notion that mothers imprinted their babies smoldered along in the Middle Ages, but it was forged into medical doctrine with the revival of learning in Western Europe. At this time, the power of maternal fancy or phantasia was often called *imaginatio gravidarum*. It was used to explain not only phenotypic variation but also the birth of malformed children. The skeptical essayist Montaigne (1533–1592), whose thought distilled itself into the eternal question, "Que sais-je?" ("What do I know?"), had no doubts about the origin of congenital cutaneous stains:

We know by experience that women impart the marks of their fancy to the bodies of the children they carry in their womb (Montaigne, 1902).

Ambroise Paré (1510–1590), the premier surgeon of the Renaissance, considered a wayward maternal imagination as one of his 13 causes of monsters, and remarked on the timing of the teratogenic effect:

There are some who think the infant once formed in the Womb, which is done at the utmost within two and forty days after the conception, is in no danger of Mother's imagination.

However, he cautiously concluded, "Truly I think it best to keep the woman all the time she goeth with child, from the sight of such shapes and figures" (Paré, 1634) (Fig. 1–1). Shakespeare was well aware that a mother, suddenly frightened, might disturb her unborn child. In the third part of *Henry VI*, the pregnant queen learns that her husband, Edward IV, has been defeated and has lost his crown to the Earl of Warwick. She replies to these painful tidings thus:

And I the rather wean me from despair
For love of Edward's offspring in my womb:
This is it that makes me bridle passion,
And bear with mildness my misfortune's cross;
Ay, ay, for this I draw in many a tear
And stop the rising of blood-sucking sighs,
Lest with my signs or tears I blast or drown
King Edward's fruit, true heir to the English crown.
Henry VI, Third Part, Act IV, Sc. iv, 17.

Belief in the teratogenic powers of maternal imagination reigned supreme in the sev-

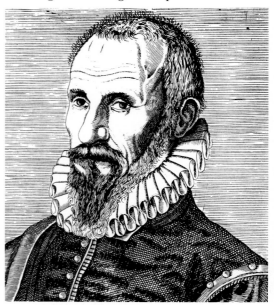

Figure 1–1. Ambroise Paré (1510–1590), 16th century wood engraving. Although the surgeon nonpareil of the Renaissance, he shared many of the ancient superstitions of his age. He wrote a curious treatise on monsters, terrestrial and marine (1573), embellished with drawings of strange, hypothetic creatures that could result from maternal impressions. (Courtesy of Francis A. Countway Library of Medicine.)

enteenth and well into the eighteenth century. It was also a simple explanation for the origin of the common mother's marks, or *naevi materni*. Descartes (1596–1650) reasoned thus:

The image of a given object is sometimes transmitted by the arteries of a woman to one or other part of the foetus and imprints there, marks known as birth-marks, which provoke the astonishment of the learned (Descartes, 1955).

The concept was that if a woman's emotions were sufficiently stirred during pregnancy, the fetus may feel the shock and register it as a skin blemish. Thus, the birthmark resembled the object or circumstance that produced the mother's emotional state. Robert Boyle (1627–1691), who brilliantly conceived the relationship between pressure and volume for a gas, repeated the tale about a speckled child, whose mother had gazed too intently at the red pebble-stones at St. Winifred's Well (Boyle, 1744).

Pregnant women were especially warned not to look upon the scene of an accident or the slaughter of animals. The fact that vascular birthmarks were commonly found on the face and scalp was attributed to the pregnant woman's tendency to touch these locations in a gesture of fright. Woe betide the gravid woman who longed for anything and simultaneously touched her body, for the fetus could be marked by the thing desired on the very anatomic area that had been in contact with her hand (chirapsy). Sir Kenelm Digby (1603–1665), English naval commander and diplomat-author, was fascinated by birthmarks, those "marvelous marks of longing" that pregnant women inflict on their offspring while under the influence of powerful fancies. In his *Two Treatises*, Digby explains that when a mother is stricken by some longing, "the like happening to the child, the violence of that sudden motion, dyeth the mark or print of the thing in the tender skin of it" (Digby, 1658). His treatises were reprinted in 1669, along with an essay, *The Powder of Sympathy*, in which he cites several examples of mother's marks (Digby, 1669). Daniel Turner, in his 1714 work, *De Morbis Cutaneis: A Treatise of Disease Incident to the Skin*, Chapter XII, detailed the mechanism for these sympathetic birthmarks (Fig. 1–2):

We shall take notice of some montrous Births, or otherways deform'd and blemish'd by Marks from the strong Imagination or disappointed

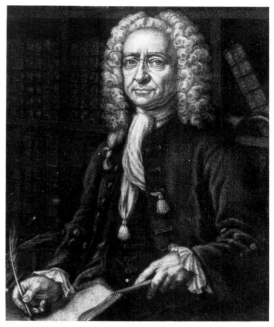

Figure 1–2. Daniel Turner, M.D. (honorary) (1667–1740) of the College of Physicians, mezzotint from his 4th edition of *De Morbis Cutaneis*, 1731. (Courtesy of Francis A. Countway Library of Medicine.)

Longings of the Mother; which have had not only Power sufficient to pervert and disturb what the Ancients called the *Plastick*, or formative Faculty, in drawing forth the *prima Stamina*, or first Lines from the then ductile and pliable Matter, but to stamp its Characters, to dismember and dislocate, and to make large and bloody Wounds upon the Body of the Foetus, conceived long since and formed completely (Turner, 1714).

Turner also described how vascular birthmarks often resembled various fruits, and how these lesions "have their times of bloom, ripening and languishing," a rather accurate description of the life cycle of the common hemangioma. John Maubray, M.D., author of *The Female Physician* (1724), agreed how common it was for a mother to mark her unborn child with fruit, even "after the infant is entirely formed, by the strength of her imagination only" (Maubray, 1724).

The eighteenth century also ushered in a new critical spirit and emancipation of thought; it was known as the Age of Enlightenment. Public skepticism on the subject of maternal impressions was dramatically heightened in late 1726 by the incredible case of Mary Toft, a woman said to have given birth to 16 rabbits (Wall, 1985). It seems that

Mrs. Toft, who was "five weeks gone with child," developed a powerful craving for rabbit, and one day was seen chasing two of these furry creatures across the field of Godlyman (Surrey). Over the ensuing weeks, she occasionally suffered intense abdominal pains and thereafter would periodically expel parts of tiny rabbits. London obstetricians insisted that she be evaluated in town, and in time, the ruse was exposed. For reasons not apparently clear, Mrs. Toft had been stuffing her vagina with newborn rabbit tissue and even hog's bladder. The entire farce was well-publicized in the London newspapers in ballads, and by the satirical drawing pen of Hogarth (Fig. 1–3).

Within a year after the Toft case, another blow to the doctrine of maternal impressions was struck by a French expatriate physician living in London, J.A. Blondel. His first treatise was anonymously published in 1727, entitled *The Strength of Imagination in Pregnant Women Examined, etc.* (Fig. 1–4). He mustered a satirical and convincing argument against Daniel Turner and the other "imaginationists," stating "How can anybody believe, with-

out reflecting upon the Wisdom of God, that it is left to her to disfigure the child, and to spoil the regular Work of Heaven?" (Blondell, 1727). Turner discovered that Blondel, also a licentiate of the College of Physicians, was the author of these words. Turner, therefore, quickly appended a defense of maternal impressions to his treatise on gleets in 1729 (Turner, 1729). Blondel, now out in the open, wrote another exposé on the fallacies of Dr. Turner's opinions (Blondel, 1729), to which Turner replied the next year with *The Force of the Mother's Imagination...Still Farther(sic) Considered* (Turner, 1730). Before libel laws, these pamphlet wars were commonplace among physicians.*

---

*Daniel Turner should also be remembered as the recipient of the first medical degree given in the English colonies of North America. He began his medical career as a member of the Barber-Surgeon Company, but he switched allegiance in 1711. That same year, he was admitted as a licentiate of the College of Physicians; he could not be a Fellow because he did not have a doctoral degree. In 1723, the nascent Yale College conferred upon Turner an honorary medical degree in appreciation for his gift of 32 books, including *De Morbis Cutaneis*, given the preceding year (Lane, 1919).

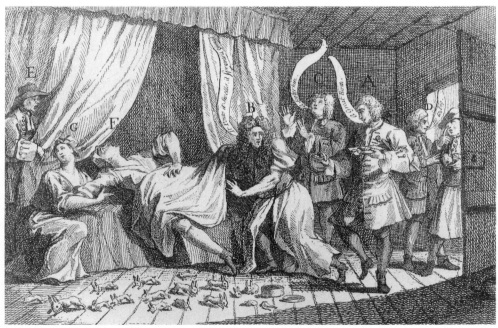

Figure 1–3. *Cunicularii, or, The Wise Men of Godliman in Consultation*, by William Hogarth, 1726. The principal characters are identified in the legend to this etching (Wall, 1985): A. Dr. Nathaniel St. André, surgeon-anatomist to His Majesty King George I, who exclaims, "A Great Birth." B. Samuel Molyneux, noted amateur astronomer, saying, "It Pouts, it Swells, it Spreads, it Comes." C. Dr. John Maubray, who says, "A Sooterkin," a monstrous little creature; he claimed in his book *The Female Physician* (1724) that these monsters often accompanied births in Holland. D. Dr. John Howard, the surgeon who delivered Mrs. Toft's first rabbit, shown rejecting a bunny for sale by saying, "It's too big." E. "The Rabbit getter." F. "The Lady in the straw," Mary Toft. G. "The Nurse or Rabbit Dresser." (By permission of the Trustees of the British Museum.)

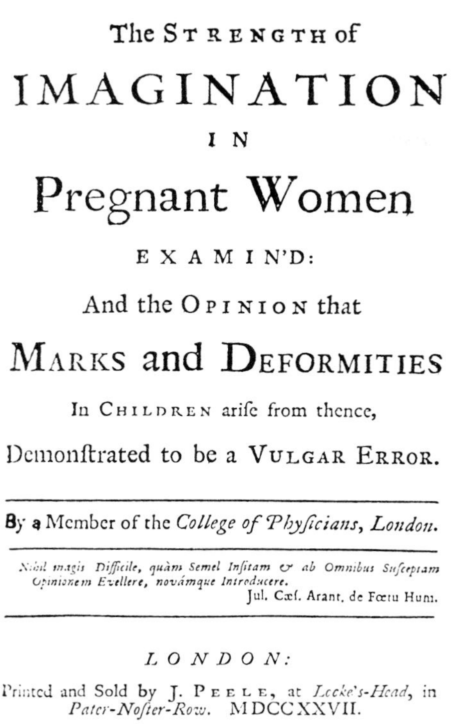

The S T R E N G T H of

IMAGINATION

I N

Pregnant Women

E X A M I N'D:

And the O P I N I O N that

MARKS and DEFORMITIES

In CHILDREN arife from thence,

Demonftrated to be a VULGAR ERROR.

By a Member of the *College of Phyficians, London.*

Nihil magis Difficile, quàm Semel Infitam & ab Omnibus Sufceptam Opinionem Evellere, novámque Introducere.
Jul. Cæf. Arant. de Fœtu Hum.

L O N D O N:

Printed and Sold by J. P E E L E, at *Locke's-Head,* in *Pater-Nofter-Row.* MDCCXXVII.

Figure 1–4. Title page from an anonymously published booklet of 1727. Its author was soon revealed to be Dr. James Augustus Blondel (1666–1734). With wit and sarcasm, he openly waged a pamphlet war against Dr. Daniel Turner and the doctrine of maternal impressions.

Blondel's challenge to the concept of maternal impressions had a great effect on medical opinion throughout Europe. The cudgel was taken up by no less than Alexander Monro *primus*, first Professor of Anatomy, Edinburgh University. He offered a physiological explanation for the impossibility of maternal impressions:

The Liquors sent into the *Foetus* by the umbilical Vein not having their propelling Force communicated from the Mother, the State of Mother's Pulse cannot affect the Child (Monro, 1734).

About the same time, William Smellie, the father of British obstetrics, also doubted whether his patients could mark their babies (Fig. 1–5). In his *Treatise on Midwifery* he noted:

I have delivered many women of children who retained no marks, although the mothers had been frightened and surprised by disagreeable objects, and were extremely apprehensive of such consequences (Smellie, 1754).

It was Smellie's one time pupil William Hunter who completed the first prospective

clinical investigation on the subject. The results of this study were related by Erasmus Darwin to his son Charles (Darwin, 1868). Hunter asked prospective mothers in a large London lying-in hospital about psychic traumas prior to confinement and found no correlation between the women's answers and congenital anomalies in the children. It was his brother, John Hunter, who deserves the credit for demonstrating in 1754 that there was no direct communication between the circulatory system of the mother and that of her fetus (Meyer, 1939). Thereafter, some physicians began to question whether maternal emotional signals could be transmitted through the vascular system.

Yet the doctrine of maternal impressionism seemed to flourish anew in the nineteenth century. Desgranges wrote a syllogistic argument in support of this theory and advised the local magistrate of police to protect the curious public from exposure to "bizarre" animals and to prohibit the sale of "unnatural" paintings and sculpture (Desgranges, 1801). In the third year of the French Republic, an infant was born with a vascular anomaly on the left breast, which so resembled the Phrygian cap of liberty that the mother was awarded 400 francs per annum for her patriotic thoughts (Geoffrey Saint-Hilaire, 1832). Vascular birthmarks were typ-

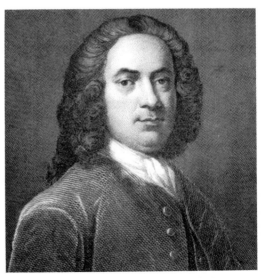

Figure 1–5. William Smellie (1697–1763), the greatest man-midwife of the 18th century, observed that his patients were frequently shocked by terrifying sights and yet their babies were not impressed. (Engraving from his self-portrait of 1719, in Royal College of Surgeons of Edinburgh. Courtesy of Francis A. Countway Library of Medicine.)

ically ascribed to a mother's cravings or excessive engorgement of vividly colored fruits, particularly strawberries, raspberries, and red currants. Even Dr. Arthur Conan Doyle, in his story *The Doctors of Hoyland*, described a certain Mrs. Crowder as a person "who had always regarded the birthmark upon her second daughter, Eliza, as a sign of the indignation of the Creator at a third helping of raspberry tart which she had partaken of during a critical period" (Doyle, 1894).

W.A. Hammond, erstwhile Surgeon-General of the U.S. Army and pioneer neurologist, wrote that he doubted whether transient longing for fruit could impress an image on an unborn child (Hammond, 1868). However, he strongly believed that "incessant mental occupation or excitement" could cause deformities in a fetus. He explained that mother's blood is the "medium that all impressions from her mind to her offspring must pass" and that these impressions cross through the placental membranes by "endosmosis and exosmosis." Yet, there were other voices calling from the darkness that followed the Civil War; one was from Augusta, Georgia. L.A. Dugas, Professor of Surgery at the University of Georgia, in a remarkable paper, systematically exposed the fallacies of belief in maternal impressions (Fig. 1–6). In 1866, he wrote:

> Hideous objects have been known to frequent the thoroughfares of London for many months without giving rise to a solitary well-authenticated instance of deformity in anywise resembling them, although they must have been seen by thousands of women, at all stages of gestation (Dugas, 1866).

This surgeon went on to note, "Was there ever a woman who, under the influence of the derangement of the functions of the stomach, and the capricious appetite peculiar to pregnancy did not ardently desire some article of diet she could not obtain?" If the impression theory was correct, why were not more children born with marks of mothers' dietary indiscretion? Aware of advances in embryology, Dugas believed that it would be "physiologically impossible" for a mother's emotion to destroy tissues and organs that had already formed. He concluded that if mental emotions were to reach the embryo, it would have to be via the nervous system, and indeed, no such neural connection between uterus and fetus had ever been demonstrated. G.J. Fisher, a surgeon and noted bibliophile in Sing Sing, New York, had a

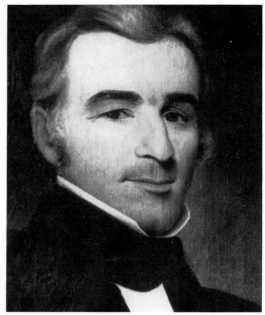

Figure 1–6. Lewis Alexander Dugas, M.D. (1806–1884), Professor of the Principles and Practice of Surgery, the Medical College of Georgia. While president of the Medical Society of Augusta, he presented a paper in 1866 that logically dismissed the power of maternal impressions, and also noted that *naevi materni* could spontaneously regress. (Courtesy of Library of the Medical College of Georgia.)

special interest in the new science of teratology. In 1870, he wrote a scathing rebuttal to the eminent Dr. Hammond's article and concluded that malformations were the result of faulty embryological development, and not maternal impressions (Fisher, 1870). As for birthmarks, Fisher believed the fault lay not with the mother's mind:

> The alleged resemblances of various congenital maculae to fruits and animals, are either accidental, as in the case of rocks, the outlines of mountains, and the forms of clouds, which exhibit the profile of the human head and face; or they are the result of pure imagination and fancy on the part of the observer.

Thus, belief in the power of maternal imprinting was on the wane by the end of the nineteenth century, but the concept was by no means moribund. In Keating's *Cyclopedia of Diseases of Children*, published in 1890, W.C. Dabney wrote a chapter entitled *Maternal Impression*, in which he tabulated 90 recorded cases of "photographic" effects of mothers' fancy (Dabney, 1890). He pointed out that for skin marks, the impression was often made comparatively late in pregnancy and was "almost certainly produced by some disturbance of the circulation." He also noted that it was unnecessary for the woman to be conscious of the impression, or to expect a defect or anomaly to occur. Dabney concluded in his retrospective study that "it is the duty of every physician to warn his pregnant patients of the necessity for guarding against emotional disturbances of any kind." A contemporary physician agreed with Dabney, that vascular birthmarks were the result of maternal impressions caused by "local circulatory stasis, apoplexy, or inflammation...induced by deviation from the normal chemistry or circulation of maternal blood" (Work, 1894).

Pregnancy taboos exist in slightly different forms in every culture and in every corner of the world. Perhaps it is not surprising that the superstitious belief in maternal marking should persist. For example, there remains a folk tradition that claret or port-wine stains are due to conception having taken place during menstruation. This explanation can be traced to the ancient Hebrew legislation prohibiting coitus during or immediately after the period of impurity, for it was believed that such activity may result in a malformed infant (Ballantyne, 1897; Rosner, 1983). Pregnant women are still reminded by older relatives that when a food craving occurs, every effort should be made to consume the desired viand, thus to satisfy the appetite before the fetus is damaged. At a large meal, the pregnant woman may be obligated to taste each item for fear of marking her child. It is said that if the woman has a craving for a certain food and is unable to satisfy her desire, she must touch a hidden part of her body so that should a birthmark appear on her child, it would at least be concealed.

In a study of current opinions about the cause of facial deformities, maternal impression was considered an etiological factor only in cases of port-wine stain, in contrast to other facial deformities such as cleft lip and prognathism. One fourth of 200 Welsh women interviewed believed that a port-wine stain is related to maternal consumption of strawberries or red cabbage, to an unsatisfied craving for such foods, or to contact with blood during the pregnancy (Shaw, 1981). Thus, belief in maternal impressions lingers on to this day, perhaps reinforced by paternal convictions.

History

What he sees often, he does not wonder at, even if he does not know why it is. If something happens which he has not seen before, he thinks it is a prodigy.
Cicero

INTRODUCTION

Maternal impression was not the only possible explanation for a birthmark. A belief in the pureness of God's own works led to a suspicion that the Devil or his agents may have had a part in the conception of such imperfect children (Glenister, 1964). As a consequence of this belief, birth defects were not infrequently assumed to indicate that the child or the mother was in some way a morally or socially unsatisfactory person. The resemblance of some vascular birthmarks to smears of blood upon the skin has also led the primitive but creative mind to assume traits of violence or lustfulness. In the light of this, it is hardly surprising that history records few remarkable people who had birthmarks. Was this deliberate, or did such people fail to achieve prominence in a superstitious society? Nevertheless, three statesmen are known to have had vascular birthmarks and they stand out, neatly straddling the centuries: Marcus Tullius Cicero, King James II of Scotland, and Mikhail Gorbachev.

CICERO'S RIDDLE

In 1672, George Hieronymous Velsch (1624–1677) wrote a provocative essay suggesting that the famous Roman orator and poet Marcus Tullius Cicero (106–43 B.C.) had a vascular birthmark. In a rather convoluted literary style, Velsch said that Cicero had a conspicuous anomaly below his left eye similar in appearance to a chick-pea that was secondary to his mother Helvia's imagination during her pregnancy (Velsch, 1681). In fact, the Latin word cicer means chick-pea, and the writer implied that Cicero owed his family name to this "chick-pea" birthmark. It is highly improbable that this cheek anomaly had any relation to Cicero's name, which can be traced back to well before this consummate Roman. The Elder Pliny, in his *Natural History*, notes that the family name Cicero initiated with an ancestor who specialized in the cultivation of chick-peas (Plinius). Plutarch's largely anecdotal *Life of Cicero* states that the first member of the family was so surnamed because he had a dent at the tip of his nose, like the cleft of a chick-pea. Cicero himself was, in fact, proud of his name; as Plutarch relates, he had a silver plate inscribed with *Marcus Tullius* in front of an engraved chick-pea (Plutarch).

Seventeenth century physiognomists believed that a vascular blemish on the left side of the face portended a violent death, brought on by the subject's misdeeds. Velsch concluded that this prediction was fulfilled in the case of Cicero, who during the civil turmoil in Rome failed to join the stronger faction and was beheaded by the triumvirate in December 43 B.C.

Velsch observed that the absence of a birthmark on the coins and statues depicting Cicero cannot be construed to mean that such a blemish did not exist. He explained that artists tended to conceal such unflattering marks in their renditions. Nevertheless, a statue of Cicero, located in the Capitoline Museum in Rome, clearly shows a hemispherical swelling beneath his left eye (Fig. 1–7). Is this an inclusion cyst or a lipoma, or did Cicero, indeed, have a localized vascular birthmark?

A deliberate exclusion of Cicero's birthmark from most representations of him is not surprising. Throughout history, artists and sculptors have for preference done their best to show their sitters in the best light—a prudent move for an artist living by commissions. It was, in fact, necessary for Oliver Cromwell to demand of the artist for whom he was sitting that the painting show him "warts and all." Birthmarks, like warts, were usually omitted in the interest of aesthetics as well as prudence and good taste.

We know from contemporary accounts that

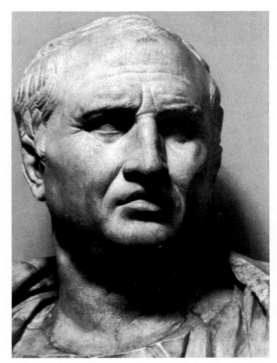

Figure 1–7. Bust of Cicero, The Capitoline Museum, Rome.

James II of Scotland had a red birthmark, probably a port-wine stain in the second division of the trigeminal area on the left side of his face. Indeed, he was known as "James of the fiery face." Few portraits of him exist, and none for certain shows that mark (Fig. 1–8). We have already noted that folklore has it that one born with a blood-colored birthmark will be of a violent temperament and will meet with a terrible death. If ever there was a man to confirm this notion, it was James II.

JAMES II OF SCOTLAND

James II was born on October 16, 1430 and at the age of 7, on the murder of his father, James I, succeeded to the throne. His father's assassins were caught, tortured, and executed with a barbarity that was deemed unusual even in that day. Because the child James was too young to govern, power was held by two feuding nobles, Sir William Crichton and Sir Alexander Livingstone. Fearing the violence of the former, James' mother smuggled the boy in a chest from Edinburgh to Stirling Castle, where she placed him under the protection of Livingstone. Unfortunately, she had misjudged Livingstone, for he had her locked away in the castle, releasing her only when he was given sole wardship of James. At this point, Crichton kidnapped the boy and took him back to Edinburgh. William, Sixth Earl of Douglas and a close friend of James, joined in the feuding, only to be tricked into coming peacefully to Edinburgh, where, to the King's distress, Crichton had him and his brother arrested and beheaded. Acrimony degenerated into protracted civil war. At the age of 19, James, already worldly wise and battle scarred, was married to Mary Gueldres, on the recommendation of Philip The Good. Having gained his emancipation from tutelage by this marriage, James truly became the king and was able to restore some stability to Scotland. The Livingstones were imprisioned or executed, and Crichton became Chancellor. The Douglas' allegiance was, however, never entirely to be trusted. At one lull in the smoldering unrest, James offered William The Eighth, Earl of Douglas, a safe conduct to parlay. After entertaining him at supper on Shrove Thursday, 1452, James demanded that the Earl break his ties with his confederates; Douglas replied that he could not and would not; whereupon James fell upon him, screaming, "Since you will not, I shall!" and stabbed him to death with a dagger.

The accounts of James' reign are repetitive recitals of violent and protracted struggles hither and thither across the Highlands and Lowlands of Scotland, as James tried to control his rebellious earls. Castles were sacked, towns razed, and resistors killed by the sword or the gallows. The thread of violence runs strongly through his whole life, and his end was no less bloody. At war with England, he was about to storm the castle at Roxburgh, when his own cannon exploded, killing him instantly. James of the fiery face was 30. His wife, who was with him, continued the siege and took the castle the next day.

The Scottish historian John Prebble credits James with a ruthless character "moulded by terror, by the murder of his father, his friends, by lonely isolation and night-riding dreams" (Prebble, 1971). His biographer in the National Biography shed a more objective and charitable light on James' short life, noting that he was "vigorous, politic and singularly successful," and commented also that his extensive legislative program had a markedly popular character. He concluded that "the manner of the death of Douglas leaves a stain on the memory; but it was an age when violence and treachery were regarded as lawful weapons" (Dict. of Nat. Biography).

MIKHAIL GORBACHEV

From James of the fiery face, we must leap to the twentieth century to find another prominent person so marked. In 1984, Mikhail Gorbachev became the most powerful man in the Communist world. In spite of his past as head of the KGB, the state security service, Western opinion greeted this appointment, seeing Gorbachev as a steady and reasonable man. However, Andrei Gromyko, when nominating Mr. Gorbachev as leader of the Communist Party, observed that he

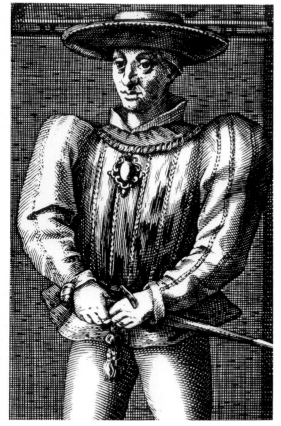

Figure 1–8. James II of Scotland (1430–1460), from the Diary of Georg von Ebingen, c. 1450. This crude woodcut suggests that he, indeed, had a port-wine stain on the left side of his face. (Original in the Scottish National Portrait Gallery.)

had a nice smile, but that it hid iron teeth (Owen, 1985).

Communist publications have carefully airbrushed out the rather unusual vascular anomaly that stains the right side of the leader's forehead (Fig. 1–9), a birthmark that looks as if blood had been tipped onto him (Fig. 1–10). If it were only that easy to treat a capillary dermal malformation in the flesh.

Birthmarks were once judged to be a clue to the bearer's personality. We have remarked on the notion that the bearers of blood-colored birthmarks are of a violent and vigorous disposition. It is but a short step to claims for lustfulness, and there is also the curious corollary belief of coexistent genital marks in those who have red facial birthmarks. If there is "a red mole on the nose of a man or a woman, then there will be another

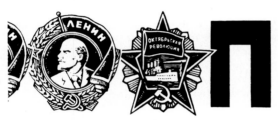

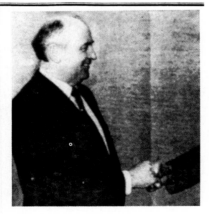

Во время встречи.

Figure 1–9. Mikhail Gorbachev as depicted on the front page of Pravda, October 25, 1985. The birthmark on his forehead has been airbrushed out. Of 200 consecutive 1985 issues of Pravda reviewed, 24 showed pictures in which the vascular mark would be expected to show—it could be discerned in none. (Courtesy of A. E. Young.)

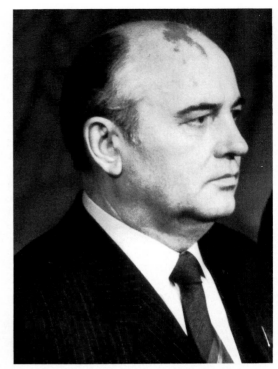

Figure 1–10. Mikhail Gorbachev, the General Secretary of the Communist Central Committee of the Soviet Union. (Courtesy of Time Magazine, March 25, 1985.)

on the most secret parts, sometimes on the ribs, and it denotes great lechery" (Lean, 1903). The most celebrated such association was Chaucer's Wyf of Bath (1387):

Yet have I Martes marke upon my face
and also in another privee place.
(Wyf of Bath, prol., 619)

Although unsubstantiated, it has been suggested that the famous writer, traveler, charletan, and lover Casanova was so marked. However, no relevant illustrations or paintings are known to be extant!

A visible vascular birthmark affects not only how others view the bearer but also how he sees himself. As for any asymmetrical deformity, the stained side of the face is constantly compared with the normal side. Each of us can imagine how such a blemish might affect our personality. Perhaps one would tend to be withdrawn or possibly overcompensate for the deformity in some way, hopefully with productive behavior. A glimpse of how a facial vascular birthmark can modify life and career is seen in the following sketch of an influential leader of the academic world.

THE CRIMSON STAIN ON A HARVARD UNIVERSITY PRESIDENT

No other president did so much to change and direct Harvard University as Charles W. Eliot during his 40 year tenure. He took a special interest in upgrading the medical curriculum, and he played a pivotal role in moving the Harvard Medical School from Boston's Back Bay to the Longwood area at the turn of the century. The school's quadrangle of neoclassical buildings and grassy enclosure was officially dedicated on September 25, 1906. As President Eliot rose to give the final consecration, no one could help but notice that the right side of his face was distorted and colored a deep crimson hue (Fig. 1–11).

Charles William Eliot was the third of five children, born on March 20, 1834 to a long-established patrician family of Eliots and Lymans. The novelist Henry James describes that day in the house on Beacon Street across from the Common:

His entrance upon the scene brought a shock to a family which was justified in expecting its men and women to be good-looking. The new child carried an ugly and unconcealable birthmark, a swollen, liver-colored welt that occupied most of the right side of his face down to his mouth. It was impossible to overlook the naevus, or to see it and forget it (James, 1930, Vol. I, p. 12).

It was said that Eliot's mother taught the boy that his vascular birthmark "was a cross which he must carry to his grave and which he must bear manfully" (James 1930, Vol. I, p. 13). Looking back on his youth, Eliot said those days were "not as rich and bright as later days...are we not to forget how vivid and real are the pains, griefs and fears of childhood" (James, 1930, Vol. I, p. 15). There are stories of young Eliot's problems playing with the North End boys on the Common. According to an elder cousin, he

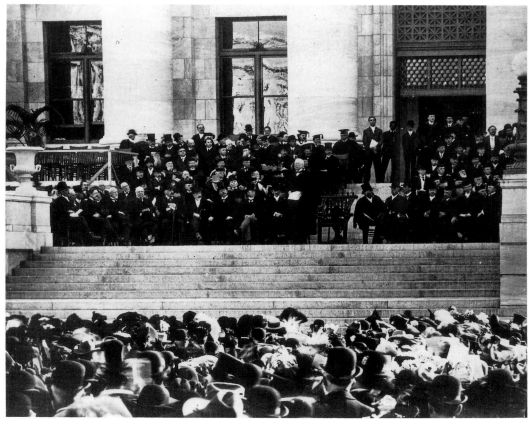

Figure 1–11. President Charles W. Eliot addressing the crowd from the marble steps of Building A at the dedication of the new Harvard Medical School quadrangle, September 25, 1906. (Courtesy of Francis A. Countway Library of Medicine.)

was once "hooted off the Boston Common because of his face" (James, 1930, Vol. I, p. 14). Undoubtedly, the birthmark contributed to Eliot's natural shyness and made him feel more comfortable with those he knew well; he had only a few boyhood pals outside the family circle. Years later, Dr. Francis G. Peabody, Eliot's brother-in-law, recalled a time upon which young Eliot alluded to his birthmark. Apparently, his grandfather had given him a special gift of money, and when Peabody asked why, Eliot replied, "Because of this," pointing to the right side of his face (James, 1930, Vol. I, p. 13).

His parents emphasized that it was not one's appearance but what one did that mattered. Throughout his life Eliot was fond of quoting the precepts of American Unitarian minister and author Edward Everett Hale: "Look forward and not backward—look out and not in" (James, 1930, Vol. II, p. 309). In the beginning, Eliot found little pleasure in attending the rigorous Boston Latin School. In time, he discovered the ancient poets and found joy in oratory. At graduation, he delivered the salutatory address in Latin. His successful declamations suggest that he was overcoming his sensitivity. By age 15, Eliot was ready for Harvard College.

The undergraduate Eliot was not well known by his classmates. He was introverted and bookish, and his scholarly habits carried him into the top four of his class by his junior year (James, 1930, Vol. I, p. 41). Eliot was a high myope, a handicap in being unable to recognize his classmates at a walking distance—just one more cross to bear. During his junior year, his eyes failed and he had to have his textbooks read aloud to him (James, 1930, Vol. II, p. 41). This is a rather curious happening, unlikely in someone who is merely nearsighted. Eliot's port-wine stain was localized to the second trigeminal division, and therefore it is unlikely he suffered with the ophthalmic complications of Sturge-Weber syndrome. Moreover, this was a transient and bilateral amblyopia. It is likely that Eliot had a central or macular loss of vision secondary to bilateral optic neuritis. This temporary amblyopia had its compensation in the camaraderie generated from having his classmates help with his studies.

In his junior year, Eliot came under the care of the formidable Dr. Henry J. Bigelow at the Massachusetts General Hospital. In a letter written years later to Bigelow's son, Eliot recalled:

He wanted to try an experiment on the naevus on my face, having read of successful operations by a Viennese surgeon on similar blotches. I was glad to have the experiment tried, but was much surprised to discover that your father did not know how to make the powerful freezing mixture which was required. He did not know the difference between chloride of lime and calcium chloride. The experiment failed, though pushed to a point beyond which your father said he did not dare to go. (James, 1930, Vol. II, p. 314).

Eliot graduated second in his class of 88; a photograph of a handsome young man appeared in the Harvard Class of 1853 album (Fig. 1–12A). The poignancy of this photograph is appreciated only when it is compared with another taken in the fall of 1854, after Eliot was appointed Tutor in Mathematics (Fig. 1–12B). Note that in the 1853 photograph, the part in Eliot's hair is on the opposite side and his shirt buttons are incorrectly placed. The sensitive Eliot had his class photograph printed in reverse in order to hide the right side of his face.

Eliot's academic career was off to a good start. In 1858, the College made him Assistant Professor in Mathematics and Chemistry, and in October of that year, he married Ellen Peabody, daughter of the minister of King's Chapel. In 1863, the Eliot family, including two young children, were off to Europe. There, he would dabble in chemistry and primarily concentrate on the organization of the continental educational systems. He preferred Paris to London; he was uncomfortable in England, where his port-wine stain was constantly stared at (James, 1930, Vol. I, p. 135).

In 1865, after 2 years in Europe, Eliot became Professor of Analytical Chemistry in the newly established "Boston Tech" (later to become the Massachusetts Institute of Technology). In the spring of 1869, the Harvard Corporation voted to offer Eliot the presidency; he was only 35. In a touching account in the diary of his cousin Theodore Lyman, Eliot asked for advice on whether or not to accept the position. He wondered whether his facial birthmark might detract from the dignity of such a public office (James, 1930, Vol. I, p. 104). After some opposition, his election was confirmed on May 19, 1869; the news came to Eliot alone, for his wife had died just a few weeks before.

Eliot had a keen interest in physical fitness. He was an oarsman in college, and throughout his life he was fond of long walks, horse-

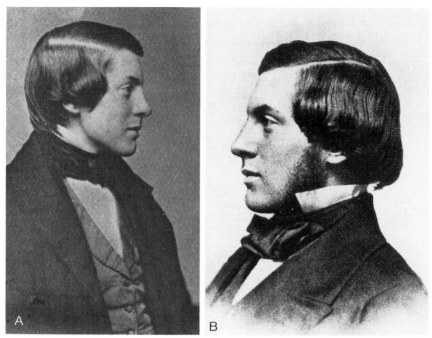

Figure 1–12. *A,* Salt print of the 19 year old Charles W. Eliot in the 1853 Harvard Class Album. The buttons are on the incorrect side of his waistcoat, betraying the fact that the photograph was printed in reverse. *B,* Photograph taken in 1854 of Eliot as newly appointed Tutor in Mathematics. Note that the profile is the same as in *A,* including part of the hair; now he has sideburns. (Courtesy of Harvard University Archives.)

back riding, bicycling, and yachting. According to one biographer, Eliot's facial birthmark "only served to heighten the total impression created by his bodily vigor, tall and erect figure, resonant voice and strong, clean-cut features" (Perry, 1931). Yet whenever he was photographed, Eliot would turn his head so as to hide the port-wine stain from the camera. This strong left side of his face would forever be the public view of Eliot (Fig. 1–13).

Perhaps Charles Eliot's vascular birthmark caused him to be particularly interested in medical education. He was the driving force in upgrading the Harvard Medical School's admission and curriculum standards. As the result of Eliot's prodding, after 1892, the Medical School required 4 years attendance, and finally, by 1900, an undergraduate degree was necessary for admission.

In October 1877, Eliot remarried. His new wife was Grace Mellon Hopkinson. Her nephew Charles Hopkinson was an artist and a Harvard man (A.B. degree, 1891). Hopkinson made a specialty of portraying educators, and many colleges possess his works. The Hopkinson and Eliot families were very close, often summering together at Northeast Har-

bor, Mt. Desert Island, Maine. It is not surprising that the artist-in-law was able to intimately portray the retired president. The Hopkinson painting of 1909, which hangs at

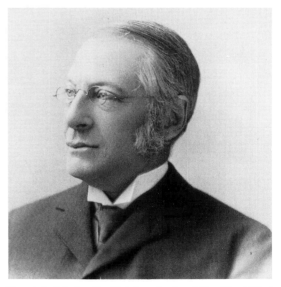

Figure 1–13. In all official portraits of President Eliot, such as this photograph of 1893, the head is turned to the right. There is hypertrophy of the right upper lip. (Courtesy of Harvard University Archives.)

the Harvard Medical School, clearly shows the port-wine stain, although it is in a shadow. Interestingly, the portraits of Eliot by the collector-artist Denman W. Ross of the same year and the John Singer Sargent portrait of 1907 still depict Eliot's face turned to his right, hiding the birthmark. By the time Eliot was 87, Hopkinson was able to portray him in unabashed full-face (Fig. 1–14). Hopkinson was known for his unusual techniques, and this painting artfully disguises the port-wine stain on the right cheek. However, it is impossible to turn from the sculpturer's eye, and the numerous busts of Eliot done by Lewis Potter clearly depict the asymmetry and droop of President Eliot's face (Fig. 1–15).

This brief sketch of Charles Eliot's life suggests that the vascular birthmark on his right cheek caused some pyschosocial problems during his childhood. Nevertheless, with the support of his family and by strength of character, he was able to overcome this handicap and grow from a shy boy to a leader of men. He was a man characterized by remark-

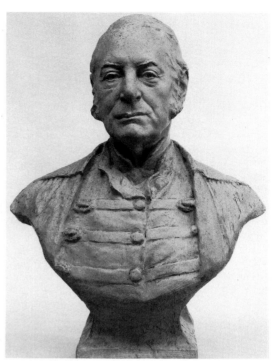

Figure 1–15. Bust of Charles Eliot, in academic gown, by Lewis Potter, 1910. (Courtesy of Harvard University Portrait Collection.)

able qualities of integrity, joy in hard work, and talent for organization. A full and successful life of service to Harvard would have occurred even if her most influential president had not been born with a port-wine stain.

The connection of Boston with the chronicle of birthmarks does not rest solely with Charles Eliot. For just a short distance from the Eliot home, over Beacon Hill, is the Massachusetts General Hospital. There, in the fall of 1846, was admitted another young man with a facial vascular birthmark who was destined to walk into the spotlight of surgical history.

EDWARD GILBERT ABBOTT'S FAMOUS CERVICAL VASCULAR ANOMALY

On September 25, 1846, a tall, thin, rather sickly 20 year old Boston printer named Edward Gilbert Abbott was admitted to the Massachusetts General Hospital for treatment of a tumor located in the left neck. His family history disclosed a tubercular heredity. The admission physical examination was re-

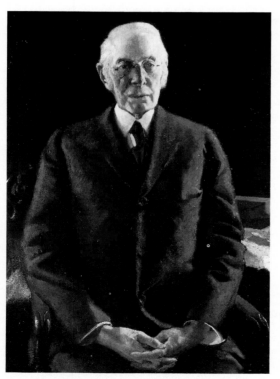

Figure 1–14. President Eliot at age 87; oil portrait done in 1921 by Charles S. Hopkinson. Subject is seen full-face, but the stain and facial asymmetry are artfully disguised. (Courtesy of Fogg Art Museum, Harvard University.)

corded by house surgeon Dr. Charles G. Heywood: "This man had come with a tumor under the jaw on the left side. It occupies the left neck, bounded on the inside by median line—on outside is even with the edge of jaw—below on a level with Pomum Adami—and in front tapers gradually as far as anterior edge of jaw" (Case of Gilbert Abbott, M.G.H., 1846). The skin overlying the mass was of normal color and moved freely over the lump. The tumor was soft and was "readily emptied by slight pressure, but filled again on one or two seconds." Heywood palpated the lower edge of the left mandible and felt that it had an irregular contour. On intraoral examination, he found the lower lip mucosa and tongue to be a "dark purple color." There was a hemispheric swelling of the left tongue, which also was a purplish hue. Heywood carefully described the extent of the cutaneous vascular anomaly:

For the distance of 5 lines* from the angle of mouth on Rt side the lower lip is of a livid hue—this seems to be a continuation of a stripe, similar in appearance which extends from angle of jaw on Rt side about on a level with lower teeth—it is about 4 lines wide and is slightly raised—its color seems to depend upon small spots, like granulations, of a livid color set on mucous membrane of ordinary appearance.

The operation on Abbott's neck was originally scheduled for Tuesday, October 13, but the surgeon, Dr. John C. Warren, asked his patient's permission to delay the procedure. Warren was anxious to try a medicine said to relieve pain that had just been discovered by William Green Morton, a recent graduate of Harvard Medical School. Morton received Dr. Warren's message on Wednesday, October 14, inviting him to come to the Massachusetts General Hospital that Friday at 10 A.M.

On Friday, October 16th, the amphitheatre at the hospital was crowded with some of Boston's most eminent physicians. Morton arrived embarrassingly late—he explained that he had been delayed in preparing his apparatus. He composed himself and poured a clear liquid into a glass globe containing a sponge. Abbott was strapped down to the operating chair. Morton took Abbott's hand and spoke a few encouraging words to him. "Are you afraid?" he asked. "No," replied Abbott, "I feel confident and will do precisely

what you tell me" (Rice, 1859). Morton lifted the neck of the inhaler to his patient's lips. Within 4–5 minutes, Abbott was asleep (Fig. 1–16). Dr. Warren stepped forward and made a 4 inch incision over the tumor in the left neck; to his surprise, the patient did not move or cry out. He then cut through the subcutaneous tissue and fascia, exposing "congeries of large veins and small arteries." The hemorrhage was slight. Warren passed a curved needle armed with a heavy suture through the base of the wound and tied the ligature down to decompress the vascular lesion. The wound was left open and was filled with lint compresses. After completion of the dressing, Abbott aroused and was asked if he had felt any pain; he replied that he had felt nothing. Dr. Warren turned to the audience and proclaimed, "Gentlemen, this is no humbug" (Rice, 1859; Truax, 1968). Within a few days, ether was successfully used in other cases and the news spread from Boston across the Atlantic. This dramatic first public demonstration of ether anesthesia was for ligation of a venous vascular birthmark.

On the first postoperative day, the lint dressing was removed and the wound was filled with potassa cum calce (potassium hydroxide and calcium salt or lime water). Venous bleeding began; this continued for 3–4 hours before it was finally stopped with more lint compresses. With the repeated application of various caustics and poultices, an eschar eventually separated from the wound and granulation tissue began to appear by late October. Potassa Fasa was often sprinkled on the wound. With daily dressings and periodic touches of silver nitrate, the wound eventually healed by secondary intention. Abbott's hospital stay was a prolonged one, but was probably acceptable by standards of that time. Only one postoperative note was written in his record during that November; it read, "Doing well" (Case of Gilbert Abbott, M.G.H., 1846). Seven weeks postoperatively, on December 7, Abbott was finally released from the hospital. Heywood wrote his discharge summary in the record:

Cicatrix perfect. Tumor of same size as on entrance but no vessels to be decteckted(sic) in it—Tumor on Tongue not altered—nor is the appearance on inside of Rt. cheek. General health much improved. Discharged.

Thus, Abbott's venous malformation was little changed by the famous operative procedure.

---

*Five lines equals 5/12 inch.

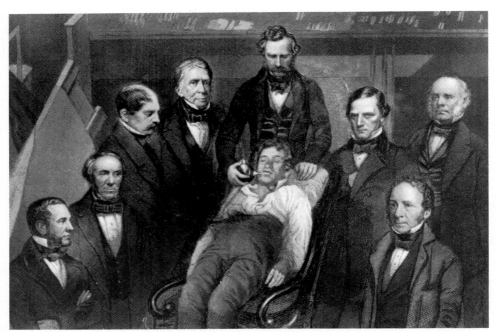

Figure 1–16. The first public demonstration of etherization at the Massachusetts General Hospital, October 16, 1846. The patient, Edward Gilbert Abbott, is seen semi-recumbent in a chair. There is a vascular swelling in the left anterior neck; the lips are somewhat prominent and perhaps stained. The physicians around Abbott are reputed to be (from left to right): H.J. Bigelow, A.A. Gould, J. Mason Warren, J. Collins Warren, W.T.G. Morton, Samuel Parkman, George Hayward, and S.D. Townsend. A steel engraving by H.H. Hale from *Trials of a Public Benefactor* (Rice, 1859).

Edward Gilbert Abbott became an assistant editor of the *The Boston Herald* and later was proprietor and editor of *The Cambridge Mercury*. He married Mary Dunbar Fuller of Osterville, Massachusetts in 1850, and they lived in the Maplewood section of Malden, Massachusetts. He died of pulmonary tuberculosis on Tuesday, November 27, 1855 at age 30 years and 2 months, leaving his widow and two children (Vandam and Abbott, 1984).

Art

In our search for depicted birthmarks, we have approached custodians of many portrait galleries in Europe and the United States and found that at least in this context, the much-worn claim that "art mirrors life" has no validity. The result of our quest was an almost uniform blank. No such marks are known on portraits, although it becomes frankly impossible in much twentieth century art to determine whether distortions represent physical defects in the sitter, or mere artistic license. There are, for example, several portraits painted by Picasso in 1906 that show a woman who appears to have a lymphatic anomaly ("cystic hygroma"), perhaps even complete with a surgical scar (Fig. 1–17).

Literature

Although artists may have been shy of making anything of birthmarks, writers have felt no such restraint. From the hump of Richard III to the blue eyes of Hollywood heroes, it is a familiar trick of the written and dramatic arts to illustrate some defect or virtue of character using physical attributes as a hieroglyph. However, we are not familiar

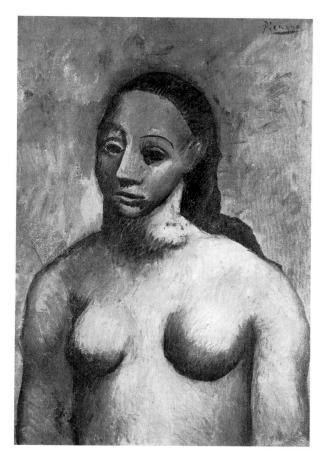

Figure 1–17. Picasso, *Bust of a Woman,* 1906. The swelling in the left neck is anatomically typical of a cystic lymphatic malformation. There is even a hint of a biopsy scar. Picasso made several other renderings of this same model in which the anomaly is not so obvious. (Courtesy of the Art Institute of Chicago.) (See Fig. 12–11A.)

with any story in which a vascular birthmark is used for that purpose, but the presence of such blemishes is the core of the plot in three stories, one by Shakespeare, one by Nathaniel Hawthorne, and one by V.S. Pritchett. Each bears retelling.

THE TRAGEDIE OF CYMBELINE BY WILLIAM SHAKESPEARE (FOLIO OF 1623)

Shakespeare cleverly employed a hidden vascular birthmark in his tragicomedy *Cymbeline*. The play begins as a gentleman named Posthumus has presumptuously married Imogen, the daughter of Cymbeline, the King of Britain. Posthumus is sent into exile, and arriving in Rome, he encounters a rascal called Iachimo. The Italian casts aspersions on the chastity of all women, and wagers that he can expose the dishonor of Imogen. Posthumus has such confidence in his wife's integrity that he consents to the trial. Iachimo

travels to the English court, but he fails in his initial overtures to Imogen. He must resort to stealth. One night, Iachimo gains admittance to Imogen's bedchamber by having himself carried there hidden in a trunk. While the heroine sleeps, Iachimo removes her bracelet and takes mental notes of her room and "some natural notes about her body" (Fig. 1–18):

On her left breast
A mole cinque-spotted, like the crimson drops
I' the bottom of a cowslip: here's a voucher,
Stronger than ever law could make: this secret
Will force him think I have pick'd the lock and
  ta'en
The treasure of her honour. (Act II, Sc. ii, 38)

Armed with this circumstantial evidence, Iachimo returns to Rome to convince Posthumus of Imogen's guilt.

Posthumus' confidence is shaken by Iachimo's detailed description of his wife's bedroom and by the presentation of her bracelet. As he demands still more evidence, Iachimo complies:

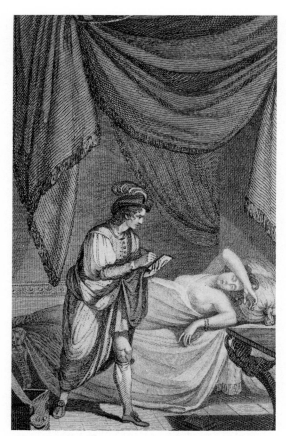

Figure 1–18. In this depiction of Shakespeare's *The Tragedie of Cymbeline,* the rogue Iachimo has inveigled his way into Imogen's chamber and in order to convince her husband of her infidelity, he writes down "such and such pictures." The five spotted vascular stain on her left breast is not shown in this engraving by M. Liart, in *John Bell's Edition of Shakespeare's Plays,* 1773. (Courtesy of the Trustees of the Boston Public Library.)

If you seek
For further satisfying, under her breast—
Worthy the pressing—lies a mole, right proud
Of that most delicate lodging: by me life,
I kiss'd it, and it gave me present hunger
To feed again, though full. You do remember
This stain upon her? (Act II, Sc. iv, 134)

Posthumus answers: "Ay, and it doth confirm, another stain, as big as hell can hold, were there no more but it." Enraged by another man's knowledge of Imogen's vascular birthmark, the misguided husband orders that his wife be put to death.

THE BIRTHMARK
BY NATHANIEL HAWTHORNE

In July 1842, young Nathaniel Hawthorne brought his fragile bride Sophia Peabody to Concord, Massachusetts, to live in the parsonage called The Old Manse (Fig. 1–19*A* and *B*). While there, the reclusive Hawthorne wrote some of his best short stories and later published 17 of them in a book entitled *Mosses from an Old Manse* (Hawthorne, 1846). During their 3½ years in Concord, the newlyweds were incredibly happy; their rented home became Paradise on Earth (Hawthorne, J., 1885; French, 1957; Brooks, 1983). Yet the stories penned during this period tell of human frailty and potential for evil. Herman Melville was profoundly impressed by *Mosses from an Old Manse.* In those tales, Melville found the "great power of blackness" that derived from the Puritan past and "from whose visitations, in some shape or other, no deeply thinking mind is always and wholly free" (Melville, 1850).

The first story in this collection, *The Birthmark,* probes the psychological problems caused by a facial vascular stain. The tale centers around Alymer, a late eighteenth century man of science—"an eminent proficient in every branch of natural philosophy" and whose "accomplishments aroused the learned societies in Europe." The alchemist falls in love with beautiful Georgiana, and his devotion to science becomes enmeshed with his affection for her. Soon after their wedding, Alymer becomes obsessed by a tiny red birthmark located on his beloved's left cheek. He feels it is a type of the "brute" in her, "a visible mark of earthly imperfection and a symbol of his wife's liability to sin, sorrow, decay and death."

At first, Georgiana is hurt by her husband's aversion to the birthmark. She had always thought it was a mark of beauty. It resembles a little hand, and former lovers often said that a tiny fairy had made an imprint upon Georgiana's cheek and thus given her magical power over another's heart. However, all too quickly, Georgiana comes to share her husband's obsession over the vascular stain. It is unclear whether she does so out of vanity, perfectionism, or to please Alymer. She foreshadows the outcome:

I know not what may be the cost to both of us, to rid me of this fatal birthmark. Perhaps its removal may cause cureless deformity. Or, it may be, the stain goes as deep as life itself. Again, do we know that there is a possibility, on any terms, of unclasping the firm grip of this little Hand, which was laid upon me before I came into the world?

Alymer is convinced that he can remove the birthmark from his wife's cheek, but says the

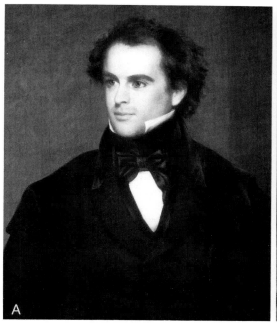
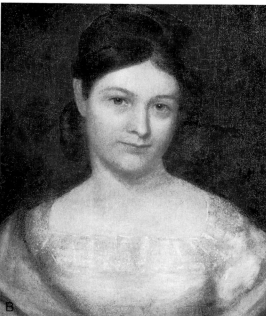

Figure 1–19. *A,* Nathaniel Hawthorne in 1840, two years prior to his marriage. Painting by Charles Osgood. (Courtesy, Essex Institute, Salem, Mass.) *B,* Sophie Amelia Peabody, artist unknown, circa 1842. (Courtesy of the House of Seven Gables, Salem, Mass.)

case calls for no easy remedy, nothing superficial. Georgiana is now a "fascinated participant," completely caught up in the scheme, and extolls her husband's scientific powers. The reader is still uncertain whether she actually wants the birthmark removed or is innocently trying to please her husband. She is impressed by his record book of laboratory experiments, by its thoroughness and its illustration of her husband's superior mind. Yet the book also documents that "his most splendid successes were almost invariably failures, if compared to the ideal at which he aimed . . . ."

Soon, Alymer's experiments result in a "perfect draught," one that cannot fail. He demonstrates for his wife the power of this elixir to bring forth fresh leaves to a dying geranium. Georgiana now agrees to take the potion, even if it is poisonous, so that she "might put off the birthmark of mortality by relinquishing mortality itself." She drinks the liquor, colorless as water, and her husband begins to methodically observe her physiological changes in his laboratory notebook. Within a few hours, the mark begins to fade, more so with each breath. Alymer cries, "Success!" But soon he notes Georgiana's pale complexion. His wife is dying. As the life fades from her body, Alymer's brutish laboratory assistant chuckles:

Thus ever does the gross Fatality of Earth exult in its invariable triumph over the immortal essence, which, in this dim sphere of half-development, demands the completeness of a higher state. Yet, had Alymer reached a profounder wisdom, he need not thus have flung away the happiness, which would have woven his mortal life on the self-same texture with the celestial. The momentary circumstance was too strong for him; he failed to look beyond the shadowy scope of Time, and living once for all in Eternity, to find the perfect Future in the present.

As in many of Hawthorne's stories, *The Birthmark* reveals what he called "the truth of the human heart." The tale briefly questions what might cause such a vascular blemish, and it accurately describes typical reactions of others to such an anomaly, particularly in loved ones. But it is the moral issue, the tragedy of Alymer, the perfectionist, his inordinate pride and self-confidence, that most concerns Hawthorne. For the author, hubris is the unpardonable sin. Alymer becomes an irresponsible medical researcher, for his work fails to take human consequences into account. He attempts to erase a mark of human imperfection, and in so doing unintentionally destroys the most precious thing he had. Today, medical science still does not have a satisfactory treatment for Georgiana's vascular birthmark. Yet, like Alymer, we must continue, in a scientific spirit, to find remedies. We cannot accept the laboratory technician's view that a birthmark should not be removed, a Calvinistic orthodoxy of unquestioned acceptance of man's imperfection. However, Hawthorne's tale also instructs us never to lose human contact as we struggle to care for patients with vascular anomalies.

BLIND LOVE AND OTHER STORIES BY V.S. PRITCHETT

The emotional issues engendered by a visible congenital deformity usually become integrated into the personality from an early age. However, the bearer of a hidden deformity may not so easily resolve the struggle for self-assurance. The psychological havoc wrought by a secret vascular birthmark is perceptively addressed in a short story by V.S. Pritchett entitled *Blind Love* (Pritchett, 1969).

Helen Johnson was born with a vascular stain on her chest. She always wears a high blouse to cover the mark. She is proud of her adroitness, over the years, in keeping her secret so that no one would know "the inhabitant of the ragged island on her body." If someone notices the birthmark, showing "like a red leaf over the collar," Helen quickly dismisses them with the remark, "Mother went mad with wanting plums when she was carrying me."

At age 36, her day of exposure came. On her wedding night, her husband first sees the birthmark and recoils with a look of shocked disgust on his face:

From the neck over the left shoulder down to the breast and below, and spreading like a red tongue to the back was this ugly blob—dark as blood, like a ragged liver on a butcher's window, or some obscene island with ragged edges. It was as if a bucket of paint had been thrown over her.

Helen cries out, "What do you think? Do you think I got it done, that I got myself tattooed in the Waterloo Road? I was born with it." A week later, her husband leaves her.

She is ashamed and depressed and feels punished for the deception she has carried on over the years. Somehow, she manages to find a job as a secretary and housekeeper to a Mr. Armitage, a wealthy English country gentleman. He, too, has been punished, for his wife left him 22 years ago, after he went blind. As the reader might anticipate, one

day Helen Johnson and her employer become intimate. Now she is almost vain about her stain, often displaying it, almost taunting him with what he cannot see. Yet, sometimes, she wonders whether her lover can see into her mind. Is it blind love, or can love be blind?

References

Folklore

Adams, F.: *The Genuine Works of Hippocrates*. XLI. *On Superfoetation*. New York: William Wood and Co., 189? p. 94.

Ballantyne, J. W.: *Teratogenesis: An Inquiry into the Causes of Monstrosities*. Edinburgh: Oliver and Boyd, 1897, p. 15.

Ballantyne, J. W.: *Manual of Antenatal Pathology and Hygiene. The Embryo*. New York: William Wood and Co., 1905, pp. 96–127.

Blondel, J. A.: *The Strength of Imagination in Pregnant Women Examin'd: And the Opinion that Marks and Deformities in Children Arise from Thence, Demonstrated to Be a Vulgar Error*. London: J. Peele, 1727, p. 106.

Blondel, J. A.: *The Power of the Mother's Imagination over the Foetus Examin'd. In answer to D. Turner's book, intitled* (sic) "A Defence of the XIIth Chapter of the First Part of a Treatise, De Morbis Cutaneis." London: J. Brotherton, 1729, p. 143.

Boyle, R.: Experiments and considerations touching colours, 1664. In *The Works of Robert Boyle*, edited by Thomas Birch, London, 1744, Vol. II, p. 37.

Dabney, W. C.: Maternal impressions. In Keating, J. M. (ed.): *Cyclopedia of the Diseases of Children*, Vol. I. Philadelphia: J. B. Lippincott, 1890, pp. 191–216.

Darwin, C. R.: *The Variation of Animals and Plants under Domestication*, Vol. III. London: J. Murray, 1868, p. 264.

Descartes, R., quoted by Sendrail, M.: Sur l'origine des monstres. Concours Med. 77:305, 1955.

Desgranges: Dans lequel il établit, par plusieurs observations, que les taches des enfants, naevi materni, sont produites par l'imagination de la mère. Rec. d. Actes Soc. de Santé de Lyon 2:83, 1801.

Digby, K.: *Two Treatises of Bodies and of Mans Soul, to Discover the Immortality of Reasonable Souls*. Paris: Gilles Blaizat, 1658.

Digby, K.: *Two Treatises of Bodies and of Mans Soul to Discover the Immortality of Reasonable Souls with Two Discourses of the Powder of Sympathy and of Vegetation of Plants*. London: Printed by S.G. and B.G. for J. Williams, 1669, pp. 186–189.

Doyle, Sir A. C.: The Doctors of Hoyland. The Idler Magazine (London) 5(April):227, 1894.

Dugas, L. A.: Remarks upon the supposed influence of the mother in the production of naevi materni, or congenital "marks," and other deformities. South. Med. Surg. J. 1:317, 1866.

Fisher, G. J.: Are malformations or monstrosities of the foetus in utero ever produced by the power of maternal mental emotions? Amer. J. Insanity 26:241, 1870.

Geoffrey Saint-Hilaire, M. I.: *Histoire Générale et Particulière des Anomalies de l'Organization chez L'Homme et les Animaux*, Vol. I. Paris: J. B. Ballière et fils, 1832, p. 332.

Hammond, W. A.: On the influence of the maternal mind over the offspring during pregnancy and lactation. Quart. J. Psychol. Med. Jurisprud. 2:1, 1868.

Lane, J. E.: Daniel Turner and the first degree of doctor of medicine conferred in the English colonies of North America by Yale College in 1723. Ann. Med. Hist. N.Y. 1:367, 1919.

Maubray, J.: *The Female Physician, Containing all the Diseases Incident to that Sex, in Virgins, Wives and Widows.* London: James Holland, at the Bible and Ball, in St. Paul's Church-yard, 1724, p. 368.

Meyer, A. W.: Truth overtakes "Doctor Hunter." California and West. Med. 50:120, 199, 275, 1939.

Monro, A.: *Med. Essays and Observ,* Vol. II. Edinburgh: T. and W. Ruddimans, 1734, p. 238.

Montaigne, M. E.: On the force of imagination. In *Essays* Translated by C. Cotton, Hazlitt, W. C. Editor, Vol. I. London: Reeves and Turner, 1902, p. 94.

Paré, A.: *The Workes of the Famous Chirurgion Ambrose Parey,* Book 25. Translated by Thomas Johnson. London: Thomas Cotes and R. Young, 1634, p. 979.

Plinius, Gaius Secundus: *Historia Naturalis* Libro VII, 52.

Rosner, F. (trans. and ed.): *Julius Preuss' Biblical and Talmudic Medicine.* New York: Hebrew Publishing Co., 1983, p. 123.

Shaw, W. C.: Folklore surrounding facial deformity and the origins of facial prejudice. Brit. J. Plast. Surg. 34:237, 1981.

Smellie, W.: *Treatise on Midwifery and Practice of Midwifery,* Vol. II, Cases 89 and 90, 3rd ed. London: D. Wilson, 1754.

Turner, D.: *De Morbis Cutaneis. A Treatise of Diseases Incident to the Skin.* London: R. Bonwicke, W. Freeman, T. Goodwin, etc., 1714, pp. 102–128.

Turner, D.: *A Discourse Concerning Gleets . . . Containing Some Remarks upon a Discourse . . . Entitled, The Strength of Imagination in Pregnant Women* Examin'd (*By J.A.B.*). London: Printed for John Clarke, 1729, pp. 52, 162.

Turner, D.: *The Force of the Mother's Imagination upon Her Foetus in Utero Still Farther Considered: In the Way of a Reply to Dr. Blondel's Last Book.* London: J. Walthoe, 1730, p. 192.

Turner, D.: *Des Morbis Cutaneis. A Treatise of Diseases Incident to the Skin,* 4th ed. London: J. Walthoe, 1731, pp. 169–170.

Wall, L. L.: The strange case of Mary Toft (who was delivered of sixteen rabbits in 1726). Med. Heritage 1:199, 1985.

Work, H.: Maternal impressions. Med. News. 65:451, 1894.

History

Case of Gilbert Abbott, Surgical Rounds, Massachusetts General Hospital 30:1, 1846.

Dictionary of National Biography (compact Edition), Vol. 1: James II of Scotland. Oxford Univ. Press, 1975, p. 1059.

Glenister, T. W.: Fantasies, Facts and Foetuses. The interplay of fancy and reason in teratology. Med. History 8:15, 1964.

James, H.: *Charles W. Eliot, President of Harvard University 1869–1909,* Vols. I and II. Cambridge, MA: The Riverside Press, 1930.

Lean, V. C.: *Collectanea,* Vol. II, Part 1. Bristol, England: J.W. Arrowsmith, 1903, p. 312.

Owen, R.: The Times (London), No. 62, 244, 16 September 1985, p. l.

Perry, R. B.: *Dictionary of American Biography,* Vol. 6. New York: Scribner's Sons, 1931, pp. 71–78.

Plinius, Gaius Secundus: *Historia Naturalis* Libro XVIII, 10.

Plutarch: *The Lives of the Noble Grecians and Romans.* Translated by John Dryden. New York: Random House, 1948, p. 1041.

Prebble, J.: *The Lion in the North,* London: Secker and Warburg, 1971, p. 141.

Rice, N. P.: *Trials of a Public Benefactor as Illustrated by the Discovery of Etherization.* New York: Pudney and Russel, 1859, pp. 91–93.

Truax, R.: *The Doctors Warren of Boston.* Boston: Houghton Mifflin, 1968, pp. 190–193.

Vandam, L. D., and Abbott, J. A.: Edward Gilbert Abbott: Enigmatic figure of the ether demonstration. N. Engl. J. Med. 311:991, 1984.

Velsch, D. G. H.: Observation de naevorum varietate et cicere in facie M.T. Ciceronis. In *Miscellanea Curiosa Medico-Physica Academiae Naturae Curiosorum sive Ephemeridum Medico-Physicarum Germanicarum Annus Tertius,* 1672. Leipzig und Frankfort: J. Fritzsch, 1681, p. 53.

Art and Literature

Brooks, P.: *The Old Manse and the People Who Lived There.* Privately printed by the Trustees of Reservations, 1983, pp. 48–68.

French, A.: *Hawthorne at the Old Manse.* Concord, MA: Blackburn Printing Co., 1957.

Hawthorne, J.: *Nathaniel Hawthorne and His Wife,* Vol. I. Boston: James R. Osgood and Co., 1885, pp. 48–63.

Hawthorne, N.: The Birthmark. In *Mosses from an Old Manse.* New York: Wiley and Putnam, 1846, pp. 32–51.

Melville, H.: Hawthorne and His Mosses (1850). In *The Golden Age of American Literature,* Edited by P. Miller. New York: Braziller, Inc., 1959, p. 410.

Pritchett, V. S.: *Blind Love and Other Stories.* London: Chatto and Windus, 1969, pp. 9–57.

CHAPTER TWO

Classification of Vascular Birthmarks

John B. Mulliken

*. . . Those difficulties which have hitherto
amused philosophers, and blocked up the way
to knowledge, are entirely owing to ourselves.
That we have first raised a dust and then
complain we cannot see.*
Bishop George Berkeley (1685–1753)
(Berkeley, 1710)

INTRODUCTION

Nomenclature is the major obstacle to our understanding and management of vascular birthmarks. The confusion is iatrogenic, for the bewildering nosologic systems have evolved from ignorance of pathophysiology. Textbook classifications offer an array of admixed histologic and descriptive words. Unfortunately, the same word is often used for entirely disparate vascular lesions. *Hemangioma* has become a generic term, used to describe a variety of vascular lesions, both congenital and acquired, and with different etiologies and natural histories. For example, hemangioma, the most common tumor of infancy, known by the specific epithets "capillary," "juvenile," and "strawberry," predictably undergoes involution. Yet, the port-wine stain, which never regresses, also has been injudiciously labeled a "capillary hemangioma" (Popkin, 1977; Thomson, 1979). The term *naevus flammeus* has been used synonymously for the permanent port-wine stain, as well as for the common infantile forehead and nuchal stains that fade during the first year of life. The same adjective "cavernous" has been clinically applied to hemangiomas that predictably involute (Walter, 1953; Lampe and Latourettte, 1956; Simpson, 1959), to those that never involute (Costello, 1949; MacCollum and Martin 1956; Andrews et al., 1957), and to those that can occasionally pale, although more rarely than capillary lesions (Matthews, 1968). The most common tumor of infancy and a rare type of vascular malformation have both been called "hypertrophic hemangioma." Terms with hyphenated modifiers, such as "capillary-cavernous hemangioma," and hybrid words, such as "lymphangiohemangioma" or "hemangiolymphangioma," permeate the medical literature and further add to the confusion.

The classifications used in the past, like those for other diseases, have reflected the methodological obsessions of the time and, in this context, follow the historically familiar sequence of descriptive, anatomicopathological, embryological, and biological.

DESCRIPTIVE CLASSIFICATION

From ancient times, the doctrine of maternal impressions was the basis for the descriptive classification of vascular birthmarks. The mother who had longed for strawberries, raspberries, or cherries or who had been terrified by frogs or mice found her hapless babe stigmatized with these mental experiences. Nosology, based on brightly colored edibles, continues to the present day, e.g., "strawberry hemangioma," "cherry angioma," "port-wine stain," and "salmon patch."

Physicians have always preferred Latin to the vernacular terms, and for centuries, vascular birthmarks or mothers' marks were called *macula materna, macula matricis, naevus maternus*, or *stigma metrocelis* (Hooper, 1841). William Hunter first properly described acquired arteriovenous aneurysm in 1757 (Hunter, 1757). John Hunter studied the formation of collateral circulation following arterial ligation and, in 1785, successfully performed this procedure to cure atherosclerotic popliteal aneurysm (Home, 1793). Aware of the Hunters' contributions, the talented John Bell of Edinburgh realized that not all pulsating vascular lesions were the same (Fig. 2–1). In his monumental *Principles of Surgery*, he accurately described arteriovenous malformation, calling it "aneurysm by anastomosis," and realized that this was a separate entity from the common *naevus maternus* of infancy (Bell, 1815). His case reports offer a wealth of clinical description and shrewd comment and are embellished by his own beautiful engravings (Fig. 2–2). J.L. Petit warned about bleeding problems following excision of vascular lesions that consist of dilated veins with a normal sized arterial pedicle. He named these venous anomalies "tumerus variqueuses" (Petit, 1774). More commonly, vascular anomalies were called by picturesque cognomens such as "sanguineous fungus" or "fungus haematodes." Alibert, the founder of French dermatology, pleaded for his "natural method" of classifying diseases. He used the general term "angioses," or affections of the vascular system, for a wide variety of congenital and acquired skin lesions (Alibert, 1817). He called some congenital cutaneous vascular anomalies *ecchymoma congeniale*; others were labelled *haematoncus*, or "blood tumor." He divided the latter into three types: *haematoncus fongoïdes* (like a

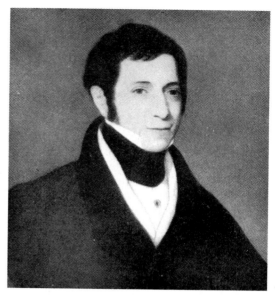

Figure 2–1. John Bell (1763–1820), Edinburgh surgeon, anatomist, and artist of considerable talent, first used the term "aneurysm by anastomosis" to describe arteriovenous malformation. Along with Desault and John Hunter, he is regarded as a founder of modern vascular surgery (Walls, 1964). (Courtesy of the Wellcome Museum.)

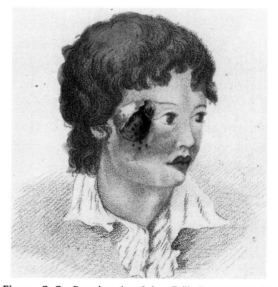

Figure 2–2. Drawing by John Bell: "aneurysm by anastomosis" in a 5 year old boy; it was the size of a sixpence at birth. Bell remarked that "when puberty arrives I am apprehensive there will be a very unfavorable change." (From J. Bell's *The Principles of Surgery*, 1815.)

mushroom), *haematoncus framboesia* (like a raspberry), and *haematoncus tuberosus* (like a potato). Alibert prided himself upon the fact that he was the first to use burin and palette to illustrate skin diseases (Garrison, 1929) (Fig. 2–3). In 1818, James Wardrop published a paper that differentiated "subcutaneous vascular naevus" from "cuticular naevus." This was the same year he was appointed Surgeon Extraordinary to the Prince Regent of England (Fig. 2–4). Wardrop correctly emphasized that both the cuticular and subcutaneous lesions were *naevi materni* and keenly observed that either "could diminish in size" (Wardrop, 1818). Wardrop, always one to be in the arena of controversy, chided his French colleagues for confusing the terminology of vascular birthmarks because they used the expression "fungus haematodes" for both *naevus maternus* and "anastomosing aneurysm," regarding them as two species of the same disease.

Thus, by the mid-nineteenth century, critical physicians and surgeons were aware of the differences between the commonplace *naevus maternus, naevus vascularis,* or *naevus sanguineous* and the less common, more dangerous forms of vascular birthmark. This latter type was variously known as "aneurysm by anastomosis," "circoid aneurysm," or what Baron Dupuytren called "erectile tumor" or "pulsatile fungus haematode" (Dupuytren, 1839). Nevertheless, any classification of disease based on *descriptive* terminology is predisposed to inaccuracy and confusion, because lesions that look very similar may be quite different in etiology and behavior. The microscope heralded the ascendency of pathological anatomy over simple clinical description. Would this instrument provide a more accurate classification of vascular birthmarks?

ANATOMICOPATHOLOGICAL CLASSIFICATION

Rudolf Virchow, the father of cellular pathology, decreed *"omnis cellula e cellula,"* that

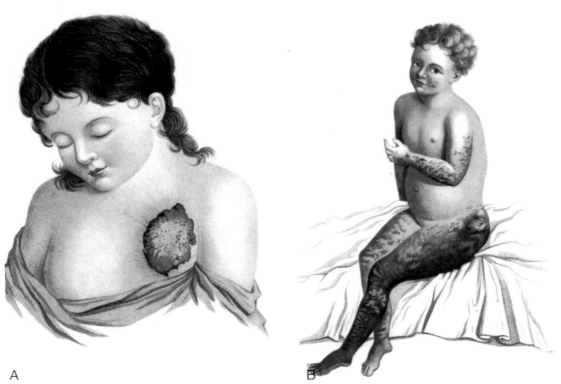

A

B

Figure 2–3. *A,* "L'Hématoncie framboisée" in a 2½ year old girl, drawn in bust form. According to Alibert, the blood tumor was present since birth and became darker at times, particularly during the "chaleurs de la canicule" (sultry days of summer). She has a hemangioma; the signs of involution are more clearly seen in the frontispiece. (From Alibert's *Nosologie Naturelle,* 1817.)

B, "L'Ecchymome congénial," colored engraving from Alibert's expensive and lavishly illustrated dermatologic text of 1817. He remarked that the surface of the vascular anomaly was rough, like a "pile of little lichens" commonly seen on the bark of old trees.

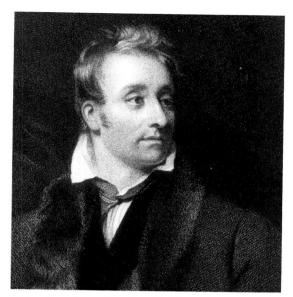

Figure 2–4. James Wardrop (1782–1869), Edinburgh-trained London surgeon, recognized the differences between true hemangiomas, called *naevi materni*, and vascular malformations. He is best remembered as an early specialist in ophthalmic surgery and for successful distal ligation for aneurysm. (Courtesy of Francis A. Countway Library of Medicine.)

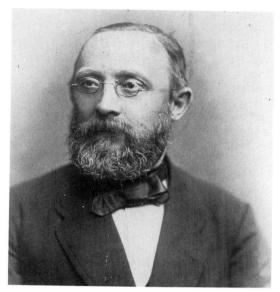

Figure 2–5. Rudolf Virchow (1821–1902), founder of cellular pathology, classified vascular anomalies as simple, cavernous, or racemose angioma. (Photograph of 1872, courtesy of Francis A. Countway Library of Medicine.)

pathological cells derive from pre-existing cellular elements. He called all vascular birthmarks "angiomas" and categorized them, based on channel architecture, as *angioma simplex, angioma cavernosum*, and *angioma racemosum* (Virchow, 1863) (Fig. 2–5). *Angioma simplex* was a tumor in which the tissue consisted of capillaries; *angioma cavernosum* was the replacement of normal vasculature with large channels; and *angioma racemosum* was a pathologic tissue consisting of markedly dilated interconnected vessels. He felt that Bell's "aneurysm by anastomosis" was a combination of cavernous and racemose angioma. Virchow conceived that one type of vascular lesion could transform into another by either cellular proliferation or vessel dilatation. Thus, he believed that angiomas were truly tumors, involving growth and extension of new blood vessels. Wegner, once a student with Virchow at the Berlin Pathological Institute, proposed a histomorphic division of lymphatic swellings remarkably similar to that of his professor: *lymphangioma simplex, lymphangioma cavernosum*, and *lymphangioma cystoides* (Wegner, 1877). These Teutonic classifications were to be perpetuated in textbooks and influence thinking about vascular birthmarks for the next century. Virchow's *angioma simplex* became synonymous with

"capillary hemangioma" or "strawberry mark"; only later was the term misapplied to the port-wine stain with its capillary sized channels (Fig. 2–6). The microscopic desig-

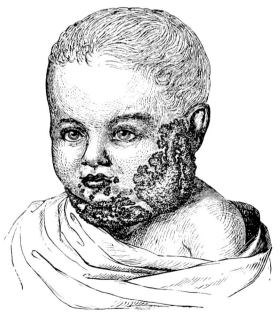

Figure 2–6. Drawing of *angioma simplex*, taken from Virchow's text of 1863 (Virchow, 1863). Unfortunately, this designation evolved into "capillary hemangioma," a term now used to describe not only the common "strawberry" mark, but also port-wine stain, as well as various acquired vascular lesions.

nation "cavernous," in time, came to be indiscriminately assigned to lesions that involute as well as to those that do not. Some vascular swellings were even called "cavernomas."

At the turn of this century, the pathologist J.G. Adami insisted on the need for a sharp demarcation between variocosities or aneurysmal enlargements of blood vessels and true vascular tumors (Adami, 1908). With remarkable insight, Adami discussed the terminology of vascular birthmarks:

Here once more we must dwell on the meaning of words. A cell rest or inclusion within a tissue is not a blastoma so long as it lies latent and is not growing; similarly a mass of tissue which, owing to developmental defects, is aberrant in structure is not a blastoma so long as it strictly respects physiological laws and at most grows coincidently with the rest of the organism. Independent growth is the test of what constitutes a tumor of this order. Does this mean that we are to remove most of the conditions now included under the heading of angiomas, and place them under the class of, say, telangiectases? Frankly, this would be the better course; it would make for precision. We must be governed here by our conception of the meaning of the word *angioma*. If that is to be taken as meaning simply a swelling composed of blood vessels, then all these remain as angiomas. If we restrict it to mean a tumor, due to independent growth of vessels, they must be cast out of this class.

Fraser defined "haemangioma" as "a tumor in which there is an actual new formation of vessels or proliferation of the vessel walls." He divided them into compact, capillary, and cavernous types, the compact type representing a more cellular or malignant stage (Fraser, 1919). However, the conceptual confusion persisted between a true tumor (neoplasm) of vascular origin and a vascular malformation or ectasia, in which there is no cellular proliferation. For example, Cushing and Bailey felt obvious discomfiture in trying to resolve whether lesions that appeared to be vascular malformations of the brain were capable of neoplastic growth (Cushing and Bailey, 1928). The waters of terminology were further muddied by Albrecht's introduction of a new word, "hamartoma" (Albrecht, 1907). *Hamartia* (Greek, hamartia, to sin or err) denoted a birth defect, whereas *hamartoma* designated a lesion of developmental origin, but one with the capacity for benign cellular proliferation. The term "hamartoma" is still indiscriminately applied to

diverse soft tissue lesions such as neurofibroma, lymphatic malformation, port-wine stain, and the common infant hemangioma.

The words continued to be jumbled around as pathologists struggled to understand tumors derived from the vascular system. In the 1940 edition of Ewing's textbook, "angioma" was redefined as a true neoplastic process of vascular tissue that could give rise to two classes of tumors: "hemangioma" and "lymphangioma" (Ewing, 1940). In the same year, Watson and McCarthy, in a monumental study of 1056 vascular lesions, failed to separate new vascular growths from malformations (Watson and McCarthy, 1940). Harvey and coworkers stated that "it is not possible to lay down where an angiectatic malformation ends and an angiomatous tumour begins" (Harvey, Dawson, and Innes, 1940).

The word "endothelium" was introduced by His in 1865 to describe the flat cells that line blood and lymphatic vessels, as well as the meninges, pleura, pericardium, and joint spaces (His, 1865). The term "endothelioma" was proposed by Golgi in 1869 as being synonymous with Virchow's "psammoma," a vascular tumor of the meninges containing sand-like material (Golgi, 1903). This term soon further stirred up the clouds of confusion that surrounded vascular lesions. Atypical and exuberant vascularity often accompanies both epithelial and mesenchymal malignancies. Thus, as MacCallum noted, every unusual tumor not immediately recognizable was likely to be labeled an "endothelioma" (MacCallum, 1936). Pulford reviewed 290 cases of vascular neoplasms at the Mayo Clinic from 1907 to 1922 and was convinced that "haemangiomas and lymphvascular angiomas, although usually benign, are potentially malignant endotheliomas" (Pulford, 1925). Thus, he correctly concluded that there are, indeed, malignant vascular tumors, but he muddled the field by insisting on an intermediate stage tumor, called "angio-endothelioma," which is "relatively benign but definitely malignant." However, behind the clouds was a "silver lining"; in 1943, A.P. Stout introduced reticulin staining to demonstrate basement membrane patterns in the various vascular lesions (Stout, 1943). He preferred the term "hemangioendothelioma" for tumors in which clusters of endothelial cells were located within the reticulin sheath. Thus, Stout preferred the designation "benign hemangioendothelioma" for the common soft tissue tumor of infancy, in contrast to the rare "malignant hemangioendothelioma" (Stout, 1943). Nevertheless, the term "hemangioendothelioma" connoted possible malignant behavior, and this notion was mistakenly applied to the common hemangioma of infancy that spontaneously regresses (Andries and Kaump, 1944; Schwartz, 1945). Another tumor, "hemangiopericytoma," also described by Stout, consists of pericyte proliferation outside the reticulin network and with each pericyte surrounded by reticulum fibers (Stout and Murray, 1942; Stout, 1949). Both benign and malignant forms of "hemangiopericytoma" are recognized, and there is also a rare, benign, "infantile hemangiopericytoma" (Enzinger and Smith, 1976). For the Armed Forces Institute of Pathology fascicles, Stout and Lattes gathered all vascular lesions under a single heading, entitled "hemangiomatoses and lymphangiomatoses" (Stout and Lattes, 1967). Whatever its anatomicopathologic merits, this classification is difficult to translate into clinical care of children with vascular birthmarks. For example, the term "angioma" in Stout and Lattes' classification is applied to both congenital lesions (e.g., *naevus flammeus*, hereditary telangiectasia) and acquired lesions (e.g., spider nevus and pyogenic granuloma). The Stout-Lattes system also lists benign and malignant neoplastic lesions under the same headings as congenital vascular anomalies. This agglomeration of vascular lesions of various etiology has been perpetuated by other authors (Pack and Miller, 1950).

The pathologist's preference for the word "hemangioma" in its broadest sense is further exemplified in Enzinger's text *Soft Tissue Tumors* (Enzinger and Weiss, 1983). He defines hemangioma as a "benign but nonreactive process in which there is an increase in the number of normal or abnormal-appearing blood vessels" (Enzinger and Weiss, 1983). Enzinger's classification of vascular "tumors" of soft tissue is given in Table 2–1. Once again, lesions of disparate clinical behavior and etiology are gathered together as "hemangiomas," whereas the term "endothelioma" is rightfully restricted to vasoformative tumors of malignant behavior. Enzinger, however, admits that an "arteriovenous hemangioma" could just as appropriately be considered a vascular malformation.

Any strictly histopathological classification, without clinical correlation, has not proved to be useful

Table 2–1. A CLASSIFICATION OF VASCULAR TUMORS OF SOFT TISSUE

I. Benign vascular tumors
  A. Localized hemangioma
    1. Capillary hemangioma (including juvenile type)
    2. Cavernous hemangioma
    3. Venous hemangioma
    4. Arteriovenous hemangioma (racemose hemangioma)
    5. Epithelioid hemangioma (angiolymphoid hyperplasia, Kimura's disease)
    6. Hemangioma of granulation tissue type (pyogenic granuloma)
    7. Miscellaneous hemangiomas of deep soft tissue (synovial, intramuscular, neural)
  B. Angiomatosis (diffuse hemangioma)
II. Vascular tumors of intermediate or borderline malignancy (hemangioendothelioma)
  A. Epithelioid hemangioendothelioma
III. Malignant vascular tumors
  A. Angiosarcoma (including lymphangiosarcoma)
  B. Kaposi's sarcoma
  C. Malignant endovascular papillary angioendothelioma
  D. Proliferating angioendotheliomatosis

Reproduced by permission from Enzinger, F. M., and Weiss, S. W.: *Soft Tissue Tumors.* St. Louis, 1983, The C. V. Mosby Co.

in the diagnosis and management of patients with vascular birthmarks. This approach, despite the best efforts of all concerned, has befuddled pathologist and clinician alike. The confusion is perhaps best illustrated by descriptions of "hemangiomas" behaving in a "malignant" fashion, with the potential for invasion and metastasis (Robinson and Castleman, 1936; Ward and Jonas, 1938; Brown and Byars, 1938; Byars, 1943; Andries and Kaump, 1944; Hoehn et al., 1970).

EMBRYOLOGICAL CLASSIFICATION

With increasing knowledge of cardiovascular embryology, researchers envisioned vascular birthmarks as problems of faulty development. Woollard described the morphogenetic process of coalescence within the primordial vascular system of the pig limb bud (Woollard, 1922). Both Lewis and Sabin studied the development of the lymphatic system (Savin, 1902; Lewis, 1905). The common hemangiomas of childhood were conceived as being embryonic rests of angioblastic cells (Fraser, 1919). Stimulated by the work of Sabin and encouraged by his chief, W.S. Halsted, W.F. Reinhoff studied vascular development in pig embryos and chickens (Reinhoff, 1924). He concluded that vascular anomalies were the result of faulty embryogenesis and could be arterial, venous, or combined arteriovenous in type. Limb vascular anomalies seemed the most easily explained by these embryologic studies as arrests at various stages of channel development (DeTakats, 1932; Szilagyi et al, 1976). It was hypothesized that arrested development at the capillary network stage would result in formation of a "capillary" hemangioma, whereas a "cavernous" hemangioma resulted if the insult to the primitive vascular network occurred deep in the skin. Arteriovenous fistulae resulted if there was faulty vascular morphogenesis during the later retiform stage. If the aberration affected still later development, more mature venous ectasias could result. Professor Edmondo Malan spent his lifetime studying vascular anomalies, or "angiodysplasias," as he preferred to call them (Fig. 2–7). His 1974 monograph is a monument to his scholarly and unremitting quest to understand vascular birthmarks. He struggled with an embryonic classification of

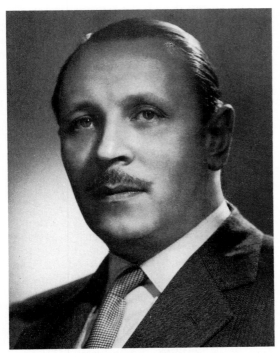

Figure 2–7. Edmondo Malan (1910–1978), Professor of Surgery at the University of Milan, devoted his career to the study of "angiodysplasias." (Photograph courtesy of the wife of Professor Malan.)

"angiomas," subdividing them as follows: (a) venous, (b) troncular (sic) arteriovenous fistula, (c) arteriovenous, and (d) capillary (Malan, 1974). However, in the final analysis, Malan endorsed the anatomicopathological classification of Stout and Lattes.

These attempts at an embryological classification, albeit fanciful, are conceptually appealing and superficially logical. However, when put to the test of clinical usefulness, the embryological classifications fail to differentiate between involuting and non-involuting lesions and offer little to guide clinical management of the wide variety of vascular birthmarks. The embryological approach has also had heuristic faults, failing to stimulate investigation into the molecular mechanisms underlying vascular morphogenesis.

BIOLOGICAL CLASSIFICATION

In 1975, a prospective study was undertaken by Mulliken and Glowacki to define the cellular features of the various vascular lesions seen in infancy and childhood and to correlate the findings with physical examination and natural history. Surgical specimens were analyzed by selected histochemical, autoradiographic, and electron microscopic techniques. This investigation demonstrated that, on the basis of cell kinetics, there are two major types of vascular birthmarks: *hemangiomas*, those demonstrating endothelial hyperplasia; and *malformations*, those with normal endothelial turnover (Mulliken and Glowacki, 1982).

Hemangiomas

The Greek noun suffix *-oma* denotes a swelling or tumor. For example, Hippocrates used the terms *carcinoma* ("crab swelling") and *condyloma* ("knobby swelling"). In modern usage, the suffix *-oma* usually signifies a tumor that is characterized by hyperplasia. Therefore, the unmodified noun *hemangioma* should be restricted to a vascular tumor that enlarges by rapid cellular proliferation. It is critical that, at the present state of our knowledge, the infant hemangioma should not be labelled a "vascular malformation" (or badly formed vessels). It is, in fact, much more biologically similar to a neoplasm. This common tumor of infancy, during its rapid growth phase, is characterized by hypercellularity and endothelial multiplication as documented by thymidine incorporation (Mulliken and Glowacki, 1982). These data confirm that a hemangioma is not a collection of dilated or malformed vessels. Endothelial cells normally show very few mitotic figures and very long doubling times.

Hemangiomas can proliferate to establish a large cell mass, which *pari passu* necessitates the dilatation and formation of new draining and feeding vascular channels. These subordinate vessels, within and around the perimeter of hemangiomas, do not represent an accompanying vascular malformation. The flow through these feeding and draining vessels can, in large hemangiomas and particularly those in the liver, give a clinical and angiographic picture of arteriovenous shunting, thus mimicking a high-flow vascular malformation.

The term *hemangioma* can also be applied to hypercellular tumors of vascular origin seen in adults; for example, there are rare examples of "hemangioma of muscle," as well as other benign synovial and neural hemangiomas. The skeletal muscle hemangiomas usually present in the lower limb, manifesting before age 30. There is no gender predilection. Histologically, plump proliferating endothelial cells infiltrate between muscle fibers and within nerve sheaths and intraluminal papillary projections (Allen and Enzinger, 1972; Enzinger and Weiss, 1983). There is also another rare tumor of adulthood of intermediate or borderline malignancy, called "epithelioid hemangioma" (angiolymphoid hyperplasia with eosinophilia, histiocytoid hemangioma) (Kimura's disease) (Wells and Whimster, 1969; Rosai et al., 1979; Enzinger and Weiss, 1983).

Until further cellular studies are forthcoming, several other entities, e.g., "spider angioma," "senile hemangioma" (cherry spot), and "hemangioma of pregnancy," appear to be anomalies secondary to vascular dilatation, rather than true tumors, and therefore should not be called "-omas." They can be referred to as cutaneous ectasias.

Vascular Malformations

The second major category of vascular birthmarks is properly designated *malformations*, lesions that exhibit a normal rate of endothelial cell turnover throughout their natural history (Mulliken and Glowacki, 1982). These lesions are true structural anomalies, inborn errors of vascular morphogenesis. The molecular mechanism underlying the abnormal pattern formation for these anomalies is unknown; however, it is unlikely that endothelial hyperplasia plays a role. Of course, a transient cellular hyperplasia does occur in these lesions, just as in normal tissues, during the healing phase following trauma or surgical intervention. Vascular malformations are, by definition, congenital (i.e., present at birth), and many are obvious at that time. Some vascular anomalies are undetected at birth and manifest themselves during adolescence or adulthood. Thus, the designation "acquired" vascular lesion must be used with caution. A vascular malformation might be a subtle abnormality of the vessel wall that only, in time, presents as the result of progressive ectasia.

Vascular malformations grow commensurately with the child, although they may gradually or suddenly expand because of changes in blood or lymphatic flow/pressure, collateral formation, or hormonal modulation. Vascular malformations can be subdivided into the following groups: *capillary, venous,* and *arterial* abnormalities, with or without fistulae and *lymphatic* anomalies. A single type of channel anomaly may predominate; however, there are often combined channel anomalies (Fig. 2–8). It is clinically important

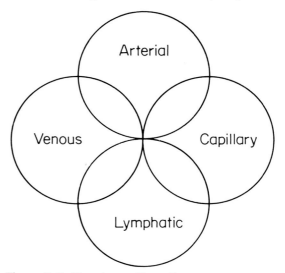

Figure 2–8. Vascular malformations can occur as a single channel conformation. Often these anomalies are *combined* with overlapping of anatomic types, simplistically represented in this diagram.

Table 2–2. TRANSLATION FROM OLD TERMINOLOGY FOR VASCULAR BIRTHMARKS INTO *HEMANGIOMA* OR *MALFORMATION*

Hemangioma	Old Terminology	Malformation
←	Capillary	
←	Strawberry	
	Port-wine	→ CAPILLARY
←	Capillary-cavernous	
	Cavernous	→ VENOUS
	Venous	
	Hemangio-lymphangioma	→ LYMPHATIC
	Lymphangioma	
	Arteriovenous	→ ARTERIOVENOUS

to separate the vascular anomalies into "low-flow" (capillary, venous, lymphatic, or a combination) or "high-flow" (arteriovenous) categories.

Translation of Terminology

The terminology for vascular birthmarks used in this text can be translated from older nomenclature (Table 2–2). "Hemangioma" is restricted to the common tumor of infancy; this is synonymous with the older terms, including "capillary," "cellular," "hypertrophic" and "juvenile hemangioma," or "benign hemangioendothelioma." The hyphenated histologic designation "capillary-cavernous" is unhelpful, for it does not denote a special type of hemangioma or one that differs in its superficial and deep layers or in its behavior from other hemangiomas. Hemangiomas may be superficial, lying in the papillary dermis or deep in the reticular dermis, fat, and muscle (Fig. 2–9A). It is incorrect to assume that a particular hemangioma has mixed superficial ("immature," "capillary") and deep ("mature," "cavernous") elements. Differences in color of the overlying skin reflect the extent of invasion into the papillary dermis. At any point in time, a particular hemangioma has its own microscopic pattern, and this is quite consistent throughout the depth of the lesion. Every hemangioma has an initial *proliferating phase*, which is followed by a prolonged *involuting phase*.

The histologic term "cavernous" causes particular confusion; for example, medical literature can be cited to indicate that "cavernous" hemangiomas usually involute (Simpson, 1959), involute slowly (Andrews et al., 1957), or never involute (MacCollum and Martin, 1956). The so-called "cavernous" lesions that never involute are mislabelled—they are, in fact, venous malformations of a particularly spongy architecture (Fig. 2–9B). The clinically diagnosed "cavernous" hemangiomas that proceed to involute are, in fact, deep-seated hemangiomas with little penetra-

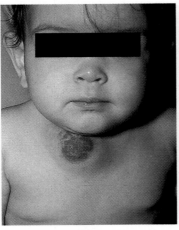 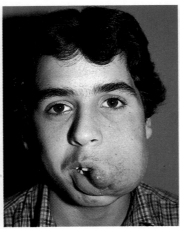 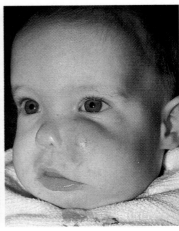

A   B   C

Figure 2–9. Examples of *past* confusion using the term "cavernous" and the *present* nomenclature.
  A, Three month old child with vascular tumor of the chest, which appeared shortly after birth and grew rapidly. Past: "capillary-cavernous" hemangioma; present: *hemangioma*.
  B, Fifteen year old male with vascular lesion of the face, present since birth. Past: "cavernous hemangioma"; present: *venous malformation*.
  C, Infant with enlarging mass in cheek. Past: "cavernous" hemangioma; present: *hemangioma*.

tion of the overlying skin (Fig. 2–9C). The histologic features of a hemangioma during its life cycle also add to the confusion over the term "cavernous." As the typical infant hemangioma undergoes involution, endothelial hyperplasia diminishes while fibrous tissue appears to separate vascular spaces. Some of the densely packed channels enlarge, and the lining endothelium begins to flatten. Thus, the once "capillary" hemangioma now assumes a more "cavernous" appearance, particularly in lesions excised and examined in the 2–5 year old age group. This histologic picture is partially responsible for the confusing phrase "mixed capillary-cavernous hemangioma." The remainder of the blame can be placed on the clinical use of this hyphenated expression to describe a hemangioma that is located in both the superficial and deep layers of the skin. In the final analysis, the term "cavernous" is not useful and should be avoided in any discussion of vascular birthmarks.

Fat laden parenchyma, characteristic of an involuting phase hemangioma, has also caused terminological confusion. This fatty infiltration can be quite prominent, and the term "angiolipoma" has been incorrectly applied to these surgical specimens. More precisely, an "angiolipoma" is a subcutaneous tumor, often multiple and frequently painful, that typically appears in the forearm of young adults. "Sclerosing hemangioma" is another unfortunate term for an acquired tumor of young adulthood, better known as "dermatofibroma" or "histiocytoma." There are a myriad of other acquired cutaneous lesions, mostly ectasias, that have been inaccurately called "angiomas," e.g., "cherry angioma" ("senile angioma"), "spider angioma," and "angioma serpiginosum." These entities are only briefly mentioned in this book.

The port-wine stain, which is composed of dilated capillary-like vessels, has been incorrectly listed as a "capillary hemangioma." It is also called *naevus flammeus*, which confuses it with the commonplace fading macular stain of the forehead, eyelids, and nose. Port-wine stain is a well-accepted descriptive term; the lesion is more precisely designated as a capillary malformation or dermal vascular malformation (Fig. 2–10A). A dermal capillary malformation with hyperkeratosis is often inaccurately called "verrucous hemangioma."

"Lymphangioma" and "cystic hygroma" are terms that imply that these lymphatic lesions grow by cellular proliferation. In fact, most investigators agree that these lesions are really lymphatic malformations, consisting of anomalous channels and cysts of various size, shape, and extent of tissue involvement (Fig. 2–10B and C). Lymphangiectasia is an accurate histologic term that signifies an intraembryonic origin. If capillaries or veins are combined with anomalous lymphatic channels, the lesion should be called capillary-lymphatic or venous-lymphatic malformation, respectively, and not "hemangiolymphangioma" (Table 2–2) (Fig. 2–10D and E). A dermal capillary-lymphatic malformation often evidences hyperkeratosis (hence the old term "verrucous hemangioma").

Eponyms have, all too often, obscured our thinking about complex vascular anomalies. With the system outlined herein, these malformation syndromes can be anatomically delineated. One example is the Klippel-Trenaunay syndrome; it is best envisioned as a combined capillary-venous-lymphatic malformation with skeletal overgrowth (Fig. 2–10F).

SUMMARY

Einstein once said that "explanation of natural phenomena should be as simple as possible but not one bit simpler." This counsel also applies to our attempts to explain abnormal phenomena. The conceptual separation of vascular birthmarks into "hemangiomas" and "malformations" is employed throughout this text (Table 2–3). This terminology is not just a question of semantic precision. A classification of disease is successful only if it has diagnostic applicability, helps in planning therapy, and guides studies of pathogenesis. This simplified classification of vascular birthmarks can be called "biological" because it combines cellular features with clinical behavior. At the same time, it is a practical system—one that *does not* necessitate complicated diagnostic studies; nor is biopsy a requisite. An accurate medical history, physical examination, and, if necessary, repeated clinical evaluation permit accurate classification of vascular birthmarks in the vast majority of patients (Finn et al., 1983). Therapeutic planning can be rationally formulated once the cellular basis of a particular lesion is understood (Mulliken, 1984). For example, prednisone can be useful in controlling rapidly growing hemangiomas, but steroids have no place in the treatment of enlarging lym-

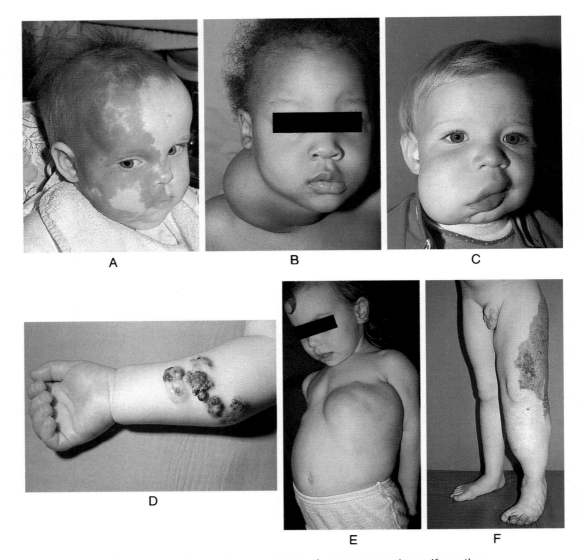

Figure 2–10. Examples of *past* and *present* nomenclature of common vascular malformations.

A, Infant with diffuse vascular birthmark of face and scalp. Past: "naevus flammeus," "capillary hemangioma"; present: *capillary malformation* (port-wine stain).

B, One year old boy with swelling in right neck present since birth. Past: "cystic hygroma"; present: *lymphatic malformation.*

C, One year old boy with swelling in right cheek, enlarging proportionately. Past: "lymphangioma"; present: *lymphatic malformation.*

D, Five month old infant with firm, raised vascular lesions of forearm that bleed intermittently, present since birth. Note verrucous or hyperkeratotic surface. Past: "hemangio-lymphangioma" or "verrucous hemangioma"; present: *capillary-lymphatic malformation.*

E, Five year old girl with vascular lesion of chest wall, which has grown commensurately since birth. Past: "lymphangio-hemangioma"; present: *venous-lymphatic malformation.*

F, Seven year old boy with vascular anomaly of lower extremity with soft tissue and bone enlargement. Note raised hemorrhagic vesicles within the port-stained area. Past: "mixed hemangioma, phlebectasia" with skeletal overgrowth, or "nevus vasculosus osteohypertrophicus"; present: *combined capillary, lymphatic,* and *venous malformation* with skeletal overgrowth (Klippel-Trenaunay syndrome).

Table 2–3. BIOLOGICAL CLASSIFICATION OF VASCULAR BIRTHMARKS BASED ON CELLULAR AND CLINICAL STUDIES

Hemangiomas	Malformations
Proliferating phase	Capillary
Involuting phase	Lymphatic
	Venous
	Arterial
	Combined

From Mulliken, J. B., and Glowacki, J.: Plast. Reconstr. Surg. *69*:412, 1982.

phatic, venous, or arteriovenous malformations.

The characteristics that distinguish *hemangioma* from vascular *malformation* during infancy and childhood are summarized in Table 2–4 and in the following discussion.

Clinical Differences

The clinical criteria are, by far, the most important in making a proper diagnosis. A hemangioma is usually not seen in the newborn nursery. Some 30% of hemangiomas are present as a small macular red spot, and, rarely, a fully grown hemangioma is seen at birth. Hemangiomas are characterized by rapid postnatal growth and very slow involution. Females are more commonly affected; the gender ratio is 3:1.

All cutaneous vascular malformations, by definition, are present at birth. Most of them are plainly seen. However, lymphatic, venous, and arteriovenous anomalies can first appear later in childhood and the early adult period. A vascular malformation grows proportionately with the child; it may expand secondary to sepsis, trauma, or hormonal changes. Vascular malformations have no gender predilection.

Cellular Differences

The nosologic system described has stimulated cellular studies of pathogenesis, particularly for hemangiomas. Early in its life cycle, a hemangioma is composed of plump, proliferating endothelial cells. Mast cells, known to play a role in neoangiogenesis, increase thirty-fold during a hemangioma's proliferating phase (Glowacki and Mulliken, 1982). Mast cells fall to normal levels as involution is completed. Ultrastructural analysis of young hemangiomas reveals multilamination of the basement membrane (Mulliken and Glowacki, 1982) and interactions between mast cells and local macrophages, fibroblasts, and multinucleated giant cells (Dethlefsen et al., 1986).

There is no evidence for hyperplasia in tissue specimens of enlarging vascular malformations. The microscopic findings show

Table 2–4. CHARACTERISTICS OF VASCULAR BIRTHMARKS

Hemangioma	Malformation
Clinical	
Usually nothing seen at birth, 30% present as red macule	All present at birth; may not be evident
Rapid postnatal proliferation and slow involution	Commensurate growth; may expand as a result of trauma, sepsis, hormonal modulation
Female:male 3:1	Female:male 1:1
Cellular	
Plump endothelium, increased turnover	Flat endothelium, slow turnover
Increased mast cells	Normal mast cell count
Multilaminated basement membrane	Normal thin basement membrane
Capillary tubule formation *in vitro*	Poor endothelial growth *in vitro*
Hematological	
Primary platelet trapping: thrombocytopenia (Kasabach-Merritt syndrome)	Primary stasis (venous); localized consumptive coagulopathy
Radiological	
Angiographic findings: well-circumscribed, intense lobular-parenchymal staining with equatorial vessels	Angiographic findings: diffuse, no parenchyma Low-flow: phleboliths, ectatic channels High-flow: enlarged, tortuous arteries with arteriovenous shunting
Skeletal	
Infrequent "mass effect" on adjacent bone; hypertrophy rare	Low-flow: distortion, hypertrophy, or hypoplasia High-flow: destruction, distortion, or hypertrophy

progressive ectasia of structurally abnormal vessels. The anomalous channels are lined by a flat endothelium lying on a thin basal lamina. Mast cells are not increased on histologic examination of resected vascular malformations.

Studies document *in vitro* behaviorial differences between hemangiomas and vascular malformations. Capillary endothelium derived from infant hemangioma forms capillary tubes in tissue culture (Mulliken, Zetter, and Folkman, 1982). Capillary endothelium from vascular anomalies is difficult to culture.

Hematological Differences

There are also hematological dissimilarities between the two major categories of vascular birthmarks. A large hemangioma can cause platelet trapping, shortened platelet half-life, and profound thrombocytopenia (Kasabach-Merritt syndrome). A hemangioma may also evidence consumptive coagulopathy, but this is probably a secondary phenomenon. Vascular malformations, particularly the venous type, induce a true intravascular coagulation defect with only mild thrombocytopenia and slightly decreased platelet survival.

Radiological Differences

The dichotomy between hemangioma and malformation can also be seen angiographically (Burrows et al., 1983). A hemangioma appears as a well-circumscribed mass, with intense, prolonged tissue staining that is usually organized in a lobular pattern. The feeding arteries often form an "equatorial" network at the periphery of the tumor. Vascular malformations, although angiographically variable depending on the predominant channel type, are diffuse lesions consisting entirely of vessels without intervening parenchymal stain.

Skeletal Differences

There are differences in the skeletal changes associated with vascular birthmarks (Boyd et al., 1984). Growing hemangiomas only very rarely cause bone distortion or hypertrophy. Hemangiomas can give a localized mass effect, e.g., depression of the outer table of the skull, shift of the nasal skeleton,

or secondary enlargement of the orbit. On the other hand, low-flow vascular anomalies are frequently associated with diffuse bone hypertrophy, distortion, or elongation; high-flow lesions may cause destructive interosseous changes.

The classification of vascular birthmarks into *hemangiomas* and *malformations* is justified on both a clinical and an heuristic basis. This system is also flexible enough to accept newer concepts as our knowledge of vascular birthmarks increases.

References

Adami, J. G.: *The Principles of Pathology*. Philadelphia: Lea & Febiger, Vol. I, 1908, pp. 748–759.

Albrecht, E.: Die Grundprobleme der Geschwülstlehre. I. Teil. Frank. Z. Pathol. *1*:221, 1907.

Alibert, J. L.: *Nosologie Naturelle ou Les Maladies Du Corps Humain Distribuées par Familles*. Paris: Caille and Ravier, 1817, pp. 349–351.

Allen, P. W., and Enzinger, F. M.: Hemangioma of skeletal muscle. Cancer *29*:8, 1972.

Andrews, G. C., Domonkos, A. N., Torres-Rodriguez, V. M., and Bembenista, J. K.: Hemangiomas—treated and untreated. JAMA *165*(9):1114, 1957.

Andries, G. H., and Kaump, D. H.: Multiple malignant hemangiomas of the liver. Amer. J. Clin. Path. *14*:489, 1944.

Bell, J.: *The Principles of Surgery*. London: Longman, Hurst, Rees, etc., 1815, pp. 456–489.

Berkeley, G.: *A Treatise Concerning the Principles of Human Knowledge*. Dublin: Jeremy Pepyat, 1710, p. 4.

Boyd, J. B., Mulliken, J. B., Kaban, L. B., Upton, J., and Murray, J. E.: Skeletal changes associated with vascular malformations. Plast. Reconstr. Surg. *74*:789, 1984.

Brown, J. B., and Byars, L. T.: The interstitial radiation treatment of hemangiomata. Amer. J. Surg. *39*:452, 1938.

Burrows, P. E., Mulliken, J. B., Fellows, K. E., and Strand, R. D.: Childhood hemangiomas and vascular malformations: Angiographic differentiation. Amer. J. Roentg. *141*:483, 1983.

Byars, L. T.: The "malignant" hemangioma. Surg. Gynec. Obstet. *77*:193, 1943.

Costello, M. J.: Management of vascular nevi. Pediatrics *4*:825, 1949.

Cushing, H., and Bailey, P.: *Tumors Arising from the Blood Vessels of the Brain*. Springfield, IL: Chas. C Thomas, 1928, pp. 211–212.

DeTakats, G.: Vascular anomalies of the extremities. Surg. Gynec. Obstet. *55*:227, 1932.

Dethlefsen, S. M., Mulliken, J. B., and Glowacki, J.: Ultrastructural study of mast cell interactions in hemangiomas. Ultrast. Path. *10*:175, 1986.

Dupuytren, G.: *Leçons Orales de Clinique Chirurgicale Faites à l'Hôtel-Dieu de Paris*. Paris: G. Baillière et Fils, Vol. III, 1839, p. 225.

Enzinger, F. M., and Smith, B. H.: Hemangiopericytoma, an analysis of 106 cases. Human Path. *7*:61, 1976.

Enzinger, F. M., and Weiss, S. W.: *Soft Tissue Tumors*. Chapter 16, Benign tumors and tumor-like lesions of blood vessels. St. Louis: C.V. Mosby, 1983, pp. 379–421.

Ewing, J.: *Neoplastic Diseases*, 4th ed. Philadelphia: W.B. Saunders Co., 1940, p. 249.

Finn, M. C., Glowacki, J., and Mulliken, J. B.: Congenital vascular lesions: Clinical application of a new classification. J. Pediatr. Surg. *18*:894, 1983.

Fraser, J.: The haemangioma group of endothelioblastomata. Brit. J. Surg. *7*:335, 1919–1920.

Garrison, F. H.: *An Introduction to the History of Medicine*, 4th ed. Philadelphia,: W.B. Saunders Co., 1929, p. 417.

Glowacki, J., and Mulliken, J. B.: Mast cells in hemangiomas and vascular malformations. Pediatrics *70*:48, 1982.

Golgi, C.: Sulla struttura e sullo sviluppo degli psammomi. In *Patologia Generale e Isto-Patologia*, Vol. III of *Opera Omnia*. Milan: Ulrico Hoepli, 1903, p. 797.

Harvey, W. F., Dawson, E. K., and Innes, J. R. M.: Endothelioma. Edinburgh Med. J. *47*:513, 1940.

His, W.: Akad. Programm, Basel, 1865, quoted by Lewis, D., and Geschickter, C. F.: Endothelial tumors. Trans. West. Surg. Assoc. *45*:447, 1935.

Hoehn, J. G., Farrow, G. M., Devine, K. D., and Masson, J. K.: Invasive hemangioma of the head and neck. Amer. J. Surg. *120*:495, 1970.

Home, E.: An account of Mr. Hunter's method of performing the operation for the cure of the popliteal aneurism. Trans. Soc. Impr. Med. Chirg. Know. Vol. I, p. 138, 1793.

Hooper, R.: *Lexicon Medicum (Medical Dictionary)*, Vol. 1. New York: Harper and Brothers, 1841.

Hunter, W.: The history of an aneurysm of the aorta, with some remarks on aneurysms in general. Med. Observ. Inquir. *1*:323, 1757.

Lampe, I., and Latourette, H. B.: The management of cavernous hemangiomas in infants. Postgrad. Med. *19*:262, 1956.

Lewis, F. J.: The development of the lymphatic system in rabbits. Am. J. Anat. *5*:95, 1905.

MacCallum, W. G.: *Textbook of Pathology*, 6th ed. Philadelphia: W.B. Saunders Co., 1936, p. 1055.

MacCollum, D. W., and Martin, L. W.: Hemangiomas in infancy and childhood. A report based on 6479 cases. Surg. Clin. North Am. *36*:1647, 1956.

Malan, E.: *Vascular Malformations (Angiodysplasias)*. Milan: Carlo Erba Foundation, 1974, pp. 15–26.

Matthews, D. N.: Hemangiomata. Plast. Reconstr. Surg. *41*:528, 1968.

Mulliken, J. B., and Glowacki, J.: Hemangiomas and vascular malformations in infants and children: A classification based on endothelial characteristics. Plast. Reconstr. Surg. *69*:412, 1982.

Mulliken, J. B., Zetter, B. R., and Folkman, J.: In vitro characteristics of endothelium from hemangiomas and vascular malformations. Surgery *92*:348, 1982.

Mulliken, J. B.: Cutaneous vascular lesions of children. In Serafin, D., and Georgiade, N. G. (eds.): *Pediatric Plastic Surgery*. St. Louis: C.V. Mosby Co., 1984, pp. 137–154.

Pack, G. T., and Miller, T. R.: Hemangiomas, classification, diagnosis and treatment. Angiology *1*:405, 1950.

Petit, J. L.: *Traité des Maladies Chirurgicales et Opérations*. Paris: Chez P. Fr. Didot, 1774, Tome Premier, Chap. VII, p. 223.

Popkin, G. L.: Tumors of the vascular system. In Converse, J. M. (ed.): *Reconstructive Plastic Surgery*, 2nd Ed., Vol. 5. Philadelphia: W.B. Saunders Co., 1977, p. 2865.

Pulford, D. S., Jr.: Neoplasms of the blood-lymph-vascular system with special reference to endotheliomas. Ann. Surg. *82*:710, 1925.

Reinhoff, W. F., Jr.: Congenital arteriovenous fistula, an embryological study, with the report of a case. Bull. Johns Hopkins Hosp. *35*:271, 1924.

Robinson, J. M., and Castleman, B.: Benign metastasizing hemangioma. Ann. Surg. *104*:453, 1936.

Rosai, J., Gold, J., and Landy, R.: The histiocytoid hemangiomas: A unifying concept embracing several previously described entities of skin, soft tissue, large vessels, bone and heart. Hum. Path. *10*:707, 1979.

Sabin, F. R.: On the origin of the lymphatic system from the veins and the development of the lymph hearts and thoracic duct in the pig. Am. J. Anat. *1*:367, 1902.

Schwartz, A. R.: Multiple malignant hemangioendothelioma in an infant. Report of a case. Arch. Pediat. *62*:1, 1945.

Simpson, J. R.: Natural history of cavernous haemangiomata. Lancet *2*:1057, 1959.

Stout, A. P.: Hemangio-endothelioma: A tumor of blood vessels featuring vascular endothelial cells. Ann. Surg. *118*:445, 1943.

Stout, A. P.: Hemangiopericytoma: A study of twenty-five new cases. Cancer *2*:1027, 1949.

Stout, A. P., and Lattes, R. S.: Tumors of the soft tissues. Washington, D.C., 1967, Armed Forces Institute of Pathology, fascicle 1, second series.

Stout, A. P., and Murray, M. R.: Hemangiopericytoma. A vascular tumor featuring Zimmerman's pericytes. Ann. Surg. *116*:26, 1942.

Szilagyi, D. E., Smith, R. F., Elliott, J. P., and Hageman, J. H.: Congenital arteriovenous anomalies of the limbs. Arch. Surg. *111*:423, 1976.

Thomson, H. G.: Hemangioma, lymphangioma, and arteriovenous fistula. In Grabb, W. C., and Smith, J. W. (eds.): *Plastic Surgery: A Concise Guide to Clinical Practice*, 3rd ed. Boston: Little, Brown, 1979, p. 518.

Virchow, R.: Angiome. In *Die krankhaften Geschwülste*. Berlin: August Hirschwald, 1863, Vol. 3, pp. 306–425.

Walls, E. W.: John Bell, 1763–1820. Med. Hist. *8*:63, 1964.

Walter, J.: On the treatment of cavernous haemangioma with special reference to spontaneous involution. J. Fac. Rad. *5*:13, 1953.

Ward, G. E., and Jonas, A. F., Jr.: Metastasizing hemangioma simulating an aneurysm. Arch. Surg. *36*:330, 1938.

Wardrop, J.: Some observations on one species of naevus maternus with the case of an infant where the carotid artery was tied. Medico-Chirurgical Trans. *9*:199, 1818.

Watson, W. L., and McCarthy, W. D.: Blood and lymph vessel tumors: A report of 1,056 cases. Surg. Gynecol. Obstet. *71*:569, 1940.

Wegner, G.: Ueber lymphangiome. Arch. Klin. Chir. *20*:641, 1877.

Wells, G. C., and Whimster, I.: Subcutaneous angiolymphoid hyperplasia with eosinophilia. Br. J. Dermatol. *81*:1, 1969.

Woollard, H. H.: The development of the principal arterial stems in the forelimb of the pig. Contrib. Embryol. *14*:139, 1922.

PART TWO

Hemangiomas

CHAPTER THREE

Diagnosis and Natural History of Hemangiomas

John B. Mulliken

And the blots of Nature's hand
Shall not in their issue stand;
Never mole, hare-lip, nor scar,
Nor mark prodigious, such as are
Despised in nativity,
Shall upon their children be.

Shakespeare, A Midsummer Night's Dream
(Act V, Sc. i., 406)

Hemangiomas are the most common tumors of infancy. About one third are first noted in the nursery (Simpson 1959; Finn et al., 1983); the incidence is reported to be 1.0–2.6% (Pratt, 1967; Jacobs and Walton, 1976). There may be a small punctate or macular spot, although occasionally a hemangioma in full bloom is seen at birth. The majority of hemangiomas (70–90%) appear during the first to fourth week of life. By age 1 year, approximately 10–12% of white children have a hemangioma (Holmdahl, 1955; Jacobs, 1957). In Japanese infants, an incidence of 0.8% can be calculated from the report of Hidano and Nakajima (Hidano and Nakajima, 1972). In our institution, hemangiomas are uncommon in black children; however, Pratt reports an incidence of 1.4% in black infants examined during the first week of life (Pratt, 1967). Hemangiomas occur in an equal frequency (approximately 12%) in premature and full-term infants (Greenhouse, 1955; Holmdahl, 1955). These studies included only premature infants weighing in the 1500–2500 gm range. In our newborn nursery, we recently noted that hemangiomas appeared in 30% of tiny premature infants, those weighing less than 1000 gm. However, those premature infants with a birth weight greater than 1500 gm had the same frequency of hemangiomas (10%) as that noted in Holmdahl's report. Hemangiomas are more common in females than in males, in a 3:1 ratio (Bowers, 1960; Finn et al., 1983). Hemangiomas are not familial, although they occur frequently in fair-skinned families. Margileth and Museles elicited a family history of hemangioma in 10% of their infant patients (Margileth and Museles, 1965).

The first sign of a nascent hemangioma is an erythematous macular patch, a blanched spot, or a localized telangiectasia, surrounded by a pale halo (Payne et al., 1966; Hidano and Nakajima, 1972) (Fig. 3–1). Telangiectases later appear throughout the well demarcated pale area. Hidano and Nakajima describe two such lesions that failed to form

41

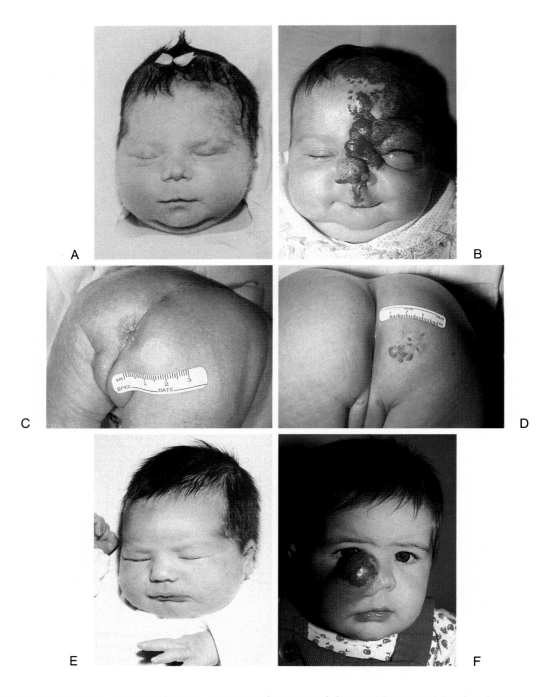

Figure 3–1. First signs of hemangioma. *A,* Macular stain on the left forehead is barely visible in this photograph taken on the day of birth. *B,* By 4 months, the child in *A* has a large hemangioma infiltrating the left face and obstructing the eye. *C,* Pale spot noted on the right buttock at 2 days post-birth. *D,* Hemangioma appeared in same area 3 weeks later; this photograph taken at age 4 months. (Courtesy of Arthur R. Rhodes, M.D.) *E,* Nursery photograph shows no signs of impending hemangioma; however, a macular area on the right cheek was seen "a few days" after birth. *F,* Hemangioma at apogee of growth, age 10 months.

vascular papules and were judged to be abortive hemangiomas (Hidano and Nakajima, 1972). A hemangioma may grow as an extensive tumor in a local area or may simultaneously proliferate in multiple sites anywhere in the body. Eighty per cent of hemangiomas are present as a single lesion; 20% of affected infants have more than one hemangioma (Margileth and Museles, 1965). There are exceptional cases of multiple tiny cutaneous hemangiomas; Lunsford observed a 6 day old neonate with 834 lesions (Lunsford, 1932). The head and neck region is the most commonly involved (60%), followed in frequency by the trunk (25%) and the extremities (15%) (Finn et al., 1983). This regional distribution is slightly skewed by the natural tendency for parents to bring children with facial hemangiomas to medical attention. Hemangiomas have been found in lymph nodes, spleen, liver, thymus, gastrointestinal tract, lung, urinary bladder, gallbladder, pancreas, and adrenal glands (Kundstadter, 1933; Andries and Kaump, 1944; Edmondson, 1956; Cooper and Bolande, 1965; Burman et al., 1967; Holden and Alexander, 1970).

It is rare for an infant with visceral system hemangiomatosis not to have cutaneous involvement or to manifest just a few lesions. The corollary is also true, that some infants with multiple cutaneous lesions do not have hemangiomas of internal organs (Fig. 3–2). There are also reported cases of hemangiomas in the meninges, brain, and spinal cord (Burke, 1964; Burman et al., 1967; Cooper and Bolande, 1965). In all cases of documented intracranial hemangiomas, there were also multiple cutaneous lesions.

In the past, the term "disseminated hemangiomatosis" was incorrectly applied to cases with cutaneous and intracranial visceral involvement, thus implying that they are malignant tumors (Kundstadter, 1933; Schwartz, 1945). Multiple hemangiomas should be regarded as multicentric new growths, and not as "metastases."

Rapid growth during the neonatal period is the hemangioma's hallmark. If the lesion begins in the superficial dermis, cellular proliferation causes the skin to become raised and finely bosselated with a vivid crimson color. Parents often comment that the hemangioma changes color during the day. Most hemangiomas remain as well-circumscribed lesions 0.5–5.0 cm in diameter, whereas some spread in a localized geographic pattern. It is common to note two or three large superficial veins radiating from the lesion. A hemangioma may proliferate in the lower dermis and subcutaneous tissue layer with little involvement of the superficial or papillary dermis. These lesions may be slightly raised with a bluish hue, or the overlying skin can be smooth and of normal color. The covering skin may also exhibit several faint, dilated veins or tiny telangiectatic vessels. These deeper lesions were once labelled "cavernous" hemangiomas. When a hemangioma involves both deep and superficial skin layers, it has been called a "mixed, capillary-cavernous" hemangioma. In fact, histologic examination of hemangiomas with this morphologic appearance shows that the proliferative endothelial pattern is remarkably consistent throughout the depth of any particular tumor (Mulliken and Glowacki, 1982) (Fig. 3–3A to C). The microscopic terms "capillary" and "cavernous" are clinically confusing and should not be used in clinical parlance. Instead, it is more accurate to refer to a bright red hemangioma as "superficial," and to refer to a lesion with normal overlying skin as a "deep" hemangioma (Fig. 3–3D). Hemangiomas commonly present with both superficial and deep cutaneous as well as subcutaneous proliferation.

DIFFERENTIAL DIAGNOSIS

Clinical Differences

The initial, and perhaps most critical, determinant in differentiating hemangioma

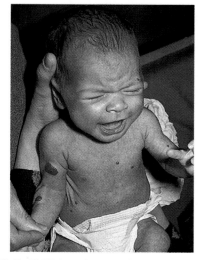

Figure 3–2. Multiple cutaneous hemangiomas. These lesions have a characteristic dome shape. They often are associated with visceral hemangiomas; however, this was not the case in this child.

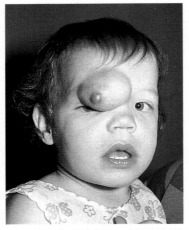

Figure 3–3. Fallacy of the old term "capillary-cavernous" hemangioma. *A*, One year old child with supraorbital hemangioma. The lesion was excised because the mass caused astigmatism. *B*, Microscopic section of the superficial (red) portion of this specimen shows endothelial proliferation with admixed large and small channels (H&E × 38). *C*, Microscopic section of the deep (blue) portion of this specimen shows the same proliferative pattern with large and small channels. Note parenchymal fat and large feeding-draining vessels (H&E × 38). *D*, Drawing illustrates that the "strawberry" hemangioma's location in the skin determines the color and configuration of the tumor.

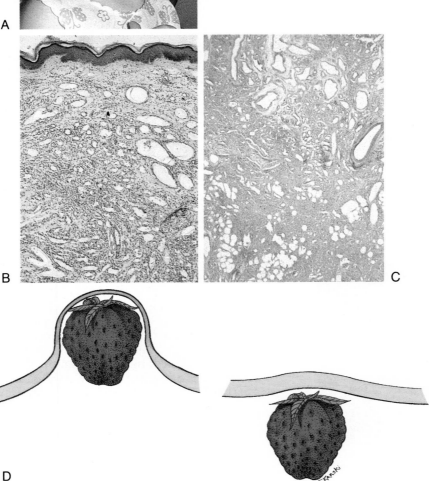

from malformation is the clinical history of the lesion. Usually hemangiomas are not seen at birth; they characteristically proliferate rapidly, at a rate beyond the child's growth, during the first 2–3 weeks after birth. Vascular malformations, on the other hand, are usually noted at birth and expand commensurately with the child. The color of a vascular birthmark is particularly helpful in the differential diagnosis. A superficial hemangioma, during the first few months of life, has a bright scarlet color that gradually deepens during the first year. Malformations have a persistent colored hue, depending on the arterial, venous, capillary, and lymphatic components.

It is important to remember two axioms that help to distinguish hemangioma from vascular malformation. The first is that *not all hemangiomas look like strawberries*. The tumor may lie deep within subcutaneous tissue or muscle, giving the overlying skin a faint bluish color or a normal complexion (Fig. 3–4A). In rare cases, the skin may be elevated and have a pale color with scattered tiny tortuous vessels (Fig. 3–4B). It is also possible for a hemangioma to infiltrate the skin densely without elevating it, giving an appearance similar to that of a port-wine stain (Fig. 3–4C and D). The corollary axiom is that *not all strawberries are hemangiomas*. A cutaneous venous or capillary-venous malformation can look remarkably similar to a hemangioma (Fig. 3–5). It is helpful to imagine the microscopic appearance of the hemangioma, a dense cellular tumor with relatively

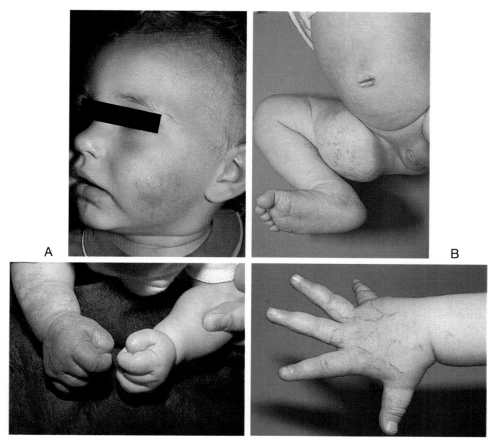

Figure 3–4. Axiom I: *Not all hemangiomas look like strawberries. A,* Tumor in left cheek with ecchymosis-like chin discoloration; appeared at one month of age. *Diagnosis:* hemangioma. *B,* One month old girl with vascular tumor on the right medial thigh, which was present at birth. The skin is raised, pale, and punctuated with tiny serpiginous vessels. This lesion underwent rapid involution during the first year. *Diagnosis:* hemangioma. *C,* Hemangioma of the right hand and forearm that was present at birth, infiltrating the dermis and giving a crimson hue without elevation of the skin. Appearance in this 3 month old child is deceptively similar to that of a port-wine stain. *D,* The child's hand at 3 years of age. Only a few dilated vessels remain to mark the site of the involuting hemangioma.

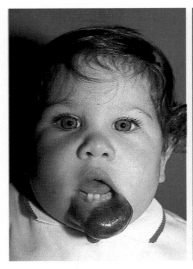 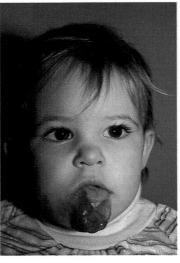

Figure 3–5. Axiom II: *Not all strawberries are hemangiomas. A,* One year old girl with vascular lip lesion that appeared after birth and grew rapidly. It has a doughy consistency and cannot be completely compressed. *Diagnosis:* hemangioma. *Prognosis:* involution. *B,* One year old girl with vascular lip lesion that was present at birth. It is easily compressible and refills rapidly. Thrombi can be palpated. *Diagnosis:* venous malformation. *Prognosis:* commensurate growth with child, likely expansion, and dentoalveolar distortion.

A   B

little luminal area, versus the malformation, a sponge-like anomaly of dilated channels and sparse parenchyma. Palpation is also useful in differentiating these lesions. The hemangioma feels firm or rubbery and rather dense in comparison with the soft and easily compressible vascular malformation. A hemangioma cannot be completely emptied of blood with compression, quite unlike a portstain or a protuberant venous malformation.

In most instances, hemangiomas can be differentiated from vascular malformations without resorting to invasive diagnostic techniques (Finn et al., 1983; Mulliken, 1984). An accurate history, often with the help of the baby's photographs, and a physical examination should confirm the diagnosis. In some instances, the physician must willingly admit that he or she cannot be certain of the exact nature of the vascular birthmark. This situation may prompt a consultation with a colleague. Alternatively, the physician can honestly explain to the parents that another visit in 2–3 months will be necessary before their infant's vascular birthmark can be accurately diagnosed. Usually parents will accept a clear explanation of the most likely diagnoses and the fact that immediate therapy is usually not required. Clearly, this kind of consultation must be carried out with concern and confidence and without signs of a sympathicoadrenal response on the part of the physician.

Uncertainty is most likely to occur in the differential diagnosis between a deep heman-

gioma and a localized lymphatic malformation. In particular, confusion may arise with swelling in the cheek or preauricular (parotid) region. In fact, hemangioma is the most common benign tumor affecting the parotid gland (50%), followed in frequency by pleomorphic adenoma (29%) and intracapsular or juxtaparotid lymphatic anomalies (7%) (Welch, 1986). A history of rapid growth within the first week of life favors a diagnosis of hemangioma. However, lymphatic anomalies may not be recognized at birth, and then they seem to suddenly appear "almost overnight." Palpation is useful—a lymphatic anomaly feels soft, cystic, or flabby, and often this lesion can be transilluminated. Hemorrhage within a lymphatic malformation may explain the sudden appearance of a firm subcutaneous mass with dark blue skin discoloration and the failure of transillumination. Hemangiomas have a more doughy or spongy consistency, and if the overlying skin is penetrated, giving the typical bright red color, the diagnosis is secure. Within a few weeks, an unequivocal diagnosis between deep hemangioma and lymphatic malformation usually becomes obvious; each lesion has its own characteristic natural history. In most cases, time is not crucial for immediate diagnosis and therapy, although the parents will need constant reassurance.

One must always be wary. There are very rare instances when an infant presents with a rapidly growing subcutaneous mass that feels unusually firm; in this situation, a sarcoma must be considered in the differential diagnosis. Radiographic study, particularly computed tomography, can be helpful, and a biopsy may be necessary.

Radiographic Differences

To reiterate, history and physical examination are usually all that are needed to make a correct diagnosis of hemangioma. However, in certain cases of deep hemangiomas without the telltale cutaneous signs, *computed tomography* with dye injection can be used to help differentiate hemangioma from a lymphatic or venous malformation. The proliferative phase hemangioma demonstrates a well-circumscribed homogeneous density and homogeneous enhancement (Figs. 3–6A and 3–7A). However, a hemangioma in its involuting phase has a more variegated density and lobular architecture.

Computed tomography of vascular malformations shows a heterogeneous density. Venous anomalies occasionally have calcifications and enhance in a heterogeneous pattern. Pure lymphatic anomalies are seen as multilocular cysts, which may show enhancement in the septa with intravenous contrast (Figs. 3–6B, 3–7B, and 3–7C). Minor

skeletal deformation can occur with a hemangioma; however, bone hypertrophy and distortion are more typically seen near a lymphatic malformation. A soft tissue sarcoma must be considered if the tomographic pattern does not fit a diagnosis of either hemangioma or lymphatic malformation (Figs. 3–6C, 3–7D, and 3–7E).

Arteriography is rarely indicated in the evaluation of hemangiomas. It may be necessary when embolization is contemplated in a child with a giant hemangioma or hepatic hemangioma that causes platelet trapping with or without congestive heart failure. There are radiographic characteristics that will differentiate the tumor mass of hemangioma from a vascular malformation (Burrows et al., 1983). The two angiographic features that distinguish hemangioma are the following: (1) it is a well circumscribed mass; and (2) there is intense, persistent tissue staining, usually organized in a lobular pattern. Seen radiographically, this lobular organization is most pronounced during the involution phase (Fig. 3–8A and B). Hemangiomas are often supplied by multiple (2–4) enlarged branches of normal adjacent systemic arteries. These feeding arteries often form an equatorial network around the periphery of the tumor mass, sending smaller feeding ar-

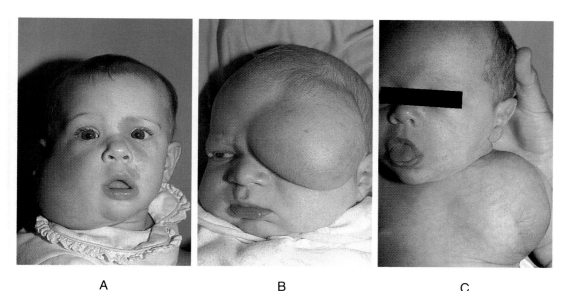

A   B   C

Figure 3–6. Differential diagnosis aided by computed tomography. *A*, One year old child with port-wine stain of left face and large subcutaneous mass in right cheek. *Diagnosis*: deep hemangioma versus lymphatic malformation. *B*, Cystic mass of the forehead and upper eyelid, present at birth and enlarging with the child. *Diagnosis*: venous-lymphatic or lymphatic anomaly. *C*, Two month old child with mass of left chest, growing rapidly. It is firm to palpation and does not clearly transilluminate. *Diagnosis*: hemangioma versus lymphatic anomaly (with hemorrhage).

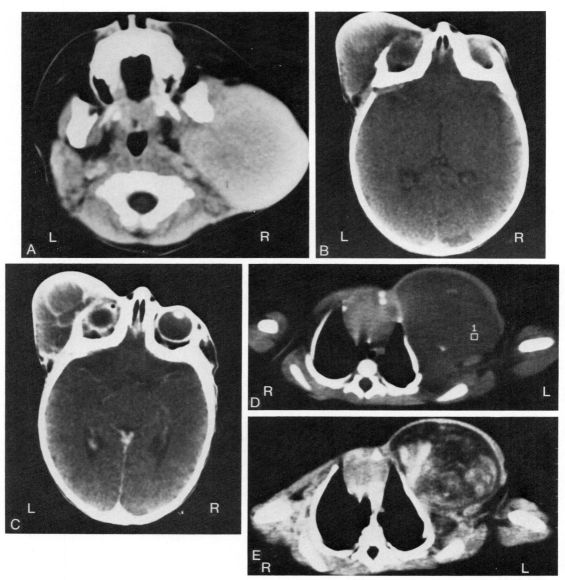

Figure 3–7. Computed tomographic studies of cases in Figure 3–6. *A,* See Figure 3–6*A*: CT scan demonstrates homogeneous contrast enhancement, confirming clinical diagnosis of *hemangioma.* Since these are the most common tumors of childhood, it is not surprising that one could arise coincidentally with a vascular malformation. *B,* CT scan of child in Figure 3–6*B*: note homogeneous, low density mass in frontal region with intraorbital involvement. *C,* With dye injection, the axial CT scan shows a non-enhanced, honeycombed configuration with a few vessels in the septa; the lesion also involves the retrobulbar orbital cone. This is the typical CT appearance of *lymphatic malformation. D,* See Figure 3–6*C*: Axial CT scan through upper thorax, without contrast, shows homogeneous extrathoracic mass. *E,* With contrast, the lesion is enhanced in a heterogeneous pattern that is non-characteristic of either hemangioma or lymphatic anomaly. Biopsy revealed *infantile fibrosarcoma.*

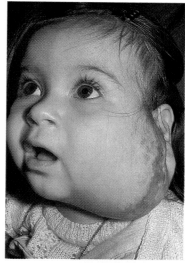

A

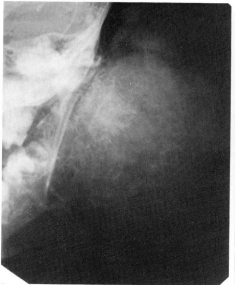

B

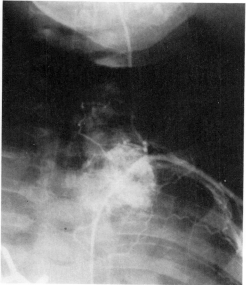

C

Figure 3–8. Angiography of hemangioma. *A,* Two year old girl with large hemangioma of the left face. *B,* Common carotid arteriogram (frontal view) shows homogeneously staining, well-circumscribed mass, faint lobular architecture, and no arteriovenous shunting. *C,* Selective left subclavian angiogram in the patient in *A* and *B* demonstrates an additional separate hemangioma in the mediastinum supplied by several thyrocervical branches. Note equatorial feeding vessels.

teries into the lesion at right angles to the peripheral vessels (Fig. 3–8*C*). In contrast, vascular malformations consist of collections of abnormal vessels without a parenchymal or staining component. Hemangiomas can have high blood flow and an angiographic pattern suggesting arteriovenous shunting. This feature may not be clearly distinguishable from true shunting seen in arteriovenous malformations (Azzolini et al., 1973).

Hemangiomas and Morphogenetic Syndromes

Hemangioma is often said to occur in association with a wide variety of birth defects.

However, in these dysmorphic conditions, the "hemangioma" referred to is usually a port-wine mark or telangiectatic stain. It is also important to emphasize that true hemangiomas are common lesions, and therefore it would be likely to find one in an infant who also happens to have a rare dysmorphic condition. One example in which such a link may exist is the reported combination of a large facial hemangioma with a sternal cleft (Hersh et al., 1985) or a supraumbilical midabdominal raphe (Igarashi et al., 1985).

Pyogenic Granuloma

Pyogenic granuloma is a reactive proliferative vascular lesion frequently confused with hemangioma, since both, unfortunately, share the common histologic designation "capillary hemangioma." Clinically, pyogenic granuloma (also called *granuloma telangiectaticum*) is an acquired vascular lesion, and therefore cannot be called a birthmark. Pyogenic granulomas appear quite suddenly; rarely is a history of trauma to the particular area elicited from the parents. Typically, the patient is a young child, although these lesions also occur in adults. The typical location for a pyogenic granuloma is on the skin of the cheek, eyelids, or extremities. These lesions also often occur on the lips, oral mucosa, tongue, and nasal cavity (Mills et al., 1980). Curiously, pyogenic granulomas frequently emerge as a superimposed growth within an area of obvious port-wine stain, either intra- or extraorally (Fig. 3–9A).

When seen early, the epidermis over a pyogenic granuloma may be intact, and the lesion will bear some resemblance to a tiny hemangioma (Fig. 3–9B). An early pyogenic granuloma often has a pedunculated shape with a tiny neck. The stalk may be remarkably small in comparison with the florid tip of the lesion. Often, by the time medical care is sought, the epidermis is gone, and a brown-black crust or bright red granular surface is seen. Repeated episodes of bleeding, refractoriness to pressure, and repeated trials of cautery or caustics constitute a common presenting history. Frequently the child will arrive with an adhesive bandage on the cheek, a sign of frequent bleeding episodes and multiple visits to the emergency room. This prompted H.G. Thomson to call the entity "Band-Aid disease."

Pyogenic granulomas may grow 1 cm in diameter. Histologically, proliferating endothelial cells are seen, admixed in an edematous stroma filled with a variable population

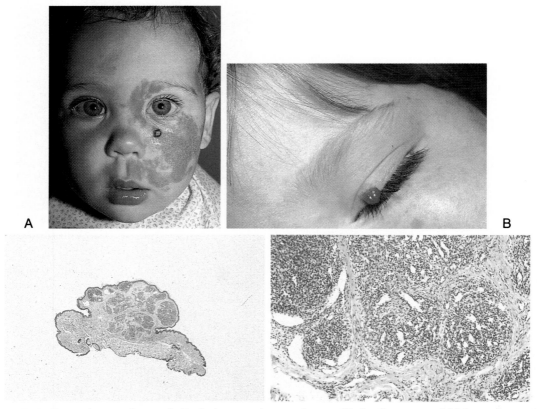

Figure 3–9. Pyogenic granuloma. *A,* Typical pyogenic granuloma with fragile scar and history of repeated bleeding episodes. Curiously, these lesions often occur in port-wine stained skin. *B,* Five year old girl with a vascular lesion that suddenly appeared on her eyelid. *Diagnosis:* pyogenic granuloma with intact epithelium. *C,* Low power photomicrograph of the lesion in *B* demonstrates lobular architecture, tiny stalk, and epidermal collarette (H&E × 1). *D,* High power view of same lesion shows congeries of differing sized capillary-like vessels lined by plump endothelium and surrounded by perivascular stromal cells and edematous septa. There is minimal to absent inflammation. Pyogenic granuloma can be difficult to differentiate histologically from "capillary hemangioma" (H&E × 100).

of inflammatory cells; there may also be epidermopoiesis. A characteristic feature is the "epidermal collarette," located where the covering epithelium meets the surrounding skin at the base of the lesion (Davies and Marks, 1978) (Fig. 3–9C). The character of the stroma and the nature of the inflammatory infiltrate depend on both the depth of the section through the lesion and the presence or absence of ulceration. Deep sections through a pyogenic granuloma demonstrate a dense fibrous stroma surrounding compact lobules of proliferating endothelium. At this level, there is only slight inflammatory cell infiltration and edema (Fig. 3–9D). However, the superficial portion of the lesion is usually more edematous, with few neutrophilic cells. If the excised lesion is ulcerated, the microscopic pattern can be indistinguishable from that of ordinary granulation tissue (Mills et al., 1980). Often a pathologist will designate the lesion as "capillary hemangioma, granuloma type." Sometimes, it is difficult to make a microscopic differentiation between a true hemangioma of infancy and a pyogenic granuloma.

An infectious cause is implied by its name, but scientific evidence for this pathogenesis is lacking. Although they can occur at the sites of small wounds or repeated irritation, most pyogenic granulomas seem to appear without an inciting cause. Tritiated thymidine studies have shown high labelling indices in both epidermis and endothelium in pyogenic granulomas (Davies and Marks, 1978).

Sometimes, a pyogenic granuloma undergoes necrosis and healing without medical ministrations. Repeated bleeding usually requires therapy. The base of the lesion can be cauterized with a silver nitrate stick, although recurrence is not uncommon with this approach because the vascular proliferation extends into the deep dermis. Electrocoagulation or laser removal gives more predictable results. If these measures fail and the lesion continues to bleed interminably, excision and closure are necessary.

THE PROLIFERATIVE PHASE COMPLICATIONS

Ulceration

As a hemangioma grows beneath the cuticular basement membrane, the epidermis may slough and cause ulceration or annoying bleeding. This happens in less than 5% of hemangiomas (Margileth and Museles, 1965). Ulceration can occasionally be seen in a hemangioma at birth. Usually, however, ulceration occurs at the height of the proliferative phase in tense, distended lesions (Bowers et al., 1960) (Fig. 3–10A). However, it is also common in hemangiomas located on the lips and genitoanal areas, where abrasion is common. Secondary infection invariably accompanies ulceration. Venous oozing from an ulcerated hemangioma is usually not worrisome. Episodic bleeding from a tiny punctate area can frighten the parents and be an annoyance to emergency room physicians. There are rare instances in which an ulcerated hemangioma and secondary infection cause extensive necrosis and destruction of facial soft tissues, the so-called "wildfire hemangioma" (Fig. 3–10B).

Obstruction

Visual

A growing hemangioma may impinge on a critical anatomical structure. The best known example is obstruction of the visual axis, causing deprivation amblyopia and failure to develop binocular vision (Robb, 1977; Stigmar et al., 1978; Thomson et al., 1979; Haik et al., 1979) (see Figs. 3–1B and 3–10B). Any interruption of vision, even for 1–2 weeks, can result in permanent damage to the visual system; longer periods of obstruction are even more injurious. Periorbital hemangiomas can also cause anisometropia, resulting in amblyopia, even though the vision is not apparently occluded. The mass effect of a periorbital tumor in infants can distort the growing cornea and thus produce refractive errors, both astigmatic and myopic (Robb, 1977). Hemangiomas exert pressure on the eye in a direction perpendicular to the axis of the astigmatism (see Fig. 3–3A). Robb documented that the axis of greatest corneal curvature could be predictably accounted for by the location of the hemangioma. The other ophthalmological complication of hemangioma is strabismus; this may be either paralytic (secondary to extraocular muscle infiltration by hemangioma) or secondary to the amblyopia (Stigmar et al., 1978). Thus, all children with periorbital hemangiomas should be refracted, using reti-

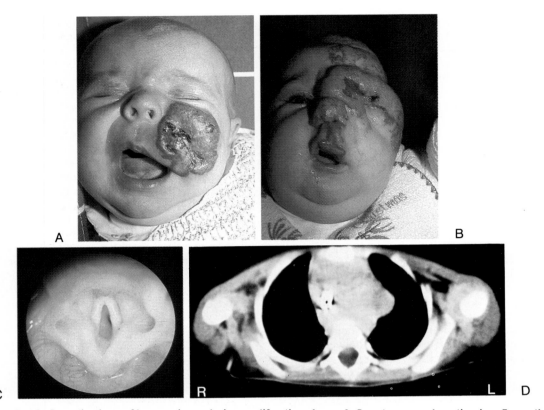

Figure 3–10. Complications of hemangioma during proliferative phase. *A,* Spontaneous ulceration in a 3 month old girl. In the past, this was interpreted as a danger sign or as an indication of ensuing involution. *B,* Ulceration and secondary infection causing destruction of medial canthal tissue. See Figure 3–1*A* and *B* for earlier photographs of this child. *C,* Photograph, taken via laryngoscope, showing left subglottic hemangioma in a 2 month old infant admitted with biphasic stridor. (Courtesy of Trevor McGill, M.D.) *D,* Enhanced axial CT scan through upper chest in a 7 month old child who required tracheostomy for circumferential subglottic hemangioma. Note extension around trachea and upper mediastinum and dislocation of the tracheostomy tube.

noscopy with cycloplegia. When the lesion is within the upper eyelid, frequent periodic refraction is mandatory. Large hemangiomas of the lower eyelid and cheek region must be followed closely, but these lesions are less likely to cause visual disturbances. The absence of an asymmetrical refractive error is a favorable prognostic sign for normal vision after involution of a periorbital hemangioma (Robb, 1977). Later residual complications of periorbital and adnexal hemangiomas include globe proptosis, blepharoptosis, and even optic atrophy (Stigmar et al., 1978).

Nasal or Laryngeal

A hemangioma may block the nasal air passages early on, when the infant is an obligatory nose breather. Nevertheless, the obstruction of the nasal airway usually occurs so slowly that the infant adapts and breathes through the oral passage. More insidious is hemangiomatous proliferation in the subglottic airway, a rare but potentially life-threatening occurrence. Characteristically, these infants are asymptomatic at birth, but within 6–8 weeks they develop biphasic stridor, accompanied by varying degrees of respiratory distress. The common clinical presentation is either a protracted episode of laryngotracheitis or recurrent bouts of "croup" (Healy et al., 1980). Approximately one half of infants with subglottic hemangioma will have associated cutaneous hemangiomas, usually in the cervicofacial area (Ferguson and Flake, 1961). The appearance of the cutaneous lesion is not necessarily an accurate indication of whether or not an infant who presents with stridor has a laryngeal hemangioma. There may be signs of early involution in the skin hemangioma (e.g., softening and a dull gray color change) at the same time that a subglottic hemangioma begins to obstruct the airway.

Any infant who is suspected of having laryngeal hemangioma should have anteroposterior and lateral radiographs, looking for an eccentric subglottic swelling. The diagnosis is confirmed by direct laryngoscopy. The typical finding is a smooth, compressible mass in the posterior subglottic area, often extending around either lateral wall (Fig. 3–10C). Usually the mucosal surface contains a few telangiectatic vessels; sometimes, it is stained a bright red by the submucosal hemangioma. Only rarely does subglottic hemangioma proliferate circumferentially or encroach on the trachea or true vocal cords (Healy et al., 1980) (Fig. 3–10D). In the past, this entity had a high mortality rate, approaching 50% in some series (Ferguson and Flake, 1961).

Auditory

Obstruction of the external auditory canal, unilateral or bilateral, can occur with hemangiomatous involvement of the parotid regions. This causes a mild to moderate conductive hearing loss. The blockage is relieved with regression of the hemangioma. This should not be a problem unless bilateral obstruction persists beyond 1 year, when auditory conduction is necessary for normal speech development.

The child shown in Figure 3–11, in addition to having bilateral auditory obstruction, had hemangiomatous narrowing of the nasopharynx, documented by axial computed tomography. She presented with moderately severe sleep apnea at age 5 months.

Bleeding

Spontaneous bleeding from a punctate area within a small, florid hemangioma is a very unusual occurrence; sometimes there is associated skin ulceration. However, one must be alert to the possibility of a generalized clotting disorder that usually manifests with petechiae, ecchymoses, or internal bleeding. This condition was first documented in 1940 by Kasabach and Merritt, who described thrombocytopenic purpura and prolonged bleeding time in a 2 month old infant with a large and rapidly growing hemangioma of the left thigh (Kasabach and Merritt, 1940). We recommend that the term "Kasabach-Merritt syndrome" be reserved for the generalized bleeding disorder that results from a profound thrombocytopenia (as low as 2000–40,000 per cubic millimeter) and that is associated with either a large hemangioma or an extensive hemangiomatosis (Dargeon et al., 1959; Levin et al., 1960; Sutherland and Clark, 1962; Shim, 1968). It is not known what constitutes a "giant" hemangioma, or what the mass of hemangioma must be, to trigger this bleeding complication. There is one documented case of intrauterine and perinatal bleeding in an infant born with a 5×7 cm hemangioma (Bowles et al., 1981). A number of authors report that radiolabelled platelets have a shortened survival time in patients with large or extensive hemangiomas (Kontras et al., 1963; Propp and Scharfman, 1966; Ardissone et al., 1980; Bona et al., 1980; Koerper et al., 1983; Sondel et al., 1984). Scintillation counting, after infusion of radioactive chromium labelled platelets, demonstrates maximal activity over the hemangioma as well as the spleen, suggesting sequestration of platelets in this organ (Kontras et al., 1963). Platelet thrombi have also been seen in microscopic sections of excised hemangiomas (Good et al., 1955; Hill and Longino, 1962; Kontras et al., 1963). Platelet trapping appears to be a primary event in a hemangioma's proliferative phase. There may also be turbulent flow leading to activation of platelet aggregation and sequestration of clotting factors within the abnormal vascular channels.

Heparin is normally bound to endothelium. Perhaps hemangiomatous endothelial proliferation results in heparin saturation, which, in turn, stimulates localized intravascular coagulation. On the other hand, it is possible that mast cells, abundant in the young hemangioma, may release heparin and thus affect the local coagulant milieu.

Evidence for consumptive coagulopathy can also be seen with hemangioma; it is more likely when infection complicates the clinical presentation (Ardissone et al., 1980; Cartwright and Van Coller, 1981; Esterly, 1983; Koerper et al., 1983; David et al., 1983). Ogle and colleagues report the case of an infant with a giant hemangioma and disseminated intravascular coagulopathy who died from unrecognized septicemia (Ogle et al., 1976). Postmortem examination showed diffuse infiltration of the hemangioma with gram-negative bacilli.

The Kasabach-Merritt syndrome classically occurs during the early postnatal period of

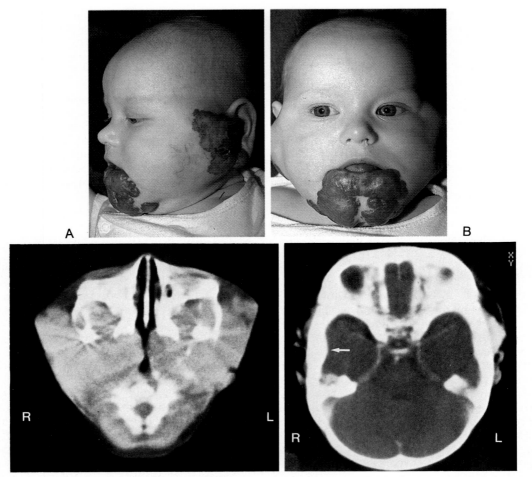

Figure 3–11. Hemangioma is commonly located in the parotid region. *A,* Infant with bilateral preauricular and chin hemangiomas was presented with obstructive sleep apnea at 5 months of age. *B,* Lateral view shows hemangiomatous obstruction of the ear canal (this is bilateral). *C,* Transverse computed tomograph (with dye enhancement) demonstrates total obstruction of the eustachian tubes and hemangioma encroaching on the nasopharynx. *D,* Calvarial CT section of same patient reveals dural thickening (soft tissue density) in lateral aspect of right temporal fossa, anterior to petrous bone (arrow). This finding was interpreted as hemangiomatous extension in meninges, projecting into temporal fossa.

rapid growth of the hemangioma. In a review of 74 cases, Shim noted that the median age of admission to hospital was 5 weeks (Shim, 1968). The clinical dangers of this syndrome are the onset of acute hemorrhage (gastrointestinal, pleural, peritoneal, or central nervous system) and a rapid increase in the size of the hemangioma with possible compression of vital structures, secondary to intralesional bleeding into the tumor. The hemangioma may become tense and the overlying skin may be shiny and discolored, suggesting cellulitis. Petechiae and ecchymoses are initially seen overlying and adjacent to the hemangioma; later, other skin areas are involved.

A complete blood count, with a review of the peripheral blood smear for evidence of microangiopathy, and a platelet count or estimate should be performed in high risk infants, including a child with a large hemangioma (over 5 cm diameter); multiple hemangiomas; or signs suggesting a bleeding tendency, e.g., petechiae, bruising, gastrointestinal bleeding, or unexpected anemia. If thrombocytopenia is present, or if an operative procedure is planned (whether related to the hemangioma or not), further coagulation studies should be performed, including prothrombin time (PT), activated partial thromboplastin time (aPTT), fibrinogen, fibrin degradation products, and fibrinopeptide A, for evidence of consumptive coagulopathy. If this is documented and the lesion is infected, wound and blood cultures are indicated.

Congestive Heart Failure: Multiple Cutaneous and Hepatic Hemangiomas

Congestive heart failure is another potentially lethal complication in an infant with multiple cutaneous and visceral hemangiomas. The earlier descriptions of this entity considered the liver as a primary focus for "hemangioendothelioma," a malignant tumor with metastatic potential (Kundstadter, 1933; Edmondson, 1956). This condition has also been incorrectly labelled "disseminated hemangiomatosis." Probably the best term is "multiple neonatal hemangiomatosis" (Crocker and Cleland, 1957; Robbins and Castle, 1965; Cooper and Bolande, 1965; Touloukian, 1970; McLean et al., 1972). These infants present at 2–8 weeks of life with the triad of congestive heart failure, hepatomegaly, and anemia. Usually there are multiple hemangiomas of the skin; they are often quite small (5–10 mm diameter) and hemispherical (Fig. 3–12A). The most common sites of visceral involvement are, in order, the liver, lungs, and gastrointestinal tract. High output cardiac failure can also occur with large cutaneous hemangiomas in the absence of liver hemangiomas (Stern et al., 1981).

Hepatic hemangiomas occur more commonly in girls, just as do cutaneous lesions, with a reported 2:1 ratio (deLorimier, 1977). This condition can masquerade as congenital heart disease (Levick and Rubie, 1953). The hepatomegaly typically is out of proportion to the degree of congestive heart failure. Frequently, there is a systolic bruit heard over the enlarged liver. Less common presenting features are transient obstructive jaundice (Sardemann and Tygstrup, 1974; Wishnick, 1978), intestinal obstruction, and portal hypertension (Helikson et al., 1977; Larcher et al., 1981). There are also reported cases of rupture in the newborn that produces massive intra-abdominal hemorrhage (Hendrick, 1948; Stone and Neilson, 1965). A platelet-trapping coagulopathy (Kasabach-Merritt syndrome), the well-recognized complication of large cutaneous hemangiomas, may also complicate hepatic lesions and manifest with alimentary tract hemorrhage (Alpert and Benisch, 1970).

The liver hemangioma may be single or multiple and of any size (Larcher et al., 1981). Hemangiomatous proliferation within the highly vascular liver parenchyma results in a far more hemodynamically active tumor than is usually seen with cutaneous hemangiomas. The hemangioma, with its low-resistance sinusoids and channels, perhaps lacking smooth muscle control, and its newly formed feeding/draining vessels, acts as a large arteriovenous shunt. This does not mean that a hemangioma contains arteriovenous malformations or fistulae. The hemodynamic changes observed at cardiac catheterization reflect the response of the cardiovascular system to a large left-to-right shunt, viz., an increased cardiac output, a small systolic pressure gradient across the pulmonary outflow tract, and a mild elevation of the pulmonary artery pressure (Rocchini et al., 1976). The serum bilirubin level is elevated in one third of cases; otherwise, the liver function tests are typically normal (Ishak, 1976).

Radiographic studies of liver hemangiomas include ultrasonography, computed tomography, radionuclide scanning, and angiography. Ultrasonography is a non-invasive method of documenting the presence of hepatic hemangiomas (Fig. 3–12B). Sonograms are also particularly useful in monitoring the course of hepatic hemangiomas. Abramson and coworkers noted a distinctive sonographic appearance for liver hemangiomas in infants, viz., a complex mass with large, draining veins and dilated proximal abdominal aorta (Fig. 3–12C). The latter finding indicates arteriovenous shunting within the hemangioma. Hepatoblastomas and hepatomas, although usually quite vascular, do not have such extensive arteriovenous shunting to produce detectable changes in the caliber of nutritive and draining vessels (Abramson et al., 1982). Computed tomographic scan with enhancement and 99m-Tc scanning are also accurate ways to diagnose and document the extent of liver hemangiomas.

Embolic therapy or surgical intervention is considered if efforts to control congestive heart failure by medical measures are unsuccessful. The use of selective celiac angiography or the more recent digital angiography is particularly valuable in determing the configuration, size, and blood supply of the le-

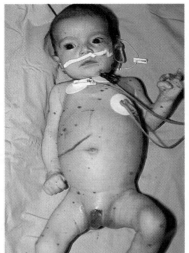

Figure 3–12. Visceral hemangioma. *A*, Three month old girl with multiple cutaneous hemangiomas, hepatomegaly, anemia, and congestive heart failure. *B*, Transverse ultrasonogram of her right upper abdomen shows multiple echolucent areas (hemangiomas) throughout the liver. S = spine. *C*, Ultrasonographic section higher through the liver shows large hepatic vein draining periphery of hemangioma (arrow). (Courtesy of Rita L. Teele, M.D.) *D* and *E*, Selective hepatic arteriogram. (Courtesy of Kenneth E. Fellows, M.D.) *D*, Arterial phase showing enlarged common hepatic artery and branches supplying densely staining vascular tumors throughout the liver. *E*, Venous phase demonstrating persistent homogeneous staining and discrete tumor margins, typical of hemangioma.

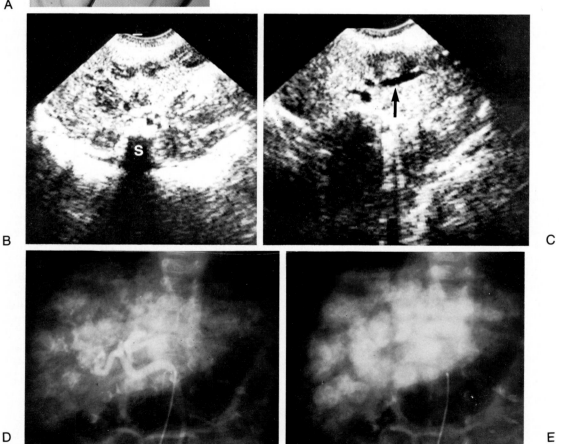

sions in preparation for embolization or operative therapy, e.g., ligation of a feeding artery, local excision, or lobectomy. Angiography typically shows rapid filling through enlarged hepatic arteries with dense staining of multiple tumors and early filling of hepatic veins (Moss et al., 1971). On the venous phase, there is persistent staining and accentuation of the multiple hepatic hemangiomas (Fig. 3–12*D* and *E*).

The radiological literature on this subject is frequently confusing because of a failure to clearly differentiate between infant hemangioma and adult venous anomalies ("cavernous hemangioma") of the liver (Pantoja, 1968; Jensen and Klinge, 1976). It is far more important to discriminate between hepatic hemangioma and hepatic arteriovenous malformation in a critically ill infant who presents with a liver mass and congestive heart failure. Absence of cutaneous lesions is not helpful because both of these entities may present in this manner. Often, angiographic findings of a liver hemangioma are interpreted as arteriovenous malformation because of the rapid flow. Hepatic hemangioma can usually be differentiated from vascular malformation by angiographic criteria, as shown by Fellows and colleagues (Fellows, 1986). Hepatic hemangioma shows a more diffuse pattern of tumors or nodules. In contrast, a liver arteriovenous malformation is a more localized lesion with dense filling of vascular spaces, enlarged collateral vessels, and impressive extrahepatic arterial supply with prominent arteriovenous shunting (Fig. 3–13).

Histologic diagnosis is rarely necessary to exclude hepatoblastoma. Percutaneous needle biopsy should never be performed, because of the great risk of intraperitoneal hemorrhage. When necessary, open liver biopsy is preferred but frequently must be deferred in these critically ill infants (Touloukian, 1970). The clinical triad of hepatomegaly, congestive heart failure (in the absence of congenital cardiac disease), and cutaneous hemangiomas, in conjunction with positive radiographic data, is sufficient to institute treatment (Touloukian, 1970).

Although there is spontaneous regression with visceral and hepatic hemangiomas, just as with cutaneous hemangiomas, the overall mortality rate is as high as 54% (Berman and Lim, 1978). Death is usually the result of congestive heart failure, infection, or hemorrhage. These mortality data may be distorted because of past failure to differentiate cases of liver hemangioma from cases of arteriovenous malformation. Management is discussed in Chapter Five.

Skeletal Distortion

Skeletal changes are very unusual with hemangiomas. In over 300 cases from our clinic, only 3 instances of minor bone deformation were seen, specifically (1) deviation of an infant's nasal pyramid, (2) orbital enlargement, and (3) a minor deformation of the outer calvaria (Boyd et al., 1984). Similar cases of orbital enlargement are reported by Williams and colleagues (Williams, 1979). The mechanism of skeletal distortion is presumed to be a mass effect on the underlying growing bone. This is clearly demonstrated experimentally, whereby an enlarged orbit can be produced by expansion of ocular volume (Sarnat and Shanedling, 1974). There are also rare cases of enlargement of the auricular cartilage and overgrowth of the facial skeleton in children with a massive hemifacial hemangioma.

THE INVOLUTION PHASE

After a period of rapid expansion, the hemangioma stabilizes and, for a time, seems to grow at the same rate as the child. This change in a hemangioma usually becomes evident between the sixth and tenth month of life. It is important to note that proliferation and involution are not distinct phases in the life cycle of a hemangioma. Both clinically and histologically, proliferation continues as involution slowly begins to predominate. One of the first signs of regression is fading of the shiny crimson color to a dull purple. The surface of the hemangioma assumes a mottled, grayish mantle, and on close examination, tiny white flecks can be seen. The lesion softens, it is less tense to palpation, and the involved skin becomes slightly wrinkled; now it is a lilac hue. Bleeding and ulceration cease to be a problem. Whereas a young, tense hemangioma is often tender to the touch, with the onset of involution, the parents may remark that the hemangioma seems less tender and that their child is not so fussy. The parents may also notice that when the child

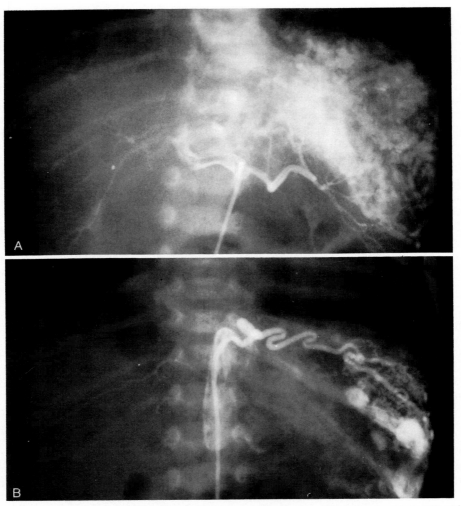

Figure 3–13. Arteriographic study of hepatic arteriovenous malformation of the liver in a 1 month old child who was presented in severe congestive heart failure with a mass in the right upper quadrant. Calcifications in upper abdomen noted on plain radiograph. (Courtesy of Kenneth E. Fellows, M.D.) *A,* Celiac arteriogram shows enlarged tortuous left hepatic artery supplying a poorly defined vascular anomaly of the left lobe of the liver. Early venous filling signifies arteriovenous shunting. *B,* Selective left intercostal arteriogram reveals large tortuous collateral vessels supplying the mass in the left lobe. Diagnosis of liver arteriovenous malformation was confirmed histologically following successful left hepatectomy.

sions in preparation for embolization or operative therapy, e.g., ligation of a feeding artery, local excision, or lobectomy. Angiography typically shows rapid filling through enlarged hepatic arteries with dense staining of multiple tumors and early filling of hepatic veins (Moss et al., 1971). On the venous phase, there is persistent staining and accentuation of the multiple hepatic hemangiomas (Fig. 3–12D and E).

The radiological literature on this subject is frequently confusing because of a failure to clearly differentiate between infant hemangioma and adult venous anomalies ("cavernous hemangioma") of the liver (Pantoja, 1968; Jensen and Klinge, 1976). It is far more important to discriminate between hepatic hemangioma and hepatic arteriovenous malformation in a critically ill infant who presents with a liver mass and congestive heart failure. Absence of cutaneous lesions is not helpful because both of these entities may present in this manner. Often, angiographic findings of a liver hemangioma are interpreted as arteriovenous malformation because of the rapid flow. Hepatic hemangioma can usually be differentiated from vascular malformation by angiographic criteria, as shown by Fellows and colleagues (Fellows, 1986). Hepatic hemangioma shows a more diffuse pattern of tumors or nodules. In contrast, a liver arteriovenous malformation is a more localized lesion with dense filling of vascular spaces, enlarged collateral vessels, and impressive extrahepatic arterial supply with prominent arteriovenous shunting (Fig. 3–13).

Histologic diagnosis is rarely necessary to exclude hepatoblastoma. Percutaneous needle biopsy should never be performed, because of the great risk of intraperitoneal hemorrhage. When necessary, open liver biopsy is preferred but frequently must be deferred in these critically ill infants (Touloukian, 1970). The clinical triad of hepatomegaly, congestive heart failure (in the absence of congenital cardiac disease), and cutaneous hemangiomas, in conjunction with positive radiographic data, is sufficient to institute treatment (Touloukian, 1970).

Although there is spontaneous regression with visceral and hepatic hemangiomas, just as with cutaneous hemangiomas, the overall mortality rate is as high as 54% (Berman and Lim, 1978). Death is usually the result of congestive heart failure, infection, or hemorrhage. These mortality data may be distorted because of past failure to differentiate cases of liver hemangioma from cases of arteriovenous malformation. Management is discussed in Chapter Five.

Skeletal Distortion

Skeletal changes are very unusual with hemangiomas. In over 300 cases from our clinic, only 3 instances of minor bone deformation were seen, specifically (1) deviation of an infant's nasal pyramid, (2) orbital enlargement, and (3) a minor deformation of the outer calvaria (Boyd et al., 1984). Similar cases of orbital enlargement are reported by Williams and colleagues (Williams, 1979). The mechanism of skeletal distortion is presumed to be a mass effect on the underlying growing bone. This is clearly demonstrated experimentally, whereby an enlarged orbit can be produced by expansion of ocular volume (Sarnat and Shanedling, 1974). There are also rare cases of enlargement of the auricular cartilage and overgrowth of the facial skeleton in children with a massive hemifacial hemangioma.

THE INVOLUTION PHASE

After a period of rapid expansion, the hemangioma stabilizes and, for a time, seems to grow at the same rate as the child. This change in a hemangioma usually becomes evident between the sixth and tenth month of life. It is important to note that proliferation and involution are not distinct phases in the life cycle of a hemangioma. Both clinically and histologically, proliferation continues as involution slowly begins to predominate. One of the first signs of regression is fading of the shiny crimson color to a dull purple. The surface of the hemangioma assumes a mottled, grayish mantle, and on close examination, tiny white flecks can be seen. The lesion softens, it is less tense to palpation, and the involved skin becomes slightly wrinkled; now it is a lilac hue. Bleeding and ulceration cease to be a problem. Whereas a young, tense hemangioma is often tender to the touch, with the onset of involution, the parents may remark that the hemangioma seems less tender and that their child is not so fussy. The parents may also notice that when the child

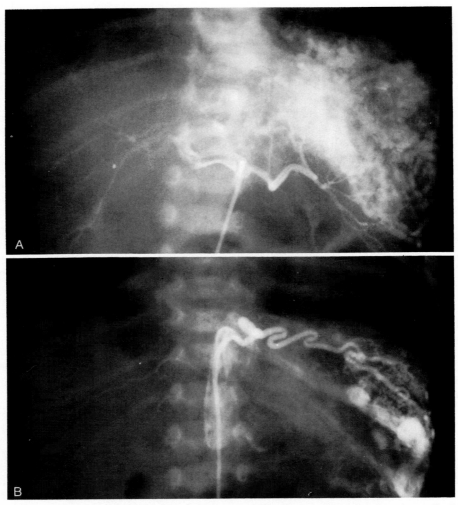

Figure 3–13. Arteriographic study of hepatic arteriovenous malformation of the liver in a 1 month old child who was presented in severe congestive heart failure with a mass in the right upper quadrant. Calcifications in upper abdomen noted on plain radiograph. (Courtesy of Kenneth E. Fellows, M.D.) *A,* Celiac arteriogram shows enlarged tortuous left hepatic artery supplying a poorly defined vascular anomaly of the left lobe of the liver. Early venous filling signifies arteriovenous shunting. *B,* Selective left intercostal arteriogram reveals large tortuous collateral vessels supplying the mass in the left lobe. Diagnosis of liver arteriovenous malformation was confirmed histologically following successful left hepatectomy.

cries and strains, the hemangioma does not swell up the way it did at first. These signs and symptoms are sufficiently accurate to predict the subsequent behavior of a particular vascular birthmark. Bingham describes how a Doppler ultrasonic flowmeter may be used to monitor a hemangioma's clinical course (Bingham, 1979).

In time, it becomes obvious that the child's growth is proportionately greater than that of the hemangioma. The tumor begins to shrink and soften; by this time, involution is well under way. The cutaneous signs of involution, which begin centrally, seem to spread in a centrifugal fashion toward the periphery of the hemangioma. Usually, the last traces of color are gone by the fifth year (Fig. 3–14). If ulceration complicated the proliferative phase, this healed area eventually becomes a yellow-white scar. This scarred area will never have quite the skin quality that results from involution without intercedent ulceration. Typically, the skin that remains after involution exhibits mild atrophy; has a wrinkled quality, with a few telangiectatic vessels; and is slightly paler than the normal skin.

Most clinical studies confirm that complete resolution of hemangiomas occurs in over 50% of children by age 5 years and in over 70% by the age of 7 years, with continued improvement in the remaining children until age 10–12 (Lister, 1938; Simpson, 1959;

Bowers et al., 1960; Pratt, 1967). In general, neither sex, race, site, size, presence at birth, duration of proliferative phase, nor clinical appearance of the hemangioma appears to influence the involution (Finn et al., 1983). Some authors suggest that large hemangiomas are less likely to involute than smaller ones. However, our experience in the Vascular Anomalies Clinic at The Children's Hospital in Boston confirms the unexpected finding noted by Bowers, that the rate and completeness of resolution are unrelated to the size of the lesion (Bowers et al., 1960; Finn et al., 1983). In addition, to our surprise, we found that lesions that began *in utero* and were quite large at birth did not seem to involute any earlier than lesions that appeared after birth. Simpson also found no significant relationship between the final result of regression and the age at which the lesion appeared (Simpson, 1959). It is often stated that these deep or subcutaneous hemangiomas (previously called "cavernous") involute more slowly than superficial ("capillary") lesions. This observation probably results from our inability to monitor regression of a deep hemangioma, in which softening of the tumor can be appreciated more easily than diminishing volume. Our clinical studies indicate that involution proceeds on the same time schedule for both deep and superficial hemangiomas (Bowers et al., 1960; Finn et al., 1983) (Figs. 3–14 to 3–16).

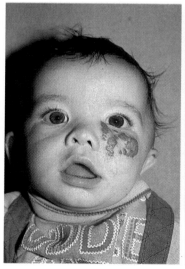 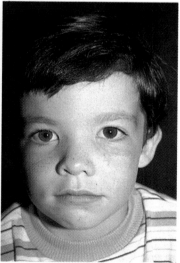

Figure 3–14. Involution in a superficial hemangioma. *A,* Hemangioma in cheek of an infant boy. *B,* At age 5 years; very little residual fibrous tissue remains.

A   B

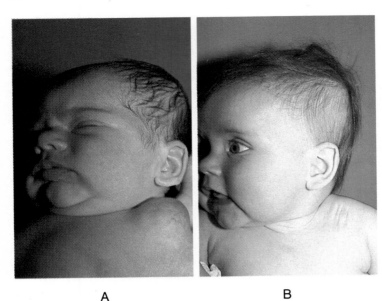

A   B

Figure 3–15. Involution of a deep hemangioma. *A,* One week old infant with rapidly growing deep hemangioma of supraclavicular area; present at birth. *B,* Remarkable regression by 6 months of age. Clinical studies fail to confirm that hemangiomas that are present at birth necessarily involute earlier than those that appear postnatally.

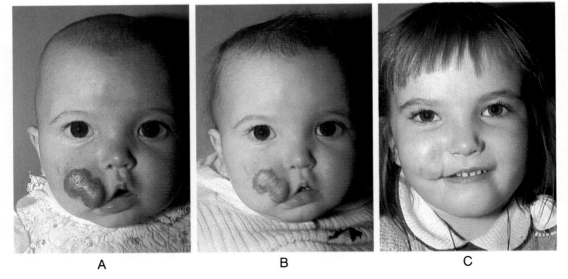

A   B   C

Figure 3–16. Involution in a deep-superficial hemangioma. *A,* Seven month old girl with facial hemangioma in dermis and subcutaneous tissue. The color is not quite so intense, nor is the tumor as tense as it was earlier. *B,* By 1 year of age, there is flattening of the tumor and graying of the surface. *C,* By age 5, the skin color is almost normal. There will be further regression of the residual hemangioma.

The hemangioma may gradually expand the overlying tissue to such a degree that, despite eventual involution, excess skin will surely remain. There is a lingering impression that, in some locations, involution seems to proceed more slowly, particularly on the nose and lips (Bowers et al., 1960). In some cases, we have documented foci of continued cellular proliferation in these apparently slowly involuting hemangiomas. However, the deposition of fibrofatty tissue that replaces the hemangiomatous parenchyma is the most likely explanation for a persistent soft tissue mass. Indeed, it is this variable amount of fibrofatty tissue residuum that accounts for the persistent "tumor" seen following cessation of involution.

References

Abramson, S. J., Lach, E. E., and Teele, R. L.: Benign vascular tumors of the liver in infants: Sonographic appearance. Amer. J. Roent. *138*:629, 1982.

Alpert, L. L., and Benisch, B.: Hemangioendothelioma of the liver associated with microangiopathic hemolytic anemia. Amer. J. Med. *48*:624, 1970.

Andries, G. H., and Kaump, D. H.: Multiple malignant hemangiomata of the liver. Amer. J. Clin. Pathol. *14*:489, 1944.

Ardissone, P., Pecco, P., and Italiano, F.: Attuali aspetti patogenetici e terepeutici della sindrome de Kasabach-Merritt. Min. Ped. *32*:1047, 1980.

Azzolini, A., Rossi, L., and Chinelli, C.: Gli aspetti angiografici degli angiomi in maturi dell'infanzia. Minerva Chir. *28*:1240, 1973.

Berman, B., and Lim, H. W. P.: Concurrent cutaneous and hepatic hemangiomata in infancy: Report of a case and a review of the literature. J. Dermatol. Surg. Oncol. *4*:869, 1978.

Bingham, H. G.: Predicting the course of a congenital hemangioma. Plast. Reconstr. Surg. *63*:161, 1979.

Bona, G., Mussa, G. C., Mora, P., and Silvestro, L.: Studio della sequentrazione piastrinica con piastrine marcate con 99m-Tc in un caso di sindrome di Kasabach-Merritt. Min. Ped. *32*:215, 1980.

Bowers, R. E., Graham, E. A., and Tomlinson, K. M.: The natural history of the strawberry nevus. Arch. Dermatol. *82*:667, 1960.

Bowles, L. J., Kostopoulos-Farri, E., and Papageorgiou, A. N.: Perinatal hemorrhage associated with Kasabach-Merritt syndrome. Clin. Pediat. *20*:428, 1981.

Boyd, J. B., Mulliken, J. B., Kaban, L. B., Upton, J., and Murray, J. E.: Skeletal changes associated with vascular malformations. Plast. Reconstr. Surg. *74*:789, 1984.

Burke, E. C., Winkelmann, R. K., and Strickland, M. K.: Disseminated hemangiomatosis. Amer. J. Dis. Child *108*:418, 1964.

Burman, D., Mansell, P. W. A., and Warin, R. P.: Miliary hemangiomata in the newborn. Arch. Dis. Child. *42*:193, 1967.

Burrows, P. E., Mulliken, J. B., Fellows, K. E., and Strand, R. D.: Childhood hemangiomas and vascular malformations: Angiographic differentiation. Amer. J. Roent. *141*:483, 1983.

Cartwright, J. D., and Van Coller, J. D.: Conservative management of the Kasabach-Merritt syndrome (cavernous haemangioma and thrombocytopenia). S. Afr. Med. J. *60*:670, 1981.

Cooper, A. G., and Bolande, R. P.: Multiple hemangiomas in an infant with cardiac hypertrophy. Pediatrics *35*:27, 1965.

Crocker, D. W., and Cleland, R. S.: Infantile hemangioendothelioma of liver: Report of three cases. Pediatrics *19*:596, 1957.

Dargeon, H. W., Adiao, A. C., and Pack, G. T.: Hemangioma with thrombocytopenia. J. Pediatr. *54*:285, 1959.

David, T. J., Evans, D. K., and Stevens, F. R.: Haemangioma with thrombocytopenia (Kasabach-Merritt syndrome). Arch. Dis. Child. *58*:1022, 1983.

Davies, M. G., and Marks, R.: Dermo-epidermal relationships in pyogenic granuloma. Brit. J. Dermat. *99*:503, 1978.

deLorimier, A. A.: Hepatic tumors of infancy and childhood. Surg. Clin. North Am. *57*:443, 1977.

Edmondson, H. A.: Differential diagnosis of tumors and tumor-like lesions of liver in infancy and childhood. Amer. J. Dis. Child. *91*:168, 1956.

Esterly, N. B.: Kasabach-Merritt syndrome in infants. J. Amer. Acad. Dermatol. *8*:504, 1983.

Fellows, K. E.: Hepatic hemangioma in infancy: Angiographic differentiation. Presented at the 6th International Workshop for the Study of Vascular Anomalies, Boston, June 14, 1986.

Ferguson, C. F., and Flake, C. G.: Subglottic hemangioma as a cause of respiratory obstruction in infants. Ann. Otol. Rhinol. Laryngol. *70*:1095, 1961.

Finn, M. C., Glowacki, J., and Mulliken, J. B.: Congenital vascular lesions: Clinical application of a new classification. J. Ped. Surg. *18*:894, 1983.

Good, T. A., Carnazzo, S. F., and Good, R. A.: Thrombocytopenia and giant hemangioma in infants. Am. J. Dis. Child. *90*:260, 1955.

Greenhouse, J. M.: In discussion of a paper by B. Yaffe. A. M. A. Arch. Dermat. *72*:89, 1955.

Haik, G. R., Jakobiec, F. A., Ellsworth, R. M., and Jones, I. S.: Capillary hemangioma of the lids and orbit. An analysis of the clinical features and therapeutic results in 101 cases. Ophthalmology *86*:760, 1979.

Healy, G. B., Fearon, B., French, R., and McGill, T.: Treatment of subglottic hemangioma with the carbon dioxide laser. Laryngoscopy *90*:809, 1980.

Helikson, M. A., Shapiro, D. L., and Seashore, J. H.: Hepatoportal arteriovenous fistula and portal hypertension in an infant. Pediatrics *60*:920, 1977.

Hendrick, J. G.: Hemangioma of the liver causing death in a newborn infant. J. Pediat. *32*:309, 1948.

Hersh, J. H., Waterfill, D., Rutledge, J., et al.: Sternal malformation/vascular dysplasia association. Amer. J. Med. Genet. *21*:177, 1985.

Hidano, A., and Nakajima, S.: Earliest features of the strawberry mark in the newborn. Brit. J. Dermatol. *87*:138, 1972.

Hill, G. J., and Longino, L. A.: Giant hemangioma with thrombocytopenia. Surg. Gynec. Obstet. *114*:304, 1962.

Holden, K. R., and Alexander, F.: Diffuse neonatal hemangiomatosis. Pediatrics *46*:411, 1970.

Holmdahl, K.: Cutaneous hemangiomas in premature and mature infants. Acta Paediatrica *44*:370, 1955.

Igarashi, M., Uchida, H., and Kajii, T.: Supraumbilical midabdominal raphe and facial cavernous hemangiomas. Clin. Genet. *27*:196, 1985.

Ishak, K. G.: Primary hepatic tumours in childhood. In

Popper, H., and Schaffner, F. (eds.): *Progress in Liver Diseases*. New York: Grune and Stratton, Vol. 5, 1976, p. 536.

Jacobs, A. H.: Strawberry hemangiomas: The natural history of the untreated lesion. Calif. Med. *86*:8, 1957.

Jacobs, A. H., and Walton, R. G.: The incidence of birthmarks in the neonate. Pediatrics *58*:218, 1976.

Jensen, J. T., and Klinge, T.: Hemangioma of the liver. Acta Radiology Diag. *17*:61, 1976.

Kasabach, H. H., and Merritt, K. K.: Capillary hemangioma with extensive purpura. Amer. J. Dis. Child. *59*:1063, 1940.

Koerper, M. A., Addiego, J. E., deLorimier, A. A., Lipow, H., Price, D., and Lubin, B. H.: Use of aspirin and dipyridamole in children with platelet trapping syndromes. J. Pediatr. *102*:311, 1983.

Kontras, S. B., Green, O. C., King, L., and Duran, R. J.: Giant hemangioma with thrombocytopenia. Amer. J. Dis. Child *105*:188, 1963.

Kundstadter, R. H.: Hemangio-endothelioma of the liver in infancy: Case report and review of the literature. Amer. J. Dis. Child *46*:803, 1933.

Larcher, V. F., Howard, E. R., and Mowat, A. P.: Hepatic hemangiomata: Diagnosis and management. Arch. Dis. Child. *56*:7, 1981.

Levick, C. B., and Rubie, J.: Haemangioendothelioma of the liver simulating congenital heart disease in an infant. Arch. Dis. Child. *28*:49, 1953.

Levin, E. R., Holcomb, T. M., and Lutzner, M. A.: Hemangioma associated with thrombocytopenia. Arch. Derm. *82*:148, 1960.

Lister, W. A.: The natural history of strawberry naevi. Lancet *1*:1429, 1938.

Lunsford, C. J.: Multiple disseminated angiomas: Report of a case. Arch. Derm. Syph. *25*:344, 1932.

Margileth, A. M., and Museles, M.: Cutaneous hemangiomas in children: Diagnosis and conservative management. JAMA *194*:523, 1965.

McLean, R. H., Moller, J. H., Warwick, W. J., Satran, L., and Lucas, R. V., Jr.: Multinodular hemangiomatosis of the liver in infancy. Pediatrics *49*:563, 1972.

Mills, S. E., Cooper, P. H., and Fechner, R. E.: Lobular capillary hemangioma: The underlying lesion of pyogenic granuloma. A study of 73 cases from the oral and nasal mucous membranes. Amer. J. Surg. Path. *4*:471, 1980.

Moss, A. A., Clark, R. E., Paulubinskas, A. H., and deLorimier, A.: Angiographic appearance of benign and malignant hepatic tumours in infants and children. Amer. J. Roentgenol. *113*:61, 1971.

Mulliken, J. B., and Glowacki, J.: Hemangiomas and vascular malformations in infants and children: A classification based on endothelial characteristics. Plast. Reconstr. Surg. *69*:412, 1982.

Mulliken, J. B.: Cutaneous vascular lesions of children. In Serafin, D., and Georigade, N. G. (eds.): *Pediatric Plastic Surgery*. St. Louis: C. V. Mosby Co., 1984, pp. 137–154.

Ogle, J., Hope, R. R., and Watson, C.: Kasabach-Merritt syndrome with terminal gram negative infection. N. Zeal. Med. J. *83*:441, 1976.

Pantoja, E.: Angiography in liver hemangioma. Amer. J. Roent. *104*:874, 1968.

Payne, M. M., Moyer, F., Marcks, K. M., and Trevaskis, A. E.: The precursor to the hemangioma. Plast. Reconstr. Surg. *38*:64, 1966.

Pratt, A. G.: Birthmarks in infants. Arch. Dermatol. *67*:302, 1967.

Propp, R. P., and Scharfman, W. B.: Hemangioma-thrombocytopenia syndrome associated with microangiographic hemolytic anemia. Blood *28*:623, 1966.

Robb, R. M.: Refractive errors associated with hemangiomas of the eyelids and orbit in infancy. Amer. J. Ophthal. *83*:52, 1977.

Robbins, B. H., and Castle, R. F.: Hemangiomas, hepatic involvement, congestive failure. Pediatrics *35*:868, 1965.

Rocchini, A. P., Rosenthal, A., Issenberg, H. J., and Nadas, A. S.: Hepatic hemangioendothelioma: Hemodynamic observations and treatment. Pediatrics *57*:131, 1976.

Sardemann, H., and Tygstrup, I.: Prolonged obstructive jaundice and haemangiomatosis. Arch. Dis. Child *49*:665, 1974.

Sarnat, B. G., and Shanedling, P. D.: Increased orbital volume after periodic intrabulbar injections of silicone in growing rabbits. Am. J. Anat. *140*:523, 1974.

Schwartz, A. R.: Multiple malignant hemangioendothelioma in infant: Report of a case. Arch. Pediatr. *62*:1, 1945.

Shim, W. K. T.: Hemangiomas of infancy complicated by thrombocytopenia. Amer. J. Surg. *116*:896, 1968.

Simpson, J. R.: Natural history of cavernous haemangiomata. Lancet *2*:1057, 1959.

Sondel, P. M., Ritter, M. W., Wilson, D. G., Lieberman, L. M.: Use of 111In platelet scans in the detection of treatment of Kasabach-Merritt syndrome. J. Pediatr. *104*:87, 1984.

Stern, J. K., Wolf, J. E., Jr., and Jarratt, M.: Benign neonatal hemangiomatosis. J. Amer. Acad. Dermat. *4*:442, 1981.

Stigmar, G., Crawford, J. S., Ward, C. M., and Thomson, H. G.: Ophthalmic sequelae of infantile hemangiomas of the eyelids and orbit. Amer. J. Ophthalmol. *85*:806, 1978.

Stone, H. H., and Neilson, I. C.: Hemangioma of the liver in the newborn. Arch. Surg. *90*:319, 1965.

Sutherland, D. A., and Clark, H.: Hemangioma associated with thrombocytopenia. Report of a case and review of the literature. Amer. J. Med. *33*:150, 1962.

Thomson, H. G., Ward, C. M., Crawford, J. S., and Stigmar, R.: Hemangiomas of the eyelid: Visual complications and prophylactic concepts. Plast. Reconstr. Surg. *63*:641, 1979.

Touloukian, R. J.: Hepatic hemangioendothelioma during infancy: Pathology, diagnosis, and treatment with prednisone. Pediatrics *45*:71, 1970.

Welch, K. J.: The salivary glands. In Welch, K. J., Randolph, J. G., Ravitch, M. M., et al. (eds.): *Pediatric Surgery*, 4th ed. Chicago: Year Book Medical Publishers, Inc., 1986, p. 487.

Williams, H. B.: Facial bone changes with vascular tumors in children. Plast. Reconstr. Surg. *63*:309, 1979.

Wishnick, M. M.: Multinodular hemangiomatosis with partial biliary obstruction. J. Pediatr. *92*:960, 1978.

CHAPTER FOUR

Pathogenesis of Hemangiomas

John B. Mulliken

*It is in her moments of abnormality that
Nature reveals her secrets.*
                                        Goethe

EARLY THEORIES

"Maternal impression" was the accepted explanation for hemangiomas until the turn of this century. This theory assumes that the hemangioma is the product of the mother's emotion that caused her, during the pregnancy, to be alarmed by the sight of blood or affected with a whimsical desire for certain fruits (see Chapter One). Virchow, eschewing such fanciful proposals, pondered the critical issue: When does a hemangioma begin? He asked the question that is still not fully answered to this day: Is hemangioma a localized growth of sequestered embryonic mesoderm, or does it arise *de novo* as a postembryonic tumor? Can either hypothesis explain the hemangioma's rapid neonatal appearance, its simultaneous proliferation in multiple locations, and its predictable slow involution?

Virchow believed that "angioma simplex" (hemangioma) involved the growth of new blood vessels and was not just a simple, passive dilatation of pre-existing channels (Virchow, 1863). He speculated that the mechanism was a progressive irritation of tissue, and that this reaction was particularly likely to occur about the margins of fetal clefts, which are well-supplied with blood vessels. The hemangioma thus remained latent for a time before it appeared: Virchow called these lesions "fissural angiomas." Ribbert tested Virchow's teachings by injecting angioma specimens. He concluded that they were true neoplasms that arose independently from normal existing channels of the invaded tissue and were later connected by efferent and afferent vessels (Ribbert, 1898). These same prominent afferent and efferent vessels were later demonstrated in facial hemangiomas by Walsh and Tompkins (Walsh and Tompkins, 1956). Their injection studies led these investigators to conclude that hemangiomas secure their nourishment from a single afferent arterial vessel. Walsh and Tompkins hypothesized that a given hemangioma's potential for rapid growth was dependent upon the tumor's location over a normally situated subcutaneous artery.

Intuitive theories citing an embryonic origin for hemangiomas abound. Laidlow and Murray suggested that hemangiomas are phylogenetic remnants of vascular tufts that served as accessory lungs in the skin of primitive amphibia (Laidlow and Murray, 1933). Malan proposed that "dormant angioblasts" become activated to form hemangiomas—a delayed expression of genetically programmed growth and involution of the embryonic capillary network (Malan, 1974). Rather than representing recrudescence, Pack and Miller envisioned hemangiomas as "embryonic sequestrations of unipotent angioblastic cells" (Pack and Miller, 1950). Kaplan agreed, stating that hemangioma is a failure of normal morphogenesis from the stage of undifferentiated capillary network, as described by Woollard in the 20 day pig embryo (corresponding to the 13 day human embryo) (Woollard, 1922). Kaplan cites the immature appearance of the endothelial cells, namely, large nuclei and scant cytoplasm, as evidence for this theory (Kaplan, 1983).

Reese and Blodi (1951) and Andrews and Domonkos (1953) suggested that hemangiomas were analogous to retrolental fibrovascular proliferation as seen in premature infants who had received oxygen therapy. The prediction that hemangiomas would therefore be more frequent in premature babies was not confirmed by Holmdahl's data (Holmdahl, 1955). In addition, in a small group of premature babies with retrolental fibroplasia, Holmdahl found the same frequency of hemangiomas as for healthy premature infants. Nevertheless, the concept that neoangiogenesis can occur during the first weeks of extrauterine life deserves further investigation. Studies from our neonatal unit confirm the data, presented by Amir and coworkers, that hemangioma occurs in 22.9% of preterm infants with a birth weight below 1000 gm and in 15.6% of babies weighing less than 1500 gm, in comparison with the expected frequency of 10% in full-term infants (Amir et al., 1986).

ANIMAL MODELS

A scientific approach to the pathogenesis of the common human hemangioma has been handicapped, in no small way, by our failure to find or develop a suitable model in lower animals. Most vascular lesions in animals, e.g., swine, chickens, and dogs, are developmental malformations. They are noted at birth and remain stable throughout the life of the animal (Cordy, 1979; Munro et al., 1982; Wells and Morgan, 1982). True neoplasms of vascular origin are also seen in animals (Moulton, 1961; Waller and Rubarth,

1967). Multiple malignant angiomatous tumors have been documented in the neck skin of certain young chickens (Monlux and Delaplane, 1952; Darcel and Franks, 1953). There is an angioblastic tumor that can be passed in an inbred A/Jax mouse strain (Jackson Laboratories, Bar Harbor, Maine). In our laboratory, full-thickness human skin grafts with proliferating hemangioma were transplanted to nude mice. Despite successful skin graft take, the hemangioma tissue disappeared within 2 weeks.

Several carcinogens, benzanthracene (Howell, 1963), nitrosamine (Toth et al., 1964; Takayama and Octa, 1965), and dimethylhydrazine (Toth and Wilson, 1971), produce both benign and malignant vascular tumors within soft tissues and livers of rodents. Some induced tumors regress, but most prove to be sarcomas that metastasize and kill the host. Inoculation of newborn rats and hamsters (Kirsten et al., 1962; Stanton, 1965) with polyoma virus produces malignant angiomatous tumors of the liver and subcutaneous tissues, depending on the route of infection. Repeated topical application of methylcholanthrene to the skin of white Peking ducks produces hemangiomatous tumors, and some of these spontaneously regress (Rigdon, 1954; Rigdon, 1955; Rigdon et al., 1956).

None of these examples seems to be truly comparable with human hemangioma of infancy. Until a suitable animal model is forthcoming, investigation into the pathogenesis of hemangiomas must rely on analysis of available tissue specimens and on general studies of the biology of vascular neogenesis.

CELLULAR INTERACTIONS IN HEMANGIOMAS

Proliferating Phase

Light Microscopy

Light microscopic examination demonstrates that the hallmark of the growing hemangioma is a proliferation of endothelial cells, forming syncytial masses, with and without lumens. In the earliest stage, the lesion consists of solid masses of proliferating cells where lumen formation is difficult to appreciate (Fig. 4–1A). Occasional mitotic figures are seen; however, the nuclei are benign appearing without exhibiting pleomorphism.

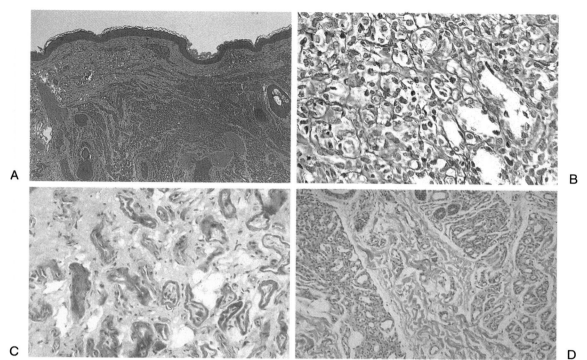

Figure 4–1. Hemangioma histology: proliferating phase. *A,* Hemangioma, 4 month specimen, showing proliferating endothelial masses within the papillary and reticular dermis. Tiny lumens can barely be discerned at this power (H & E × 16). *B,* Silver stain demonstrates nests of endothelial cells within baskets of reticulin fibers (basement membranes), specimen from a 1 year old infant (silver-reticulin stain × 100). *C,* Periodic acid–Schiff stain to show glycoproteins within thickened basement membranes in this specimen from a 2 year old child (PAS × 82). *D,* Later in the proliferation stage, lobule formation is more obvious. The vascular channels are larger; there are still foci of endothelial proliferation in this specimen from a 2 year old child. Feeding-draining vessels are seen in the fibrous septa (H & E × 40).

Later in the proliferative phase, vascular channels are not so compressed, and capillary-sized lumens may be seen lined by plump endothelial cells. Reticulin staining confirms that the endothelial proliferation is within a limiting reticulin sheath, i.e., each group of endothelial cells is surrounded by a limiting membrane of reticulin fibers (Fig. 4–1B). Periodic acid–Schiff (PAS) staining demonstrates a thickened basement membrane beneath the proliferating endothelial channels (Fig. 4–1C). In time, the hemangioma seems to become more organized, as lobular compartments are separated by fibrous septa. Large calibered feeding and draining vessels are seen within these fibrous septa (Fig. 4–1D).

Autoradiography demonstrates incorporation of tritiated thymidine into replicating

endothelial DNA (Fig. 4–2A and B) (Mulliken and Glowacki, 1982). The endothelium produces Factor VIII during the proliferative phase, as shown by both peroxidase and fluorescent antibody techniques (Fig. 4–2C). Histochemical staining for alkaline phosphatase reveals cytoplasmic granules within the hemangioma endothelium (Fig. 4–2D). Thus, the hemangioma is differentiated to the extent that its endothelium is able to make these proteins.

Mast cells are also abundant within proliferating hemangioma tissue (Glowacki and Mulliken, 1982) (Fig. 4–3A). Quantitative analysis shows a 30–40 fold increase in the number of mast cells aligned along hemangioma vessels compared with normal tissues, age and site matched. In tissue judged to be involuted hemangioma, the mast cell count

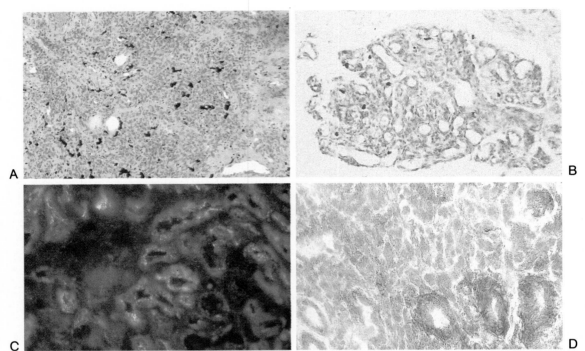

Figure 4–2. Other specialized light microscopic studies of proliferating hemangioma. *A,* Autoradiograph of a tissue specimen from a 1 year old patient; 3H thymidine grains document incorporation into replicating cellular DNA (× 64). *B,* Autoradiograph of a 2 year old involuting phase hemangioma showing persistent foci of proliferation (× 100). *C,* Immunofluorescent antibody stain demonstrates Factor VIII in hemangioma tissue from a 1 year old infant (× 100). *D,* Histochemical identification of alkaline phosphatase (marker of adult endothelium) in hemangioma specimen from a 2 year old infant (× 100).

is within normal levels (Glowacki and Mulliken, 1982) (Fig. 4–3B). These observations have been confirmed by other investigators (Pasyk et al., 1984). Pasyk and colleagues also report increased numbers of mast cells in fibrous regions of hemangiomas and propose that these cells are implicated in the fibrous involution (Pasyk et al., 1984). The role of mast cells in the evolution of hemangiomas is not yet fully understood. Mast cells are known to align along arteries, venules, and capillaries in normal tissues. Pathologists have noted mast cells in highly vascular tumors since the early twentieth century (Fromme, 1906; Greggio, 1911; Riley, 1959; Baroni, 1964; Dalion, 1965). Mast cell granules contain amines, such as serotonin; other vasoactive substances, e.g., prostaglandins and leukotrienes; as well as acid hydrolases and neutral proteases. They are also responsible for production of the highly sulfated glycosaminoglycan heparin. This is of partic-

ular relevance in light of increasing laboratory evidence that mast cells play an intermediary role in vasoproliferation for tissue repair and for tumor neovascularization. Mast cells accumulate prior to neovascularization in two animal model systems: when xenografts are implanted in rabbit corneas (Smith and Basu, 1970) and when tumors are placed onto chick chorioallantoic membranes (Kessler et al., 1976). *In vitro* studies show that mast cell conditioned medium stimulates the migration, but not the proliferation, of capillary endothelial cells (Azizkhan et al., 1980). Of all the mast cell's products, heparin is the most potent stimulus for migration of cultured capillary endothelium. Thornton and coworkers demonstrated that heparin can potentiate the proliferation of endothelium by endothelial cell growth factor (ECGF) (Thornton et al., 1983). Thus, the evidence suggests that although mast cells are probably not the direct cause of heman-

genesis of hemangiomas. The proliferating phase hemangioma is composed of plump endothelium with the ultrastructural characteristics of intracellular activity: convoluted nuclear membrane, swollen mitochondria, membranes of rough endoplasmic reticulum, and clusters of free ribosomes (Höpfel-Kreiner, 1980). The luminal surface of these endothelial cells exhibits thin projections, whereas the basal side has thicker, club-like projections (Fig. 4–4A).

Multilamination of the basement membrane is a pathological characteristic of the proliferative phase hemangioma (Fig. 4–4B) (Höpfel-Kreiner, 1980; Iwamoto and Jakobiec, 1979; Mulliken and Glowacki, 1982). Similar laminar changes are seen in skeletal-muscle capillaries of diabetic patients (Siperstein et al., 1968; Vracko and Benditt, 1970), in scleroderma, and in Raynaud's disease (Camilleri et al., 1984). It is proposed that cyclical endothelial proliferation and death cause the multilamination of the basal membrane.

Electron microscopy provides a close look at the cells involved in the hemangioma drama. Mast cells appear to play a major role. Their long microvillous projections can be seen aligned along the vessel walls in proliferative hemangiomas. These projections are parallel to the laminations of the basement membrane (Dethlefsen et al., 1986) (Fig. 4–4B). As proliferation and early involution proceed, the mast cells interact with macrophages and fibroblasts. One such interaction, termed "transgranulation," represents a specialized form of cell-to-cell communication involving secretion and transfer of exocytosed mast cell granules to the cytoplasm of adjacent cells (Greenberg and Burnstock, 1983). The intimate cell-to-cell contacts along apposing membranes are markers of incorporation of soluble factors into a cell (Fig. 4–4C). Coated vesicles can be found along the periphery of the membranes in regions of close apposition with the mast cell projections. The granules of the mast cells appear to be in various stages of degranulation and seem to form blebs that separate from the cell surface (Fig. 4–4D). As fibrosis occurs, cytoplasmic bridges between mast cells and fibroblasts can be seen (Fig. 4–5).

In summary, our evidence for release of mast cell material and subsequent uptake by adjacent cells includes the following: (1) close alignment of the mast cell projections along

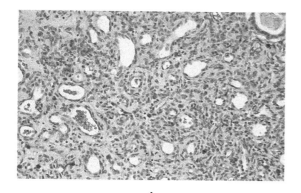

A

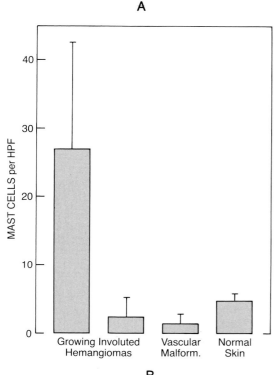

B

Figure 4–3. Mast cells in hemangiomas. *A,* Mast cells, stained red, seen surrounding endothelial cells in a proliferating phase hemangioma (Safranin-O × 64). *B,* Mast cell counts per high power field (× 450) of growing and involuted hemangiomas, vascular malformations, and normal skin specimens. Values are expressed as means ± SD.

giomatous endothelial proliferation, they play a central part in the growth and involution of these tumors.

Electron Microscopy

Electron microscopic studies provide further clues to our understanding the patho-

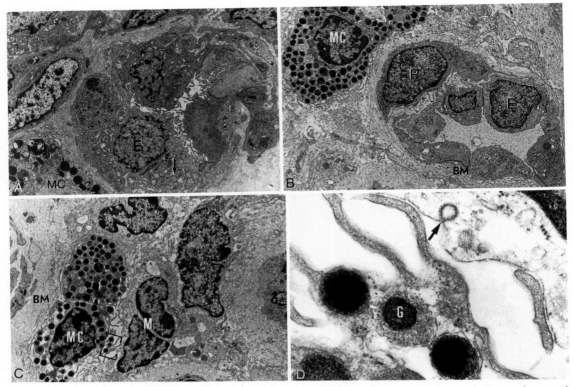

Figure 4–4. Electron microscopic studies of proliferating hemangioma. *A,* Hemangioma electron micrograph from an 8 month old child. Note plump endothelium (E) with signs of intracellular activity: convoluted nuclear membranes, swollen mitochondria (arrow), rough endoplasmic reticulum, and free ribosomes. Note also a mast cell (MC) aligned along a multilaminated basement membrane that surrounds the vessel (× 7700). *B,* Hemangioma specimen from a 2 year old. The large endothelial cells (E) surround the multilaminated basement membrane (BM). Pericytes (P) and mast cells (MC) align along the vessel wall (× 6500). *C,* Two year old hemangioma: two mast cells (MC) lined along a thickened basement membrane (BM). Both mast cells are interacting with a macrophage (M). Brackets indicate detachment of mast cell granules from the cell surface (× 5200). *D,* High power view of *C* showing coated vesicle (arrow) and partially disrupted mast cell granules (G) with membranes. The clean intercellular areas suggest pinocytic activity between the mast cell and macrophage (× 59,000). (*B, C,* and *D* from Dethlefsen, S. M., Mulliken, J. B., and Glowacki, J.: An ultrastructural study of mast cell interactions in hemangiomas. Ultrastruct. Path. *10*:175, 1986.)

the apposing cell surfaces; (2) the localization of mast cell granules in the extreme periphery of the cell and alteration of their contents; (3) the presence of fibroblasts, macrophages, and multinucleated cells in close contact with mast cells; (4) existence of cytoplasmic bridges between mast cells and fibroblasts; and (5) intercellular spaces devoid of electron dense material as well as numerous pinocytic vesicles along the periphery of apposing cells (Dethlefsen et al., 1986).

Involuting Phase

The most curious biological characteristic of the common childhood hemangioma is natural regression. Some writers have assumed *a priori* that involution is the result of thrombosis and infarction (MacCollum and Martin, 1956; Watson and McCarthy, 1940; Matthews, 1968). Yet there is no microscopic evidence for such a mechanism of involution. Hemangiomas from children aged 2–5 years exhibit diminishing endothelial cellularity and progressive deposition of perivascular and inter- and intralobular fibrofatty tissue (Fig. 4–6A). The vascular channels seem to diminish in number as fibrosis increases and, *pari passu*, the remaining vessels dilate with flattening of the endothelial lining (Fig. 4–6B). In time, the dilatation of vessels within an involuted hemangioma gives a "cavernous" appearance that can be histologically

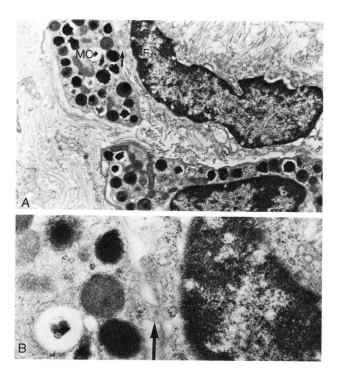

Figure 4–5. Ultrastructural evidence for mast cell–fibroblast interaction. *A,* Mast cell (MC) and fibroblast (F) aligned; fibrosis is conspicuous in this 5 year old specimen (× 15,600). *B,* An intercellular bridge noted in this area (arrow) magnified from *A* (× 50,000).

confused with a venous malformation (Fig. 4–6C and D).

Ultrastructural observations on tissue from involuting hemangiomas at age 3 reveal signs of endothelial discontinuity and vessel degradation. The lumens contain endothelial cell remnants, often lined by only one or two endothelial cells (Fig. 4–7A). Few mast cells are evident in the older specimens, and the prominent interactions with other cell types are not seen. The end-stage, involuted hemangioma is composed of thin-walled vessels that resemble normal capillaries. The basement membrane is still multilaminated, although it is thin and disordered. In the perivascular areas, there are islands of fat deposition intermingled with dense collagen and reticular fibers (Fig. 4–7B).

THE HEMANGIOMA: A PLAY IN THREE ACTS

The hemangioma life cycle can be envisioned as a play in three overlapping Acts: I, proliferation; II, early involution; and III, late involution (Fig. 4–8). Proliferation is the predominant theme early in the drama, whereas involution becomes the controlling force in the dénouement. Proliferation and involution run concurrently. Even when involution is well under way, there are scattered proliferative foci, seen at the microscopic level. In lesions less than 1 year old, tritiated thymidine incorporation measured 27 ± 1 labelled cells/high power field. In hemangioma specimens 1–2 years of age, the labelled cell count dropped to 9 ± 3 cells/high power field and diminishes further thereafter (Mulliken and Glowacki, 1982). Thus, as the drama is viewed through the light microscope, whatever stimulus triggered endothelial mitoses gradually diminishes.

The actors in the hemangioma play can be seen more clearly with electron microscopy. The "Dramatis Cellae" include endothelial cell, pericyte, mast cell, macrophage, and fibroblast. As Act I begins, an unknown stimulus incites the normally quiescent endothelial cells to multiply and migrate. In time, the thin basement membrane begins to thicken beneath the plump dividing endothelial cells. Later, the pericytes become trapped, perhaps innocently, in the multilaminated basement membranes. Mast cells are introduced in Act I. They seem to promote and direct the migration of endothelial cells. Macrophages and fibroblasts enter the stage with Act II

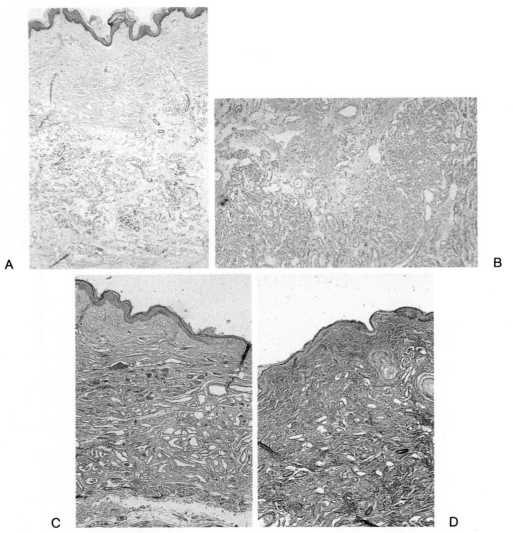

Figure 4–6. Involuting phase: light microscopy. *A,* Age 2 year old skin specimen; the involuting hemangioma is surrounded by loose fibroadipose tissue (H & E × 10). *B,* Higher power of 2 year old skin hemangioma specimen shows progressive inter- and intralobular fibrosis and channel dilatation. A few large thick-walled feeding-draining vessels are also seen (H & E × 25). *C,* Age 8, final stage of involution. Large thin-walled channels remain throughout the dermis, giving a "cavernous" look; not to be confused with a venous malformation (H & E × 16). *D,* Same specimen as in *C,* stained to highlight the extent of dermal fibrosis (van Gieson × 16).

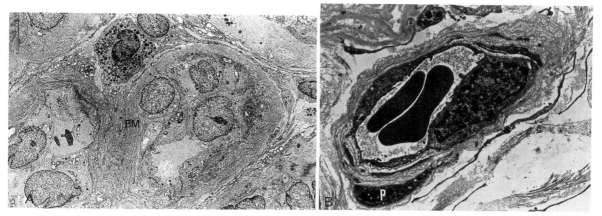

Figure 4–7. Involuting phase: electron microscopy. *A,* Three year old hemangioma: the endothelial cell lining is disrupted and the degenerating endothelial cells partially obstruct the vessel lumen. The basement membrane (BM) is still multilaminated and contains cellular debris and pericytic processes (× 2800). *B,* Involuted hemangioma from a 13 year old child. The vessel has reverted to a more normal architecture and resembles a dilated capillary. The wall contains a single endothelial cell and is surrounded by a pericyte (P). The multilaminated basement membrane is thinner and disorganized. Interstitial collagen fibers are prominently seen (× 9180).

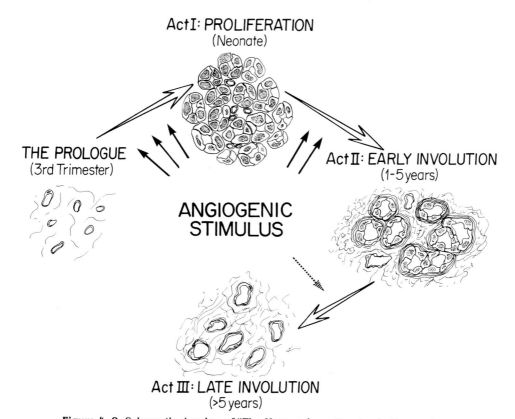

Figure 4–8. Schematic drawing of "The Hemangioma," a play in three acts.

and carry on a dialogue with the mast cells. These cell-to-cell interactions may involve the transfer of biologically active granules from the mast cells.

By Act III, only a few thin-walled vascular channels remain on the stage now cluttered with fibrous tissue. The channels are similar to normal capillaries or venules; however, they still have a telltale thin multilaminated basement membrane.

Clearly, more must be known about the roles of the cellular players before the hemangioma scenario can be fully understood.

ANGIOGENESIS CONCEPT: THE REGULATION OF ENDOTHELIAL CELL GROWTH

The first step in trying to solve any biological problem is to ask the proper question of Nature. The key to unlocking the hemangioma's secret is the answer to the query, "What normally regulates the proliferation of endothelial cells?" It is known that endothelium in normal tissue has an exceedingly low mitotic rate, which only can be measured in years (Denekamp, 1984). Yet endothelial cells can proliferate within 24 hours after a tissue is wounded. If a hemangioma is envisioned as a problem of endothelial growth control, the question remains: What turns on the program? It is possible to theorize that proliferation could result from (1) an external stimulus to mitosis, (2) a deficiency of an inhibitor, or (3) an intrinsic biochemical defect in a localized endothelial cell population. The rapidly growing hemangioma is, in many ways, reminiscent of capillary proliferation as seen during wound healing and neovascularization associated with tumor growth. The hypothesis that tumors are *angiogenesis-dependent*, first proposed by Folkman, provides new insights into the pathogenesis and life cycle of hemangiomas (Folkman, 1974; Folkman, 1976).

The angiogenesis concept proposes that capillaries are normally prevented from growing by physiological regulation of *angiogenic factors*. These angiogenic factors are found in neoplastic tissue but also seem to be present in normal tissue where neovascularization is not occurring. Release of stored angiogenic factors occurs in the short bursts of capillary proliferation during wound heal-ing and, in the female, during ovulation and menstruation. Folkman and Klagsbrun have reviewed the investigative trail leading to the discovery of angiogenic factors; several have been purified, their amino acid sequences determined, and their gene structure known (Folkman and Klagsbrun, 1987). These angiogenic factors appear to fall into two main groups: (1) those that act directly on vascular endothelium to stimulate locomotion or mitosis, and (2) those that act indirectly by mobilizing host helper cells (e.g., macrophages and mast cells) to release endothelial growth factors. Folkman also proposes that there are non-neoplastic "angiogenic diseases," characterized by persistent angiogenesis, e.g., diabetic retinopathy, retrolental fibroplasia, and neonatal hemangioma (Folkman and Klagsbrun, 1987).

A nascent hemangioma may result from endothelial proliferation secondary to increased levels of growth-stimulating factors or to a decreased level of a normally present growth-inhibitory factor. An attempt to assay for angiogenic factors in hemangioma tissue was reported by Wolf and Hubler (Wolf and Hubler, 1975). Transparent acrylic chambers placed in the hamster cheek pouch were used to observe the vascular response to various benign and malignant skin tumors. Transplanted human hemangiomas were noted to produce venous ectasia and neovascularization with capillary proliferation. These findings were interpreted as being evidence for an angiogenic response to the hemangioma transplants. However, since the transplants were xenografts, albeit in a relatively privileged site, the observed vascular response may indicate graft rejection. Inflammatory cells, particularly activated macrophages and lymphocytes, are known to be strongly angiogenic (Polverini et al., 1977; Auerbach and Sidky, 1979; Hunt et al., 1984). That is to say, if the transplant caused an inflammatory response, the experiment fails to distinguish between an angiogenic stimulus produced by the transplanted cells and possible angiogenic capacity of the tested material. Nevertheless, the concept that hemangiomas may stimulate their proliferation by autosecretion of growth-promoting factors into the microenvironment deserves further investigation (Sporn and Todaro, 1980). Recently, Klagsbrun and coworkers showed that tumor cells can synthesize their own angiogenic factors (Klagsbrun et al., 1986).

HEMANGIOGENESIS: POSSIBLE HORMONAL EFFECT

Several observations suggest that endogenous hormones may play a role in the development and growth of hemangiomas. For example, hemangiomas are known to be more commonly diagnosed in fair-skinned female infants. Cutaneous vascular ectasia is frequently seen during pregnancy, e.g., palmar erythema and vascular spiders, called, incorrectly, "hemangiomas" of pregnancy. Sasaki and Pang hypothesize that hemangiomas contain steroid hormone receptors that mediate hemangioma proliferation (Sasaki et al., 1984). These investigators measured elevated serum 17β estradiol levels in infants with proliferating hemangiomas and found them to be four fold higher than in control samples or in patients with port-wine stains and other vascular anomalies. Using a receptor assay system, they also found that biopsy specimens exhibited abnormally high levels of specific 17β estradiol binding sites, compared with normal skin and vascular malformation tissue. An alternate interpretation of these data is that the elevated estradiol binding activity within hemangioma tissue reflects the high density of endothelial cells. These investigators also demonstrated that the *in vitro* estrogen binding capacity of young hemangioma explants was inhibited by both high and low doses of cortisone. Furthermore, when infants were treated with systemic prednisone, serum estradiol levels diminished in those patients whose hemangiomas seemed to clinically respond to steroids. This exciting investigative work points the way to future studies, such as the source of elevated serum estradiol, possible estrogen effects on endothelial mitosis, and nature of steroid and estrogen interaction.

ANGIOGENESIS

Morphological Sequence

Even though we know nothing about the trigger mechanism controlling hemangiomas, we can learn something about the earliest morphological events from studies of tumor angiogenesis. The sequence of capillary proliferation in response to implanted tumor has been observed using scanning electron microscopy (Ausprunk and Folkman, 1977;

Ausprunk et al., 1978). All new capillaries arise from capillaries or venules. Once the signal for angiogenesis is processed, endothelial cells begin to make collagenase, which allows them to break through the underlying basement lamina. The endothelial cells migrate in tandem, at approximately 0.2 mm/day, elongating and aligning with one another to form a solid sprout. A lumen forms by a curvature occurring within each endothelial cell. Then, a number of hollow sprouts join up with one another to establish capillary loops. All that is needed is a signal, a stimulus—the construction of tubes and channels is already programmed within the endothelium. This fact was elegantly demonstrated by Folkman and coworkers, who were the first to isolate and culture capillary endothelium (Folkman et al., 1979). Capillary endothelium, derived from fetal and adult tissue, is capable of forming tubules in culture— "angiogenesis in vitro" (Folkman and Haudenschild, 1980). Using the same techniques, capillary endothelium can be isolated from specimens of proliferating hemangioma; these cells grow easily in culture, and in time, they form capillary tubes (Mulliken et al., 1982) (Fig. 4–9). Proliferating hemangiomas also demonstrate rapid outgrowth of tubular structures from plasma clot cultures. On the other hand, capillary endothelium isolated from vascular malformation specimens is difficult to culture and does not form capillary tubes in medium designed to potentiate growth.

Modulation and Inhibition

Folkman's laboratory studies suggest that helper cells may be involved in the proliferation of endothelium. One of the most likely candidates for this role is the mast cell. Kessler and coworkers showed that there is a 40 fold increase in the mast cell population in the chick chorioallantoic membrane model prior to ingrowth of new capillaries (Kessler et al., 1976). Capillary endothelial cells move slowly or not at all when growing in ordinary culture medium. Zetter showed that when mast cell–conditioned medium or when a tumor-conditioned medium is added, the cells begin to migrate and their migratory patterns can be quantitated by area mensuration using the colloidal gold assay technique (Zetter, 1980). The mast cell product heparin

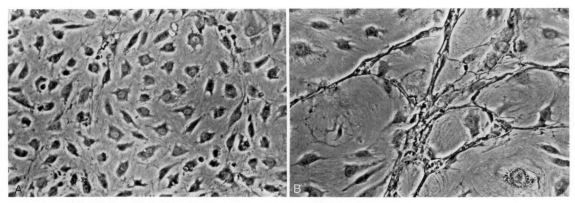

Figure 4–9. Hemangioma in tissue culture. A, Tissue culture at 1 month of a 2 month old hemangioma specimen contains confluent capillary endothelial cells (phase contrast × 230). B, Photomicrograph of the same culture as in A, taken 3 months after primary culture (passage 4). There are endothelial cells surrounding a tubular structure that they have produced—"hemangiogenesis in vitro" (phase contrast × 230). (From Mulliken, J. B., Zetter, B. R., and Folkman, J.: *In vitro* characteristics of endothelium from hemangiomas and vascular malformations. Surgery 92:348, 1982.)

is known to bind to endothelium and enhance migration. This migration can be selectively blocked by protamine. The antiangiogenesis action of protamine can also be demonstrated using the chick chorioallantoic membrane model (Taylor and Folkman, 1982). These studies from Folkman's laboratory confirm that mast cells potentiate angiogenesis, although they cannot initiate the process. Other groups of investigators report that mast cell granules cause proliferation of cultured human endothelial cells (Thornton et al., 1983; Marks et al., 1986). The angiogenesis phenomenon becomes even more intriguing with the finding of increased numbers of mast cells in proliferating hemangiomas (Glowacki and Mulliken, 1982).

The concept of angiogenesis inhibition is a potentially fruitful approach to pharmacologic control of growing hemangiomas. Folkman's laboratory has shown that there are potent inhibitors of angiogenesis: (1) a constituent factor in viable cartilage (Brem and Folkman, 1975), (2) protamine (Taylor and Folkman, 1982), and (3) angiostatic steroids (Crum et al., 1985). Corticosteroids are known to accelerate involution in some infants with rapidly growing hemangiomas. When cortisone was tested in the rabbit iris–tumor model, there was no effect on angiogenesis response, although inflammation was suppressed (Gimbrone et al., 1974). However, heparin, which stimulates capillary migration *in vitro*, when given in combination with steroid surprisingly brings angiogenesis

to a halt. It is the hexasaccharide component of heparin that inhibits angiogenesis (Folkman et al., 1983). Furthermore, cortisone and hydrocortisone, but not dexamethasone, are antiangiogenic in the presence of heparin and heparin fragments (Folkman et al., 1983). Thus, there appear to be two parts of the heparin molecule: one that turns on angiogenesis and another, that in combination with steroids, turns off angiogenesis. Folkman and collaborators have also shown that certain tetrahydrocortisone analogs, which lack glucocorticoid and mineralocorticoid activity, are more potent "angiostatic" drugs than the parent hormone, hydrocortisone (Crum et al., 1985). Other structural determinants critical to steroid angiostatic activity include an alpha hydroxyl configuration at C11 and a hydroxyl at C17. It seems likely that there are natural inhibitors to angiogenesis. It is possible that steroids in plasma could be acting with heparin to maintain the normal quiescent state of endothelium.

For the past 15 years, systemic and local prednisone has been known to hasten the involution of hemangiomas unpredictably. Perhaps very soon, more specific and effective angiostatic drugs will be available to treat the infant with a destructive hemangioma.

References

Amir, J., Metzker, A., Krikler, R., and Reisner, S. H.: Strawberry hemangioma in preterm infants. Ped. Dermatol. *3*:331, 1986.

Andrews, G. C., and Domonkos, A. N.: Skin hemangioma and retrolental fibroplasia. A. M. A. Arch. Dermat. *68*:320, 1953.

Auerbach, R., and Sidky, Y. A.: Nature of the stimulus leading to lymphocyte-induced angiogenesis. J. Immunol. *123*:751, 1979.

Ausprunk, D. H., and Folkman, J.: Migration and proliferation of endothelial cells in preformed and newly formed blood vessels during tumor angiogenesis. Microvasc. Res. *14*:53, 1977.

Ausprunk, D. H., Falterman, K., and Folkman, J.: The sequence of events in the regression of corneal capillaries. Lab. Invest. *38*:284, 1978.

Azizkhan, R. G., Azizkhan, J. C., Zetter, B. R., and Folkman, J.: Mast cell heparin stimulates migration of capillary endothelial cells in vitro. J. Exp. Med. *152*:931, 1980.

Baroni, C.: On the relationship of mast cells to various soft tissue tumors. Brit. J. Cancer *18*:686, 1964.

Brem, H., and Folkman, J.: Inhibition of tumor angiogenesis mediated by cartilage. J. Exp. Med. *141*:427, 1975.

Camilleri, J. P., Fiessinger, J. N., Debure, C., Bruneval, P., Tricottet, V., Kazandjian, S., and Houseet, E.: Fine structural capillary changes and basal lamina thickening in scleroderma (progressive systemic sclerosis) and Raynaud's disease. Path. Res. Pract. *178*:230, 1984.

Cordy, D. R.: Vascular malformations and hemangiomas of the canine spinal cord. Vet. Pathol. *16*:275, 1979.

Crum, R., Szabo, S., and Folkman, J.: A new class of steroids inhibits angiogenesis in the presence of heparin or a heparin fragment. Science *230*:1375, 1985.

Dalion, J.: Mastocytes et tumeurs vasculaires. J. Sc. Méd. de Lille *83*:683, 1965.

Darcel, C. le Q., and Franks, L. M.: Angiomatoid lesions of the skin in young chicks. J. Path. Bact. *66*:499, 1953.

Denekamp, J.: Vasculature as a target for tumour therapy. Angiogenesis. In Hammersen, F., and Hudlicka, O. (eds): *Progress in Applied Microcirculation.* Basel: Karger, 1984, Vol. 4, pp. 28–38.

Dethlefsen, S. M., Mulliken, J. B., and Glowacki, J.: An ultrastructural study of mast cell interactions in hemangiomas. Ultrastruct. Path. *10*:175, 1986.

Folkman, J.: Tumor angiogenesis factor. Cancer Res. *34*:2109, 1974.

Folkman, J.: The vascularization of tumors. Scient. Amer. *234*:58, 1976.

Folkman, J., and Haudenschild, C.: Angiogenesis *in vitro.* Nature *288*:551, 1980.

Folkman, J., and Klagsbrun, M.: Angiogenic factors. Science *235*:442, 1987.

Folkman, J., Haudenschild, C. C., and Zetter, B. R.: Long-term culture of capillary endothelial cells. Proc. Natl. Acad. Sci. U.S.A. *76*:5217, 1979.

Folkman, J., Langer, R., Linhardt, R. J., Haudenschild, C., and Taylor, S.: Angiogenesis inhibition and tumor regression caused by heparin or a heparin fragment in the presence of cortisone. Science *221*:719, 1983.

Fromme, H.: Demonstration über das Verhalten der Mastzellen beim Karzinom. Zentralbl. Gynaekol. *30*:1146, 1906.

Gimbrone, M. A., Cotran, R. S., and Folkman, J.: Human vascular endothelial cells in culture. J. Cell Biol. *60*:673, 1974.

Glowacki, J., and Mulliken, J. B.: Mast cells in hemangiomas and vascular malformations. Pediatrics *70*:48, 1982.

Greenberg, G., and Burnstock, G.: A novel cell-to-cell interaction between mast cells and other cell types. Exp. Cell Res. *147*:1, 1983.

Greggio, H.: Les cellules granuleuses (mastzellen) dans les tissues normaux et dans certaines maladies chirurgicales. Arch. Med. Exp. *23*:323, 1911.

Holmdahl, K.: Cutaneous hemangiomas in premature mature infants. Acta Paediat. *44*:370, 1955.

Höpfel-Kreiner, I.: Histogenesis of hemangiomas—an ultrastructural study on capillary and cavernous hemangiomas of the skin. Path. Res. Pract. *170*:70, 1980.

Howell, J. S.: The experimental production of vascular tumours in the rat. Brit. J. Cancer *17*:663, 1963.

Hunt, T. K., Knighton, D. R., Thakral, K. K., Goodson, W. H., and Andrews, W. S.: Studies on inflammation and wound healing: Angiogenesis and collagen synthesis stimulated in vivo by resident and activated wound macrophages. Surgery *96*:48, 1984.

Iwamoto, T., and Jakobiec, F. A.: Ultrastructural comparison of capillary and cavernous hemangiomas of the orbit. Arch. Ophth. *97*:1144, 1979.

Kaplan, E. N.: Vascular malformation of the extremities. In Williams, H. B. (ed.): *Symposium on Vascular Malformations and Melanotic Lesions.* St. Louis: C. V. Mosby Co., 1983, p. 144.

Kessler, D. A., Langer, R. S., Pless, N. A., and Folkman, J.: Mast cells and tumor angiogenesis. Int. J. Cancer *18*:703, 1976.

Kirsten, W. H., Anderson, D. G., Platz, C. E., and Crowell, E. B.: Observations on the morphology and frequency of polyoma tumors in rats. Cancer Res. *22*:484, 1962.

Klagsbrun, M., Sasse, J., Sullivan, R., and Smith, J. A.: Human tumor cells synthesize an endothelial cell growth factor that is structurally related to basic fibroblast growth factor. Proc. Natl. Acad. Sci. U.S.A. *83*:2448, 1986.

Laidlow, G. F., and Murray, M. R.: Melanoma studies. III. A theory of pigmented moles. Their relation to the evolution of hair follicles. Am. J. Pathol. *9*:827, 1933.

MacCollum, D. W., and Martin, L. W.: Hemangiomas in infancy and childhood: A report based on 6,479 cases. Surg. Clin. North Am. *36*:1647, 1956.

Malan, E.: *Vascular Malformations (Angiodysplasias).* Milan: Carlo Erba Foundation, 1974, p. 4.

Marks, R. M., Roche, W. R., Czerniecki, M., Penny, R., and Nelson, D. S.: Mast cell granules cause proliferation of human microvascular endothelial cells. Lab. Invest. *55*:289, 1986.

Matthews, D. N.: Hemangiomata. Plast. Reconstr. Surg. *41*:528, 1968.

Monlux, W. S., and Delaplane, J. P.: Hemangiomas in the skin of the chicken. Cornell Vet. *42*:193, 1952.

Moulton, J. E.: *Tumors in Domestic Animals.* Berkeley, CA: University of California Press, 1962.

Mulliken, J. B., and Glowacki, J.: Hemangiomas and vascular malformations in infants and children: A classification based on endothelial characteristics. Plast. Reconstr. Surg. *69*:412, 1982.

Mulliken, J. B., Zetter, B. R., and Folkman, J.: *In vitro* characteristics of endothelium from hemangiomas and vascular malformations. Surgery *92*:348, 1982.

Munro, R., Head, K. W., and Munro, H. M. C.: Scrotal haemangiomas in boars. J. Comp. Path. *92*:109, 1982.

Pack, G. T., and Miller, T. R.: Hemangiomas, classification, diagnosis, and treatment. Angiology *1*:405, 1950.

Pasyk, K. A., Cherry, G. W., Grabb, W. C., and Sasaki,

G. H.: Quantitative evaluation of mast cells in cellularly dynamic and adynamic vascular malformations. Plast. Reconstr. Surg. *73*:69, 1984.

Pasyk, K. A., Grabb, W. C., and Cherry, G. W.: Cellular hemangioma. Light and electron microscopic studies of two cases. Virch. Arch. Pathol. Anat. Histol. *396*:103, 1982.

Polverini, P. J., Cotran, R. S., Gimbrone, M. A., Jr., and Unanue, E. R.: Activated macrophages induce vascular proliferation. Nature *269*:804, 1977.

Reese, A. B., and Blodi, F. C.: Retrolental fibroplasia. Amer. J. Ophth. *34*:1, 1951.

Ribbert, V. A.: Ueber Bau, Wachsthum und Genese der Angiome, nebst Bemerkungen uber Cystenbildung. Arch. F. Pathol. Anat. *151*:381, 1898.

Rigdon, R. H.: Spontaneous regression of neoplasma: An experimental study in the duck. South. Med. J. *47*:303, 1954.

Rigdon, R. H.: Spontaneous regression of hemangiomas, an experimental study in the duck and chicken. Cancer Res. *15*:77, 1955.

Rigdon, R. H., Walker, J., and Teddlie, A. H.: Hemangiomas. An experimental study in the duck. Cancer *9*:1107, 1956.

Riley, J. F.: *The Mast Cells*. Edinburgh: E & S Livingston Ltd., 1959, pp. 23–24.

Sasaki, G. H., Pang, C. Y., and Wittliff, J. L.: Pathogenesis and treatment of infant skin strawberry hemangiomas: Clinical and in vitro studies of hormonal effects. Plast. Reconstr. Surg. *73*:359, 1984.

Siperstein, M. D., Unger, R. H., and Madison, L. L.: Studies of muscle capillary basement membrane in normal subjects, diabetic, and prediabetic patients. J. Clin. Invest. *47*:1973, 1968.

Smith, S. S., and Basu, P. K.: Mast cells in corneal immune reaction. Can. J. Ophthalmol. *5*:175, 1970.

Sporn, M. G., and Todaro, G. J.: Autocrine secretion and malignant transformation of cells. N. Engl. J. Med. *303*:878, 1980.

Stanton, M. F.: Transplantability, morphology, and behavior of polyoma virus–induced hepatic hemangiomas of hamsters. J. Nat. Ca. Inst. *35*:201, 1965.

Takayama, S., and Oota, K.: Induction of malignant tumors in various strains of mice by oral administration of N-nitrosodimethylamine and N-nitrosodiethylamine. Gann *56*:189, 1965.

Taxy, J. B., and Gray, S. T.: Cellular angiomas of infancy. An ultrastructural study of two cases. Cancer *43*:2322, 1979.

Taylor, S., and Folkman, J.: Protamine is an inhibitor of angiogenesis. Nature *297*:307, 1982.

Thornton, S. C., Mueller, S. N., and Elliot, E. M.: Human endothelial cells: Use of heparin in cloning and long-term serial cultivation. Science *222*:623, 1983.

Toth, B., Magee, P. N., and Shubik, P.: Carcinogenesis study with dimethylnitrosamine administered orally to adult and subcutaneously to newborn BALB/C mice. Cancer Res. *24*:1712, 1964.

Toth, B., and Wilson, R. B.: Blood vessel tumorigenesis by 1,2-dimethyl-hydrazine dihydrochloride (symmetrical). Amer. J. Pathol. *64*:585, 1971.

Virchow, R.: Angiome. In *Die Krankhaften Geschwülste*. Berlin: August Hirschwald, 1863, Vol. 3, p. 306.

Vracko, R., and Benditt, E. P.: Capillary basal lamina thickening. Its relationship to endothelial cell death and replacement. J. Cell Biol. *47*:281, 1970.

Waller, T., and Rubarth, S.: Haemangioendothelioma in domestic animals. Acta Vet. Scand. *8*:234, 1967.

Walsh, T. S., Jr., and Tompkins, U. N.: Some observations on the strawberry naevus of infancy. Cancer *9*:869, 1956.

Watson, W. L., and McCarthy, W. D.: Blood and lymph vessel tumors: A report of 1,056 cases. Surg. Gynec. Obstet. *71*:569, 1940.

Weibel, E. R., and Palade, G. E.: New cytoplasmic components in arterial endothelia. J. Cell Biol. *23*:101, 1964.

Wells, G. A. H., and Morgan, G.: Multifocal haemangioma in a pig. J. Comp. Path. *90*:483, 1980.

Wolf, J. E., and Hubler, W. R., Jr.: Tumor angiogenic factor and human skin tumors. Arch. Dermatol. *111*:321, 1975.

Woollard, H. H.: The development of the principal arterial stems in the forelimb of the pig. Contrib. Embryol. *14*:139, 1922.

Zetter, B. R.: Migration of capillary endothelial cells is stimulated by tumor-derived factors. Nature *285*:41, 1980.

CHAPTER FIVE

Treatment of Hemangiomas

John B. Mulliken

Our whole attitude to the treatment of strawberry naevi must be based on the knowledge of their invariable tendency to spontaneous retrogression.

W. A. Lister

HISTORICAL METHODS

The rapidly growing, bright red hemangioma beckons us to do something—to try anything. A guilt-ridden mother might attempt to erase a birthmark from her baby by rubbing it with the afterbirth (Hand et al., 1981). There is another folk belief that the hand of a corpse should be touched to the birthmark in order to make it disappear and that this should be done in secret (Hand et al., 1981). Saliva is an instinctive medicine from time immemorial; there is an old remedy, attributed to Flemish peasants, that to remove a vascular birthmark from a newborn, the mother must lick the lesion on nine consecutive postpartum mornings (Cantero, 1929).

Physicians, too, have been remarkably resourceful in their attempts to treat hemangiomas, notwithstanding their ignorance of the pathogenesis of these tumors. Medical reports of bygone days often failed to differentiate whether a vascular lesion was congenital or acquired, a tumor or a malformation. Nevertheless, it is possible to construe what kind of remedies were once used for hemangioma, as the lesion is defined in this text. This summary of older therapeutic methods is given as a perspective—for only by an appreciation of the past can we properly manage our present problems and endeavor to improve care in the future.

Ligation and Excision

In his 1714 *Treatise*, Daniel Turner dismissed as reprehensible the treatment of vascular birthmarks by rubbing the lesion with "blood of the secundine." He favored surgical resection, cautery, ligation, and caustics for "Currans (sic), Cherry, Raspberry, Mulberry or Similitudes of the lesser fruits; and those only when they have been seated securely, and have had their surface not too much spread" (Turner, 1714). He warned against treating vascular anomalies that "have large *Plexus* of Vessels to supply them, there is Danger of great Haemorrhage or Flux in their Extirpation: And if they cannot be eradicate (sic) entirely, they will rise again and

77

become more rebellious and troublesome than before they were undertaken."

Turner recounts the successful removal of a hemangioma using excision, ligature, and escharotics by Wilhelm Fabry of Hildanus, called Fabricius de Hilden (1560–1624). The lesion was on the nose of a 3 year old boy; at first it was no bigger than a lentil and then grew to resemble a cherry. Turner also related two cases from his own practice: a raspberry mark near the eyebrow and a currant-like excrescence on the internal canthus, both of which he treated with ligature and sundry caustics. Turner recommended the hot iron for a third case, the "mark of a shrimp" on the cheek of a maidservant (supposedly impressed by her mother's longing for this crustacean). The frightened girl went to another physician.

There are isolated reports from the early nineteenth century telling of the profuse hemorrhage that occurs during excision of even small hemangiomas, sometimes with a fatal outcome (Lawrence, 1827). Cabot honestly communicated his case of a 7 month old child who died the day following removal of a scalp lesion (Cabot, 1864). Nevertheless, surgeons were expected to treat the large, ulcerated, or rapidly growing *naevus maternus*. Always fearful of hemorrhage, they devised ingenious methods of interrupting the vascular supply to the tumor. Wardrop tried removing large cervical hemangiomas in two children. In one instance, he first tied the carotid artery; nevertheless, both children died (Wardrop, 1818). He later reported a successful outcome with proximal ligation, without excision, in a 5 month old child (Wardrop, 1826). Wardrop wisely advised, whenever possible, to cut outside the border of the hemangioma to minimize bleeding. Brodie recommended cutting through the base of the hemangioma, then introducing a caustic, such as silver nitrate, with a spoonlike probe. He called his technique "subcutaneouis cauterization" (Brodie, 1846). Hall proposed "subcutaneous laceration"—passing a small tenotome or cataract needle through the skin in eight to ten different directions, thus severing the subcutaneous vessels supplying the hemangioma (Hall, 1831). White, in 1827, was one of the first authors to report several cases in which double-armed ligatures were passed around the base of the hemangioma to strangle its blood supply (White, 1827). In some instances, the morbid hemangioma sloughed and the ulcerated base healed by scar contraction; or the surgeon would amputate the tumor above the ligatures. John Collins Warren recommended tying off the base of the *naevus maternus* in quarters, and noted: "The more closely the ligature is tied, the sooner will the patient cease to suffer" (Warren, 1839). Samuel Gross advised that when the skin overlying the hemangioma was not involved, flaps could be elevated and transfixion sutures placed through the tumor under direct vision (Gross, 1859) (Fig. 5–1). Garrotting suture techniques for subcutaneous hemangiomas continued to be popular throughout the nineteenth century. Surgeons endorsed figure-of-eight, spiral, or interlocking subcutaneous sutures of catgut, wire, or silk (Curling, 1850; Murray, 1864; Bobbs, 1870–1871; Barwell, 1875; Beck, 1903). Even today, selective subcutaneous ligation is still recommended by some authors (Walsh, 1969; Bingham, 1979).

Until the natural involution of hemangiomas was appreciated in the second quarter of this century, surgical excision and irradiation were the primary modes of therapy. In

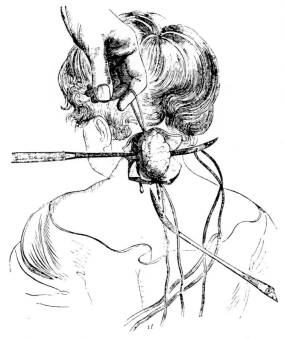

Figure 5–1. Illustration from Gross' textbook *System of Surgery* (1859). Skin flaps elevated to expose deep hemangioma of the neck; "transfixion" sutures passed prior to ligation and removal of the tumor.

1934, J.S. Davis reported over 200 cases of hemangioma treated by excision at The Johns Hopkins Hospital; he often utilized a tourniquet or loop of flexible lead wire on the skin to minimize bleeding (Davis and Wilgis, 1934). J.B. Brown, another forefather of plastic surgery, commenting on this paper, agreed that hemangiomas should be excised early to prevent pain, ulceration, hemorrhage, or destruction of normal tissue.

Artificial Ulceration

The old observation that a hemangioma that ulcerates eventually heals to form skin of a pale color suggested that artificially induced ulceration would imitate this process. To "excite inflammation," a litany of astringents, caustics, and refrigerants have been applied to superficial hemangiomas, including caustic potash (potassium hydroxide), potash and lime (Vienna paste), fuming nitric acid, liquor arsenical, tartrate of antimony, collodian, liquor plumbi subacetatis (lead subacetate), and croton oil (Wardrop, 1818; Gross, 1859; Kingston, 1862; Beatty, 1883; Forster, 1860; Gazzo, 1875; Blair, 1884). As an alternative, an escharotic, e.g., tincture of iodine, zinc chloride, or perchloride of iron, was drawn through the hemangioma with needles and setons of silk or worsted.

Inoculation of a superficial hemangioma with hospital pus was suggested by Ollivier in 1822 (Pouley, 1873); thankfully, there is no documentation that it was ever tried. In 1830, Marshall described using a lancet daubed in "vaccine lymph" to incite vesiculation and crusting, noting eventual healing of the hemangioma so treated (Marshall, 1830). Jonathan Mason Warren, in a letter to his father, told of his friend Dr. George Washington Norris of Philadelphia, who would inoculate the circumference of a *naevus maternus* with vaccine matter. Thus, the eruption "in drying up carries the tumor off with it" (Jones, 1978). The influential Nélaton advised passing setons soaked in vaccine, impaling the infant's hemangioma, a procedure he called "subcutaneous vaccination," as recounted by Harris (Harris, 1871).

Efforts to freeze hemangiomas to death became popular early in this century (Pusey, 1907; Morton, 1909–1910; Bunch, 1911). Carbon dioxide slush or solid crayon techniques were used until recently (Semon,

1934; MacCollum, 1935; Blaisdell, 1936). The slush was made by adding a little acetone to powdered CO_2 snow in an insulated container; the mixture was swept over the hemangioma with a small brush or with an absorbent cotton swab twisted around an orange stick (Brain and Calnan, 1952). The other method involved whittling CO_2 ice into an applicator of proper size and shape, which was then held in contact against the tumor for 10–20 seconds. The treatments were repeated at intervals of 2–3 weeks until an effect was seen. Local anesthesia was usually not necessary. The development of the modern liquid nitrogen apparatus offered another opportunity to congeal hemangiomas.

Electrolysis and Thermocautery

Hemangiomas were not overlooked in the rush to find medical applications for galvanic electricity during the late Victorian era (Dawson, 1874; Knott, 1875; Duncan, 1888). Eight to ten galvanic cells were joined in a series; the number of batteries adjusted the voltage for electrolysis (Clutton, 1882). A red-hot wire of silver or platinum was placed directly on the hemangioma, or needles were inserted subcutaneously prior to activation of the direct current (called "Galvano-puncture") (Coombs, 1881). Battery-powered electrolysis for hemangiomas was quickly replaced by radium therapy at the turn of the century.

Another attempt at producing inflammation in hemangiomas was to pierce the tumor in various directions with long sewing needles heated to a white heat; this technique was known as "ignipuncture" (Warren, 1839). A fancier thermocautery device was introduced by Paquelin in 1876 and had a brief bloom in the treatment of subcutaneous hemangiomas (Owen, 1883, Parker, 1886) (Figs. 5–2 and 5–3). The contemporary electrical diathermy unit was used with a needlepoint attachment to puncture deep hemangiomas, a technique called "endothermy coagulation" (MacCollum, 1935), or for surface coagulation (Matthews, 1953; Matthews, 1968). These modalities are the direct antecedents of today's sophisticated laser technology as a source of thermal energy to destroy hemangiomas (Apfelberg et al., 1981; Hobby, 1983).

One must question the need to use heat to destroy a tumor that appears to be the result of deranged cellular turnover and one that

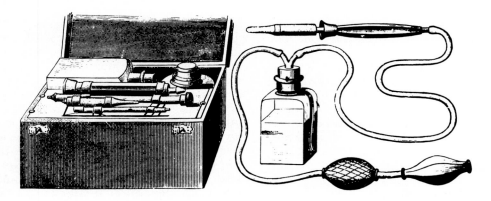

The apparatus consists of a hollow handle, insulated with wood, to protect the hands from the heat. It is furnished with three movable hollow platinum cauteries; into these, after they have been heated to blackness in a flame of a spirit lamp, a blast of benzine vapor is introduced by means of a Richardson's spray bellows, which at once rises to and maintains them at a state of vivid incandescence. The heat thus produced can be kept up for an indefinite time by slightly compressing the bellows occasionally. The apparatus, in a morocco case, imported directly from the manufacturer in Paris $50.00

Figure 5–2. Thermocautery apparatus introduced by C. A. Paquelin (1835–1905) was used to treat hemangiomas. It consisted of a hollow platinum tip, filled with platinum sponge through which a heated hydrocarbon was blown. Details noted in the catalogue of G. Tiemann and Co., *The American Armamentarium Chirurgicum,* New York, C. H. Ludwig, 1879, p. 134.

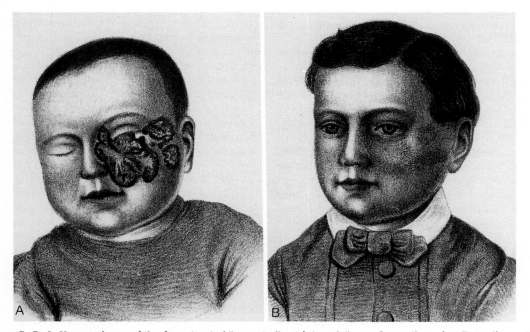

Figure 5–3. *A,* Hemangioma of the face, treated "repeatedly at intervals" over 2 months using Paquelin cautery; a case report by Sir Jonathan Hutchinson. *B,* Portrait drawing several years later. Hutchinson assures the reader that this post-treatment illustration is not exaggerated. Compare this with the expected appearance that would have resulted after natural regression. Illustrations from Hutchinson's *Archives of Surgery,* London, 5:192, 1893.

has a predictable course of natural regression. Thermal coagulation, including argon laser, is not specifically directed at a hemangioma's proliferating cell population and, perforce, causes unnecessary tissue damage and scarring.

Sclerosant Therapy

Injection of "stimulating solutions" for treatment of hemangiomas had its shadowy beginnings in the early nineteenth century. The results were occasionally fatal, as in the case, reported by Paget in 1837, of a 2 year old child with a hemangioma that had been injected with nitric acid and liquor ammoniae (Paget, 1837). A wide variety of sclerosants were tried: ergot (Hammond, 1876), tannic acid, carbolic acid (recommended by Lord Lister, according to Bradley, 1876), perchloride of iron (Hodges, 1864), dilute HCl, tincture of iodine, hypertonic Cl, sodium and potassium ethylate (Brunton, 1878; Richardson, 1879–1881), and 95% alcohol (Holgate, 1889). In this century, 5% sodium morrhuate (a mixture of sodium salts of codliver oil) has been intermittently popular (Watson and McCarthy, 1940; Owens and Stephenson, 1948; Lewis, 1957), along with several other sclerosants: quinine hydrochloride; ethyl carbamate (urethan); 30% sodium citrate; hypertonic saline, with and without dextran (Andrews and Kelly, 1932; Kaessler, 1938; Crawford, 1948; Matthews, 1968); ethamolin froth (monoethanolamine oleate, one of the major constituents of the fatty acids in sodium morrhuate diluted with benzyl alcohol) (Matthews, 1953); and sodium tetradecyl sulfate (a synthetic anionic detergent) (Walsh and Tompkins, 1956).

Injection of boiling water, introduced by Wyeth in 1903 (Wyeth, 1903), was used to treat hemangiomas for several years (Reder, 1920). A well-insulated syringe was necessary so that the operator would not burn himself!

Metal sutures of magnesium are known to cause sclerosis, and Nicoladoni, in 1893, was the first investigator to use this approach for vascular anomalies. His assistant, von Payr, continued to endeavor with this therapeutic modality. He inserted magnesium foil "arrows" into vascular lesions and reported salutary regression in all of his cases (von Payr, 1902). Wilflingseder and colleagues revived magnesium sclerotherapy and described this approach in troublesome, rapidly proliferating hemangiomas (Wilflingseder et al., 1981). They inserted tiny arrows cut from magnesium foil into the hemangioma with a hemostat forceps, or rods cut from magnesium wire (0.25–1.0 mm diameter) and embedded via hypodermic needles.

Radiation

The lowly, benign hemangioma could not escape the new "x-rays," as Roentgen modestly called them. In fact, radiation therapy for hemangiomas proved to be remarkably successful, reaching its heyday in the 1930–1950 era. Thorium-X varnish was tried (Bowers, 1951), as well as interstitial gamma irradiation (gold radon seeds and radium needles) (Brown and Byars, 1938; Edwards, 1941; Bailey and Kiskadden, 1942), radon brass plaques (Montgomery and Culver, 1920; Watson and McCarthy, 1940), and external beam irradiation (Newcomet, 1917; Dana and Beyer, 1966, Paterson and Tod, 1939). Conway reported a case of a 7 month old infant who received a single dose of radiation (2800 R) to a parotid hemangioma via an open exploration wound (Conway, 1951).

A proliferating hemangioma is exquisitely sensitive to even small doses of radiation. Sometimes a hemangioma would begin to show signs of involution just after the child was taken through the door of the radiotherapy department. As little as 300–600 rads was the usual empirical dose. Unfortunately, radiation was also used to treat vascular malformations, particularly port-wine stains, tissues with a stable, non-radiosensitive cell population. Repeated courses of irradiation for these vascular anomalies resulted in severe consequences: radiation burns (Straatsma, 1930), bone and soft tissue atrophy (Benedek, 1950), and late development of tumors (Cannon et al., 1959). There is no question that early radiation therapy was not well controlled, and that late tissue sequelae are minimized with modern techniques. Long-term follow-up analysis of children given radiation (300–600 rads) for hemangiomas showed that, up to 20 years later, the rate of tumor incidence was no greater than that for sarcoma in the general pediatric population (Li et al., 1974). Nevertheless, there are well-documented cases of hemangiosarcoma de-

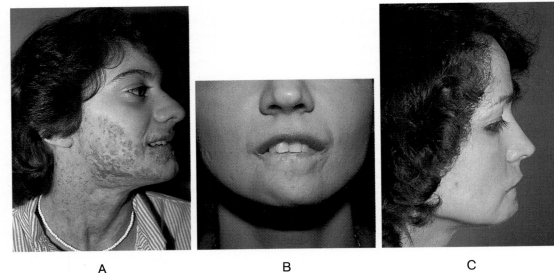

Figure 5–4. Late consequences of irradiation for hemangioma. *A,* Eighteen year old woman treated in infancy with tracheostomy and irradiation for cervicofacial hemangioma. She received 450 rads at 2½ months and another 400 rads at 6 months of age. The atrophy, pigmentation, and telangiectasiae are more prominent than would be expected with natural involution. These skin changes are difficult, if not impossible, to correct. This patient takes thyroxine for hypothyroidism and is followed closely for possible thyroid or salivary gland tumor. *B,* Thirty year old woman had hemangioma of lower lip, which was treated in infancy with insertion of 22 radon seeds. She has had numerous reconstructive procedures for scarring of the mucosa, skin, and musculature. *C,* Lateral photograph of patient in *B* demonstrates atrophy and contracture of the lower lip. Alloplastic chin implant corrects the microgenia, but not the lip posture.

veloping 20–30 years after small radiation doses for hemangioma (Ward and Buchanan, 1977; Bennett et al., 1978). Patients treated with radiation therapy to the neck region have a cumulative risk for developing carcinoma of the thyroid, parathyroid dysfunction, and salivary gland tumors. Cataract can be a late complication of contact roentgen therapy for eyelid hemangioma (Bek and Zahn, 1960). Mammary hypoplasia is a particularly disturbing problem for the young woman treated with irradiation as an infant for breast hemangioma (Gregl and Weiss, 1961; Skalkeas et al., 1972). I have seen a 38 year old woman who developed breast carcinoma in the site where radium implants were inserted for hemangioma of the chest. Even small amounts of radiation can cause stenosis of large intracranial vessels in young children. There are three reported cases of radiation-induced internal carotid artery occlusion resulting from therapy for facial hemangiomas during infancy (Wright and Bresnan, 1976). It is difficult to treat the late skin changes that follow irradiation for hemangioma, e.g., atrophy, contracture, pigmentation, and telangiectasia (Fig. 5–4).

The advent of systemic steroid therapy for hemangiomas has, thankfully, limited the need for irradiation. Yet, there are some investigators who maintain that the risk/benefit ratio indicates that judicious use of irradiation is still an alternative treatment modality for hepatic hemangiomas that are unresponsive to steroids, or for those lesions that interfere with vision or obstruct vital structures, e.g., the subglottic airway (Order, 1979).

Compression

John Abernathy, the popular surgeon-lecturer of St. Bartholomew's Hospital, was probably the first physician to try compression therapy for hemangioma (Abernathy, 1811). Presented with a 2 month old infant with a vascular birthmark of the forearm resembling "the entrails of a pig," he noted that he could force blood from the lesion, and that the limb had increased heat. Abernathy recommended roller banding with a "many-tailed bandage of sticking plaster" and constant wetness "to regulate its temperature." Within 6 months, the hemangioma had diminished in size, while the overlying skin was pale with a shrivelled appearance. Baron Boyer described how an extensive hemangioma of the upper lip slowly disappeared after the mother assiduously followed his advice to moisten the child's lip frequently with alum-water and apply digital pressure for several hours each day (Boyer, 1815). Pressure also was advocated by Forster in the mid-nineteenth century: for a scalp hemangioma, he used a lead plate, plaster of Paris, and elastic bands for 6 weeks to 2 months (Forster, 1860). There are more recent reports of success using compressive elastic garments for hemangiomas of the extremities (Moore, 1964; Miller et al., 1976; Mangus, 1972). However, given a hemangioma's predictable regression, it is difficult to document the efficacy for any proposed remedy. To date, there are no controlled prospective studies to document the value of compression therapy for hemangiomas.

Waiting for Involution

Descriptions of spontaneous involution of *naevi materni* can be found scattered throughout the nineteenth century medical literature (Abernathy, 1811; Wardrop, 1818; Warren, 1839; Gay, 1857; Bobbs, 1870; Duncan, 1870; Marshall, 1893; Patterson, 1894). The natural course of hemangioma, however, like that for other diseases, often escaped notice because medical reports of this period usually consisted of single case histories. In 1923, because of the persistent confusion over the disposition of hemangiomas, Traub mailed a questionnaire, asking whether these lesions should be treated, to all the members of the American Dermatological Association. Of the respondents, less than 10% had observed spontaneous disappearance of a hemangioma in "more than a very few instances" (Traub, 1933). W.A. Lister was the first to design a careful, prospective study of the natural history of hemangiomas (Lister, 1938) (Fig. 5–5). From 1931 to 1938, he observed, with a keen eye, 93 strawberry birthmarks in 77 children. Lister concluded that "no exception has been found to the rule that naevi which grow rapidly during the early months of life, subsequently retrogress and disappear of their own accord, on the average about the fifth year of life" (Lister, 1938). Lister's findings were corroborated by other investigators

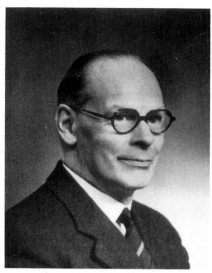

Figure 5–5. William A. Lister, M.B., B.Chir., M.D., FRCP (1897–1981), Consultant Physician to the Prince of Wales' Hospital, Plymouth, was the great-nephew of Lord Lister and the son of Sir William Lister. While serving in the trenches in World War I, he was injured by shrapnel, losing an eye. Yet, it is said, "with one eye he saw more than many physicians with two" (Obit. Letter, Brit. Med. J. *284:*62, 1982). He was elected FRCP in 1938, the same year his paper was published that proved that hemangiomas spontaneously regress. (Photograph courtesy of the Royal College of Physicians, London.)

(Anderson, 1944; Brain and Calnan, 1952; Wallace, 1953; Walter, 1953; Ronchese, 1953).

Nevertheless, the adjectives used to describe hemangiomas, and resultant confusion about the diagnosis, continued to muddle these observations. In particular, there was persistent confusion regarding the potential for involution of "capillary" versus "cavernous" hemangiomas. What seemed to be extreme variability in the behavior of hemangiomas was really just a problem of accuracy in the English language. In the United Kingdom, "cavernous" lesions predictably involuted (Simpson, 1959), whereas in the United States, "cavernous" lesions rarely involuted (MacCollum and Martin, 1956). Andrews and colleagues noted improvement within 5 years in 65% of "capillary" and in only 16% of "cavernous" hemangiomas (Andrews et al., 1957). They concluded that "capillary" lesions smaller than 1 cm diameter were more likely to regress than larger "capillary" or "cavernous" hemangiomas. Obviously, there was also controversy over "mixed," or "capillary-cavernous," hemangiomas!

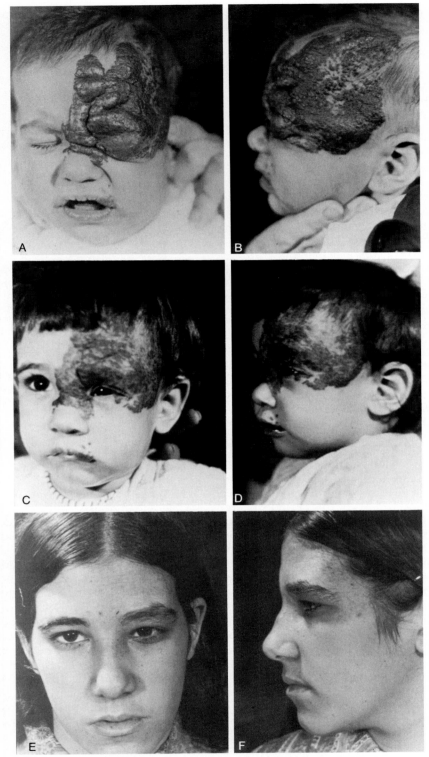

Figure 5–6. Involution of a superficial hemangioma. *A,* Newborn with extensive hemangioma of the face. *B,* Age 4 years; the lesjon is in involuting phase. *C,* Age 14 years; involution complete. The eyebrow is expanded; the skin texture is excellent.

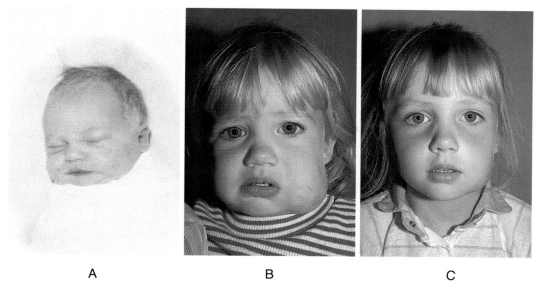

Figure 5–7. Involution of a deep hemangioma. *A,* Nursery photograph of an apparently normal infant. *B,* Age 1½ years; the child has a deep hemangioma of the cheek. *C,* Age 5 years; the hemangioma is regressing on schedule.

Thus, proper management of hemangiomas continued to be actively debated at medical gatherings (Costello, 1949; McCuistion, 1954). The exponents of active therapy persisted in their belief that involution of large, deep, or "cavernous" hemangiomas was rare; and besides, intervention during infancy (usually irradiation or surgical excision) would prevent the tumor from spreading, ulcerating, and damaging normal structures (MacFee, 1947; Matthews, 1953; Brown and Fryer, 1953; Modlin, 1955; Figi and O'Brien, 1956; Andrews et al., 1957; Kiehn et al., 1964). It took several more clinical studies to confirm the wisdom of Lister's classic paper unequivocally (Van der Werf, 1954; Bivings, 1954; Blackfield et al., 1957; Falk and Levy, 1957; Simpson, 1959; Bowers et al., 1960; Margileth and Museles, 1965). All hemangiomas spontaneously regress, whether they are located in the skin, subcutis, muscle, or viscera (Figs. 5–6 and 5–7).

CURRENT MANAGEMENT OF HEMANGIOMAS

Primum non Nocere

The physician must fully appreciate the parents' anguish during the hemangioma's early growth phase. Their child, who was normal at birth, is now becoming progressively deformed. Conflicting ideas from other physicians and relatives must be resolved in an effective manner. At the first consultation, the parents want to know what caused the hemangioma; the mother, especially, may feel that she is at fault. The physician should explain that the exact cause is unknown but should also take the time to elaborate on possible mechanisms that cause a sudden overgrowth of blood vessels. A special effort should be made to dispel blame and the preconceived notion that the mother's behavior or thoughts during the pregnancy might have produced the hemangioma. The parents will need a thorough explanation and re-explanation about the natural history of hemangioma. Repeated assurance of the benign nature of these tumors and the unlikely need for active therapy will ultimately relieve most of the parents' concerns. Some distressed parents will go to almost any lengths to find someone who would be willing to treat their child's growing tumor. As Lister cautioned: "It is easy to be stampeded into advising drastic and injudicious measures" (Lister, 1938). Photographs should be taken during the first visit so that subsequent changes in the lesion can be documented. Sometimes parents take their own photographs of the child; this is usually a healthy sign of their involvement in the child's care and confidence in the prognosis. Measurement of the size of the lesion is useful for later comparison. Some parents are too close to the problem to appreciate the rate of growth and early changes of involution. Oftentimes, however, the parents can tell whether the hemangioma is growing faster than the child, or at the same rate; or that the child is outgrowing the lesion. Textbook illustrations showing the natural course of involution and the late skin changes for a similar lesion and location are a welcome relief to the parents. The physician must be willing to spend sufficient time with each family in order to explain fully the natural history, therapy, and expected long-term result for their child's hemangioma. Needless to say, if the physician fails to gain the parents' confidence, they will search for help elsewhere.

Parents are more easily convinced of their child's prognosis if relatives have had birthmarks that regressed spontaneously. Parents also frequently find comfort in talking to other parents whose child's hemangioma has already progressed into the involution phase. However, the physician must be both discreet and precise in promoting interfamilial contacts, because of the differences in natural history and psychological trauma associated with hemangiomas of dissimilar size and location. For example, the problems encountered with even a small hemangioma of the upper eyelid or nasal tip are quite different from those encountered in a large hemangioma of the scalp or trunk.

An infant with a growing hemangioma should be seen as frequently as necessary to provide reassurance to the parents. The first 6–9 months, the proliferating phase, is the most difficult period. For the child with a small-to-medium sized hemangioma in a favorable location, visits at 3 month intervals are sufficient. Re-examination of the baby's photographs and referral to the initial measurements may only add to the parents' distress during this stage. Once the hemangioma's growth seems to plateau and early signs of regression are obvious, the parents welcome comparison with earlier measurements and pictures. Once the parents become more relaxed about their child's condition, evaluations can proceed at 6 month to 1 year intervals. More frequent office visits are necessary for infants with ulcerated, large or multiple hemangiomas, or when the physician is dealing with lesions located in critical areas, e.g., the upper eyelid or upper airway.

The physician, perhaps with the collaboration of an interested child psychologist or psychiatrist, must always be aware of the emotional issues. In the case of a highly visible hemangioma, the physician should be on the alert to the parents' problems in dealing with people outside the family. Not infrequently, strangers, when passing the baby carriage, will callously remark: "Why don't they do something about that!" or make an innuendo that the infant is a victim of parental abuse. Behavioral disturbances in the child with facial hemangioma are rare, but they can occur in the 3–5 year old age group. Patients may again press for excision during this critical preschool period. Indeed, this is a time to consider surgical resection, but only for very specific indications.

Local Complications

The complications of growing hemangioma also compel more frequent evaluation. *Ulceration* is not uncommonly seen with superficial lesions. Skin breakdown may be present at birth, but more often it occurs when the hemangioma is in its most active proliferative stage. Hemangiomas on a mucosal surface (the lips and anogenital areas) are particularly likely to develop ulceration and secondary infection (Fig. 5–8). Treatment consists of cleaning, dressing changes as necessary, and daily application of topical antibiotic ointment. Systemic antibiotics, based on bacterial culture, are indicated only when there is diffuse ulceration and cellulitis in the hemangioma. For the anogenital region, application of a petroleum jelly–based antibiotic ointment will protect the ulcerated surface from contact with urine or feces and will diminish pain. It often takes several weeks for an ulcerated hemangioma to heal by re-epithelialization. Once the ulceration heals, a characteristic smooth, slightly depressed white patch of scar remains, in clear contrast to the normal surrounding skin (Fig. 5–9A–C). Recurrent ulceration after healing is extremely rare. Ulceration is *not* an indication for excision (Fig. 5–9D).

Bleeding from a punctate area of a hemangioma is another annoying problem. Parents should be instructed to press a clean pad on

Figure 5–8. Newborn with ulceration of a nascent hemangioma of the lip. *A,* Photograph, taken in nursery, shows ulceration beginning in vermilion of upper lip. *B,* This 2 day old infant was referred with a diagnosis of "cleft lip." *C,* Hemangioma more obvious at age 1 month. *D,* At age 4 years, involution is nearly complete; note restoration of vermilion free margin and effacement of vermilion-cutaneous junction.

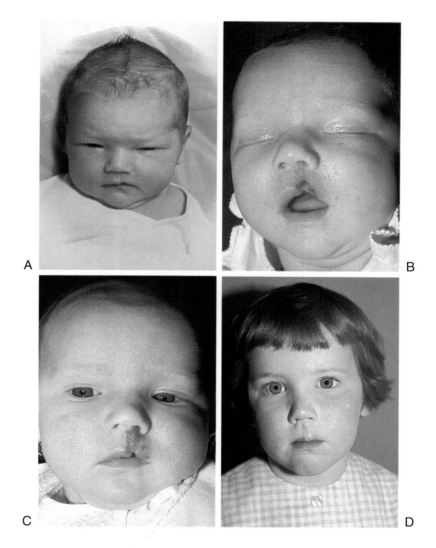

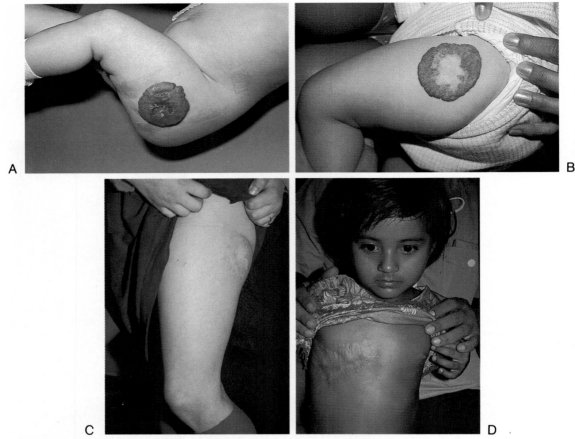

Figure 5–9. Spontaneous ulceration during proliferative phase. *A,* Deep central ulceration in a bosselated hemangioma of the thigh. *B,* Healing by epithelialization leaves a pale central scar. *C,* Involution at age 7 years; note remarkable shrinkage of skin envelope. *D,* This ill-advised wide excision of an ulcerated hemangioma of the chest included the breast anlage.

the bleeding point for 10 minutes while watching the clock. Repeated bleeding episodes, requiring visits to the local emergency service, may necessitate placement of a mattress suture. Local bleeding may be a manifestation of systemic coagulopathy and may constitute an indication for steroid administration.

Steroid Therapy

As an historical note, steroids were first given to treat hemangioma-associated thrombocytopenia, but cortisone's potential effect on the hemangioma's rate of growth was lost in the therapeutic barrage that included splenectomy, vitamins, and radiotherapy (Dargeon et al., 1959). In 1963, a serendipitous discovery was made at the Johns Hopkins

Hospital when a large facial hemangioma began to shrink coincidentally with steroid administration for thrombocytopenia (Zarem and Edgerton, 1967). Subsequent reports confirmed that prednisone may, indeed, hasten the onset and rate of involution of hemangiomas (Fost and Esterly, 1968; Brown et al., 1972). The response rate is reported to be in the range of 30% (Bartoshesky et al., 1978) to 90% (Edgerton, 1976).

Systemic steroids should be used only in selected infants with a hemangioma that is (1) a rapidly growing lesion that seriously distorts facial features; (2) a lesion causing recurrent bleeding, ulceration, or infection; or (3) a lesion that interferes with normal physiological functions (breathing, hearing, eating, or vision) (Fig. 5–10). Other situations that would justify a trial of steroids are a large hemangioma, or multicentric heman-

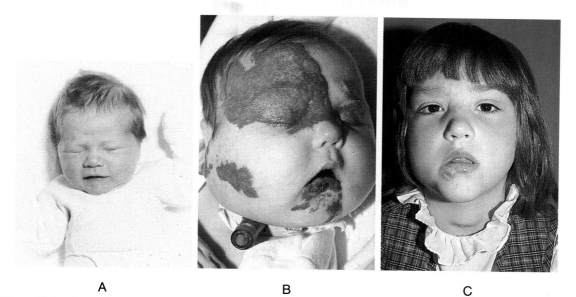

A   B   C

Figure 5–10. Systemic steroid therapy for ulcerating-obstructing hemangioma. *A,* Photograph of healthy newborn girl. *B,* At age 5 months, she is in the intensive care unit with a cervicofacial hemangioma that obstructs the upper airway and necessitated tracheostomy. Note lip ulceration. She is receiving systemic prednisone; there is already graying of the hemangioma. *C,* Involution at age 5 years; further improvement is expected.

giomatosis causing bleeding (secondary to thrombocytopenia) and/or high output cardiac failure.

The immature proliferating hemangioma is far more responsive to steroid therapy than the stable or involuting phase lesion in a child over 1 year old (Edgerton, 1976). The usual dosage is 2–3 mg/kg/day of prednisone given orally for 2–3 weeks. A sensitive hemangioma usually shows signs of responsiveness within 7–10 days, i.e., softening, lightening of color, and a diminished rate of growth. Steroid should be discontinued if there is no effect. If the hemangioma responds to steroid therapy, the dosage can be lowered to 1 mg/kg/day, or the child can be placed on an alternate day regimen, with further reduction of dosage to 0.75 mg/kg/day. The steroid level should be tapered as soon as possible; this decision depends on the tumor's sensitivity, location, and maturity. Usually, prednisone is given for a cycle of 4–6 weeks, followed by a rest period. A decision to repeat the course of steroids is made, based on the age of the child and the location and initial response of the lesion. There is no reason to continue steroids once the hemangioma is well into its involution phase.

Rebound growth may occur in young, rapidly proliferative lesions at reduced steroid dosage, and an additional 2–3 week cycle of prednisone 1 mg/kg/day, on alternate days, may have to be reinstituted. This rebound phenomenon when steroid levels fall confirms the tumor's sensitivity to endocrine modulation.

Few complications are seen with this short term, high dose course of steroids. Infants given this therapy have a temporary retardation of growth and decreased appetite. Transient facial edema also occurs, but there is no evidence for significant hypertension or salt and water retention. There is also no reported permanent effect on growth or skeletal maturation by the short term regimens. However, one study documents that even two doses of hydrocortisone, given to a neonate, may depress T cell function and cause immunologic abnormalities (Gunn et al., 1981). It is important to remember that tiny infants on prednisone are at increased risk for otitis media and pneumonia, as well as for overwhelming sepsis. They should be followed closely by the pediatrician or a pediatric endocrinologist. Thus, it is advisable to use the lowest effective dose of steroid for the shortest duration of time, until the hemangioma enters its regression phase.

Mechanism of Steroid Action

The mechanism by which corticosteroids cause accelerated involution of hemangiomas is under active investigation. Cortisone is known to cause vasoconstriction in the hamster (Wyman et al., 1953) and in the rat (Zweifach et al., 1953) in the presence of adrenal insufficiency. Edgerton suggests that the channels and sinusoids of the immature hemangioma may be very sensitive to steroids and undergo vasoconstrictive changes leading to shrinkage of the proliferating capillaries (Edgerton, 1976). There is a remarkable case report of a baby girl with a hemangioma confined to the left orbit and middle cranial fossa that totally resolved with steroid administration. Over a period of 8 months, serial angiography demonstrated that regression was accompanied by gradual occlusion of the feeding branches from the internal and external carotid arteries (Prensky and Gado, 1973). However, light and electron microscopic study of hemangiomas in various stages of involution does not show any evidence of vasoconstriction, ischemia, or thrombosis (Mulliken and Glowacki, 1982; Dethlefsen et al., 1986).

Another working hypothesis is that steroids could modulate the control of endothelial proliferation. Folkman and his coworkers have shown that certain cortisone analogs inhibit angiogenesis in the presence of heparin and heparin fragments (Folkman et al., 1983; Crum et al., 1985). The studies of Sasaki and Pang suggest that hormone receptors play a role in the influence of glucocorticoids on proliferating hemangiomas (Sasaki et al., 1984). Using a receptor assay system, these investigators demonstrated that hemangiomas contain increased estradiol binding sites, and furthermore that cortisone inhibits estrogen binding to the tissue. They also documented that infants with hemangiomas that respond to prednisone showed decreased levels of serum estradiol during therapy when compared with infants with nonresponsive hemangiomas.

Chemotherapy

There are isolated reports of using chemotherapeutic drugs for hemangiomas. In the pre-steroid era, Rush was first to publish a report of a case of a large facial hemangioma treated with intra-arterial nitrogen mustard (Rush, 1966). The alkylating agent was administered when the child was 8 months old, when the lesion may have already reached a plateau in its growth curve. More recently, cyclophosphamide has been used successfully in three infants with life-threatening pleuropericardial and liver hemangiomas that had not responded to systemic steroids or radiation therapy (Hurvitz et al., 1985).

Upper Eyelid Hemangioma

Hemangiomas of the upper eyelid present a special problem because they may potentially cause amblyopia and refractive errors (Robb, 1977; Stigmar et al., 1978). A large hemangioma located in the lower eyelid or cheek area rarely interferes with vision. However, even the smallest hemangioma in the upper eyelid can cause visual disturbance. A child with an upper eyelid hemangioma deserves serial refraction to demonstrate the presence and possible worsening of visual changes. In rare instances, an isolated hemangioma of the upper eyelid can be totally or subtotally excised (Azzolini et al., 1983). However, more often the hemangioma infiltrates the entire thickness of the upper eyelid and extends into the periorbital tissues and subconjunctiva. Steroid administration is the treatment of choice if the hemangioma is occluding the visual axis or causing astigmatism, strabismus, or anisometropia.

Intralesional steroid injection for hemangiomas was introduced in an effort to minimize the systemic effects of oral administration. This approach was first used in a series of 115 children by Azzolini and Nouvenne (Azzolini and Nouvenne, 1970). Although periorbital hemangiomas respond to oral prednisone (de Venecia and Lobeck, 1970), the intralesional route has special application for lesions in this location (Zak and Morin, 1981; Kushner, 1979; Kushner, 1985; Brown and Huffaker, 1982). The infant must be placed under light general anesthesia. The dosage is calculated based on the child's weight and the size of the hemangioma. Kushner recommends that each treatment should not exceed the injection of more than 40 mg triamcinolone acetate and 6 mg betamethasone (Kushner, 1985). A 27 gauge needle is used, and multiple punctures are necessary to distribute the steroid throughout the lesion. According to Kushner, the response rate is in the 60–80% range, although in most instances a second injection 6–8 weeks later is necessary (Kushner, 1985) (Fig. 5–11). Local steroid injections commonly re-

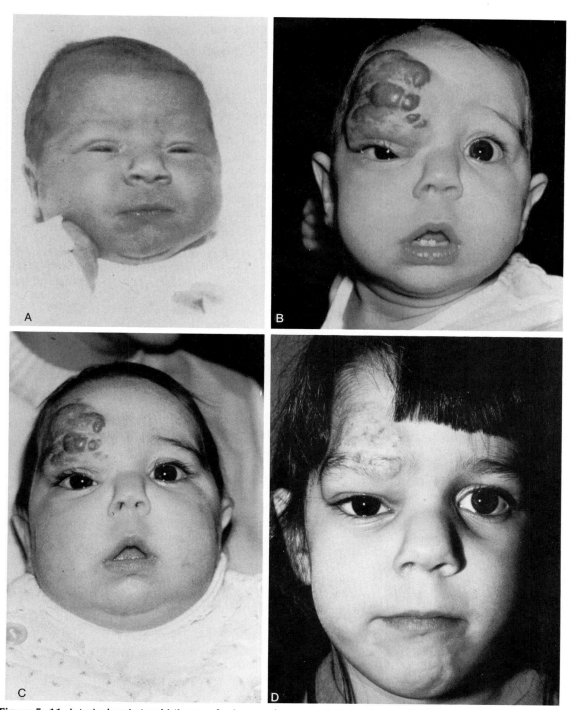

Figure 5–11. Intralesional steroid therapy for hemangioma causing visual complication. *A,* Newborn child: first sign of hemangioma appeared 2 weeks later. *B,* Age 6 months: hemangioma of upper eyelid causing astigmatism. There was equivocal response to systemic steroids; therefore, two intralesional injections were given at 2 month intervals (160 mg, 100 mg triamcinolone). *C,* Two weeks after second intralesional triamcinolone injection, there is shrinkage of the eyelid tumor and opening of the palpebral fissure. (*B* and *C* courtesy of Richard M. Robb, M.D.) *D,* At age 4, patient has residual astigmatism and fullness of the eyebrow-eyelid.

sult in cholestin plaque deposits and soft tissue atrophy; however, both of these problems seem to be temporary (Kushner, 1985).

Intralesional steroid injection for eyelid hemangioma carries an attendant risk of hemorrhage or hematoma in the retrobulbar space, which is a threat to vision. Occlusion of the central retinal artery and damage to the optic nerve can occur after retrobulbar injection of corticosteroid (Ellis, 1978), and also after injection into the nasal mucosa (Whiteman et al., 1980). There is also the danger of accidental intraocular injection of depot steroid (Zinn, 1981). Because of these possible complications, one should pause before trying intralesional injection for a hemangioma that extends posteriorly into the orbital cone. Instead, systemic steroids should be considered where there is periorbital hemangiomatous infiltration and ocular proptosis.

Patching the non-involved eye forces use of the affected eye and minimizes development of amblyopia and strabismus. In the past, radiation therapy has been used for eyelid hemangiomas. However, this modality carries a risk of causing late cataract (Bek and Zahn, 1960), and it has been superseded by steroid therapy.

Subglottic Hemangioma

An infant with cutaneous hemangioma who presents with persistent respiratory stridor is a suspect for laryngeal hemangioma. Once the diagnosis is confirmed by endoscopy, the treatment is determined by the size and extent of the subglottic narrowing. The older infant with minimal airway narrowing can be closely observed, waiting for the hemangioma to involute. Systemic steroids have been helpful in accelerating involution of subglottic hemangiomas (Cohen and Wang, 1972; Overcash and Putney, 1973). If the airway is not severely compromised, the younger infant should be given a trial of oral prednisone and watched closely. Infants who present with high grade obstruction and recurrent airway problems are candidates for tracheostomy or CO_2 laser excision. Healy and coworkers report a high rate of success using the CO_2 laser excision of obstructing subglottic hemangiomas (Healy et al., 1984). They note that intense humidification is required immediately following laser excision

in order to avoid crust formation on the denuded mucosal surface. For some infants, repeated or staged laser treatments are necessary.

There is no evidence that laser excision and coagulation cause accelerated involution of laryngeal hemangioma. The airway is physically opened by the laser excision and subsequent scarring of the remaining tissues. Healy and coworkers recommend that the rare circumferential subglottic hemangioma should not be treated by CO_2 laser excision because of the increased likelihood for subglottic stenosis (Healy et al., 1984). Also, this modality is not indicated in cases with diffuse hemangiomatous involvement of the mediastinum. Tracheostomy may be necessary in these cases of extensive airway hemangioma, or in cases that fail to respond to systemic steroids. Once the hemangioma is well into its regression phase, with or without the help of steroids, the child can be safely decannulated. External beam radiation probably no longer has a role in the management of subglottic hemangioma (Tefft, 1966); implantation of radioactive gold grains is advocated by Benjamin and Carter (Benjamin and Carter, 1983).

Cutaneous and Visceral Hemangiomas with Congestive Heart Failure

There appears to be a critical mass of hemangiomatous tissue beyond which high output congestive heart failure and systemic clotting changes are likely to develop. These rare cases usually involve combined cutaneous and liver hemangiomas, and even less frequently, an isolated giant skin hemangioma. These infants have a high morbidity and mortality rate, once bleeding and cardiac complications occur. DeLorimier reports a mortality rate of up to 50% within 2 weeks of onset of this condition (DeLorimier, 1967). However, even large hepatic hemangiomas resolve spontaneously without need for therapy (Matolo and Johnson, 1973). As emphasized in Chapter Three, an arteriovenous malformation of the liver can present in a newborn with a clinical picture that is quite similar to that of visceral hemangiomatosis. This differential diagnosis must be resolved before instituting appropriate therapy.

If systemic signs and symptoms develop

and the diagnosis is clearly visceral hemangioma, the following scheme of management is suggested, based on the reports by Larcher and colleagues (Larcher et al., 1981) and by Pereyra (Pereyra et al., 1982). Congestive cardiac failure is managed by digoxin and diuretics in conjunction with fluid restriction. An initial daily dosage of 2 mg/kg/day of prednisone should also be given. Serial determination of cardiac output by echocardiography can be used as a non-invasive method to monitor the effectiveness of steroids. Ultrasonography and/or computed tomography can be repeated in order to document shrinkage of liver hemangiomas during the course of steroid therapy. When the sporadic reports are examined in aggregate, there is diminution of hepatomegaly and control of congestive heart failure in 70% of cases treated medically (Goldberg and Fonkalsrud, 1969; Rocchini et al., 1976; Braun et al., 1975; Clemmensen, 1979; Touloukian, 1970; Pereyra et al., 1982). Observation of any cutaneous hemangiomas for signs of early "graying" and softening is a simple way to monitor the response to steroids.

Embolic Therapy

If medical management fails, i.e., there is no improvement in the infant's condition after a 2 week trial of steroids, angiography should be performed in preparation for either embolic therapy or surgical intervention. Digital arterial radiography minimizes the size of the catheter and the potential for damage to the tiny vessels and also limits the volume of contrast material. Digital radiography clearly demonstrates the rapid flow into the liver and typically enlarged hepatic arteries and other dilated intercostal and subphrenic vessels (Fig. 5–12A). In lesions over 1–2 months of age, the hypervascular nodules are clearly seen in the venous phase. In immature hemangiomas, the veins fill rapidly, reflecting the shunting through the hemangiomatous tissue. Embolization with Gelfoam has been tried for hepatic hemangiomas; however, infarction of the kidney is a potential complication (Tegtmeir et al., 1977). A remarkable example of the efficacy of Gelfoam pellet embolization is the response of a giant hemangioma of the thigh and pelvis reported by Argenta (Argenta et al., 1982). We have used tiny coils to obliterate the hepatic artery embolically proximal to the hemangioma as an adjunctive method to control congestive heart failure until involution begins (Fig. 5–12B).

Surgical Therapy

If embolic therapy is not available, or if this approach is unsuccessful in regulating the congestive heart failure, a surgical ap-

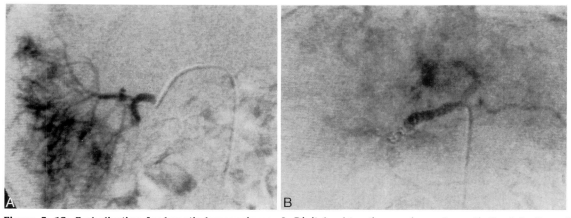

Figure 5–12. Embolization for hepatic hemangioma. *A,* Digital subtraction angiography: selective injection of right hepatic artery demonstrates enlarged branches feeding hemangioma right lobe (see Fig. 3–12A.) *B,* Repeat injection into celiac artery following embolization of right hepatic artery with 3 mini-coils. Note absent filling with reflux into left hepatic and splenic arteries. Embolization helps "buy time" until involution occurs. (Courtesy of Kenneth E. Fellows, M.D.)

proach is necessary. Hepatic artery ligation was first successfully performed by De-Lorimier (DeLorimier, 1967), and has been repeated by other investigators (Mattioli et al., 1974; Rake et al., 1970; Laird et al., 1976; Keller and Bluhn, 1979; Shannon et al., 1982). Larcher recommends that any infant less than 6 weeks of age presenting with intractable cardiac failure should be considered for immediate hepatic artery ligation (Larcher, 1981). However, arterial ligation alone may fail to control symptoms (Larcher et al., 1981). This procedure is not without its hazards; liver necrosis and abscess formation have occurred following hepatic artery ligation (Pereyra et al., 1982).

Rupture and/or intraperitoneal hemorrhage from liver hemangiomas can be treated by hepatic resection, but because the liver is usually diffusely involved, hepatic lobectomy is usually not effective (Touloukian, 1970). When the hemangioma is localized, liver resection can be performed successfully, but this is not without risk, even in the absence of overt high output congestive heart failure (Schuller et al., 1949; Wagget et al., 1969; Matolo and Johnson, 1973). There is a case report of a massive pelvic hemangioma causing intractable congestive heart failure that was treated by ligation of the hypogastric arterial supply and subtotal excision (Price et al., 1972).

Radiotherapy

Radiotherapy may be called upon to play a role in the treatment of hepatic hemangiomas (Lee et al., 1956; Park and Phillips, 1970; Dehner and Ishak, 1971; Kagan et al., 1971). However, most authors cite the associated increased mortality rate for radiation and suggest it not be employed unless other forms of therapy are contraindicated or unsuccessful (McLean et al., 1972; Larcher et al., 1981).

Berman and Lim reviewed the world literature and found the mortality rate for concurrent cutaneous and hepatic hemangiomas to be as high as 81% if no treatment was given, in contrast to a mortality rate of 29% for infants who received early aggressive therapy: steroids, hepatic irradiation, hepatic artery ligation, or lobectomy. The overall mortality rate in 59 cases of combined cutaneous and hepatic hemangiomatosis was 54% (Berman and Lim, 1978).

Coagulopathy

Infants can tolerate moderately severe thrombocytopenia without bleeding because of their relative immobility (Esterly, 1983). If thrombocytopenia does not present a clinical problem, aggressive therapy to control a low platelet count is not indicated. Kasabach-Merritt syndrome is a self-limited condition. The platelet level always returns to normal once the hemangioma undergoes regression (Wallerstein, 1961) or is simply excised (Hill and Longino, 1962). One should assess the risk of bleeding and determine whether or not there is an associated consumptive coagulopathy. If platelet trapping leading to thrombocytopenia and bleeding is the only event, this situation may be corrected by steroid therapy. For an individual infant, the decision to treat must weigh the risk of potential bleeding against the hazards of untoward steroid effects. Young infants given prednisone are at increased risk for developing life-threatening sepsis. Certainly, if there is evidence for repeated hemorrhage, a trial of steroid therapy is indicated (Evans et al., 1975). Generally, a 2–4 week period of prednisone at a dosage of 2–4 mg/kg/day is necessary for an adequate trial (Esterly, 1983).

Cyclophosphamide therapy is another alternative if the hemangioma fails to respond to steroids and life-threatening bleeding continues (Hurvitz et al., 1986). For a localized, giant hemangioma, Gelfoam embolization should also be considered (Argenta et al., 1982).

Another hematological approach is to remedy the thrombocytopenia. There is no specific platelet count that can be used as a guide for treatment in the absence of bleeding. Platelet transfusions are not likely to be beneficial, since the thrombocytopenia is secondary to increased platelet trapping and destruction. Koerper and colleagues report an increase in platelet counts in infants with platelet trapping syndromes, including hemangiomas after treatment with double agent antiplatelet therapy, namely aspirin and dipyridamole (Koerper et al., 1983). However, Sondel and coworkers found there was no benefit from antiplatelet therapy (Sondel et al., 1984).

Operative Therapy

If one postulates that *every* hemangioma begins as a localized nest of cells, it might seem that an ideal treatment should be early excision before rapid growth, extension, or possible ulceration occurs (Modlin, 1955; Andrews et al., 1957). However, there are several flaws in this logic track. First, the hemangioma that is small when first seen may well be biologically destined to remain diminutive. A linear excision and the resultant scar may be more obvious than the skin changes that follow natural involution. Second, clinical observation suggests that a particular hemangioma's size and distribution seem to be predetermined, i.e., a hemangioma begins as a field transformation. Thus, the extensive lesion is out of bounds for simple excision at the outset. Finally, from a practical point of view, most infants do not come to medical attention until after the hemangioma has reached a size when excision would be mutilating.

It must be reiterated that the vast majority of hemangiomas should be left alone, allowing the natural involution to run its course. Nevertheless, there are definite stages in the life cycle of a hemangioma when excision should be considered. These windows for surgical therapy can be conveniently divided into (1) infancy, (2) early childhood or preschool years, and (3) late childhood and early adolescence.

During Infancy

There are rare indications for operative therapy in infancy. A case in point is the isolated hemangioma of the upper eyelid causing obstruction of vision or astigmatism (Thomson et al., 1979). There are also eyelid lesions that fail to respond to steroid therapy and those unlikely to do so (Fig. 5–13). Afferent ligation for hepatic hemangiomas is another surgical consideration during infancy. Prior to 1970, parotidectomy was recommended for hemangioma, the most common parotid tumor of infancy. Perhaps the term "hemangioendothelioma," with its malignant connotation, incited surgical resection. Superficial parotidectomy for hemangioma is no longer recommended. There are excellent results following involution of pa-

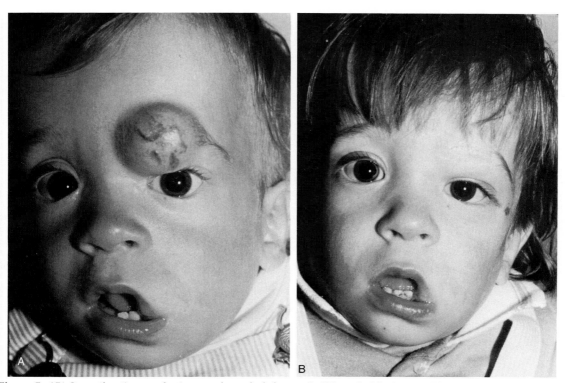

Figure 5–13. Operative therapy for hemangioma in infancy. *A,* Although this 1 year old boy's hemangioma was beginning to involute, it pressed on the upper cornea, resulting in 1½ diopters of astigmatism. The lesion is unlikely to respond to intralesional steroid therapy at this age. *B,* Nine months following subtotal excision of the hemangioma, the astigmatism has disappeared.

rotid hemangiomas, particularly considering the difficulty of complete removal and the danger of facial nerve damage, as well documented by Williams (Williams, 1975).

During Early Childhood

Excision of hemangioma may be indicated for psychosocial reasons prior to or at the time of school attendance. A hemangioma can seriously interfere with the rapidly emerging awareness of body image in a 3 to 5 year old child. Usually a child with a facial hemangioma is accepted by nursery school and kindergarten classmates. Trouble is more likely to develop when the child is exposed to older schoolmates during first grade. Another consideration for early, usu-

ally subtotal, excision is based on an appreciation of the skin expansion effect of a large hemangioma. Certain hemangiomas grow in a pendant fashion, and, even with complete involution, a sagging bag of skin will remain. In these instances, removal of the central section of the lesion may be indicated to improve contour and minimize body image distortion, rather than waiting until involution is complete (Fig. 5–14A and B). (See Chapter Twenty-Two for a discussion of the psychological issues involved in consideration of early operative intervention.) Hemangioma of the vermilion border and mucosa tends to remain bulky and may be considered for contour excision (Fig. 5–14C and D). Glabellar and eyebrow lesions also leave fibrofatty residuum, and subtotal excision may be indicated prior to the child's entry into

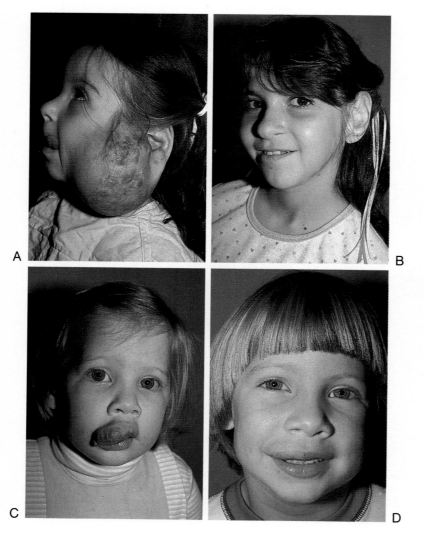

A

B

C

D

Figure 5–14. Operative therapy for hemangioma in early childhood (preschool). *A,* Large facial hemangioma in a 2½ year old girl. *B,* Although further involution was expected, excess skin and tumor were excised at age 3; the dissection was superficial to the seventh cranial nerve. Appearance at age 10; note the large auricle (this is a rare example of skeletal hypertrophy with hemangiomas). *C,* Five year old girl with regressing hemangioma of lip; she is taunted by older children. Even with complete involution, there will be excessive residual mucosa and submucosa. *D,* One year following subtotal or contour excision.

school. Whenever a procedure is performed during early childhood, there must be careful attention to placement of the excisional axis within relaxed skin tension lines. One should be cautious not to resect too much hemangioma during the early proliferative phase for fear of causing later contour defect or deformity. Residual fibrofatty tissue can always be removed when the child is older. Early contour excision of a hemangioma should only be performed in special circumstances, usually for psychological indications, and where it is obvious that skin resection will be necessary in the future, notwithstanding the final result of involution.

The nose is a psychologically sensitive focus. Nasal tip lesions are notoriously slow to evidence regression, and they often leave behind extra fibrofatty tissue. In a small series of patients with nasal tip hemangiomas,

Thomson documented that in general, the results without active treatment surpassed those managed by excision (Thomson, 1979). However, in carefully considered cases, there is a role for subtotal excision to improve nasal contour during childhood. For example, in our clinic, a 4 year old child tried to cut off her nasal hemangioma with a scissors. Excisional therapy was necessary in this acute psychological situation. Nasal hemangiomas are usually spheroidal, and there is a natural tendency to perform both a transverse and vertical wedge excision. A preferred technique is a "low flying bird" skin excision, in conjunction with subtotal removal of the hemangioma and approximation of the splayed alar genua (Fig. 5–15). Care should be taken not to remove too much tissue, which in time, and with continued involution, can result in a loss of nasal tip projection.

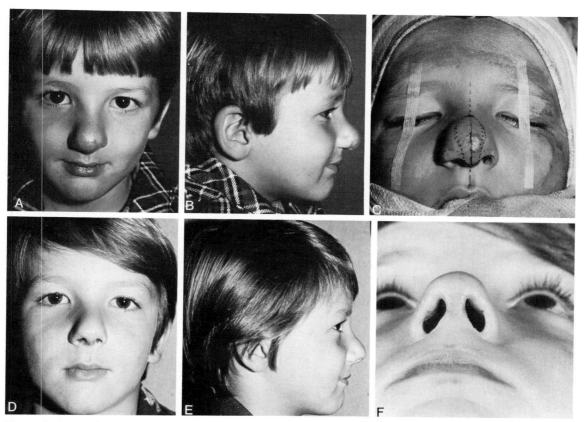

Figure 5–15. A, Six year old boy with nasal hemangioma. B, His profile view makes him the subject of jests by older schoolmates. C, Contour excision accomplished via "low flying bird" approach (solid curvilinear line over nostrils). The dotted lines denote areas for planned excision and splayed alar genua. D, Frontal view 2 years after excision and approximation of alar genua. E, Lateral view 2 years after excision. F, Submental view to show scar hidden along superior nostril margins.

During Late Childhood and Adolescence

It is usually best to wait until the child is 8–12 years of age before considering removal of the excess fibrofatty tissue and abnormal skin that remain after involution. The involved skin often looks remarkably good following involution, particularly if the hemangioma was located in the reticular dermis. Frequently the dermis is atrophic and tiny telangiectatic vessels are seen. If ulceration occurred during the lesion's proliferative phase, this area will remain a hypopigmented or yellowish-tan scar. Closure, after excision of badly scarred areas, can be aided by the newer techniques of skin expansion. Usually there is extra expanded skin left behind after involution of a distended hemangioma. Staged excisions are easily accomplished for involuted hemangiomas of the lip, cheeks, glabella, and scalp (Fig. 5–16). Blepharoplasty and rhytidoplasty type excisions are useful in tightening up the loose, crepey skin that remains after involution of large facial lesions. Ptosis correction and eyelid revision are frequently necessary after involution of upper eyelid lesions.

Important facial structures can be destroyed in infancy by an infected and ulcerated hemangioma. Although it is tempting to correct the soft tissue defect with a local flap (e.g., from the cheek or forehead), it is best to use tissue expansion techniques in order to minimize further scarring on a child's face. An anatomical defect can also be reconstructed using techniques for tissue transfer from a distant donor site (Fig. 5–17).

Laser Therapy

There are publications advocating that the argon laser be used to treat proliferating cutaneous hemangiomas (Apfelberg et al., 1981; Hobby, 1983). Argon laser penetrates the skin, and the blue-green light is absorbed by red cells within the hemangioma and normal dermal vessels. The absorbed light energy is transformed into heat, causing thrombosis or destruction of the vascular channels and perivascular tissue. Thermal damage within the skin usually causes ulceration of the hemangiomatous tissue, the papillary dermis, and epidermis; the end result is scar.

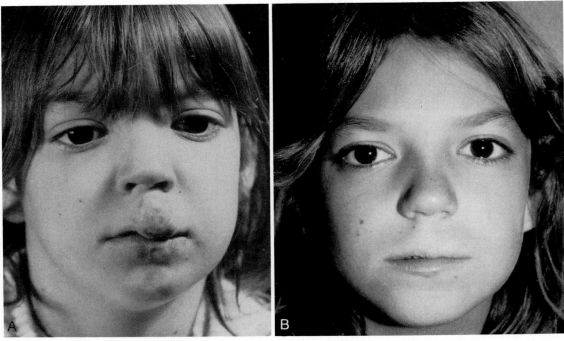

Figure 5–16. Excision of residual hemangioma during late childhood. A, Seven year old child with residual hemangioma of upper lip (despite 275 rads administered during early proliferative phase). B, Age 11, following two-stage excision in transverse and vertical axes.

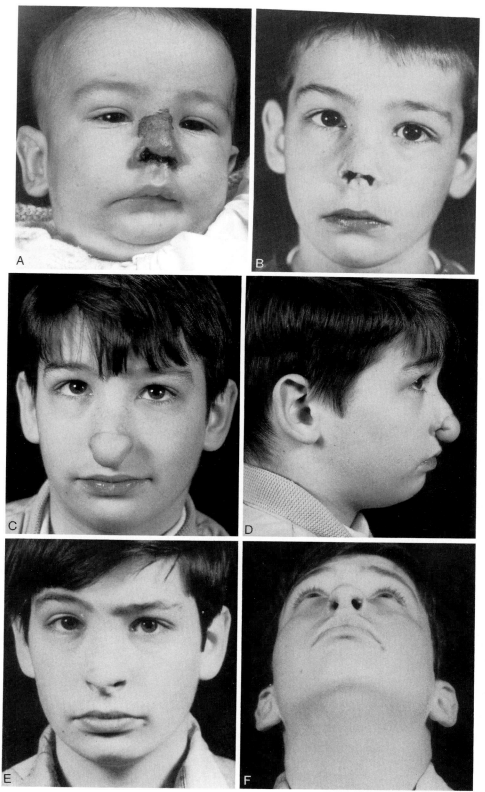

Figure 5–17. Operative reconstruction for tissue loss secondary to hemangioma. *A,* Infant with ulceration and loss of nasal tip and columella secondary to hemangioma. *B,* By age 6, the obvious nasal defect is causing psychological problems. *C,* At age 8, tissue transferred to nose with tubed flap from upper inner arm (after Tagliacozzi). *D,* Lateral view showing initial insertion of flap tissue. *E,* Age 12, following two revisions of the tubed flap. *F,* Submental view to show configuration of external nares and nasal tip.

Reappearance of persistent hemangioma has also been seen following argon laser therapy. This occurs because currently available argon lasers do not penetrate deeper than 1.5 mm into the skin, hardly enough to damage more than the upper layer of most cutaneous hemangiomas. For the present time, argon laser should be viewed as a sophisticated form of thermocautery, and it cannot be recommended for cutaneous hemangiomas. Argon laser is useful in the treatment of capillary dermal malformations (port-wine stains), as discussed in Chapter Twenty.

References

Abernathy, J.: *The Surgical Works of*. London: Longman, Hurst, Rees, Orme, and Brown, Vol. 2, Part 1, 1811, pp. 224–230.

Anderson, C. R.: Treatment of vascular naevi. J. Pediatr. *25*:148, 1944.

Andrews, G. C., Domonkos, A. N., Torres-Rodrigues, V. M., and Bembenista, J. K.: Hemangiomas—treated and untreated. JAMA *165*:1114, 1957.

Andrews, G. C., and Kelly, R. J.: Treatment of vascular nevi by injection of sclerosing solutions. Arch. Dermat. Syphil. *26*:92, 1932.

Apfelberg, D. B., Greene, R. A., Maser, R., et al.: Results of argon laser exposure of capillary hemangiomas of infancy—preliminary report. Plast. Reconstr. Surg. *67*:188, 1981.

Argenta, L. C., Bishop, E., Cho, K. J., Andrews, A. F., and Coran, A. G.: Complete resolution of life-threatening hemangioma by embolization and corticosteroids. Plast. Reconstr. Surg. *760*:739, 1982.

Azzolini, A., and Nouvenne, R.: Nuove prospettive nella terapia degli angiomi immaturi dell'infanzia, 115 lesioni trattate con infiltrazioni intralesionali di triamcinolone acetonide. Acta Bio-Medica *41*:51, 1970.

Azzolini, A., Riberti, C., Orsoni, G. J., and Porta, R.: Protocollo terapeutico combinato chirurgico-oculistico nel trattamento degli angiomi palpebrali dell'infanzia. Min. Chir. *38*:925, 1983.

Bailey, W., and Kiskadden, W. S.: Treatment of hemangiomata, with special reference to unsatisfactory results. Radiology *38*:552, 1942.

Bartoshesky, L. E., Bull, M., and Feingold, M.: Corticosteroid treatment of cutaneous hemangiomas: How effective? A report on 24 children. Clin. Pediatr. *17*:625, 1978.

Barwell, R.: On scarless eradication of naevi. Lancet *1*:642, 1875.

Beatty, W. J.: Naevus treated successfully by local application of liquor arsenicalis. Brit. Med. J. *2*:1015, 1883.

Beck, C.: A simple method of treatment of hemangioma. JAMA *41*:1575, 1903.

Bek, V., and Zahn, K.: Cataract as a late sequel of contact roentgen therapy of angiomas in children. Acta Radiol. *54*:443, 1960.

Benedek, T.: Hemiatrophy of face, sequel to treatment of an extensive nevus flammeus (port-wine mark) with X-rays and radium. Mil. Surg. *106*:466, 1950.

Benjamin, B., and Carter, P.: Congenital laryngeal hemangioma. Ann. Otol. Rhinol. Laryngol. *92*:448, 1983.

Bennett, R. G., Keller, J. W., and Ditty, J. F., Jr.: Hemangiosarcoma subsequent to radiotherapy for a hemangioma in infancy. J. Dermatol. Surg. Oncol. *4*:881, 1978.

Berman, B., and Lim, H. W. P.: Concurrent cutaneous and hepatic hemangioma in infancy: Report of a case and a review of the literature. J. Dermatol. Surg. Oncol. *4*:869, 1978.

Bingham, H. G.: Predicting the course of congenital hemangioma. Plast. Reconstr. Surg. *63*:161, 1979.

Bivings, L.: Spontaneous regression of angiomas in children. J. Pediatr. *45*:643, 1954.

Blackfield, H. M., Torrey, F. A., Morris, W. J., and Low Beer, B. V. A.: The management of hemangioma. A plea for conservatism in infancy. Plast. Reconstr. Surg. *20*:38, 1957.

Blair, J.: Naevus treated successfully by local application of liquor arsenicalis. Brit. Med. J. *1*:761, 1884.

Blaisdell, J. H.: Vascular nevi and their treatment. N. Engl. J. Med. *215*:485, 1936.

Bobbs, J. S.: Two cases of naevi in infants, treated by ligature and excision; and excision alone. Indiana J. Med. *1*:33, 1870–1871.

Bowers, R. E.: Treatment of haemangiomatous naevi with thorium X. Brit. Med. J. *1*:121, 1951.

Bowers, R. E., Graham, E. A., and Tomlinson, K. M.: The natural history of the strawberry nevus. Arch. Derm. *82*:667, 1960.

Boyer, A.: *A Treatise on Surgical Diseases and the Operations Suited to Them.* Translated by A. H. Stevens. New York: T and J. Swords, 1815, Vol. I, pp. 322–326.

Bradley, S. M.: Large veno-cutaneous naevus treated successfully by repeated injections with carbolic acid. Brit. Med. J. *1*:443, 1876.

Brain, R. T., and Calnan, C. D.: Vascular naevi and their treatment. Brit. J. Derm. *64*:147, 1952.

Braun, P., Ducharme, J. C., Riopelle, J. L., and Davignon, A.: Hemangiomatosis of the liver in infants. J. Ped. Surg. *10*:121, 1975.

Brodie, B. C.: *Lectures Illustrative of Various Subjects in Pathology and Surgery.* London: Longman, Brown, Green, and Longmans, 1846, p. 331.

Brown, B. Z., and Huffaker, G.: Local injection of steroids for juvenile hemangiomas which disturb the visual axis. Ophthalmic Surg. *13*:630, 1982.

Brown, J. B., and Byars, L. T.: Interstitial radiation treatment of hemangiomata. Amer. J. Surg. *39*:452, 1938.

Brown, J. B., and Fryer, M. P.: Hemangiomas: Role of plastic surgery in early treatment for prevention of deformities and in repair of late lesions and defects. Plast. Reconstr. Surg. *11*:197, 1953.

Brown, S. H., Jr., Neerhout, R. C., and Fonkalsrud, E. W.: Prednisone therapy in the management of large hemangiomas in infants and children. Surgery *71*:168, 1972.

Brunton, J.: Treatment of naevus by sodium ethylate. Lancet *2*:625, 1878.

Bunch, J. L.: The treatment of 300 naevi by freezing. Brit. Med. J. *1*:247, 1911.

Cabot, S.: Death following the excision of a naevus. Boston Med. Surg. J. *70*:216, 1864.

Cannon, B., Randolph, J. G., and Murray, J. E.: Malignant irradiation for benign conditions. N. Engl. J. Med. *260*:197, 1959.

Cantero, A.: Occult healing practices in French Canada. Canad. Med. Assoc. J. *20*:303, 1929.

Clemmensen, O.: A case of multiple neonatal hemangiomatosis successfully treated by systemic corticosteroids. Dermatologica *159*:495, 1979.

Clutton, H. H.: Naevi of the face treated by electrolysis. S. Thomas' Hosp. Rep. *11*:49, 1882.

Cohen, S. R., and Wang, C. I.: Steroid treatment of hemangioma of the head and neck in children. Ann. Otol. Rhinol. Laryngol. *81*:584, 1972.

Conway, H.: Cavernous hemangioma of the parotid gland treated by X-radiation at the time of operation. Plast. Reconstr. Surg. *8*:237, 1951.

Coombs, C.: A new method of treating subcutaneous naevi. Lancet *2*:374, 1881.

Costello, M. J.: Management of vascular nevi. Round table discussion of the American Academy of Pediatrics. Pediatrics *4*:825, 1949.

Crawford, G. M.: Injection therapy for angiomas. JAMA *137*:519, 1948.

Crum, R., Szabo, S., and Folkman, J.: A new class of steroids inhibits angiogenesis in the presence of heparin or a heparin fragment. Science *230*:1375, 1985.

Curling, T. B.: Observations on the treatment of naevi materni—with cases of removal of these growths from different parts of the face without deformity. London Med. Gazette XLV:133, 1850.

Dana, M., and Beyer, J.: Résultats lointains du traitement par le radium de 820 angiomes cutanés tubereux. Journ. Radiol. Electr. *47*:325, 1966.

Dargeon, H. W., Adiao, A. C., and Pack, G. T.: Hemangioma with thrombocytopenia. J. Pediat. *54*:285, 1959.

Davis, J. S., and Wilgis, H. E.: The treatment of hemangiomata by excision. South Med. J. *27*:283, 1934.

Dawson, B. F.: Treatment of vascular nevi with the galvanic cautery. Amer. J. Obstet. *7*:137, 1874.

Dehner, L. P., and Ishak, K. G.: Vascular tumors of the liver in infants and children. Arch. Path. *92*:101, 1971.

DeLorimier, A. A., Simpson, E. B., Baum, R. S., and Carlsson, E.: Hepatic artery ligation for hepatic hemangiomatosis. N. Engl. J. Med. *277*:333, 1967.

Dethlefsen, S. M., Mulliken, J. B., and Glowacki, J.: Ultrastructural study of mast cell interactions in hemangiomas. Ultrastr. Path. *10*:175, 1986.

de Venecia, G., and Lobeck, C. C.: Successful treatment of eyelid hemangiomas with prednisolone. Arch. Ophthal. *84*:98, 1970.

Duncan, J.: On Galvano-puncture of naevus. Edin. Med. J. *15*:777, 1870.

Duncan, J.: On the value of electrolysis in angioma and goitre. Brit. Med. J. *22*:984, 1888.

Edgerton, M. T.: The treatment of hemangiomas: With special reference to the role of steroid therapy. Ann. Surg. *183*:517, 1976.

Edwards, H. G. F.: Vascular birthmarks. South. Med. J. *34*:717, 1941.

Ellis, P. O.: Occlusion of the central retinal artery after retrobulbar corticosteroid injection. Am. J. Ophthalmol. *85*:352, 1978.

Esterly, N. B.: Kasabach-Merritt syndrome in infants. J. Amer. Acad. Derm. *8*:513, 1983.

Evans, J., Batchelor, A. D. R., Stark, G., and Utterly, W. S.: Haemangioma with coagulopathy: Sustained response to prednisone. Arch. Dis. Child. *50*:809, 1975.

Falk, W., and Levy, D.: Follow-up study of hemangiomas of skin treated and untreated. Amer. J. Dis. Child. *93*:165, 1957.

Figi, F. A., and O'Brien, R. W.: Treatment of angiomas. Plast. Reconstr. Surg. *18*:448, 1956.

Folkman, J., Langer, R., Linhart, R. J., Haudenschild, C., and Taylor, S.: Angiogenesis inhibition and tumor regression caused by heparin or a heparin fragment in the presence of cortisone. Science *221*:719, 1983.

Forster, J. C.: *The Surgical Diseases of Children*. London: John W. Parker & Son, 1860, pp. 206–249.

Fost, N. C., and Esterly, N. B.: Successful treatment of juvenile hemangiomas with prednisone. J. Pediatr. *72*:351, 1968.

Gay, J.: Spontaneous cure of naevi materni. Med. Times & Gazette, London *35*:146, 1857.

Gazzo, J. B. C.: Fact, relative to the action of nitrate of silver and the process of treating naevus with nitric acid. Med. Surg. Rep. Phila. *33*:343, 1875.

Goldberg, S. J., and Fonkalsrud, E.: Successful treatment of hepatic hemangioma with corticosteroids. JAMA *208*:2473, 1969.

Gregl, A., and Weiss, J. W.: Mammahypoplasie nach Roentgenbestrahlung eines Hämangioms im Säuglingsalter. Fortschr. Roentgenstr. *94*:244, 1961.

Gross, S. D.: *System of Surgery: Pathological, Diagnostic, Therapeutic and Operative*. Philadelphia: Blanchard and Lea, 1859, Vol. I, pp. 968–975.

Gunn, T., Reece, E. R., Metrakos, K., and Colle, E.: Depressed T cells following neonatal steroid treatment. Pediatrics *67*:61, 1981.

Hall, M: On a new and simple mode of operation for naevus. London Med. Gaz. *7*:677, 1831.

Hammond, W. A.: Three cases of the successful treatment of vascular tumors by injection with the fluid extract of argot. Arch. Clin. Surg. *1*:123, 1876.

Hand, W. D., Casetta, A., and Thiederman, S. B. (eds.): *Popular Beliefs and Superstitions. A Compendium of American Folklore*. Boston: G. K. Hall and Co., 1981, Vol. I, pp. 44–45.

Harris, R. P.: Case of venous erectile naevus cured by subcutaneous vaccination by means of many-eyed needles. Amer. J. Obstet. *4*:20, 1871.

Healy, G., McGill, T., and Friedman, E. M.: Carbon dioxide laser in subglottic hemangioma. An update. Ann. Otol. Rhinol. Laryngol. *93*:370, 1984.

Hill, G. L., and Longino, L. A.: Giant hemangioma with thrombocytopenia. Surg. Gynec. Obstet. *114*:304, 1962.

Hobby, L. W.: Further evaluation of the potential of the argon laser in the treatment of strawberry hemangiomas. Plast. Reconstr. Surg. *71*:481, 1983.

Hodges: Injection of a naevus with perchloride of iron. Boston Med. Surg. J. *70*:60, 1864.

Holgate, T. H.: The treatment of naevus by the intrainjection of alcohol. Arch. Ped. *6*:379, 1889.

Hurvitz, C. H., Alkalay, A. L., Sloninsky, L., Kallus, M., and Pomerance, J. J.: Cyclophosphamide therapy in life-threatening vascular tumors. J. Pediat. *109*:360, 1986.

Jones, R. M.: *The Parisian Education of an American Surgeon*. Letters of Jonathan Mason Warren (1832–1835). Philadelphia: The American Philosophical Society, 1978, Vol. 128, p. 218.

Kaessler, H. W.: Vascular birthmarks, treatment with injection of sclerosing solution. JAMA *110*:1644, 1938.

Kagan, A. R., Jaffe, H. D., and Kennamer, R.: Hemangioma of the liver treated by irradiation. J. Nucl. Med. *12*:835, 1971.

Keller, L., and Bluhm, J. F., III: Diffuse neonatal hemangiomatosis; a case with heart failure and thrombocytopenia. Cutis *23*:295, 1979.

Kiehn, C. L., DesPrez, J. D., and Kaufman, B.: Cavernous hemangiomas of the head and neck. Indications for arteriography and surgical treatment. Plast. Reconstr. Surg. *33*:338, 1964.

Kingston, S.: Treatment of naevus by adhesive or suppurative inflammation. Lancet *1*:420, 1862.

Knott, S. J.: Forty cases of naevi successfully treated with electrolysis. Lancet *1*:402, 1875.

Koerper, M. A., Addiego, J. E., DeLorimier, A. A.,

Lipow, H., Price, D., and Lubin, B. H.: Use of aspirin and dipyridamole in children with platelet trapping syndromes. J. Pediatr. *102*:311, 1983.

Kushner, B. J.: Local steroid therapy in adnexal hemangioma. Ann. Ophthalmol. *11*:1005, 1979.

Kushner, B. J.: The treatment of periorbital infantile hemangioma with intralesional corticosteroids. Plast. Reconstr. Surg. *76*:517, 1985.

Laird, W. P., Friedman, S., Koop, C. E., and Schwartz, G. J.: Hepatic hemangiomatosis. Successful management by hepatic artery ligation. Amer. J. Dis. Child. *130*:657, 1976.

Larcher, V. F., Howard, E. R., and Mowat, A. P.: Hepatic hemangiomata: Diagnosis and management. Arch. Dis. Child. *56*:7, 1981.

Lawrence, W.: On the treatment of naevi materni by ligature. Medico-Chir. Trans. *13*:420, 1827.

Lee, C. M., Jr., Newstedt, J. R., and Siddall, H. S.: Large abdominal tumors of childhood (other than Wilms' tumors and neuroblastoma). Ann. Surg. *143*:803, 1956.

Lewis, J. R., Jr.: The treatment of hemangiomas. Plast. Reconstr. Surg. *19*:201, 1957.

Li, F. P., Cassady, J. R., and Barnett, E.: Cancer mortality following irradiation in infancy for hemangioma. Radiology *113*:177, 1974.

Lister, W. A.: The natural history of strawberry naevi. Lancet *1*:1429, 1938.

Lister, W. A.: Obituary letter by ABLP. Brit. Med. J. *284*:62, 1982.

MacCollum, D. W.: Treatment of hemangiomas. Amer. J. Surg. *29*:32, 1935.

MacCollum, D. W., and Martin, L. W.: Hemangiomas in infancy and childhood. A report based on 6479 cases. Surg. Clin. North Am. *36*:1647, 1956.

MacFee, W. F.: The surgical treatment of large hemangiomas of the face in children. Surg. Clin. North Am. *27*:431, 1947.

Mangus, D. J.: Continuous compression treatment of hemangiomata: Evaluation in two cases. Plast. Reconstr. Surg. *49*:490, 1972.

Margileth, A. M., and Museles, M.: Cutaneous hemangiomas in children: Diagnosis and conservative management. JAMA *194*:523, 1965.

Marshall, J.: The naevus maternus (or mark of the mother) cured by vaccination. London Med. Surg. J. *5*:52, 1830.

Marshall, R. J.: On a case of multiple vascular nevi, with subsequent disappearance of many of them. Glasgow Med. J. *39*:105, 1893.

Matolo, N. M., and Johnson, D. G.: Surgical treatment of hepatic hemangioma in the newborn. Arch. Surg. *106*:725, 1973.

Matthews, D. N.: Treatment of hemangiomata. Brit. J. Plast. Surg. *6*:83, 1953.

Matthews, D. N.: Hemangiomata. Plast. Reconstr. Surg. *41*:528, 1968.

Mattioli, L., Lee, K. R., and Holder, T. M.: Hepatic artery ligation for cardiac failure due to hepatic hemangioma in the newborn. J. Pediatr. Surg. *9*:859, 1974.

McCuistion, C. H.: Infantile cavernous hemangiomas. Persistence into adulthood of untreated lesions. Arch. Derm. Syph. *69*:219, 1954.

McLean, R. H., Moller, J. H., Warwick, W. J., Satran, L., and Lucas, R. V., Jr.: Multinodular hemangiomatosis of the liver in infancy. Pediatrics *49*:563, 1972.

Miller, S., Smith, R., and Shochat, S.: Compression treatment of hemangiomas. Plast. Reconstr. Surg. *58*:573, 1976.

Modlin, J. J.: Capillary hemangiomas of the skin. Surgery *38*:169, 1955.

Montgomery, D. W., and Culver, G. D.: Treatment of vascular naevi with radium. Boston Med. Surg. J. *183*:412, 1920.

Moore, A. M.: Pressure in the treatment of giant hemangioma with purpura. Case report and observations. Plast. Reconstr. Surg. *34*:606, 1964.

Morton, R.: A new method of treating naevi. Clin. J. *35*:206, 1909–1910.

Mulliken, J. B., and Glowacki, J.: Hemangiomas and vascular malformations in infants and children: A classification based on endothelial characteristics. Plast. Reconstr. Surg. *69*:412, 1982.

Murray, J. J.: Removal by ligature of large subcutaneous naevi without loss of skin. Lancet *1*:321, 1864.

Newcomet, W. S.: The treatment of nevi. Amer. J. Roentgenol. *4*:605, 1917.

Order, S. E.: Hemangioma and the risk/benefit ratio. Int. J. Radiation Oncol. Biol. Phys. *5*:143, 1979.

Overcash, K. E., and Putney, F. J.: Subglottic hemangioma of the larynx treated with steroid therapy. Laryngoscope *83*:679, 1973.

Owen, E.: On the treatment of large naevi. Brit. Med. J. *2*:320, 1883.

Owens, N., and Stephenson, K. L.: Hemangioma: An evaluation of treatment by injection and surgery. Plast. Reconstr. Surg. *3*:109, 1948.

Paget, T.: Fatal convulsion during the injection of naevus. London Med. Gazette *1*:529, 1837.

Park, W. C., and Phillips, R.: The role of radiation therapy in the management of hemangiomas of the liver. JAMA *212*:1496, 1970.

Parker, R. W.: On the treatment of naevus by excision to which is appended a clinical analysis of 564 cases of naevus, together with the microscopic nature of this condition. Trans. Clin. Soc. London *19*:279, 1886.

Paterson, R., and Tod, M. C.: The radium treatment of angioma in children. Amer. J. Roentgenol. *42*:726, 1939.

Patterson, A. B.: Spontaneous cure of a naevus maternus—large vascular tumor occupying side of neck. South. Med. Rec. *24*:477, 1894.

Pereyra, R., Andrassy, R. J., and Mahour, G. H.: Management of massive hepatic hemangiomas in infants and children: A review of 13 cases. Pediatrics *70*:254, 1982.

Pooley, J. H.: Naevus. N.Y. Med. J. *17*:593, 1873.

Prensky, A. L., and Gado, M.: Angiographic resolution of a neonatal intracranial cavernous hemangioma coincident with steroid therapy. J. Neurosurg. *39*:99, 1973.

Price, A. C., Coran, A. G., Mattern. A. L., and Cochran, R. L.: Hemangioendothelioma of the pelvis. A cause of cardiac failure in the newborn. N. Engl. J. Med. *286*:647, 1972.

Pusey, W. A.: The use of carbon dioxide snow in the treatment of nevi and other lesions of the skin. JAMA *49*:1354, 1907.

Rake, M. O., Liberman, M. M., Dawson, J. L., et al.: Ligation of the hepatic artery in the treatment of heart failure due to hepatic hemangiomatosis. Gut *11*:512, 1970.

Reder, F.: Hemangioma and lymphangioma, their response to the injection of boiling water. Med. Rec. N.Y. *98*:519, 1920.

Richardson, B. W.: On sodium ethylate in the treatment of naevus and other forms of disease. Proc. Med. Soc. London *5*:257, 1879–1881.

Robb, R. M.: Refractive errors associated with hemangiomas of the eyelids and orbit in infancy. Amer. J. Ophthal. *83*:52, 1977.

Rocchini, A. P., Rosenthal, A., Issenberg, H. J., and Nadas, A. S.: Hepatic hemangioendotheliomata; hemodynamic observations and treatment. Pediatrics *57*:131, 1976.

Ronchese, F.: The spontaneous involution of cutaneous vascular tumors. Amer. J. Surg. *86*:376, 1953.

Rush, B. F., Jr.: Treatment of a giant cutaneous hemangioma by intra-arterial injection of nitrogen mustard. Ann. Surg. *164*:921, 1966.

Sasaki, G. H., Pang, C. Y., and Wittliff, J. L.: Pathogenesis and treatment of infant skin strawberry hemangiomas: Clinical and in vitro studies of hormonal effects. Plast. Reconstr. Surg. *73*:359, 1984.

Schuller, T., Rosenzweig, J. L., and Arey, J. B.: Successful removal of hemangioma of the liver in infant. Pediatrics *3*:328, 1949.

Semon, H. C.: Treatment with the carbon dioxide snow pencil. Lancet *1*:1167, 1934.

Shannon, K., Buchanan, G. R., and Votteler, T. P.: Multiple hepatic hemangiomas: Failure of corticosteroid therapy and successful hepatic artery ligation. Amer. J. Dis. Child. *36*:275, 1982.

Simpson, J. R.: Natural history of cavernous haemangiomata. Lancet *2*:1057, 1959.

Skalkeas, G., Gogas, J., and Pavlatos, F.: Mammary hypoplasia following radiation to an infant breast. Case report. Acta Chir. Plast. *14*:240, 1972.

Sondel, P. M., Ritter, W. M., Wilson, D. G., and Lieberman, L. M.: Use of 111In platelet scans in the detection and treatment of Kasabach-Merritt syndrome. J. Pediatr. *104*:87, 1984.

Stigmar, G., Crawford, J. S., Ward, C. M., and Thomson, H. G.: Ophthalmic sequelae of infantile hemangiomas of the eyelids and orbit. Amer. J. Ophthalmol. *85*:806, 1978.

Straatsma, C. R.: Plastic repair of severe radium burns and angioma. N.Y. State Med. J. *30*:9, 1930.

Tefft, M.: The radiotherapeutic management of subglottic hemangiomas in children. Radiology *86*:207, 1966.

Tegtmeier, C. J., Smith, T. H., and Shaw, A.: Renal infarction: A complication of Gelfoam embolization of hemangioendothelioma of the liver. Am. J. Roentg. *128*:305, 1977.

Thomson, H. G., and Lanigan, J.: The Cyrano nose—a clinical review of hemangioma of the nasal tip. Plast. Reconstr. Surg. *63*:155, 1979.

Thomson, H. G., Ward, C. M., Crawford, J. S., and Stigmar, G.: Hemangiomas of the eyelid: Visual complications and prophylactic concept. Plast. Reconstr. Surg. *63*:641, 1979.

Touloukian, R. J.: Hemangioendothelioma during infancy: Pathology, diagnosis and treatment with prednisone. Pediatrics *45*:71, 1970.

Traub, E. F.: Should vascular nevi be treated? Arch. Pediat. *50*:272, 1933.

Turner, D.: *De Morbis Cutaneis. A Treatise of Diseases Incident to the Skin.* London, R. Bonwicke, W. Freeman, T. Goodwin, etc., 1714, pp. 120–128.

Van der Werf, E.: Spontaneous disappearance of hemangiomata. Nederl. Tijdschr. Geneesk. *98*:676, 1954.

von Payr, E.: Über die Verwendung von Magnesium zur Behandlung von Blutgefässerkrankungen. Dtch. Z. Chir. *63*:903, 1902.

Wagget, J., Inkster, J. S., and Ashcroft, T.: Hemangioendothelioma of the liver in an infant—hypotensive crisis during resection. Surgery *65*:352, 1969.

Wallace, H. J.: The conservative treatment of hemangiomatous nevi. Brit. J. Plast. Surg. *6*:78, 1953.

Wallerstein, R. O.: Spontaneous involution of giant hemangioma. Amer. J. Dis. Child. *102*:233, 1961.

Walsh, T. S., Jr.: Giant strawberry nevi of the orbital arteries: Treatment by ligation. Surgery *65*:659, 1969.

Walsh, T. S., Jr., and Tompkins, V. N.: Some observations on the strawberry nevus of infancy. Cancer *9*:869, 1956.

Walter, J.: On the treatment of cavernous hemangioma with special reference to spontaneous regression. J. Fac. Radiol. *5*:134, 1953.

Ward, C. M., and Buchanan, R.: Haemangiosarcoma following irradiation of a haemangioma of the face. J. Maxillofac. Surg. *5*:164, 1977.

Wardrop, J.: Some observations on one species of naevus maternus with the case of an infant where the carotid artery was tied. Medico-Chir. Trans. *9*:199, 1818.

Wardrop, J.: Case of naevus on the face successfully treated by tying the carotid artery. Lancet XII:267, 1826.

Warren, J. C.: *Surgical Observations on Tumours with Cases and Operations.* Boston: Crocker and Brewster, 1839, pp. 413–427.

Watson, W. L., and McCarthy, W. D.: Blood and lymph vessel tumors. A report of 1,056 cases. Surg. Gynec. Obstet. *71*:569, 1940.

White, A.: Observations on the surgical treatment of the naevus maternus with ligature. Medico-Chir. Trans. *13*:444, 1827.

Whiteman, D. W., Rosen, D. A., and Pinkerton, R. M. H.: Retinal and choroidal microvascular embolism after intranasal corticosteroid injection. Am. J. Ophthalmol. *89*:851, 1980.

Wilflingseder, R., Martin, R., and Papp, C. H.: Magnesium seeds in the treatment of lymph- and haemangiomata. Chir. Plast. *6*:105, 1981.

Williams, H. B.: Hemangiomas of the parotid gland in children. Plast. Reconstr. Surg. 56:29, 1975.

Wright, T. L., and Bresnan, M. J.: Radiation-induced cerebrovascular disease in children. Neurology *26*:540, 1976.

Wyeth, J. A.: The treatment of vascular tumors by the injection of water at a high temperature. JAMA *40*:1778, 1903.

Wyman, L. C., Fulton, G. P., and Shulman, M. H.: Direct observations on the circulation in the hamster cheek pouch in adrenal insufficiency and experimental hypercorticalism. Ann. N.Y. Acad. Sci. *56*:643, 1953.

Zak, T. A., and Morin, D. J.: Early local steroid therapy of infantile eyelid hemangiomas. J. Pediatr. Ophthalmol. Strabismus *18*:25, 1981.

Zarem, H. A., and Edgerton, M. T.: Induced resolution of cavernous hemangiomas following prednisone therapy. Plast. Reconstr. Surg. *39*:76, 1967.

Zinn, K. M.: Iatrogenic intraocular injection of depot corticosteroid and its surgical removal using the pars plana approach. Ophthalmology *88*:13, 1981.

Zweifach, B. W., Shor, E., and Black, M. M.: The influence of the adrenal cortex on behavior of terminal vascular bed. Ann. N.Y. Acad. Sci. *56*:626, 1953.

PART THREE

Malformations

CHAPTER SIX

Pathogenesis of Vascular Malformations

A. E. Young

Vascular malformations are errors in the morphogenic processes that shape the embryonic vascular system between the fourth and tenth week of intrauterine life. These anomalies are almost all sporadic, non-familial developmental errors. There are, by contrast, a few inheritable vascular abnormalities, such as Rendu-Osler-Weber syndrome (hereditary hemorrhagic telangiectasia), in which development is normal in an embryological sense but, in time, the vessels become morphologically abnormal. In this syndrome, the genetic abnormality is revealed as structural weakness of the wall of small arteries and precapillary sphincters. Not all vascular malformations are "congenital," i.e., obvious at birth; many of these abnormalities manifest themselves years or decades postnatally.

NORMAL DEVELOPMENT OF THE PERIPHERAL VASCULAR SYSTEM

Current opinion is that the embryonic endothelium of all vascular tissue arises *in situ* directly from primitive mesenchyme (the "local origin theory"), but that the pericytes and smooth muscle cells that surround the endothelium are derived from neuroectoderm (neural crest) and not from mesoderm.

The core of our understanding of subsequent vascular development derives from the embryological studies of Sabin and Woollard in the early part of the century (Sabin, 1920; Woollard, 1922; Woollard and Harpman, 1937). Most of the work relates to the developing vertebrate limb bud, in which the following three developmental stages are recognized:

1. The undifferentiated capillary network.
2. The retiform plexus.
3. The formation of mature vessels.

The Undifferentiated Capillary Network

The earliest step in vascular development is the condensation of undifferentiated mesenchymal cells into cords. Cells on the periphery of these structures then develop into definitive angioblasts, which form primal capillary structures. By budding and branching, these capillaries extend and interconnect to form the primitive capillary retiform plexus. Insight into this process is provided by the studies of Folkman, showing that capillary-like tubules can form *in vitro* from cloned capillary endothelial cells cultured from adult tissues (Folkman and Haudenschild, 1980). These experiments demonstrate that all the information necessary to construct a capillary tube, make branches, and assemble a capillary network can be expressed in culture by a single cell type, the capillary endothelial cell. Thus, patterning of embryonic endothelium to form a plexus can also presumably occur in the absence of blood flow.

The Retiform Plexus

Through the interconnecting channels of the retiform plexus, blood begins to flow from an arterial to a venous side. A complex, ill-understood, morphogenetic patterning process now takes over, which models and remodels the plexus to form recognizable vessels. To do this, some of the plexus must disappear, some must extend and link, some must coalesce to form larger structures, and some must be spared to form adult capillaries. What influences these processes is poorly understood; blood flow seems to be important. Unlike the heart and great vessels, which will develop in the absence of flowing blood, peripheral vessels need blood flow to establish a correct pattern. Thoma was the first investigator to propose the "laws" that govern this morphogenesis (Thoma, 1893):

1. Velocity of the blood flowing through a vessel proportionately increases or decreases the vascular caliber.

2. The length of a blood vessel is determined by the pull exerted on the vascular walls by the surrounding organs and tissues.

3. The thickness of the vessel wall is determined by the pressure exerted by the blood flowing within it.

4. An increased terminal blood pressure in a given vascular area will result in the formation of new capillaries; conversely, reduced pressure will cause reduction in the size of the capillaries.

Other factors must obviously be at work, probably chemical (e.g., pH, oxygen utilization, CO_2 production), physical (Ryan and Barnhill, 1983), biochemical, and hormonal. Furthermore, the development of the vasculature cannot be shaped solely by local physiochemical events. There must also be an overall genetic control. Indeed, the patterns of capillary vascular malformation seen in the skin often resemble clone maps, suggesting that a primary genetic fault has occurred in one cell and that the vascular abnormalities are subsequently revealed in the progeny of that cell. There has been a resurgence of interest in the processes of vascular development, since it has been realized how critical vasculature is to tumor growth (Folkman et al., 1971; Folkman, 1974; Folkman and Cotran, 1976). This work has focused on the simplest processes that govern capillary development, namely angiogenesis and its converse factors that lead to the disappearance of capillaries, a process that might be called "angionemesis." A detailed review of the processes of angiogenesis can be found in the work of Hudlicka and Tyler (1986). The thrombogenic and thrombolytic capacities of vascular endothelium also may be crucial to the process of vascular development. Work by Drouet and colleagues in Paris suggests that these factors are abnormal in tissues taken from patients with vascular malformations (Drouet, 1982). If this is a primary abnormality, rather than an acquired one, it may explain why parts of the primitive retiform plexus persist, to be expressed as adult malformations. It is of interest that vascular abnormalities that show a failure of deletion of parts of the primitive rete may be associated with skeletal abnormalities that also feature failure of tissue regression, e.g., syndactyly and vertebral segmentation defects. It will be seen in Chapter Nineteen that there is a complex interaction between skeletal abnormalities and vascular ones. In this context, it is interesting that cartilage contains low molecular weight proteins that strongly inhibit endothelial cell growth (Brem and Folkman, 1975; Langer et al., 1976).

Developmental vascular anomalies may, secondarily, cause these skeletal abnormalities *in utero*. Caplan and Koutroupas have been able to study fluid flow dynamics in the developing chicken wing (Caplan and Koutroupas, 1973; Jargiello and Caplan, 1983). They find that the limb peripheral mesoderm is subcompartmentalized in an anterior-posterior fashion, whereas the limb core shows differential flow in a proximodistal manner. This suggests that differential blood flow may affect mesodermal microenvironments, e.g., specific nutrient and oxygen levels, and thus determine the critical phases of limb skeletal morphogenesis.

Development of Mature Vessels

In the limb, an axial artery develops along with a pre- and postaxial marginal vein. Further readjustments now occur. In the forearm, the axial artery may shrivel to become something as insubstantial, for example, as the interosseous artery of the forearm, while in the lower limb it persists as the femoral and popliteal arteries. The preaxial veins may persist as the cephalic vein in the arm and as the long (internal) saphenous vein in the leg.

Deep axial veins develop, and the postaxial veins of the leg disappear.

The development of the lymphatic system is less clear-cut. It develops later than the blood vascular system, and its development may be influenced by the blood vascular system.

EMBRYOLOGY OF THE LYMPHATIC SYSTEM

There is a long-standing dispute as to fundamental processes that underlie the development of the mammalian lymph system. The "centrifugal theory" postulates that lymphatics and all other parts of the embryonic vascular system develop by a process of budding from the embryonic venous system (Lewis, 1905; Sabin, 1908). The alternative explanation (Huntington and McClure, 1907; McClure, 1915; Kampmeier, 1969), the "local origin theory," is that the lymphatics develop in isolation from clefts in mesenchyme. These differences of opinion have arisen largely because the protagonists of each theory have used different techniques for their investigations. A careful study of 40 human embryos by van der Putte (1975) supports Sabin's centifugal sprouting theory. The later phases of development are, however, substantially agreed upon. Jugular, subclavian, thoracic, retroperitoneal, and ilioinguinal lymph sacs appear between the second and sixth week of intrauterine life. Peripheral lymphatic trunks probably develop as centrifugal sprouting from these sacs, a process that can be directly observed in the tail of the tadpole (Ranvier, 1895) or shown by direct injection of the embryo (Sabin, 1908). The inguinal, iliac, and lumbar lymph nodes are formed from the ilioinguinal lymph sacs, which are first divided up by connective tissue bridges; then, after invasion by lymphocytes, local condensations appear that fuse to form adult lymph node pattern (Patten, 1968). All these processes are completed by the twelfth week, though the system does not have a full set of competent valves until the beginning of the fifth month (Kampmeier, 1969).

MALDEVELOPMENTS

There are no data, histologic, embryological, or experimental, that convincingly show how, or at exactly which stage, maldevelopments occur. This has, however, not inhibited speculation about how errors at each stage might be expressed as an adult malformation (Reinhoff, 1924; Reid, 1925; deTakats, 1932; Szilagyi et al., 1976; Kaplan, 1983).

The inability of known teratogens, toxins, chemicals, or trauma to produce anything that resembles a human vascular malformation is remarkable, suggesting that simple aberrations in local physiochemical factors may not be responsible. The possibility of a primary biochemical defect in processes of *thrombosis and fibrinolysis* has already been postulated. In addition, it has been proposed that *aberrations of the autonomic nervous system* may influence the development and maldevelopment of the vascular system *in utero*.

Influence of the Autonomic Nervous System

It has already been noted that the neuroectoderm may contribute the cells that form vascular smooth muscle and pericytes (Johnston, 1966; Nozue and Tsuzaki, 1974). Abnormal development of neuroectodermal tissues might *a priori* thus be implicated in vascular malformation.

At a clinical level, the presence of hyperhidrosis over malformations and the presence of cutaneous capillary malformations in what, at first sight, seem to be "metameric" distributions that perhaps represent the distribution of the fetal nervous system point to some parallel, or even causative, autonomic nervous dysfunction. Facial patterns of portwine stains along the trigeminal nerve distribution also suggest a relationship to the developing peripheral nervous system. However, both Johnston and Nozue noted that the facial region of the developing embryo is rich in neuroectodermal cells that have migrated to contribute to perivascular and connective tissue sites.

The postulation that a primary fault in the autonomic nervous system might be the cause of vascular malformations is not new. Trélat and Monod, in the first review paper of vascular malformations ever published, espoused this theory, and many subsequent authors who accepted the "neurovegetative" theory perhaps did so because it had the appeal of linking the concept of "maternal impressions" as the causative event (see

Chapter One) to actual physical processes. Trélat and Monod cited Claude Bernard's experiment that showed that cervical sympathectomy produced hypertrophy in the rabbit's ear to support the "neurovegetative" theory (Trélat and Monod, 1869). Studies by Bevan and Tsuru show that in the rabbit ear, the sympathetic nervous system influences the composition and functional properties of the vessel wall during development (Bevan and Tsuru, 1981). Morris has confirmed Bernard's findings and has shown that interference with the sympathetic nerve supply at the time of birth increases, by a factor of 2.5, the number of arteriovenous anastomoses in the area involved (Morris, 1983). Pursuing this lead is difficult, because it is thought that the autonomic cutaneous innervation differs in the adult and the fetus (Bevan, 1983). Other clinical features suggest some neurovascular connection. Café-au-lait spots and other neuroectoderm-derived pigmentary anomalies appear to be more common in patients with vascular malformations, and Reyes has noted the association of retroperitoneal neurofibromata and venous anomalies (Reyes, 1980).

Aberrations of Normal Development Causing Malformations

As we are totally ignorant of the factors involved in vascular malformations, we cannot therefore ascribe the events to a single time or agent. However, the variety of different end points suggests not only that the causative influence can be present at any time during development but also that the influence may continue, and that once they have appeared, abnormalities may affect their own development and that of surrounding structures.

Woollard's drawings of the early development of the limb bud vasculature serve as inspiration for theories of pathogenesis. One can imagine that an error in morphogenesis during the retiform plexus stage could result in a vascular malformation (Fig. 6–1). Sequestrated and maldeveloped areas of primitive capillary rete could develop into single or multiple malformations: for example, venous malformations and combined lymphatic and venous lesions. Preservation of patches of primitive capillaries may explain the portwine stains (dermal malformations), while the failure of regression of arteriovenous communications in the primitive rete can lead to all types of arteriovenous malformations. In the later stages of development, vascular trunks may fail to develop, leaving the deep vessel aplasias and hypoplasias of the Klippel-Trenaunay syndrome, in which, in addition, embryonic vessels such as the postaxial vein of the leg may fail to regress. These processes can also be seen separately or concurrently in the lymphatic system, sequestered areas forming, for example, isolated cystic anomalies or diffuse lesions ("lymphangioma circumscriptum"). Aplasias and hypoplasias are also common. Failure of condensation of lymph tissue to form normal iliac nodes may account for the changes seen in some patients with arteriovenous malformations and in some with lymphedema associated with hyperplastic lymph trunks.

Abnormal dynamics in the developing vascular system can also be invoked to explain the particular morphology of some malformations. Thus, the anomalous superficial veins, the capillary malformation, and the limb overgrowth of Klippel-Trenaunay syndrome have been ascribed to the effects of venous hypertension, being the result of deep vein anomalies. This theory, proposed by Servelle (Servelle and Babillot, 1980), is partly confounded by the findings of other investigators, that the deep veins are most often phlebographically and hemodynamically normal in Klippel-Trenaunay syndrome (Baskerville et al., 1985), though this does not guarantee that they were normal in early intrauterine life. Another hemodynamic explanation is that failure of normal developmental control leads to delay in regression of the normal embryonic precapillary arteriovenous connections, leading to an increase in the size and number of the veins and also to the predictable histologic changes of venous intimal thickening, elastosis, and ectasia (Coget and Merlen, 1980; Leu et al., 1980), clinically apparent as skin capillary malformation and varicose veins. The increase in flow and the decreased capillary resistance would cause mild venous hypertension, which experimentally is known to cause an increase in bone growth and superficial varicosis. Such minimal changes in the timing of a normal developmental event might thus explain the whole pattern of Klippel-Tre-

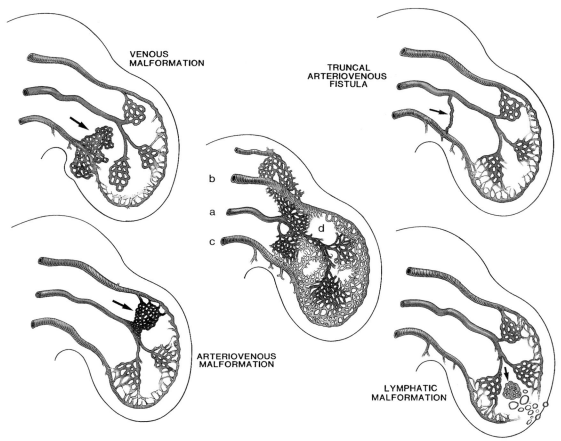

Figure 6–1. Drawing of injected 12 mm pig embryo showing early development of blood vessels in anterior appendage bud (equivalent to 6 week human embryo). (After Woollard, H. H.: Contr. Embryol. Carnegie Instit. *14*:139, 1922.) Drawing is modified to show possible vascular malformations. a = retiform central (axial) artery (persists as volar interosseous artery); b = cephalic vein; c = basilic vein; and d = primitive capillary plexus undergoing resorption.

naunay syndrome (Baskerville et al., 1985). The postulation of abnormal activity of physiological arteriovenous connections can also be tied in with the Servelle hypothesis that deep vein inadequacies may be causative. We know from the studies of Fontaine and of Lofferer that acquired deep vein obstruction (by thrombosis) causes opening of physiological arteriovenous connections and an increase in blood flow (Fontaine et al., 1968; Lofferer et al., 1969). There is no reason why this process should not occur *in utero*.

Lymphatic Malformations

The appearance of cutaneous lymphatic anomalies (e.g., "lymphangioma circumscrip-

tum") has been attributed to obstruction of deep lymph trunks in the developing embryo, the obstruction causing back-up of lymph into cutaneous lymphatics. This hypothesis emanates from the perceived similarity in the clinical appearance of cutaneous lymphatic anomalies and the skin vesicles that can occur after lymphatic obstruction as a result of an operation or radiotherapy. In spite of the similarity, lymphography in patients with lymphatic malformations invariably shows the deep lymphatics to be normal and does not show communication between them and the cutaneous lesion (Edwards et al., 1972). Cutaneous lymphatic anomalies are thus most likely to represent maldevelopment or failure of regression of sequestered parts of the developing lymphatic system.

The etiology of lymphedema of both the congenital and later appearing forms is unknown. Until recently, it was assumed, on the basis of "hypoplasia" of the lymph vessels seen on lymphography, that there was an intrinsic developmental fault in the vessels themselves. Work by Kinmonth and Eustace (1976) and Kinmonth and Wolfe (1980) found fibrosis in lymph nodes or delayed transit time of lymph through nodes, suggesting that the primary fault may be not in the lymph vessels but in the nodes themselves, hypoplasia and non-filling of distal lymphatics being merely the result of secondary obstruction and stagnation. Whether this observation will have therapeutic value remains to be seen.

References

Baskerville, P. A., Ackroy, J. A., and Browse, N. L.: The etiology of Klippel-Trenaunay syndrome. Ann. Surg. *202*:624, 1985.

Bevan, J. A.: *Development of the Vascular System.* London: Pitman 1983, p. 239.

Bevan, R. D., and Tsuru, H.: Long-term influence of the symphathetic nervous system on arterial structure and reactivity: Possible factor in hypertension. In Abboud, F. M. et al. (eds.): *Disturbances in Neurogenic Control of the Circulation.* Bethesda, MD: American Physiological Society, 1981, pp. 153–160.

Brem, H., and Folkman, J.: Inhibition of tumor angiogenesis mediated by cartilage. J. Exp. Med. *141*:427, 1975.

Caplan, A. I., and Koutroupas, S.: The control of muscle and cartilage development in the chick limb: The role of differential vascularization. J. Embryol. Exp. Morph. *29*:571, 1973.

Coget, J. M., and Merlen, J. F.: Klippel-Trenaunay, syndrome au maladie? Phlebologie *33*:37, 1980.

deTakats, G.: Vascular anomalies of the extremities. Surg. Gynec. Obstet. *55*:227, 1932.

Drouet, L.: Personal Communication, 4th International Workshop for the Study of Vascular Anomalies, Hôpital Lariboisière, Paris, 1982.

Edwards, J. M., Peachey, R. D., and Kinmonth, J. B.: Lymphangiography and surgery in lymphangioma circumscriptum. Brit. J. Surg. *59*:36, 1972.

Folkman, J.: Tumor angiogenesis factor. Cancer Res. *34*:2109, 1974.

Folkman, J., and Cotran, R. S.: Relation of vascular proliferation to tumor growth. Int. Rev. Exp. Pathol. *16*:207, 1976.

Folkman, J., and Haudenschild, C.: Angiogenesis in vitro. Nature *288*:551, 1980.

Folkman, J., Merler, E., Abernathy, C., and Williams, G.: Isolation of a tumor factor responsible for angiogenesis. J. Exp. Med. *133*:275, 1971.

Fontaine, R., LeGal, J., and Fontaine, I. L.: Aktuelle probleme in der angiologie: Band 2. Bern: H. Huber, 92, 1968.

Hudlicka, O., and Tyler, K. R.: *Angiogenesis: The Growth of the Vascular System.* London: Academic Press, 1986.

Huntington, G. S., and McClure, C. F. W.: The development of the main lymph channels of the cat in their relations to the venous system. Anat. Rec. *1*:36, 1907.

Jargiello, D. M., and Caplan, A. I.: The fluid flow dynamics in the developing chick wing. In Fallon, J. F., and Caplan, A. I. (eds.): *Limb Development and Regeneration*, Part A. New York: Alan R. Liss, Inc., 1983, pp. 143–154.

Johnston, M. C. A.: Radioautographic study of the migration and fate of cranial neural crest. Anat. Rec. *156*:143, 1966.

Kampmeier, O. F.: *Evolution and Comparative Morphology of the Lymphatic System.* Springfield, IL: Charles C Thomas, 1969.

Kaplan, E. N.: Vascular malformations of the extremities. In Williams, H. B. (ed.): *Symposium on Vascular Malformations and Melanotic Lesions.* St. Louis: C. V. Mosby Co., 1983, pp. 144–161.

Kinmonth, J. B., and Eustace, P. W.: Lymph nodes and vessels in primary lymphedema. Ann. Roy. Coll. Surg. Engl. *58*:274, 1976.

Kinmonth, J. B., and Wolfe, J. H.: Fibrosis in the lymph nodes in primary lymphedema. Ann. Roy. Coll. Surg. Engl. *62*:344, 1980.

Langer, R., Brem, H., Falterman, K., et al.: Isolation of a cartilage factor which inhibits tumor neovascularization. Science *193*:70, 1976.

Leu, H. J., Wenner, A., Spycher, M. A., and Brunner, U.: Ultrastrukturelle Veränderungen bei venöser Angiodysplasie vom Typ Klippel-Trenaunay. VASA *9*:147, 1980.

Lewis, F. T.: The development of the lymphatic system in rabbits. Amer. J. Anat. *5*:95, 1905.

Lofferer, D., Mostbeck, A., and Partsch, H.: Arteriovenöse Kurzschlüsse der Extremitäten nuclearmedizinische Untersuchungen mit besonderer Berücksichtigung des Postthrombotischen Unterschenkelgeschwürs. Zbl. Phlebol. *8*:2, 1969.

McClure, C. F. W.: The development of the lymphatic system in the light of the more recent investigations in the field of vasculogenesis. Anat. Rec. *9*:563, 1915.

Morris, J.: Cited by Bevan, R. D. in *Development of the Vascular System.* London: Pitman, 1983, p. 238.

Nozue, T., and Tsuzaki, M.: Further studies on distribution of neural crest cells in prenatal and postnatal development in mice. Okajimas Fol. Anat. Jap. *51*:131, 1974.

Patten, B. M.: *Human Embryology*, 3rd ed. New York: McGraw-Hill, 1968, pp. 532–537.

Ranvier, L.: Développement des vaisseaux lymphatiques. C. R. Acad. Sc. *121*:1105, 1895.

Reid, M. R.: Studies on abnormal arteriovenous communications, acquired and congenital: Report of a series of cases. Arch. Surg. *10*:601, 1925.

Reinhoff, W. F.: Congenital arteriovenous fistula: An embryological study, with the report of a case. Bull. Johns Hopkins Hosp. *35*:271, 1924.

Reyes, J. M.: Retroperitoneal neurofibromatosis and venous anomalies. Arch. Path. Lab. Med. *104*:646, 1980.

Ryan, T. J., and Barnhill, R. L.: Physical factors and angiogenesis. In *Development of the Vascular System.* London: Pitman, 1983, pp. 80–94.

Sabin, F. R.: Further evidence on the origin of the lymphatic endothelium from the endothelium of the blood vascular system. Anat. Rec. *2*:46, 1908.

Sabin, F. R.: Studies of the origin of blood vessels as seen in the living blastoderm. Contrib. Embryol. Carnegie Inst. 9:213, 1920.

Servelle, J., and Babillot, J.: Les malformations des veines profondes dans la syndrome de Klippel et Trenaunay. Phlebologie 33:31, 1980.

Szilagyi, D. E., Smith, R. F., Elliott, J. P., and Hageman, J. H.: Congenital arteriovenous anomalies of the limbs. Arch. Surg. 111:423, 1976.

Thoma, R.: Untersuchungen über die Histogenese und Histomechanik des Gefassystems. Stuttgart: Encke F. Publ., 1893. Cited by Malan, E.: In Malan, E.: *Vascular Malformations.* Milan: C. Erba, 1974, pp. 21–22.

Trélat, U., and Monod, A.: De l'hypertrophie unilatérale partielle ou totale du corps. Arch. Gén. Méd. 13:636, 1869.

van der Putte, S. C. J.: The development of the lymphatic system in man. Anat. Embryol. Cell Biol. 51:1, 1975.

Woollard, H. H.: The development of the principal arterial system of the forelimb of the pig. Cont. Embryol. Carnegie Inst. 14:139, 1922.

Woollard, H. H., and Harpman, J. A.: The relationship between the size of an artery and the capillary bed in the embryo. J. Anat. 72:18, 1937.

CHAPTER SEVEN

Clinical Assessment of Vascular Malformations

A. E. Young

GUIDE TO DIAGNOSIS OF MALFORMATIONS

The vast majority of clinically significant vascular birthmarks seen in infants are hemangiomas. Pratt noted such lesions in 1% of a series of 1096 neonates, and, since the majority of hemangiomas are not readily visible at birth, the true incidence is higher than 1% (Pratt, 1967). However, vascular stains, usually on the nape of the neck, glabella, or eyelids, are very much more common, but because they are thus recognized almost as "normal" by parents, they are rarely referred to physicians. Pratt noticed these macular birthmarks (*nevus flammeus nuchae*) in 42% of white neonates and in 31% of black neonates. He also found similar minor capillary marks on the eyelids, forehead, or nose in about 10% of babies. These figures are similar to those reported by other investigators. In Pratt's series, only 5 of the 1096 neonates showed a vascular malformation, indicating that such anomalies are rare. Margileth and Museles found similar proportions in a review of 210 children referred to the hospital because of vascular birthmarks (Margileth and Museles, 1965). In their series, 272 superficial ("strawberry") hemangiomas and 30 deep hemangiomas were seen. This contrasted with 24 malformations, 6 venous-lymphatic lesions, 6 port-wine stains, 6 spider nevi, and 3 venous malformations. Though numerically they are rare, malformations are more often clinical problems, for whereas hemangiomas involute and nuchal stains fade, malformations are borne through life, often a source of cosmetic distress and not infrequently requiring repeated medical attention.

Diagnosis

Diagnosis is usually clinical, and in most instances, an accurate history and an assessment of symptoms together with a careful physical examination yield a diagnosis sufficiently precise to afford a prognosis and indicate what kind of investigations, if any, are necessary. If the patient is a neonate or a very young child, clinical assessment may be difficult and it may be impossible to offer a prognosis at this stage. On these occasions, the physician should refrain from making an overconfident prognosis and should examine the child initially at monthly intervals and then less frequently. It should be possible within the first year to determine whether a vascular birthmark is likely to regress, even though it may be many years before regression is complete. Malformations are, at a histologic level, stable. They do not regress, and, for hemodynamic reasons, they may extend, enlarge, or cause problems without any obvious change in size. Problems are encountered in the presence of arteriovenous fistulae, edema, sepsis, and lymphatic leakage and where there is involvement of deep structures by vascular malformations. Where such features are present, it may be necessary to watch the patient even into the teens before it is possible to give a clear indication of how the lesion will finally affect the child. When the vascular malformation presents in an older child or in an adult, it is frequently possible to predict the future of the lesion from the first clinical examination. There are, however, additional problems encountered in assessing vascular malformations when they present late. One of these is that the range of differential diagnoses expands. Thus, for example, a metastasis from a renal carcinoma may mimic an arteriovenous malformation, anomalous leg veins may mimic venous thrombosis, and multiple nodular venous anomalies can be macroscopically indistinguishable from Kaposi's sarcoma.

The Presenting Symptoms

With the exception of arteriovenous malformations and other progressive lesions just mentioned, most vascular malformations remain stable through life. They are usually noted at birth or within the first year of life. If, after initial assessment, the vascular anomaly is seen to be a minor cosmetic problem and is unlikely to cause symptoms, it may be reasonable to discharge the patient after a thorough discussion of the problem with the parents. Therapeutic intervention may cause more disfigurement than the lesion itself. In *most* instances, however, it is best to continue to see the child with a vascular malformation at yearly intervals. Problems may well arise. These periodic visits give the parents confidence that they are doing everything possible to care for their child.

It is our experience that there is a late clinical presentation, initiated by the bearer of the malformation when he or she becomes unhappy with its appearance or when complications develop. This occurs in adolescence or adulthood. It is only at this late stage that the patients may reach a specialist center. This late presentation is particularly a feature of arteriovenous malformation, which may not cause trouble until the patient is in his fourth decade. In keeping with other authors, we have noticed presentations in the sixth decade.

In infancy, the vascular abnormality is usually noted because of *appearance, bleeding,* or *lymphatic leakage.* These complications may occur after local trauma. Later, the patient may notice *discomfort* or, less commonly, frank *pain* as a result of turgidity of the anomaly or associated vessels, to direct "invasion" of, or pressure on, other structures. *Infection* or *thrombosis* of lesions may also cause discomfort or pain. Problems caused by arteriovenous malformations are outlined in the following discussion, but it is important to remember that arteriovenous lesions may produce pain distant from the lesion, either by pressure on nerves or by stealing blood from distal vascular territories, leading to ischemic pain, ulceration, or even frank gangrene. A small minority of arteriovenous malformations may precipitate congestive cardiac failure, and this may rarely be the presenting case, with dyspnea, ankle edema, and tachycardia.

Trauma may bring an arteriovenous anomaly to light, and there has been much discussion about whether trauma can, in fact, cause progression of a latent malformation. Lawton felt that fine septa might separate the arterial and venous sides of a quiet arteriovenous malformation and be broken down by trauma, allowing new arteriovenous connections to appear and thus letting the malformation enlarge (Lawton et al., 1957).

Skeletal malformations may be associated with many types of vascular anomaly and may be noted early, but disparity in length of lower limbs and the resultant secondary scoliosis are rarely noted before the child walks. Disparity in length of the arms may go unnoticed throughout life. Deep-seated vascular malformations, particularly in the central nervous system or abdominal viscera, produce their own symptoms, and these are discussed in Chapters Fifteen and Eighteen.

Previously quiescent arteriovenous malformations may present with sudden progression following puberty or pregnancy, or even after commencement of oral contraceptive hormone therapy. Pregnancy may accentuate not only arteriovenous malformations but also venous and venous-lymphatic lesions. Although we generally regard arteriovenous malformations as being stable at a cellular level, they possess a capacity for expansion during pregnancy, presumably under the in-

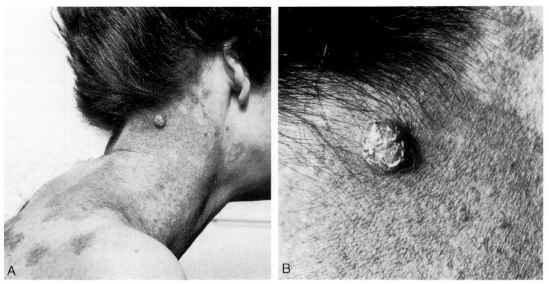

Figure 7–1. A and B, Although vascular malformations that do not contain arteriovenous fistulae are stable, changes may be seen during pregnancy. During both this woman's pregnancies, lesions erupted in her cervical (port-wine) capillary malformation: These had the histologic features of pyogenic granulomata.

fluence of some unspecified humoral agent. The increased blood volume and other hemodynamic changes associated with pregnancy may also precipitate these changes. An example is shown in Figure 7–1.

Specific Symptoms of Arteriovenous Malformations

The first abnormality noted is usually the cutaneous malformation. This may vary from a trivial pink stain (Fig. 7–2) to a mass of pulsatile vessels. The patient may complain of varices, swelling, or "disfigurement," and, in addition, certain specific symptoms:

Heaviness. The patient may be aware of a sense of heaviness in the area of the lesion that is worse with dependency and eased by elevation.

Pain. Fifty per cent of patients experience pain. This may be of a throbbing or stabbing character and is particularly experienced in hand and neck arteriovenous malformations. Lesions in the masseter and parotid may cause headache. The pain from limb malformations may be ischemic or in the territory of an identifiable nerve that is pressed upon or involved. The pain may also be due to increased pressure on glomic structures that are related to malformations and that may

themselves be abnormal. Thrombosis in complex malformations or deep-seated hematomas may lead to pain of sudden onset. In peripheral arteriovenous malformations there may also be ischemic ulcers, which are almost invariably very painful.

Pulsation. Some patients will note an uncomfortable pulsation in the lesion or in the surrounding veins.

Hyperhidrosis. Local hyperhidrosis is often marked.

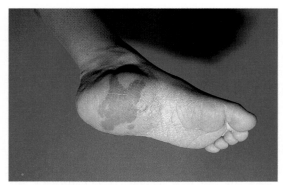

Figure 7–2. This child had a pronounced pink capillary dermal malformation of the heel at birth. Examination showed the classic clinical features of an arteriovenous malformation beneath.

Hypertrichosis. Local hypertrichosis may be a presenting sign in a case of arteriovenous malformation.

Hyperthermia. Local hyperthermia is sometimes the presenting symptom, and we have objectively documented it in 16 of 26 patients with arteriovenous malformations.

Thrill. The patients may spontaneously report that they sense a thrill in the lesion. In the head and neck malformations, this thrill will be heard by the patient as an audible bruit or buzzing in the ears. This may become very distressing by its loudness and constancy.

Other Symptoms. There may be *functional impairment* of a limb, by the mass of the malformation interfering with muscle function or by ischemia, muscle contractures, or joint deformities.

There may be *trophic changes* in the skin, typical of venous hypertension, and they may produce ulcers. These ulcers may be at unusual sites, but more often they mimic "ordinary" venous ulcers very closely (Fig. 7–3).

The patient may present with *hemorrhage* from cutaneous malformations. This is unusual with arteriovenous lesions, unless ulceration has occurred, but is encountered spontaneously in arteriovenous malformations of the mandible involving the teeth and also in malformations of the nasopharynx.

Occasionally an arteriovenous malformation is discovered incidentally during operation or examination for another reason. This is especially true of pelvic lesions.

Many writers have noted the difference in pattern of presentation between patients with localized macrofistulous lesions and those with diffuse microfistulous lesions (Lawton et al., 1957; Szilagyi et al., 1976). The former group usually present because of large veins, ischemia, pain, or local symptoms of heat. The latter group, with diffuse lesions, often only have giant limbs as initial problems, though they may progress to hemodynamic complications such as cardiac failure.

An infant who presents with congestive heart failure and with no evidence of a cardiac defect should be evaluated for an arteriovenous malformation *or* diffuse hemangioma of the liver or other viscera.

The Clinical Examination

The clinical evaluation should always begin with a complete examination of the whole patient, even if the obvious vascular mark on the surface seems trivial. A cursory look at the external lesion is insufficient for the proper assessment of vascular malformations. Many physicians fall into the trap of feeling that an impressive surface malformation, such as the port-wine stain involving a whole limb, may be the whole story; however, it is often, like the visible part of an iceberg, merely one tenth of the problem. Accurate notes about the patient should be supplemented with color photographs wherever possible, as they are invaluable for assessing progress of the lesion or for explaining subsequent problems in referring a patient to a specialist center.

The clinician may find it helpful if the examination is directed at answering the following seven primary questions with a view to understanding the natural history of the lesion.

1. *Is the lesion histologically proliferative or non-proliferative?* Is it a true hemangioma, which will predictably regress, or is it a stable malformation, a lesion that will be present for the whole of the patient's life? It is important to remember that when heman-

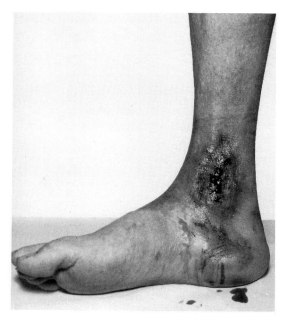

Figure 7–3. An ulcer at the ankle of a teenager with multiple arteriovenous fistulae in the leg. In position of the ulcer and the presence of surrounding induration and pigmentation, it has all the features of a venous ulcer.

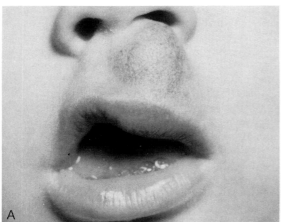
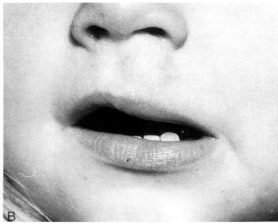

Figure 7–4. A deep hemangioma may mimic a vascular malformation but, in time, regression confirms the diagnosis. A, Hemangioma of upper lip. B, Twelve months later.

giomas are extensive, flat, or in atypical sites, they may initially mimic a vascular malformation (Fig. 7–4). A diagnosis of hemangioma must then be made from simple clinical experience, judging the consistency and texture of the lesion together with a history of rapid progression after birth. It is some- times not possible to make a definite decision that this is an involuting lesion until the child has been seen several times. The lesion should then be carefully inspected for areas of "graying" and softening and for a shrinking back of the lesion from its original outline (Fig. 7–5).

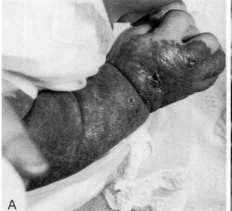
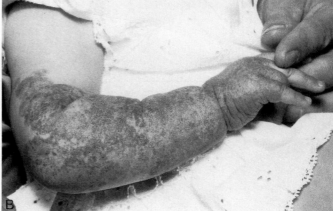

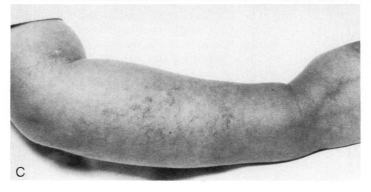

Figure 7–5. A hemangioma may, in position, outline, shape, and color, mimic a capillary dermal malformation but can be differentiated by its richer, raised texture and its redder hue. A, B, and C demonstrate its progressive resolution.

2. *Is the lesion hemodynamically stable or unstable (i.e., low flow or high flow)?* This is an easy decision to make with a classic "cirsoid" malformation, but it is more difficult with deep-seated anomalies or where there are multiple small arteriovenous fistulae. Only about 30% of patients with limb vascular abnormalities have dilated superficial veins, and many of these veins may appear to be ectatic and not obviously dilated secondary to an arteriovenous malformation. In addition, a capillary or dermal malformation may be present and distract attention from the major anomaly lying beneath the skin. Abnormal pulsations or thrill, with typical systolic accentuation or heat over a deep-seated abnormality, may assist the diagnosis in such cases, but it may not be possible to assess hemodynamic activity confidently without investigations directed at assessing the blood flow. A thrill can be a particularly misleading sign in locating a deep-seated lesion, firstly because it may be absent where the arteriovenous fistulae are small and multiple and, secondly, because when present it may be heard in the vein at some distance from the primary lesion.

3. *Is it a combined lesion?* For example, if there is an obvious venous malformation, is there a less obvious arteriovenous or lymphatic malformation also present?

4. *Is the skeleton normal?*

5. *Are there hidden, associated vascular lesions in systems other than the skin (particularly, the gastrointestinal tract, genitourinary tract, or central nervous system)?*

6. *Is the lesion possibly malignant?*

7. *Can a name be put to it?*

Histologic Stability

As already indicated, histologic stability is a clinical judgment, though in cases in which there is an urgent need to establish the diagnosis, biopsy of the lesion may be justified. In general, however, biopsy of vascular birthmarks is usually unnecessary.

Hemodynamic Stability

Some arteriovenous fistulae are hemodynamically stable and non-progressive. Active arteriovenous lesions have one or more typical clinical features. Usually such a lesion is tense and warm. The surrounding veins may be diffusely enlarged, though this may not be visible through the skin; they may be

pulsatile and difficult to compress. Not only the lesion but also the surrounding skin may be warmer than the rest of the body. Auscultation of the lesion may disclose a continuous murmur, with systolic accentuation spreading into vessels often quite far distant from the lesion and conducted along bones adjacent to them. Obstruction of the venous outflow will eliminate the diastolic portion of the murmur. Adjacent bones may also be enlarged. With proximal arteriovenous malformations in limbs, the distal part of the limb may bear the stigmata of ischemia, being cool, dusky, and edematous and showing changes of old, current, or incipient ulceration. Although rare, the signs of congestive cardiac failure should be sought in any patient with arteriovenous fistulae. Increased cardiac diameter is not uncommon, but frank high output cardiac failure is seen only in a small percentage of patients (Hyyppä and Simelä, 1971). Indeed, none of the 69 patients in the Mayo Clinic series of limb arteriovenous malformations had cardiac symptoms attributable to the presence of the fistulae (Gomes and Bernatz, 1970). By contrast, however, in a series of 156 infants with systemic arteriovenous malformations of the central nervous system, liver, and lungs reviewed by Knudson and Alden, congestive heart failure was the most common sign, occurring in 66% of central nervous system malformations, 47% of hepatic malformations, and 57% of pulmonary malformations. It was also the most common cause of death (Knudson and Alden 1979). In the limbs, the Nicoladoni test can be usefully combined with the clinical examination. In this test, the occlusion of the inflow artery to a malformation, or the main artery proximal to the malformation, produces a slowing of the heart rate. This bradycardiac reaction is probably a great vessel baroreceptor reflex precipitated by the acute hypertension that follows occlusion of the fistulae.

Is It a Combined Lesion?

Although some vascular malformations are tidily packaged syndromes, many are less readily definable. Therefore, in addition to defining the predominant lesion or part of the vasculature that is involved, the clinician should ask specifically about the other parts of the vascular system.

Is the Venous System Normal? Are there ectopic or aberrant veins (Fig. 7–6)? Are

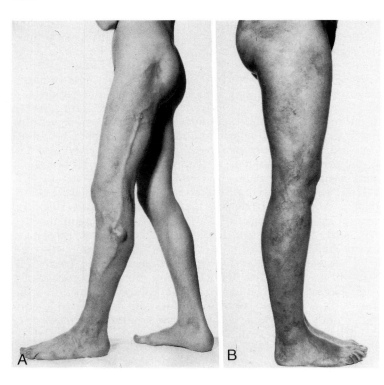

Figure 7–6. A lateral venous anomaly may exist as a visible trunk *(A)*, or as a similar pattern of capillary malformation and telangiectasiae *(B)*.

veins distended or varicose? Is there evidence of a deep venous anomaly, i.e., edema, venous claudication, or collateral veins?

Is the Lymphatic System Normal? Is there persisting edema? It is difficult to assess whether a neonate has lymphedema. If the swollen skin pits, it may not be distinguishable from the edema of other causes. If it does not pit, the rubbery swelling may be difficult to distinguish from soft tissue hypertrophy from other causes and it may mimic the fatty rolls of the healthy neonate (Fig. 7–7). Early in its history, lymphedema pits to pressure; only later does it adopt the typical appearance of subcutaneous fibrosis: square toes, keratotic skin changes, and loss of pitting to pressure (Fig. 7–8). Are there any vesicles on the skin discharging clear fluid or chyle? Sometimes this form of discharge appears to come directly from the skin without a pre-existing vesicle. Lymphatic leaks are typically found at the root of the limbs. Although the leakage of fluid may be profuse, it may also be trivial (Fig. 7–9).

Is the Arterial System Normal? Are all the pulses present and of equal size? Variations in the course and presence of arteries are not uncommon, are rarely of clinical significance, and are almost never associated with other vascular abnormalities.

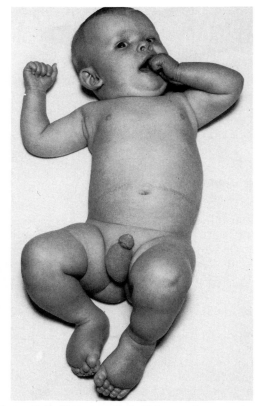

Figure 7–7. The normal chubbiness of a neonate or toddler may conceal the presence of lymphedema.

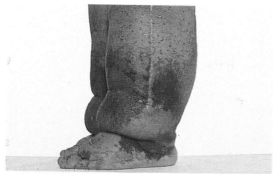

Figure 7–8. Gross edema and warty keratosis in a patient with lymphedema from infancy as a result of lymphatic hypoplasia.

Is the Skeleton Normal?

In vascular malformations, the skeleton may be affected in four different ways; each of these should be sought.

Overgrowth or Undergrowth. This is common where extensive vascular malformations affect the limbs, but overgrowth or undergrowth can affect any part of the skeleton. Where there is overgrowth, the vascular lesion is typically an arteriovenous or venous-lymphatic lesion. In arteriovenous malformations, the overgrowth is usually in proportion and related anatomically to the area affected by the arteriovenous fistulae. In venous-lymphatic anomalies, the skeletal change is usually an overgrowth, which may be disproportionate and occasionally bizarre. With venous anomalies, the toes may be particularly affected by disparate gigantism, and it has been claimed that it is usually the medial three toes that are affected, though we have seen disparate gigantism in all toes. The gigantism in venous dysplasias may be distant from the malformation itself, and it is probably the result of a parallel skeletal dysplasia rather than the direct effect of

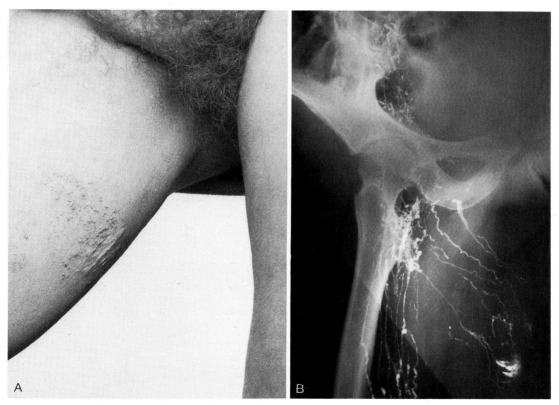

Figure 7–9. Lymphatic vesicles. Clear, multiple vesicles are usually found at or near the root of the limb. Most commonly, they are localized cystic lymphatic malformations that do not communicate with the deep lymphatics. However, when there are other abnormalities or when the vesicles discharge copious quantities of clear lymph or chyle, a connection should be suspected. A shows cutaneous lymphatic vesicles (and a biopsy scar). B, Lymphogram in the same patient, showing reflux into the cutaneous vesicles. The patient has multiple arteriovenous fistulae.

disordered hemodynamics produced by the vascular malformation. Thus, the presence of skeletal overgrowth does not definitely signify the presence of arteriovenous fistulae or deep vein obstruction.

There are other causes for limb hypertrophy or bodily hemi-hypertrophy apart from vascular lesions. Simple capillary malformations may be associated with partial gigantism without any evidence of a significant deep-seated vascular abnormality (Fig. 7–10). Yet, no matter how innocuous a diffuse dermal malformation may appear to be, such a patient should be kept under review. Later years may reveal deep venous anomalies of the extremities, viscera, or retroperitoneum.

Coexistent Skeletal Abnormalities or Malformations. A great variety of such anomalies have been documented in association with vascular malformations, and they range from simple talipes and congenital dislocations of the hip to rare conditions such as melorheostosis.

Direct Involvement of the Skeleton by the Malformation. This particularly occurs with extensive venous anomalies ("phlebangiomatoses") and becomes clinically apparent when there are pathological fractures, sometimes with malunion or delayed union, or where there is dissolution of bone.

Coexistent Enchondromas. This situation is separately described as Maffucci's syndrome in Chapter Fourteen. It may occur in a quite circumscribed fashion affecting part of a limb, but usually the whole body is affected, with gross and obvious deformity.

Assessment of Disparity in Limb Size

In the neonate and toddler, the best assessment that can be achieved is to measure

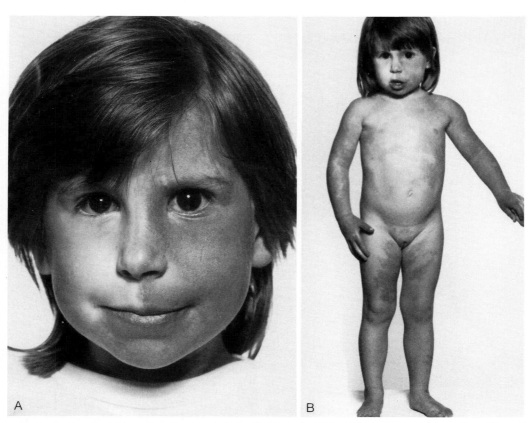

Figure 7–10. *A,* Hemifacial hypertrophy associated with trigeminal (V1–V3) capillary malformation. There is not evidence for choroidal or intracerebral vascular anomaly (Sturge-Weber syndrome). This patient should still be followed for possible development of glaucoma. *B,* Her capillary malformation involves other cutaneous areas; yet, to date, there are no other demonstrable vascular anomalies. She should be seen periodically, for, in time, deep vascular anomalies may become evident.

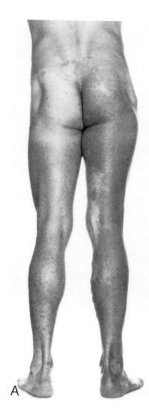

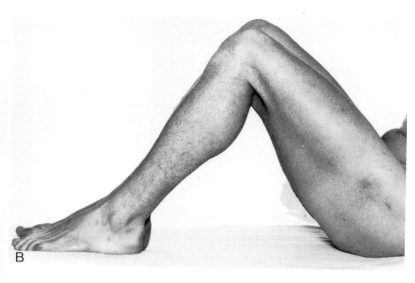

Figure 7–11. Assessment of disparity in leg length. *A*, Assuming normal hip joints, the disparity in length can be judged from pelvic tilt, difference in position of infragluteal folds, and the presence of scoliosis. *B*, With the patient lying, knees flexed and ankles together, inequality in length of the upper and lower leg is easily seen from the side. (Reproduced from Browse, N. L.: *Symptoms and Signs of Surgical Disease.* London, Edward E. Arnold, 1982.)

from bone point to bone point with a tape measure. This is also the method of choice when assessing the arms of adults for disparity of length. We have found that this is best done with the arms extended forward and parallel to the ground, and measurements are then recorded between the acromion and olecranon and between the olecranon and knuckle of the middle finger (proximal interphalangeal joint). The difference in hand size is measured with the palms together.

In the infant and adult lower limb, length disparity is easy to assess. Standing, the patient is measured from the back and the disparity in length is revealed by pelvic tilt and by a difference in the level of the subgluteal crease (Fig. 7–11A). From the front, the patellae may be seen to be at different levels. This perceived length discrepancy may be measured from the thickness of a block or book under the foot of the normal leg needed to correct asymmetry. If the patient lies supine and the hips and knees are flexed, as in Figure 7–11B, the disparity can also be seen at the knee and differential lengths of femur and tibia can be assessed. All these

measurements assume a normal hip joint and feet, and this should be confirmed. The feet are easily assessed from the plantar surface. If a disparity in limb length is noted, it should be confirmed and accurately documented radiographically by scannograms (Fig. 7–12).

Different thickness is easily measured from circumference, but it may be difficult to assess whether the difference is due to hypertrophy of all tissues or to non-pitting edema. Soft tissue radiographs or computed tomographic scans help to clarify this. Particular difficulty may also be experienced when the apparent thickness is due to diffuse venous or lymphatic malformation. For our records, we prefer a consistent anatomical place for recording limb circumferences.

Is There a Hidden Associated Lesion?

Capillary or dermal malformations of the head and neck and those overlying the spine are occasionally associated with intracranial and intraspinal vascular anomalies. These may produce neurological symptoms and are

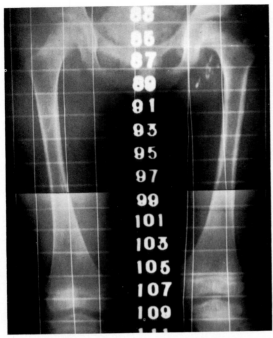

Figure 7–12. Scannograms permit accurate measurements of disparity in length of the limbs; in this instance, the 1 cm grid demonstrates a 0.6 cm difference between the lengths of the femora.

described as specific syndromes (Sturge-Weber, Wyburn-Mason, Cobb, etc.) in Chapter Fifteen.

It is rare for there to be a primary associated defect of nervous tissue; in most patients with a vascular birthmark, central nervous system signs are secondary to pressure or distortion of the nervous system by the vascular malformation. It is extremely unusual to find a patient with a vascular malformation who is mentally defective or retarded, and it is, of course, important to reassure the parents on this point early on. Before doing so, it is prudent to check

1. That the milestones have been passed satisfactorily.

2. That examination of the central nervous system is normal.

3. That there is no history of seizures.

Is the Lesion Malignant?

The answer to this question is, almost without exception, negative. This is assuming that malignancies (angiosarcoma, Kaposi's sarcoma, and hemangiopericytoma) and vascular cutaneous metastases (e.g., from a hyper-

nephroma, metastatic melanoma) have been excluded from the differential diagnosis (see following discussion). A rapidly growing "strawberry" birthmark may look malignant and an arteriovenous malformation may behave in an aggressive, destructive way, mimicking malignancy, but vascular malformations are *never* malignant in the proper sense and *do not metastasize*. There are a few scattered reports in the literature suggesting metastases from vascular malformations, but these are unconvincing (Matas, 1940).

Can a Name be Put to It?

It can be seen from the glossary to this book that named syndromes exist in profusion, often with little or no justification or clinical value. There are, however, commonly observed complex groupings of anomalies for which an eponym is justified and useful, though these compose less than a tenth of the named syndromes that exist. We have collected in the glossary as comprehensive a list of anomalies as possible and have attempted to define the majority in terms of accurate, commonly used, and helpful denominators.

Differential Diagnosis

The great variability in vascular malformations, and the fact that they are not necessarily noted at birth and may enlarge slightly during infancy, can confuse diagnosis. With some nodular lesions there may be anxiety about malignancy, but from the outset it should be noted that this is an extreme rarity.

Malignant diagnoses that may be confused with vascular malformations are the following:

1. Kaposi's sarcoma
2. Angiosarcoma
3. Infantile hemangiopericytoma
4. Cutaneous metastases of non-vascular malignancies

Malignant Lesions

Kaposi's Sarcoma. (Synonyms: angiosarcoma multiplex, hemorrhagic sarcoma, sarcoma nodulosum cavernosum, perithelioma multiplex) Kaposi's sarcoma is a vascular malignancy histologically featuring complexes of

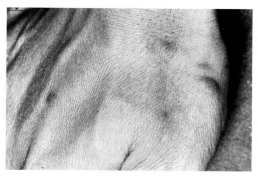 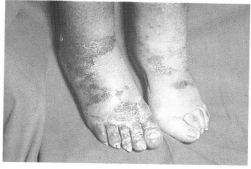

A   B

Figure 7–13. The cutaneous appearances of Kaposi's sarcoma are protean. The disease may appear as indolent bluish nodules on the hands or feet, as in this young man *(A)*, or as a more diffuse purple discoloration with swelling *(B)*.

capillaries and spindle-shaped fibrosarcoma-like cells. It may be multicentric in origin. It is usually a disease of adults, and its incidence is increasing because it is one of the malignancies associated with the acquired immune deficiency syndrome (AIDS). Four per cent of cases have in the past been reported in infants, and, as infants may be affected by AIDS, the incidence may increase (Scott et al., 1984). Where unassociated with AIDS, the disease particularly affects Africans from the Congo, Ruanda, the Sudan, and Southern Egypt. Seventy-five per cent of these patients are males. Clinically, it may present in an indolent form, with scattered, firm, bluish domed nodules (Fig. 7–13). These may have a verrucous surface. They are encountered most often in the arms and legs and can involve the head, neck, and trunk. The lesions clinically mimic multiple venous malformations and may not seem malignant, even on histologic examination, having only an inflammatory appearance. With time, the lesions enlarge and coalesce, and lymphatic involvement may produce swelling of the limb. By this stage, the lesions may have metastasized to involve lymph nodes, viscera, and bones. The prognosis is very variable; many of those patients presenting as young adults have had peripheral lesions as children. Once the disease is disseminated, the prognosis is poor, but remission may be achieved with the chemotherapy and local radiotherapy.

Pseudo-Kaposi's Sarcoma. Several reports exist of angiodermatitis with associated localized arteriovenous malformations. These lesions are clinically described as red brown macules with superimposed scaling violaceous plaques mimicking Kaposi's sarcoma (Fig. 7–14). Histologic changes also resemble Kaposi's sarcoma, with fibrovascular and neovascular proliferation but no "vascular slits" or spindle cells (Earhart et al., 1974). This is an entirely benign condition.

Angiosarcoma. (Synonyms: hemangioendotheliosarcoma, malignant hemangioendothelioma, hemangiosarcoma) Cutaneous angiosarcoma is rare and is usually seen in adults. Girard recorded that 9 of 28 patients reviewed were aged less than 20 at the time of biopsy (Girard et al., 1970). The lesions are described as raised, red to purple firm papules or nodules, often with smaller satellite lesions. The disease may begin as deep-seated painless lumps. The tumor varies in aggressiveness and tends only to be diagnosed when enlargement leads to biopsy.

Hemangiopericytoma. Most hemangiopericytomas arise in deep sites and in adults. Enzinger has, however, shown that there is a separate group of relatively benign hemangiopericytomas that occur subcutaneously in the first year of life. They are characteristically multilobulated and are usually (but not invariably) solitary. They are very rare and diagnosable only by histologic examination (Enzinger and Weiss, 1983).

Benign Lesions

Benign lesions that may be confused with vascular malformations are the following:
1. Blue marks
   a. "Mongolian blue spot"
   b. Blue nevus

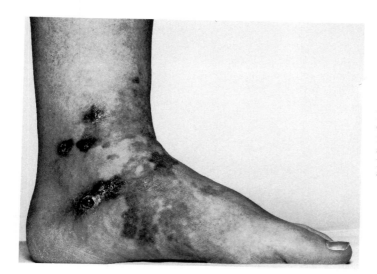

Figure 7–14. This woman has clinically discrete multiple arteriovenous fistulae involving the lower left leg. There are secondary skin changes that mimic Kaposi's sarcoma (so-called pseudo-Kaposi's sarcoma).

    c. Nevus of Ota
    d. Nevus of Ito
2. Nodular and punctate lesions
    a. Multiple glomus tumors
    b. Angiokeratoma of Fordyce
    c. Angiokeratoma circumscriptum
    d. Angiokeratoma corporis diffusum (Anderson-Fabry disease)

Blue Marks. Pratt has recorded this abnormality in half of all black children, usually involving the sacrum and buttocks but also noticed on the wrist, shoulders, knees, and ankles. Although it is claimed not to occur in white children, Pratt recorded a 0.5% incidence of this anomaly in white infants (Pratt, 1967). The lesion is purple-blue or gray in color and is melanocytic, not vascular. There are no associated anomalies. Levin has commented on the inappropriateness of the term "Mongolian blue spot," a direct translation from the first description in 1885 as "Blaue mongolische flecken" but not accurate because the disease is not confined to Mongolians, is not necessarily blue, and is not a spot, but rather a patch or mark (Levin, 1981).

Nodular Lesions

Glomus Tumors. There are hemangiopericytomas, and they may be confused with vascular malformations when multiple. Although commonly occurring under the nails, they may occur scattered throughout a limb or diffusely. They are pale and dome-shaped, though sometimes purple. The diagnostic clinical feature is pain occurring when the lesion is pressed, but often also spontaneously (Kohout and Stout, 1961). Multiple glomus

tumor is a condition that is sometimes hereditable as an autosomal dominant trait.

Angiokeratomas. The *angiokeratomas* are rare lesions but are a differential diagnosis to be considered when malformations present in adult life. The angiokeratomas are discussed in Chapter Ten.

Reticulated Lesions

There are many acquired skin lesions that might superficially be confused with reticular vascular malformations, but an account of them is outside the scope of this book. Where close examination confirms the vascular nature of the reticulation, the differential diagnosis is limited.

In children, the rare *nevus anemicus* may mimic a vascular malformation. The condition was first described by Vörner in 1906 (Vörner, 1906) and was redescribed by Parkes Weber in 1929 (Parkes Weber, 1929). Present at birth, the lesion consists of blotchy areas of pallor in otherwise pinkish skin. The pallid areas will darken with the application of heat, and the condition is a functional, not a structural, abnormality (Daniel, 1977).

Rothmund-Thomson Syndrome (Congenital Poikiloderma). Another rare skin disorder that may be confused as a vascular birthmark was first described by Rothmund, a German ophthalmologist, in 1868 (Rothmund, 1868) and by Thomson, an English dermatologist, in 1923 (Thomson, 1923). The onset of cutaneous signs is usually between 3 and 6 months of age, although lesions have been seen at birth. The earliest skin lesions are bright, red, pink, shiny, tense swellings, with reticulated patches of erythema, resembling sunburn. The cheeks are usually first involved; later, the rest of the face, ears, buttocks, and extensor surfaces of the extremities are affected. The early erythematous phase is followed by an atrophic phase, when reticulation is seen as a result of abnormally thin skin over normal blood vessels. There are also circumscribed white macules, dull red telangiectasias, and irregular areas of atrophy and scaling. Later, there may be macular or reticulated pigmentation. The irregularity and variety of the skin changes prompted Thomson to call the disorder "poikiloderma congenitale" (Thomson, 1936).

This is a systemic disorder; Silver has reviewed the literature and enumerates the features of the syndrome as follows (Silver, 1966):

1. Cutaneous atrophy with telangiectasia and pigmentation.

2. Changes noted at 3–6 months.

3. Female predominance.

4. Seventy per cent of cases show familial recessive inheritance.

5. Fifty-four per cent of patients have short stature.

6. Fifty-two per cent of patients have cataracts developing between the age of 3 and 6 years.

7. Fifty per cent have absent or sparse hair of eyebrows or lashes.

8. Thirty-nine per cent have congenital bone defects.

9. Thirty-five per cent of patients have photosensitivity.

10. Twenty-four per cent have hypogonadism.

11. Twenty-four per cent have dystrophic nails.

12. Fifteen per cent have defective dentition.

References

Daniel, R. H.: Nevus anemicus. Arch. Dermatol. *113*:53, 1977.

Earhart, R. N., Aeling, J. A., Nuss, D. D., and Mellette. J. R.: Pseudo Kaposi sarcoma. Arch. Dermatol. *110*: 907, 1974.

Enzinger, F. M., and Weiss, S. W.: *Soft Tissue Tumors*. St. Louis: C. V. Mosby Co., 1983, p. 477.

Girard, C., Johnson, W. C., and Graham, J. H.: Cutaneous angiosarcoma. Cancer *26*:868, 1970.

Gomes, N. M. R., and Bernatz, P. E.: Arteriovenous fistulas. A review and ten years experience at the Mayo Clinic. Mayo Clin. Proc. *45*:81, 1970.

Hyyppä, S., and Simelä, S.: Multiple diffuse congenital arteriovenous fistulas of the lower limb. Clin. Pediatr. *10*:282, 1971.

Knudson, R. P., and Alden, E. R.: Symptomatic arteriovenous malformations in infants less than 6 months of age. Pediatrics *64*:238, 1979.

Kohout, E., and Stout, A. P.: The glomus tumor in children. Cancer *14*:555, 1961.

Lawton, R. C., Tidrick, R. T., and Brintnall, E. S.: A clinico-pathological study of multiple congenital arteriovenous fistulae of the lower extremities. Angiology *8*:161, 1957.

Levin, S.: Mongolian spot; Afro-Asian stain; sacral stain. South African Med. J. *60*:123, 1981.

Margileth, A. M., and Museles, M.: Cutaneous hemangiomas in children. JAMA *194*:523, 1965.

Matas, R.: Congenital arteriovenous angioma of the arm. Metastases eleven years after amputation. Ann. Surg. *111*:1021, 1940.

Parkes Weber, F.: Naevus anaemicus (ischaemicus). Proc. Roy. Soc. Med. *22*:503, 1929.

Pratt, A. G.: Birthmarks in infants. Arch. Dermatol. Syph. *67*:302, 1967.

Rothmund, A.: Ueber Cataracten in Verbindung mit einer eigenthümlichen Hautdegeneration. Archiv. f. Ophth. *14*:159, 1868.

Scott, G. B., Buck, B. E., Leterman, J. G., et al.: Acquired immunodeficiency syndrome in infants. N. Engl. J. Med. *310*:76, 1984.

Silver, H. K.: Rothmund-Thomson syndrome: An oculocutaneous disorder. Amer. J. Dis. Child. *111*:182, 1966.

Szilagyi, D. E., Smith, R. F., Elliott, J. P., and Hageman, J. H.: Congenital arteriovenous anomalies of the limbs. Arch. Surg. *111*:423, 1976.

Thomson, M. S.: A hitherto undescribed familial disease. Brit. J. Derm. *35*:455, 1923.

Thomson, M. S.: Poikiloderma congenitale. Brit. J. Derm. *48*:221, 1936.

Vörner, H.: Über naevus anaemicus. Arch. Derm. u. Syph. *82*:391, 1906.

CHAPTER EIGHT

Investigation of Vascular Malformations

A. E. Young

INTRODUCTION

How, when, and, in particular, *whether* to investigate vascular malformations are frequently difficult decisions, and it must be stressed that unless there is a very clear indication that the management of the condition will be influenced by the studies, children should not be subjected to hospitalization. Unfamiliarity with these anomalies, research interests, enthusiasm of junior staff members, or a desire for an academically accurate diagnosis are all considerations that may lead to a child being admitted to the hospital for complex and painful procedures. It is customary in adult medicine to describe tests as being "invasive" or "non-invasive," a distinction that is increasingly semantic rather than real and of little interest to the child, for whom even a single blood test or half a day spent away from its mother may be a frightening or even a scarring experience. Adequate diagnosis can usually be made from the clinical examination, and for this reason we strongly urge a policy of noninterference when there are no clinical indications for interventional treatment. We take quite the opposite view in relation to patients who require active treatment, and in these circumstances investigations become mandatory, in order that the extent of the anatomical and hemodynamic lesion may be assessed. These investigations may, for example, be important in determining the volume of flow through an arteriovenous fistula or for determining the cause of edema in an affected limb. Biopsy will, very occasionally, be necessary to exclude malignancy. Special tests are appropriate for the investigation of lesions in particular areas such as the central nervous system.

The examinations described in this chapter are merely illustrations of the plethora of tests in use around the world. When the parameter to be measured or structure to be imaged is identified, it is usually best to use the appropriate locally available technique. This is particularly so with hemodynamic assessments, which rely on a locally obtained set of control values.

Investigations may be divided as follows (without regard for relative importance):

1. Clinical hemodynamic assessment
2. Plethysmography, including pulse volume recording, venous manometry, and foot volumetry
3. Doppler assessments
4. Scintigraphy
5. Thermography
6. Blood gas analysis
7. Biopsy
8. Hematological assessment
9. Angiography (see also Chapter Nine)

These tests have a multitude of applications in the context of malformations and are selected to answer specific clinical questions. For example, is there arteriovenous shunting of blood? A Nicoladoni test can show this, but plethysmography will be needed to quantify the shunting and angiography or Doppler assessments will be needed to locate the sites. Plethysmography may suggest venous anomalies, but angiography or scintigraphy may be needed to confirm them. Hematological studies may suggest excessive consumption of platelets or clotting factors, but scintigraphy is needed to elucidate the sites.

CLINICAL ASSESSMENT: THE NICOLADONI-BRANHAM TEST

The Nicoladoni-Branham test is a crude way of confirming the presence of a large arteriovenous fistula or fistulae. It is based on the principle that occlusion of the arterial inflow to a shunt will cause a reflex bradycardia. This is frequently referred to as the Branham test, after Branham's observations in 1890 of the phenomenon in a patient with a traumatic arteriovenous fistula following a femoral gunshot wound (Branham, 1890). Nicoladoni had, however, observed the same phenomenon some 15 years earlier, in a case of congenital arteriovenous malformation in the upper limb. In addition to the clinical observations, his paper included a characteristic oscillogram trace (Nicoladoni, 1875). Matas designated the phenomenon the "bradycardiac sign" (Matas, 1923). It is, in essence, only applicable to large arteriovenous fistulae in the limbs where cardiac output has risen by 50% or more. Ideally, the test is performed by occluding the arterial inflow with a pneumatic cuff. The pulse rate is measured for a full minute before and after inflation of the cuff, and a fall in pulse rate in excess of 10 per minute can be presumed to be

positive. The bradycardia is probably vagally mediated from left ventricular and aortic baroreceptors signaling the rise in arterial pressure that follows occlusion of the inflow to the fistulae; it occurs within a few seconds of occluding the inflow to the fistulae.

PLETHYSMOGRAPHY

Plethysmography is a reliable way of determining increased limb blood flow through fistulae but ideally requires a normal limb for comparison if small changes are to be assessed. Any standard method is appropriate, and studies have been undertaken using water bath displacement techniques, strain gauge, impedance, and gravimetric methods. To obtain the best results, segmental plethysmography should be performed (Bertelsen and Dohn 1953). A tracing in a patient with Klippel-Trenaunay syndrome is shown in Figure 8–1. Plethysmographic investigations are useful to chart progress, but this is only true if the technique is sufficiently trustworthy to be reliable and repeatable. This, in general, will only be true of the controlled environment of a "vascular laboratory." The techniques all determine the flow indirectly by measuring the increase of volume of the limb after occlusion of the venous outflow. Results are, at best, expressed as a ratio difference between the legs or as milliliters per gram of tissue. Plethysmography is useful in quantifying flow in a whole limb, but it is difficult to assess blood flow through circumscribed areas (Yao et al., 1973), particularly fingers, which have small soft tissue volumes

Figure 8–1. Tracings from venous occlusion plethysmography in a patient with Klippel-Trenaunay syndrome of the left leg associated with iliac vein atresia. The blood flow in ml/minute per hundred grams of tissue can be calculated from the slope of the trace after the initial cuff artifact. In this patient, the blood flow in the left calf was almost three times that in the right. Venous outflow after deflation of the cuff is seen to be normal in both legs.

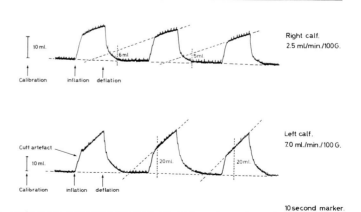

Pt.S.S. : Klippel Trenaunay Synd. L Leg : RESTING CALF BLOOD FLOWS

Right calf.
2.5 ml/min./100G.

Left calf.
7.0 ml./min./100 G.

10 second marker.

in relation to total tissue volume and also often have pre-existing venous congestion. Most techniques used for whole limb or partial limb studies are usually sufficiently sensitive to demonstrate the small and clinically unimportant arteriovenous shunting that occurs with some venous anomalies. The curves seen on plethysmography are typical of arteriovenous fistulae when they show a rapid onset, arched curve after cuff inflation and a reduced size during exercise (thus distinguishing arteriovenous fistulae from venous obstruction). Limited reporting of the effects of postocclusive reactive hyperemia shows that no useful additional information is obtained in most patients, partly because of the wide range of reported variation. In some patients, blood flow increases after arterial occlusion; in others, it decreases (Bollinger et al., 1966).

Pulse Volume Recording (PVR)

PVR has been used to demonstrate the presence of arteriovenous fistulae and will show the increased arterial pulse amplitude above and below a localized arteriovenous lesion. It is of limited quantitative value, though it is potentially useful in judging the success of therapeutic embolization.

Venous Manometry

Venous pressures may be assessed by cannulation of leg veins and connection to a transducer with a pressure recording system. This is of value in judging whether venous pressure is sufficiently raised, in relation to the general venous circulation, to allow venous reconstructive surgery to be undertaken where there is symptomatic deep vein atresia or obstruction. Venous manometry has also been used to determine the function of the deep veins of the lower limb. Foot volumetry (Nogren, 1974) or photoplethysmography (Miles and Nicolaides, 1981) can provide the same information less invasively.

Foot Volumetry

Valuable information about the function of the venous system of the lower limb can be obtained when the patient's foot and lower calf are immersed in a water bath and the patient is exercised by knee bending. Changes in tissue volume are reflected as small changes in the water level. In the normal subject, the foot volume falls during exercise and this can be easily calculated in ml per 100 ml of tissue. When exercise stops, the refilling rate can be measured. Exercise is then repeated after application of a tourniquet below or above the knee, which prevents reflux down superficial veins. This test shows, firstly, whether there is obstruction to expulsion of blood from the leg during exercise (low expelled volume) and, secondly, whether there is reflux in the deep veins (rapid refilling with tourniquet in position) or in the superficial veins (rapid refilling abolished by use of the tourniquet) (Ackroyd et al., 1984).

DOPPLER ASSESSMENTS

Doppler ultrasound transducers with pencil-sized probes operating at 5–10 MHz can be used pre- and perioperatively to detect flow. Modern machines will indicate not only velocity of flow but also direction and can thus be used accurately to locate solitary arteriovenous fistulae or small patches of microfistulae (Pisko-Dubienski et al., 1975). These units can demonstrate rapid flow in outflow veins with a typical machinery hum distinguishable from the biphasic arterial sound or the normal venous hum. The Doppler ultrasound unit can also demonstrate reverse flow in arteries distal to the malformation. The Doppler technique is, however, not good at sequential quantitative assessment. It does, nonetheless, have the virtue of inexpensiveness and portability and, in addition, sterilized probes may be used intraoperatively by the surgeon to locate arteriovenous communications at the time of operation. It does not, however, follow that therapeutic advantage will be the result. The extent and complexity of microfistulous communications are such that an operation cannot be based on the extirpation of specifically identified arteriovenous fistulae (Szilagyi et al., 1976).

Real time Doppler ultrasound is an evolving technique whereby flow in deeply placed vessels may be assessed. At the present time, only large vessels can be studied (Fig. 8–2). Future technology will probably enable this

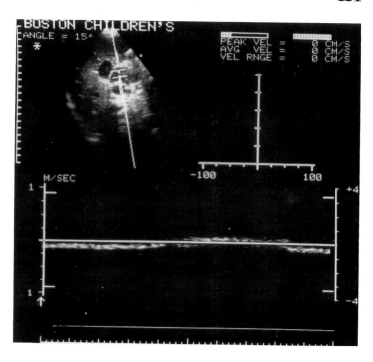

Figure 8–2. Doppler ultrasound study of a teenaged boy with a diffuse venous ectasia of limbs and intra-abdominal viscera. The cursor markers have bracketed the portal vein; the time against flow velocity line (seen below) shows indolent, to and fro flow within the vein. This gives a graphic representation of the hemodynamic status of this low-flow vascular malformation. (See Figure 18–5 for a photograph of this patient and additional ultrasonographic and computed tomographic evaluation.)

method to be used to judge flow in parenchymal structures.

RADIOLOGY

In addition to providing essential anatomical data about malformations, contrast radiology can yield hemodynamic information. Arteriography can demonstrate early venous filling and arterial enlargement, both hallmarks of arteriovenous fistulae. In the lower limbs, an intra-aortic injection allows comparison between the rates of venous filling in the two limbs. In other sites, early venous filling is more difficult to judge. It is hoped that newer techniques of digital angiography will improve the ability to localize and quantify arteriovenous fistulae and may, in particular, be sensitive to the "pooling" seen within complex malformations.

ISOTOPES

Isotopic techniques can be used to quantify the flow through arteriovenous shunts, to locate sites of thrombosis and blood loss, and to demonstrate venous and lymphatic anatomy.

Shunt Volume Measurements

Partsch and colleagues have developed a technique that uses controlled microembolization to judge the size of arteriovenous connections and flow through them (Partsch, 1974; Partsch, 1975). Macroaggregated albumen particles with a diameter greater than 10 microns will lodge in capillaries after injection. Particles of this size that bypass peripheral capillaries after intra-arterial injection may be assumed to have passed through arteriovenous shunts. If the macroaggregated albumen is isotopically labelled, the percentage of a given dose that is shunted can be measured. For example, if "shunt volumes" are to be measured in the lower limb, a dose of labelled macroaggregate is first injected into the femoral artery and the percentage of it that is initially measured in the lungs is a measure of the volume of the arteriovenous shunts (Fig. 8–3). The first injection is used merely for calibration.

The macroaggregated albumen subsequently breaks up in the capillaries and the isotopic marker slowly leaks through the capillaries, giving a second peak in the lungs. The amount of isotope that bypasses the peripheral capillary bed is a product of the size and number of the fistulae and the flow

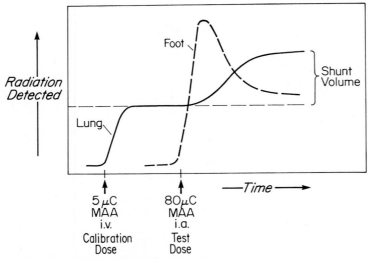

Figure 8–3. This illustrates the type of tracing that can be obtained using radioisotope labelled particles to determine the proportion of blood being shunted through arteriovenous connections. The radiation detected from the lung and from the foot is shown on the vertical axis; time is shown on the horizontal axis. Following a calibration dose of 5 μCi of radioiodine labelled macroaggregated albumin given intravenously, the count in the lung reaches a plateau level as the isotope is arrested in the pulmonary bed. Macroaggregated albumin (80 μCi) is then injected into the femoral artery of the limb under study. A rapid rise in radiation detected at the foot is seen as the particles impact in the peripheral capillary bed. Simultaneously, however, the pulmonary count rises and the foot count quickly falls

pari passu. These levels then plateau again before slowly decaying. Since the lungs have been calibrated with the initial dose, the amount of the second injected dose that has avoided lodgment in the peripheral capillary bed and passed through shunts to impact in the pulmonary bed can be calculated. The average shunt volume of normal subjects is 2.6 ± 0.4%. (Data from Lofferer, O., Mostbeck, A., and Portsch, H.: Zbl. Phlebol. 8:2, 1969.)

through them. It is thus of clinical value primarily where blood flow studies are not available or are unhelpful. The apparatus used in these isotope studies was simple, but more accurate results could be achieved by modern nuclear medicine equipment. Administration of different sized particles could be used to give more information about the size of the shunts. Lindemayr and colleagues found the "shunt volume" for normal subjects to range from 0 to 8% (Lindemayr et al., 1972).

Location of Areas of Thrombosis

When repeated thromboses occur in vascular malformations hematological abnormalities may be noted, but the presence of phleboliths in hematologically normal vascular malformations shows that thrombosis occurs even in these patients. The site of thrombosis in either type of patient can be identified and quantified by giving radiolabelled fibrinogen or radiolabelled macroaggregated albumen (Bentley et al., 1979). By this technique, it is also possible to map the extent of intralesional thrombosis occurring after therapeutic embolization. [125]I Fibrinogen is difficult to image, but ^{123}I fibrinogen has emission characteristics that allow pho-

toscans. Indium-labelled platelets can also be used to identify areas of platelet deposition in vascular anomalies (Schmidt and Lentle, 1984).

Location of Sites of Bleeding

Persistent or recurrent bleeding from gastrointestinal vascular malformations presents a difficult clinical problem, diagnostically, in situations in which the cause of recurrent iron deficient anemia may not be clear, and anatomically, in locating the level in the bowel at which hemorrhage is occurring. Barium studies are usually unhelpful, and selective mesenteric angiography is difficult and sometimes unrewarding. Endoscopy cannot visualize all the potential bleeding sites.

Angiography can only detect bleeding that occurs at a rate greater than 1 ml/min. Alavi (Alavi et al., 1977) has shown that scintigraphy can, in experimental animals, detect blood losses of 0.05–0.1 ml/min, and has found it to be more sensitive than angiography in patients (Alavi, 1980). He uses 99m-Tc sulfur colloid. The half-life of this agent is short (2–3 minutes), thus limiting its value. Labelling of red cells by 99m-Tc, as described by Pavel, avoids this problem, and images of the blood loss may be obtained for up to 24 hours, allowing preoperative localization of the bleeding point (Pavel et al., 1977; Markisz et al., 1982; Harvey et al., 1985) (Fig. 8–4).

Radionuclide Angiography

Veins

A crude assessment of the patency of deep veins can be obtained by gamma camera scanning during injection of radiolabelled macroaggregated albumen into a peripheral

vein. This is particularly useful for determining the hemodynamic significance of iliac vein compressions and for screening for the absence of deep veins in Klippel-Trenaunay syndrome (Buxton-Thomas et al., 1980). The technique does not replace contrast venography in the assessment of extensive venous malformations or prior to surgery (Fig. 8–5). Radionuclide angiography has also been used to assess vascular malformations of the spinal cord (Obayashi et al., 1980). Standard radionuclide angiography may not show localized

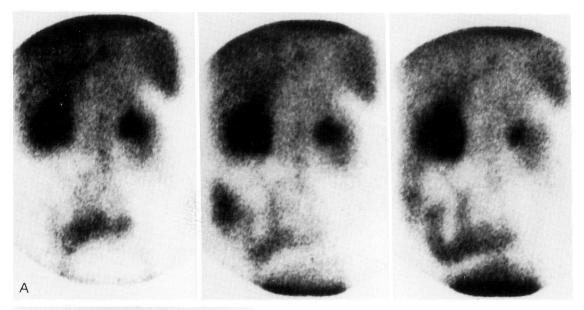

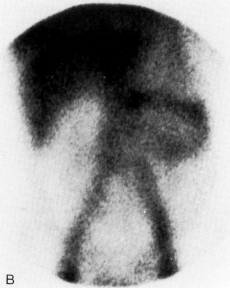

Figure 8–4. Technetium labelled red blood cell scintigraphy. *A,* Scintigraphic scans of a patient with bleeding from a vascular malformation in the cecum. The immediate scan (left) shows abnormal activity in the ileocecal region. The next scan at 10 minutes (center) shows the labelled blood passing along the ascending colon and retrogradely into the ileum. The third image at 20 minutes (right) shows labelled blood extending up to the hepatic flexure. *B,* Scintigraphic scan of a patient bleeding into the jejunum from a submucosal vascular anomaly taken 10 minutes after injection of labelled red cells. The liver, aorta, and iliac vessels are clearly shown, as is the blood that is extravasated into the upper jejunum. (Illustrations courtesy of Mr. M. H. Harvey, FRCS, and the Annals of the Royal College of Surgeons of England, 67:89, 1985.)

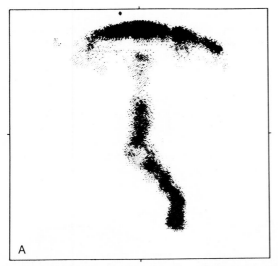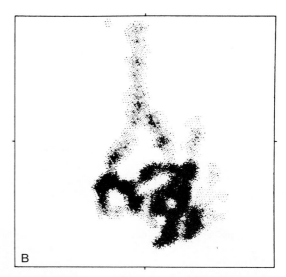

Figure 8–5. Dynamic radionuclide venography. *A,* The normal appearance of the iliac veins and vena cava following injection of 1 μCi of 99m-Tc human albumin microspheres into the veins of the left leg. *B,* The appearance of the pelvis, iliac veins, and vena cava in a patient with left iliac compression syndrome. Following injection of the isotope into the veins of the left leg, the pelvic cross collaterals are clearly demonstrated.

vascular lesions; indeed, they may show as "cold" areas. If the scintigraphic study is delayed by 1–2 hours, the lesion may be visualized by the slow-mixing between the blood pool and the blood in the malformation. This is known as "perfusion–blood pool mismatch" (Front et al., 1983).

Lymphatics

Both the function and the crude anatomy of the lymphatic system may be assessed by radioisotopes. In 1953, Sherman and Ter-Pogossian reported the diagnostic potential of radioactive colloid gold (^{198}Au) (Sherman and Ter-Pogossian, 1953). Subsequent assessment confirmed that pelvic and abdominal lymph nodes could be effectively imaged by this technique, and the range has been expanded to include the internal mammary glands. The technique has been developed with a view to identifying metastatic malignancy but is equally applicable to the investigation of vascular malformations. Colloidal substances injected intradermally or into subcutaneous tissues enter the lymphatics, are conveyed by direct transport or after phagocytosis, and lodge in the nodes. Isotopic labelling of the colloid allows both the clearance from the tissues to be measured quantitatively and the nodes subsequently to be imaged (Croll et al., 1983). A variety of

agents have been used, particularly 99m-Tc–labelled antimony sulfide (Fairbanks et al., 1972; Bergquist, 1983). Unfortunately, the images obtained are of poor quality, and nodes of less than 1 cm diameter are not visualized (Fig. 8–6*A*). Jackson and colleagues (1978) and Vieras and Boyd (1977) used the technique with benefit to investigate children with lymphedema. The technique has been shown to have a 100% specificity when used to identify lymphedema as a cause of limb edema and for distinguishing it from venous edema (Stewart et al., 1985) (Fig. 8–6*B*).

THERMOGRAPHY

All forms of vascular malformation dissipate substantial amounts of heat. Horton noted temperature increases of up to 6.5°C in areas affected by an arteriovenous fistula, and by a calorimetric technique he found a heat loss from a hand affected by an arteriovenous fistula to be 600 calories per minute, compared with the normal of 33 calories per minute (Horton, 1934). This heat loss may be mapped out by a thermoprobe, by a thermocamera, by heat sensitive plastic sheets, or by photographs taken with infrared sensitive film (Fig. 8–7). The pictures thus achieved are often impressive but are only of limited clinical value, firstly because they do not reliably differentiate between arteriovenous and purely venous anomalies, and secondly because the areas of heat loss do not correspond accurately with the anatomical lesion, as "hot" arterial blood is dissipated into essentially normal parts of the circulation.

BLOOD GAS ANALYSIS

A raised partial pressure of oxygen in the venous effluent from a limb or particular area might be expected to signify the presence of arteriovenous fistulae, but our experience has shown blood gas analysis to be largely unhelpful. This is particularly true when it is used to demonstrate hypoactive arteriovenous fistulae, as the femoral vein partial pressure of oxygen is raised in a variety of conditions, including non-congenital varicose veins in which no definite arteriovenous fistulae can be demonstrated. Szilagyi is, however, enthusiastic about this test (Szilagyi et al., 1976). If blood gas analysis is to be used, great care must be taken in the process of sampling. Blood must be taken from a vein in the immediate area of the malformation and compared with truly systemic blood taken from another limb at approximately the same time.

BIOPSY

In general, biopsy is not necessary for the evaluation and management of vascular anomalies. There are rare instances in which a sarcoma must be ruled out and unique cases in which clinical evaluation may be insufficient to make a diagnosis, e.g., the "angiokeratomas" and certain dermal lymphaticovenous anomalies. Physical examination and careful history usually suffice to differentiate a true hemangioma from a vascular malformation (Finn et al., 1983). Clinical and, if necessary, radiologic assessment permits subdivision of a particular vascular malformation into either a low flow (capillary, venous, or lymphatic) or a high flow (arteriovenous) category.

Biopsy of a port-wine stain shows dilated channels in the papillary dermis (Fig. 8–8A).

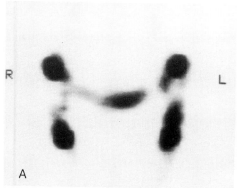

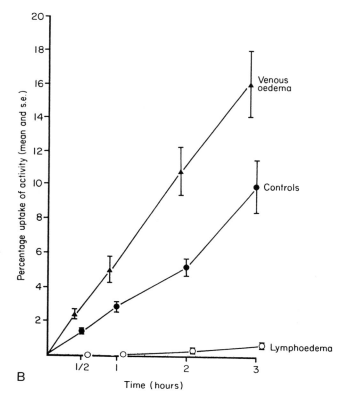

Figure 8–6. Scintilymphography. *A,* This is the 30 minute image of a normal subject following subcutaneous injection of 80 MBq of technetium labelled rhenium sulfide colloid. Although the anatomical visualization of the femoral and iliac nodes is poor, the fact that the nodes are filled half an hour after injection shows good lymph flow up the limb. The dark area between the nodes is the bladder. *B,* An isotope lymphography study measures uptake of peripherally injected 99m-Tc rhenium sulfide by ilioinguinal nodes and successfully distinguishes between venous edema (10 limbs), lymphedema (34 limbs) and controls (10 limbs). (From Stewart, G., Gaunt, J. I., Croft, T. N., and Browse, N. L.: Isotope lymphography. Brit. J. Surg. 72:906, 1985.)

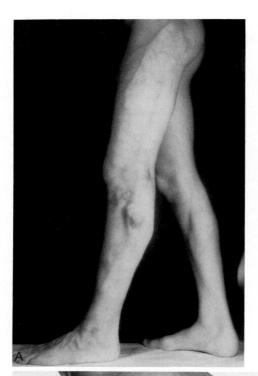

Figure 8–7. Thermography. *A,* The clinically difficult to identify lateral venous anomalies in the leg of this patient with Klippel-Trenaunay syndrome are clearly seen on an infrared photograph. *B,* The extent of this patient's venous malformation as seen with conventional photography. *C,* It is more clearly seen using infrared photography. Modern thermocameras are more sensitive but give anatomically less useful information.

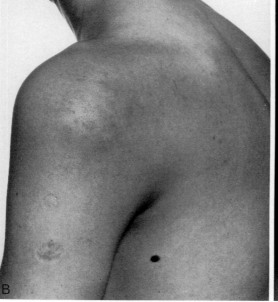

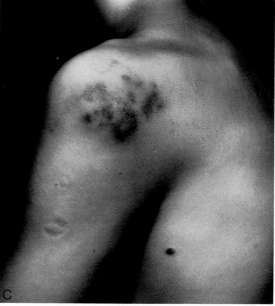

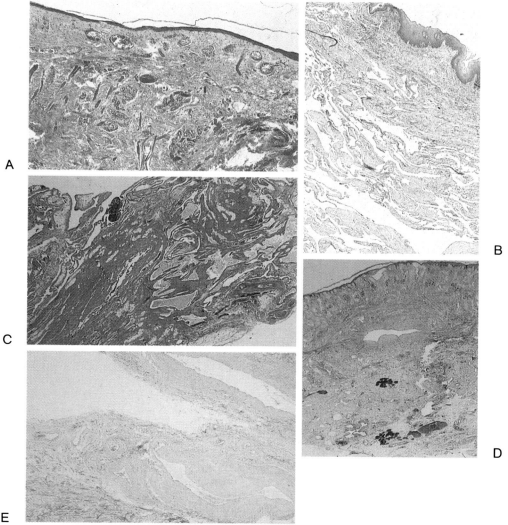

Figure 8–8. Histologic patterns of vascular malformations. *A, Capillary*: Surgical specimen of a port-wine stain excised from the face of a 19 year old female. Note the thin-walled vessels (capillary-venular size) in the upper dermis (H & E × 25). *B, Venous*: An 18 year old male with an extensive cutaneous low-flow anomaly. Note the large serpiginous channels, both thick and thin walls, very little muscle, and a lining of a single endothelial layer (H & E × 25). *C, Lymphatic*: Surgical specimen from a 1 year old boy with a cystic cervical lymphatic malformation. There are irregular, variably sized channels with thick and thin walls, sparse smooth muscle, and differing amounts of collagen. Lymphoid aggregates are also seen (H & E × 25). *D, Combined capillary-lymphatic-venous*: Skin from a distal amputation necessary in a child with Klippel-Trenaunay syndrome. There are dilated, thick-walled channels throughout the dermis and subcutaneous fat; some are blood-filled (veins), whereas others contain proteinaceous material (lymphatics). A large dysmorphic thick-walled channel is seen in the center of the field. Lymphoid aggregates and dermal fibrosis are also seen (H & E × 10). *E, Arteriovenous*: This malformation first appeared in the scalp of a 24 year old female during her second pregnancy. A dysmorphic artery is seen in the center of the field; there are multiple, large and small sclerotic veins (H & E × 25).

These thin-walled vessels become progressively ectatic with age.

Histologic examination of a venous malformation (Fig. 8–8*B*) demonstrates dilated channels, varying from capillary to cavernous dimensions. There is sparse smooth muscle and adventitial fibrosis in the larger anomalous channels. Organizing thrombi are frequently seen with dystrophic calcification (phleboliths). Lymphatic anomalies (Fig. 8–8*C*) are histologically similar to venous lesions; they frequently occur in combination (Fig. 8–8*D*). Lymphatic malformations present a wide spectrum: cystic spaces surrounded by fibromuscular thickening; honeycombed, thin-walled channels; or tiny vascular slits. The channels vary in size within the same lesion and usually contain pale eosinophilic material and a few red blood cells, which are probably artifacts. The endothelial lining in all vascular malformations is flat and shows no evidence of proliferation (Mulliken and Glowacki, 1982).

Tissue from an arteriovenous anomaly (Fig. 8–8*E*) demonstrates close juxtaposition of medium sized arteries and veins and vessels of indeterminate nature. Intimal thickening of veins suggests elevated pressure within the vasculature, the so-called "arterialized" veins. It is difficult, using routine hematoxylin and eosin staining, to determine whether any particular abnormal vascular channel is part of the original (primary) malformation or is secondarily altered because of increased flow and pressure.

HEMATOLOGICAL ASSESSMENT

Vascular malformations may have associated hemostatic abnormalities. Although this association is often called "Kasabach-Merritt syndrome" in the literature, it is different from the profound thrombocytopenia and giant hemangioma of infancy that were originally reported by Kasabach and Merritt (Kasabach and Merritt, 1940). The bleeding disorder often seen, particularly with venous malformations, is a localized consumptive coagulopathy with a normal or moderately decreased platelet count (usually in the 50,000–100,000/mm³ range) (Gilon et al., 1959; Blix and Aas, 1961; Hillman and Phillips, 1967; Lee and Kirk, 1967; Inceman and Tangün, 1969; Rodriguez-Erdmann et al., 1971;

Straub et al., 1972; Jona et al., 1974; Lang and Dubin, 1975; Phillippe et al., 1980; Neidhart and Roach, 1982).

Stasis within a low flow anomaly is probably the primary event that initiates fibrin generation. There may also be associated fibrinolysis as a result of plasminogen activation. Fibrinogen is taken up in the area of abnormal blood vessels (Hillman and Phillips, 1967; Rodriguez-Erdmann et al., 1971; Jona et al., 1974), where fibrin strands form, damaging platelets and decreasing levels of clotting factors and leading to a systemic hemorrhagic state. This complication should be considered in any patient with a vascular malformation who has a history of excessive bleeding or recurrent local thromboses. Appropriate laboratory evaluation should include a complete blood count with examination of the peripheral blood smear for evidence of microangiopathy; and clotting studies, looking for mild thrombocytopenia, increased prothrombin and partial thromboplastin times, diminished fibrinogen levels, and increased fibrin degradation products and fibrinopeptide levels. Because a low grade, well compensated consumptive coagulopathy can be exacerbated by stresses such as surgery (Gilon et al., 1959; Inceman and Tangün, 1969; Rodriguez-Erdmann et al., 1971; Lang and Dubin, 1975; Phillippe et al., 1980), it is necessary to evaluate the coagulation status of these patients preoperatively and to follow them closely after the surgical procedure. The ideal perioperative management of these patients is not clear, although a number of authors have used heparin therapy to normalize the fibrinogen level and improve hemostasis. It is most important to be aware that hemorrhage is a potential complication of a surgical procedure in these patients, even if the procedure is at a site distant from the actual malformation.

References

Ackroyd, J., Baskerville, P., Young, A. E., and Browse, N. L.: Pathophysiology of Klippel-Trenaunay syndrome. Presented at Fifth International Workshop on Vascular Anomalies, Milan, 1984.

Alavi, A.: Scintigraphic demonstration of acute gastrointestinal bleeding. G.I. Radiol. 5:205, 1980.

Alavi, A., Dann, R. W., Baum, S., and Biery, D. N.: Scintigraphic detection of acute gastrointestinal bleeding. Radiology 124:753, 1977.

Bentley, P. G., Hill, P. C., DeHaas, J. A., et al.: Radionuclide venography in the management of proximal venous obstruction. A comparison with x-ray contrast venography. Brit. J. Radiol. *52*:289, 1979.

Bergquist, L., Strand, S. E., and Persson, B. R. R.: Particle sizing and biokinetics of interstitial lymphoscintigraphic agents. Seminars Nucl. Med. *13*:9, 1983.

Bertelsen, A., and Dohn, K.: Congenital arteriovenous communications of the extremities. Clinical and pathophysiological investigations. Acta Chir. Scand. *105*:448, 1953.

Blix, S., and Aas, K.: Giant hemangioma, thrombocytopenia, fibrinogenopenia, and fibrinolytic activity. Acta Med. Scand. *169*:63, 1961.

Bollinger, A., Vogt, B., Lüthy, E., and Hegglin, R.: Flow measurements in patients with multiple arteriovenous fistulas of the extremities. Helvetica Med. Acta *33*:76, 1966.

Branham, A. A.: Aneurysmal varix of the femoral artery and vein following a gunshot wound. Internat. J. Surg. *3*:250, 1890.

Buxton-Thomas, M. S., Tonge, C. M., and Croft, D. N.: A dynamic radioisotope technique for assessing pelvic venous abnormalities. Nuc. Med. Communications *1*:66, 1980.

Croll, M. N., Brady, L. W., and Dadparvar, S.: Implications of lymphoscintigraphy in oncologic practice: Principles and differences vis-a-vis other imaging modalities. Seminars Nucl. Med. *13*:4, 1983.

Fairbanks, V. F., Tauxe, W. N., Kiely, J. B., and Miller, W. E.: Scintigraphic visualization of abdominal lymph nodes with 99m-Tc pertechnetate labelled sulfur colloid. J. Nucl. Med. *13*:185, 1972.

Finn, M. D., Glowacki, J., and Mulliken, J. B.: Congenital vascular lesions: Clinical application of a new classification. J. Ped. Surg. *18*:894, 1983.

Front, D., Israel, O., Joachims, H. Z., Brown, Y., and Eliachar, I.: Evaluation of hemangiomas with technetium 99m–labelled red blood cells. The perfusion–blood pool mismatch. JAMA *249*:1488, 1983.

Gilon, E., Ramot, B., and Sheba, C.: Multiple hemangiomata associated with thrombocytopenia: Remarks on the pathogenesis of the thrombocytopenia in this syndrome. Blood *14*:74, 1959.

Harvey, M. H., Neoptolemos, J. P., Watkin, E. M., et al.: Technetium labelled red blood cell scintigraphy in the diagnosis of intestinal hemorrhage. Ann. Roy. Coll. Surg. Engl. *67*:89, 1985.

Hillman, R. S., and Phillips, L. L.: Clotting-fibrinolysis in a cavernous hemangioma. Amer. J. Dis. Child. *113*:649, 1967.

Horton, B. T.: Some medical aspects of congenital arteriovenous fistulae: Report of 38 cases. Proc. Staff Meet. Mayo Clin. *9*:460, 1934.

Inceman, S., and Tangün, Y.: Chronic defibrination syndrome due to giant hemangioma associated with microangiopathic hemolytic anemia. Am. J. Med. *46*:997, 1969.

Jackson, F. I., Bowen, P., and Lentle, B. C.: Scintilymphangiography with 99m Tc–antimony sulfide colloid in hereditary lymphedema. Clin. Nuc. Med. *3*:296, 1978.

Jona, J. Z., Kwaan, H. C., Bjelan, M., and Raffensperger, J. G.: Disseminated intravascular coagulation after excision of giant hemangioma. Am. J. Surg. *127*:588, 1974.

Kasabach, H. H., and Merritt, K. K.: Capillary hemangioma with extensive purpura. Amer. J. Dis. Child. *59*:1063, 1940.

Lang, P. G., and Dubin, H. V.: Hemangioma-thrombocytopenia syndrome. Arch. Dermatol. *111*:105, 1975.

Lee, J. H., and Kirk, R. F.: Pregnancy associated with giant hemangiomata, thrombocytopenia, and fibrinogenopenia (Kasabach-Merritt syndrome). Report of a case. Obst. Gyn. *29*:24, 1967.

Lindemayr, W., Lofferer, O., Mostbeck, A., and Partsch, H.: Arteriovenous shunts in primary varicosis? A critical essay. Vasc. Surg. *6*:9, 1972.

Lofferer, O., Mostbeck, A., and Partsch, H.: Arteriovenöse Kurzschlüsse der Extremitäten nuclearmedizinische Untersuchungen mit besonderer Berücksichtigung des postthrombotischen Unterschenkelgeschwürs. Zbl. Phlebol. *8*:2, 1969.

Markisz, J. A., Front, D., Royal, H. D.. et al.: An evaluation of 99mTc–labelled red blood cell scintigraphy for the detection and localization of gastrointestinal bleeding sites. Gastroenterology *83*:394, 1982.

Matas, R.: On the systemic or cardiovascular effects of arteriovenous fistulae. Trans. South. Surg. Assn. *36*:623, 1923.

Miles, C., and Nicolaides, A. N.: Photoplethysmography principles and development. In Yao, J. S. (ed.): *Investigation of Vascular Disorders.* New York: Churchill Livingstone, 1981, p. 501.

Mulliken, J. B., and Glowacki, J.: Hemangiomas and vascular malformations in infants and children: A classification based on endothelial characteristics. Plast. Reconstr. Surg. *69*:412, 1982.

Neidhart, J. A., and Roach, R. W.: Successful treatment of skeletal hemangioma and Kasabach-Merritt syndrome with aminocaproic acid. Am. J. Med. *73*:434, 1982.

Nicoladoni, C.: Phlebectasie der rechten oberen extremität. Arch. Klin. Chir. *18*:252, 1875.

Nogren, L.: Functional evaluation of chronic venous insufficiency by foot volumetry. Acta Chir. Scand. Suppl. *444*:1–46, 1974.

Obayashi, T., Furuse, M., and Nakama, M.: Radionuclide angiography of vascular lesions of the spinal cord. Its efficacy in selecting patients for spinal angiography. Arch. Neurol. *37*:572, 1980.

Partsch, H.: Venenverschlussplethysmographie und Doppler-Sondenuntersuchung als Suchmethoden zum Nachweis von AV-Fisteln bei gemischten Angiodysplasien der Extremitäten. VASA *3*:39, 1974.

Partsch, H., Lofferer, O., and Mostbeck, A.: Zur Diagnostik von arteriovenösen Fisteln bei Angiodysplasien der Extremitäten. VASA *4*:288, 1975.

Pavel, D. G., Zimmer, A. M., and Patterson, V. N.: In vivo labelling of red blood cells with 99mTc: A new approach to blood pool visualization. J. Nucl. Med. *18*:305, 1977.

Phillippe, M., Acker, D., and Frigoletto, F. D.: Pregnancy complicated by the Kasabach-Merritt syndrome. Ob. Gyn. *56*:256, 1980.

Pisko-Dubienski, Z. A., Baird, R. J., Wilson, D. R., et al.: Identification and successful treatment of congenital microfistulas with the aid of directional Doppler. Surgery *78*:564, 1975.

Rodriguez-Erdmann, F., Button, L., Murray, J. E., and Moloney, W. C.: Kasabach-Merritt syndrome: coaguloanalytical observations. Am. J. Med. Sci. *261*:9, 1971.

Schmidt, R. P., and Lentle, B. C.: Hemangioma with consumptive coagulopathy (Kasabach-Merritt syndrome) detection by indium-111 oxine-labelled platelets. Clin. Nuc. Med. *9*:389, 1984.

Sherman, A. I., and Ter-Pogossian, M.: Lymph-node concentration of radioactive colloidal gold following interstitial injection. Cancer *6*:1238, 1953.

Stewart, G., Gaunt, J. I., Croft, D. N., and Browse, N. L.: Isotope lymphography: A new method of investigating the role of the lymphatics in chronic limb oedema. Brit. J. Surg. *72*:906, 1985.

Straub, P. W., Kessler, S., Schreiber, A., and Frick, P. G.: Chronic intravascular coagulation in Kasabach-Merritt syndrome. Arch. Intern. Med. *129*:475, 1972.

Szilagyi, D. E., Smith, R. F., Elliott, J. P., and Hageman, J. H.: Congenital arteriovenous anomalies of the limbs. Arch. Surg. *111*:423, 1976.

Vieras, F., and Boyd, C. M.: Radionuclide lymphangiography in the evaluation of pediatric patients with lower limb edema. J. Nucl. Med. *18*:441, 1977.

Yao, S. T., Needham, T. N., Lewis, J. B., and Hobbs, J. T.: Limb blood flow in congenital arteriovenous fistula. Surgery *73*:80, 1973.

CHAPTER NINE

Radiological Assessment of Vascular Malformations

M. Lea Thomas

Vascular malformations present a wide range of abnormalities, from small and insignificant capillary nevi to large and hemodynamically important arteriovenous fistulae. Classification of this vast range of lesions has proved extremely difficult because of the varied embryological, pathological, and angiographic features. In this chapter, the author uses the anatomical classification used throughout this text, which, of necessity, includes a number of eponymous syndromes. Only those syndromes in which there are lesions that may be usefully demonstrated by medical imaging are discussed. Many cutaneous vascular stains do not have additional associated abnormalities of the arteries, veins, or lymphatics.

From the point of view of the angiologist, the exact diagnosis of the lesion or syndrome is often not of great importance, as this is based on clinical and other observations. The object of angiography and other forms of diagnostic imaging is to show the extent and composition of the lesion to help in the diagnosis, prognosis, and management. For instance, it is important to know whether a given malformation is primarily arterial, venous, arteriovenous, or lymphatic in nature. In addition, the presence or absence of an effect on non-vascular components such as fat, soft tissues, and bone affects treatment.

Angiography is the main method of investigating congenital vascular malformations and therefore is discussed in most detail. However, other imaging techniques, such as plain films, digital subtraction angiography (DSA), ultrasound (US), computed tomography (CT), and magnetic resonance imaging (MRI), are mentioned briefly where they are considered contributory.

PLAIN RADIOGRAPHY

Plain radiographs of the affected extremity or part of the patient may be useful in showing soft tissue masses and associated abnormalities of the skeletal system (Young, 1978; Dahl and Tollefsen, 1980; Boyd et al., 1984). The clinically abnormal extremity and the normal one should be radiographed so that a comparison can be made (Figs. 9–1 to 9–3).

Fat is the most translucent of the body tissues shown by radiography and a fatty tumor may appear to be well circumscribed, suggesting that it could easily be removed surgically, or to be infiltrating into the muscle planes, so that a more complicated excision would be necessary. Phleboliths are frequently a feature primarily of venous malformations and may, from their site and extent, be a useful guide to the size of a lesion (Fig. 9–4). Bones adjacent to or involved by a vascular malformation may show rarefaction (Fig. 9–5).

Accurate measurement of bone length and girth is a useful parameter in deciding on immediate management and also as a follow-up procedure. Scannography is the term

141

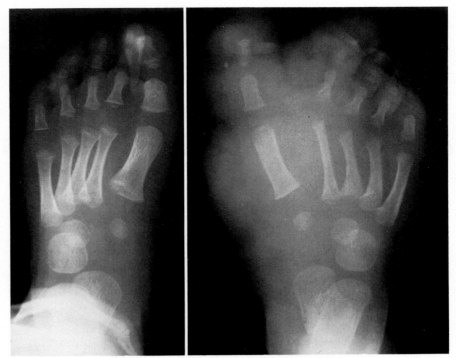

Figure 9–1. The right hand panel shows considerable soft tissue hypertrophy of the foot in a patient with a primarily venous malformation. The bones are a little osteoporotic but otherwise normal. The left hand panel shows the normal foot for comparison.

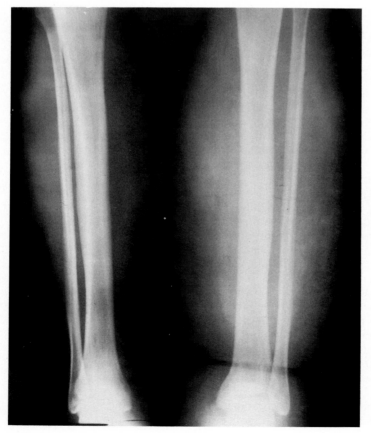

Figure 9–2. The left leg shows soft tissue hypertrophy in the calf, which was present throughout the whole limb. The patient has a combined venous and lymphatic malformation.

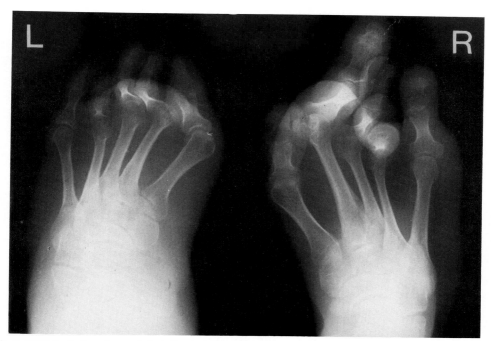

Figure 9–3. Both feet show bone deformity, but the right foot demonstrates localized gigantism of the second toe. Such bone deformities commonly occur in combined lymphaticovenous vascular malformations.

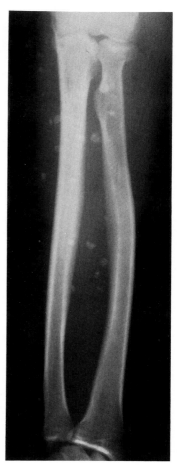

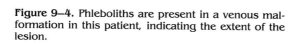

Figure 9–4. Phleboliths are present in a venous malformation in this patient, indicating the extent of the lesion.

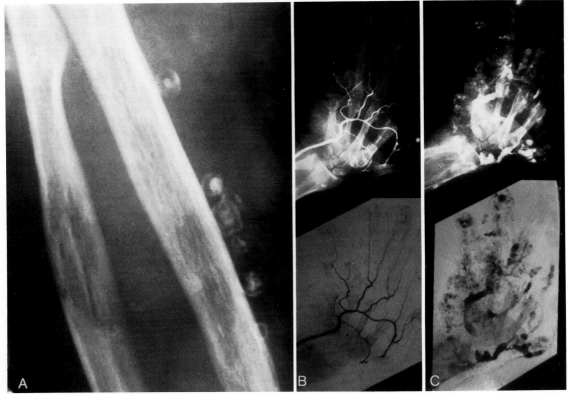

Figure 9–5. *A,* Phleboliths and soft tissue enlargement give an indication as to the size of this arteriovenous malformation. There is some rarefaction of the bones adjacent to the lesion. *B,* Arteriography identifies the arteriovenous fistulae and its venous phase. *C,* The ectatic venous system.

used for this radiographic technique. The simplest method for bone measurement is to place the affected limb, with the opposite one for comparison, on a 2 cm square wire grid that thus has the same magnification as the limb being examined; measurements are made directly from the resulting radiographs (Fig. 9–6).

ANGIOGRAPHY

Contrast angiography is the most important, and likely to remain the most important, method of investigating vascular malformations and may be the only method of diagnosing deep-seated lesions such as those in the viscera or within the skull.

The introduction in recent years of low osmolality contrast media, i.e., ioxaglate, iopamidol, and iohexol, which are virtually painless on injection, are non-thrombogenic, and have fewer allergic and other side effects, has made these investigations much safer and better tolerated. In addition, general anesthesia is virtually unnecessary except in very small children (Grainger, 1980; Lea Thomas and Briggs, 1984).

For these reasons, in the author's view, low osmolality media should *always* be used for investigating vascular malformations.

Angiography indicates the extent of the vascular involvement, shows the feeding and draining vessels, and influences the initial treatment and the response to treatment. Angiography has value in the diagnosis of lesions with atypical presentation and may allow a distinction between hemangiomas and malformations. Hemangiomas appear as organized, gland-like vascular neoplasms with vessels and a staining "parenchymal" component; malformations consist of collections of abnormal vessels without a "parenchymal" mass (Burrows et al., 1983).

Angiography has recently become a primary therapeutic method, with various techniques for embolization, thrombosis, and occlusion being employed, which are discussed in detail in Chapter Twenty-One.

Arteriography

The technique for arteriography varies with the type of lesion being investigated. In principal, it consists of the injection of contrast medium into an artery at a distance from the lesion so that supplying arteries are not missed, followed by selective catheterization to delineate the type of anomaly and its extent. Fast filming, at least 3–6 films per second, is essential to record anatomical detail, particularly if arteriovenous fistulae are suspected. A serial film changer or cine radiography may be used. The contrast material should be injected as a bolus to avoid mixing of the arterial and venous phases, which may simulate arteriovenous shunting. Hand injections are satisfactory for selective injections, but for larger arteries and when small catheters are used, a pump capable of delivering the contrast medium at 15–25 ml per second is required. The amount of contrast material used and its iodine content have to be judged by the size and position of the lesion being investigated. In infants and children and in the thinner parts of the adult patient contrast medium containing 200–300 mg/ml of iodine is satisfactory, but in the larger body parts more concentrated media are needed.

Phlebography

With venous malformations, the state of the deep venous system plays an important part in the management. A meticulous technique of ascending, descending, and other forms of phlebography is required to show the deep veins. Tight ankle tourniquets are needed to occlude the superficial veins in order to direct the contrast medium into the deep venous system; otherwise, erroneous diagnoses of absent deep veins can be made. If the percutaneous technique is not successful, intraosseous phlebography is sometimes necessary, as the deep veins adjacent to the bone marrow injected always fill if they are patent (Fig. 9–7). Also, intraosseous phlebography may be the most convenient method of demonstrating a vascular anomaly at an inaccessible site (Fig. 9–8).

In superficial and localized venous dysplasias, direct injection into the lesion with a fine needle is often the simplest way of showing the extent of the anomaly and its ramifications and connections before surgical removal (Fig. 9–9). In this respect, low osmolality contrast media are particularly useful, as they do not cause localized pain when injected and do not result in subsequent thrombophlebitis.

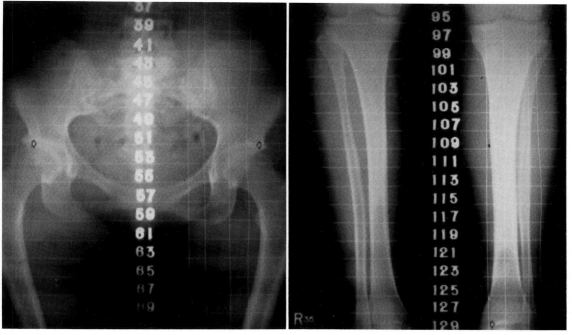

Figure 9–6. From the two centimeter square grid placed beneath the patients' limbs, the length and girth of the bones can be measured. In this patient with Klippel-Trenaunay syndrome, there is slight elongation of the left leg and also some soft tissue enlargement.

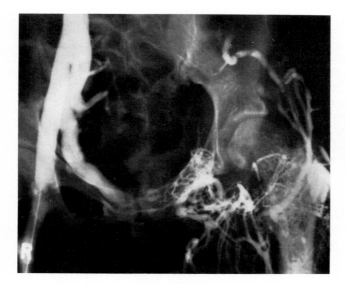

Figure 9–7. There is total occlusion of the external and common iliac veins on the left, shown conclusively by intraosseous pertrochanteric phlebography. This is the most reliable method of showing the integrity of the deep venous system.

In the more extensive angiodysplasias, injection into a feeding artery with follow-through to the venous phase (arteriophlebography) may be the only way of showing the extent of the abnormality (Figs. 9–10 and 9–11). Subtraction films to enhance the image may be used to improve definition (Fig. 9–12).

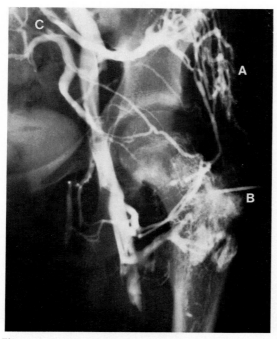

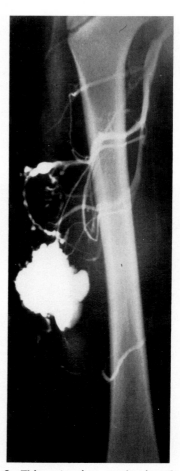

Figure 9–8. This deep malformation in the buttock (A) is most easily shown by a pertrochanteric intraosseous injection (B). The malformation drains to the internal iliac system (C).

Figure 9–9. This extensive, predominantly venous malformation of the wrist and hand is exhibited by arterial injection with a follow-through (arteriophlebography). The ulnar artery remains filled in this phase and can be seen to be a little small and certainly not enlarged. This is not an arteriovenous malformation.

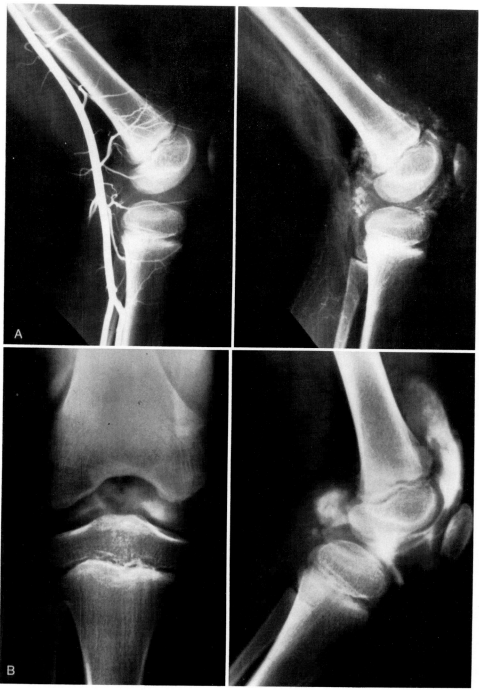

Figure 9–10. Arteriogram of a malformation of the knee. *A,* The left hand panel is the arterial phase, and the right hand panel shows the venous phase. The main femoral and popliteal arteries are not enlarged, but there are a few more branches from the artery supplying the lesion. This is a predominantly venous malformation involving the knee joint, as seen during the venous phase. *B,* An arthrogram of the same patient shows the filling defects caused by the venous malformation extending into the knee joint and into the suprapatellar pouch.

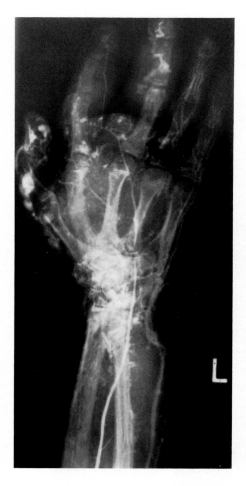

Figure 9–11. An extensive venous malformation of the wrist and hand shown by arteriography. In this late phase, the ulnar artery and some branches are still filled and can be seen to be normal in size, i.e., this is not an arteriovenous malformation.

Digital Subtraction Angiography (DSA)

Photographic subtraction has been used for many years as an adjunct to arteriography (Fig. 9–12). In 1934, Ziedes des Plantes pointed out that image subtraction could be used to separate contrast material density from those produced by bone or other surrounding structures with a resulting much clearer definition of the contrast filled vessel (Ziedes des Plantes, 1934). The use of video techniques and digital processing has made it possible to obtain dynamic computer subtracted visualization of the arterial tree, known as digital subtraction angiography (DSA). The main advantage of DSA is that because of the high contrast resolution obtainable, the arterial tree can be visualized by intravenous injections. This is particularly useful in outpatients. However, the non-selective arteriograms obtained may be difficult to interpret because of overlap of adjacent vessels. Selective arteriography using small volumes of contrast medium and very small catheters is possible, but the dangers of arterial injections, dissection by guide wires, thrombus formation and dislodgment, and hematoma formation remain. The higher incidence of allergic reactions to venous injections than to arterial ones (Rose, 1983) is not applicable to non-ionic contrast media, and the amount of contrast used becomes limited by cost rather than by safety and the comfort of the patient.

The main disadvantage of DSA is the very poor spatial resolution compared with the conventional film-screen combination, and it is frequently not sufficiently diagnostic for use in management unless supplemented by conventional angiography. Technical improvements are occurring frequently, but the inferior image quality is likely to remain (Neiman, 1985).

Thus it may well be that venous DSA should be the first investigation of a vascular anomaly to show its vascular nature and size and to give some indication about feeding arteries and draining veins, and then followed by detailed selective arteriography or phlebography according to the nature of the lesion (Fig. 9–13).

Lymphography

Because of the complex nature of many vascular malformations, associated lymphatic anomalies are frequently found.

Lymphography by the Kinmonth technique (Kinmonth, 1982), usually bipedal or of the arms, if affected, together with injections into skin vesicles, cysts, lymphoceles, or other cavities in the limb or trunk, may be required (Fig. 9–14). Before lymphography is undertaken, an injection of 0.2–0.5 ml of 10% patent blue dye is made into the web spaces or other distal structure. The purpose of this is to identify the lymphatics for cannulation. Development of surface reticulation

shows lymphatic distension but does not indicate the cause (Fig. 9–15). When a distal lymphatic cannot be identified and it is considered important to obtain a lymphangiogram, a regional lymph node may be exposed surgically and contrast material injected directly into it or into an efferent or afferent lymphatic vessel (Fig. 9–16). Successful peripheral injection lymphography allows visualization of the pelvic and retroperitoneal lymphatics and the thoracic duct. The anatomy of the lymph nodes is readily demonstrated on "lymphadenograms" taken at any time from a day to several years after the injection lymphography if an oily contrast medium has been used. In predominantly venous malformations, lymphatic hypoplasia or aplasia is the most common finding (Fig. 9–17); in mainly arteriovenous lesions, lymphatic hyperplasia is most frequent (see Fig. 9–16). In combined lymphaticovenous anomalies, there is no constant pattern and the lymphatics may be normal, aplastic, or hypoplastic (Kinmonth et al., 1976; O'Donnell, 1977).

Computed tomography can be useful in

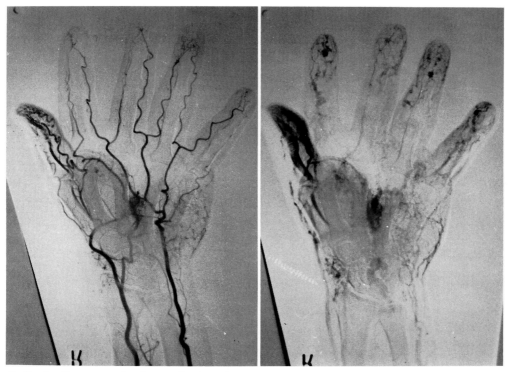

Figure 9–12. Another example of a predominantly venous anomaly of the hand and fingers, shown best by arteriography with subtraction. The left hand panel shows that the arteries are of normal size, and the right hand panel shows the venous phase.

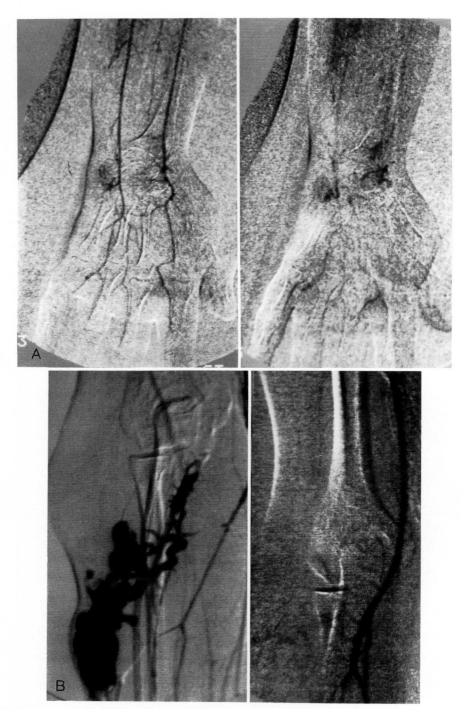

Figure 9–13. Examples of digital subtraction angiography (DSA). *A*, The left hand panel shows the arterial phase and indicates that the arteries are of normal size; the right hand panel shows pooling in a venous anomaly in the region of the wrist. *B*, The left hand panel shows an extensive venous malformation of the forearm. In the right hand panel the brachial artery is of normal size, indicating that this is not primarily an arteriovenous malformation. The spatial resolution is poor, but the examinations demonstrate the predominant nature of the lesion.

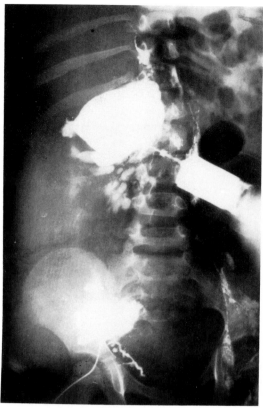

Figure 9–14. In this predominantly lymphatic malformation, semi-independent lymph cavities have been filled by separate injections into the abdomen. The lymphatic cisterns fill the right side of the pelvis and abdomen; these were later removed surgically.

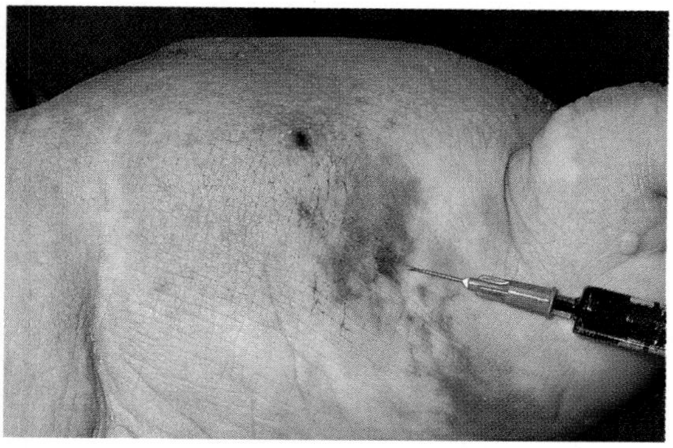

Figure 9–15. Injection of patent blue dye into the dermis of the foot with edema shows backflow into dermal lymphatics, indicating proximal lymphatic inadequacy. In this patient, a dermal capillary stain can also be seen.

Figure 9–16. Another patient undergoing investigation of lymphedema; the patent blue dye has been injected subdermally, and a femoral lymph node has been exposed surgically. The dye indicates a solitary lymphatic channel that is cannulated.

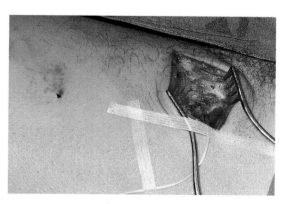

151

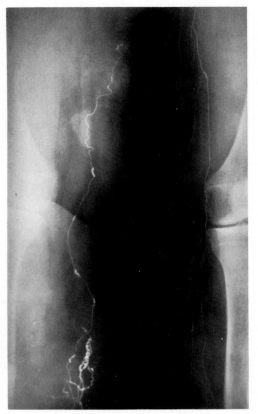

Figure 9-17. A lymphangiogram showing lymphatic hypoplasia with a solitary afferent lymphatic at the inguinal level. This patient has a combined venous-lymphatic malformation.

measuring the extent of lymphedema before or after reducing operations (Stewart et al., 1984). Lymphedema shows as multiple branching, non-enhancing, tubular structures in an enlarged subcutaneous tissue compartment.

Other Imaging Techniques

Other techniques for imaging vascular malformations include ultrasound, computed tomography, radioisotopes, and magnetic resonance. None of these methods is the definitive way of investigating vascular anomalies, but they may give some indication of the nature of a malformation, such as its size, outline, position, and tissue content and whether it is largely cystic or solid. From these findings, the most appropriate form of angiography can be initiated. Sonography is probably most useful in intravisceral malformations, where they appear as hyper- or hypoechoic masses compared with surrounding structures. In arteriovenous fistulae, appearances resembling those of angiography may be seen with enlarged feeding and draining vessels. In real time, pulsations may be appreciated. Doppler ultrasound may be useful in the analysis and measurement of blood flow in an artery supplying a malformation. Computed tomography may help in delineating angiodysplasias, whether in the viscera, the soft tissues, or the extremities (Christenson and Gunterberg, 1985). Because of the vascular nature of the lesions, contrast enhancement is particularly useful (Fig. 9-18). Radioisotope techniques may be useful in both functional and static imaging. In functional studies, blood flow can be estimated in real time; in static imaging, radioisotope techniques can be used to visualize malformations, especially when they are intravisceral in position.

Lastly, the position of magnetic resonance imaging in the diagnosis of angiodysplasias is at present uncertain, but it seems likely that because of its highly sensitive densitometry characteristics it will prove valuable in identifying the individual structures and tissues that compose a complex vascular malformation.

Angiography, however, remains the definitive method of assessing vascular malformations.

SPECIFIC VASCULAR MALFORMATIONS

As has already been pointed out, many vascular malformations are complex, and the heading of this section is intended to indicate the predominant abnormality in the particular lesion being discussed.

Arteriovenous Malformations

Congenital arteriovenous malformations are common in the central nervous system and are discussed in detail in Chapter Sixteen.

Unlike acquired arteriovenous malformations, which have a single communication, congenital ones have multiple channels, and for this reason very careful angiographic in-

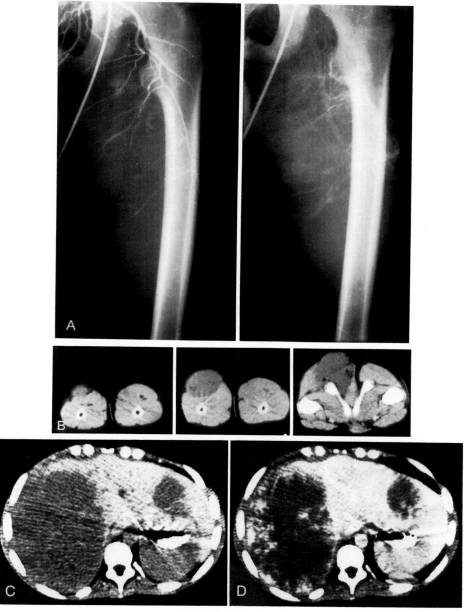

Figure 9–18. *A,* A selective arteriogram into the internal iliac artery on the left side shows that the malformation in the upper thigh is supplied by normal sized arteries; in the venous phase (right hand panel), the predominantly venous malformation is outlined by contrast medium. *B,* CT scan of the same patient, with contrast enhancement, shows that the lesion is situated posteriorly and extends from the mid-thigh to the buttock. The malformation, lying posteriorly, is slightly enhanced by the intravenous contast injection but is not as dense as would occur in an arteriovenous malformation. *C,* CT scan of the liver shows a large mass in the right lobe and a smaller one in the left. *D,* Intravenous contrast shows peripheral enhancement of the lesions shown in *C,* diagnostic of venous malformations. (Radiographs courtesy of Professor D. Allison, Royal Postgraduate Hospital.)

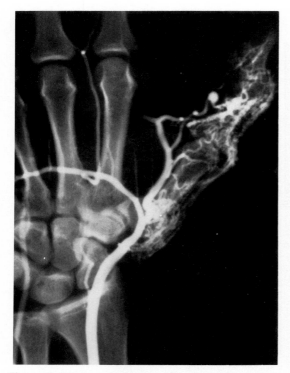

Figure 9–19. An arteriovenous malformation of the thumb, showing enlarged radial and digital arteries and also early venous filling. There is also a small aneurysm adjacent to the proximal phalanx. These are a common feature of arteriovenous malformations.

vestigation is required to show the many connections between the arteries and veins.

Arteriovenous malformations can occur literally in any region of the body, although the most common sites in the extremities are in the thigh, pelvis, arms, and hands (Erikson and Hemmingsson, 1973; Szilagyi et al., 1976; Griffin et al., 1978).

The congenital fistulae can range from capillary to macroscopic in size and can vary in appearance, number, extent, and behavior (Reinhoff, 1924). The arteriovenous fistulae, although usually small, have multiple parallel connections that can result in a large shunt.

Localized arteriovenous fistulae, sometimes called "cirsoid aneurysms," occur in skin, subcutaneous tissue, intramuscularly, or intraosseously. There are frequently associated cutaneous dysplasia, such as port-wine stains and other capillary malformations (Figs. 9–19 to 9–22).

The radiological signs of arteriovenous fistulae are early filling veins, dilated and tortuous arteries supplying the malformation, and varicose and dilated veins in the region of the fistulae. There is sometimes a localized mass, and phleboliths may be seen in plain radiographs. Arteriovenous fistulae invariably give rise to overgrowth of soft tissues and bones, as pointed out by Robertson (Robertson, 1956).

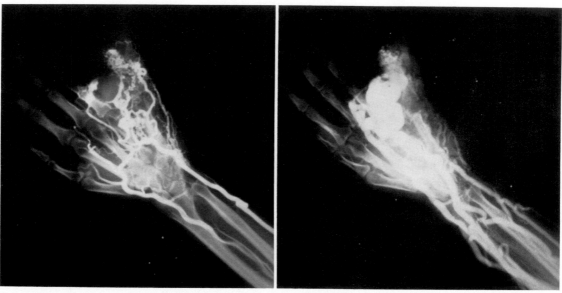

Figure 9–20. An extensive arteriovenous fistula of the ulnar aspect of the hand. Both the radial and ulnar arteries are enlarged, as is the palmar arch. Enlarged, tortuous arteries supply the malformation (left hand panel). There is early venous filling, and in the venous phase a dilated venous space can be seen (right hand panel). The index finger was amputated, but the remaining lesion re-expanded.

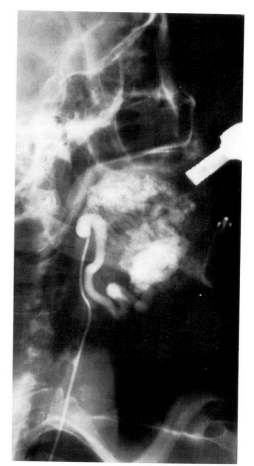

Figure 9–21. Arteriovenous anomaly of the tongue shown by selective arteriography via an enlarged lingual artery.

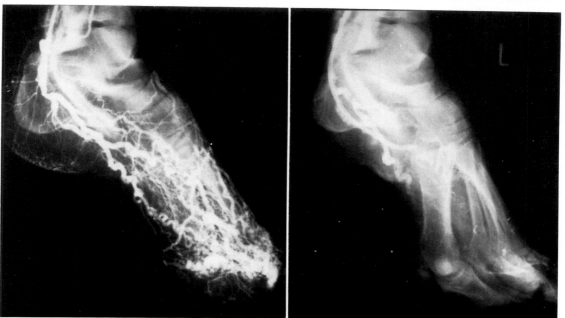

Figure 9–22. An arteriovenous malformation of the foot seen by selective arteriography of the posterior tibial artery. The lesion extends onto the plantar surface of the foot. The right hand panel shows a repeat arteriogram after embolization. The arteriovenous malformation no longer fills to any extent, and the patient has had a remission of symptoms for 3 years.

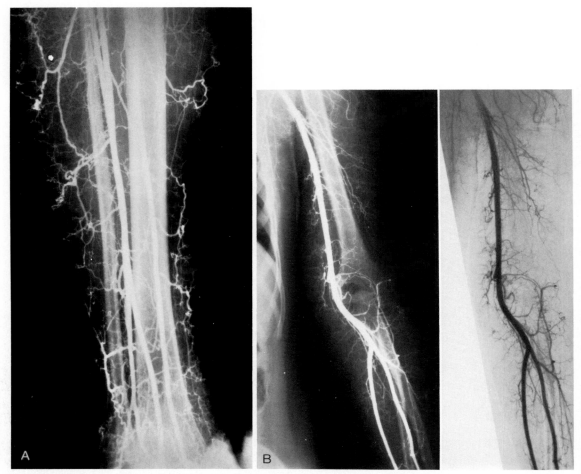

Figure 9–23. Two examples of multiple arteriovenous fistulae of the extremities in the Parkes Weber syndrome. *A,* In this leg, there are numerous tortuous arteries with early venous filling. *B,* An arm with this anomaly shows florid arterial branching (left panel); the arterial and early venous filling is more clearly seen with photographic subtraction (right panel).

Parkes Weber Syndrome

A well recognized form of diffuse arteriovenous fistulae was described by Parkes Weber (1907, 1918). The syndrome consists of a combination of circumscribed gigantism with congenital arteriovenous fistulae and usually a cutaneous capillary malformation and congenital varicose veins. These latter associated abnormalities have led to confusion with the Klippel-Trenaunay syndrome, in which there is no evidence of arteriovenous fistulae. The author considers that because of the different prognosis and treatment, each should be considered as a specific entity (Lea Thomas, 1982). Typically in the Parkes Weber syndrome, the arteriovenous fistulae are very small and multiple and are frequently confined to a single limb. Confir-

mation of these small arteriovenous fistulae can be made arteriographically (Fig. 9–23), but direct visualization is not always possible and it is difficult or impossible to demonstrate them all.

Rendu-Osler-Weber Syndrome

In hereditary hemorrhagic telangiectasia (Rendu, 1896; Osler, 1901; Weber, 1936), the telangiectasia of the skin and mucous membranes is frequently associated with multiple arterial aneurysms (Koblenzer, 1970) and arteriovenous fistulae in the lung, liver, spleen, pancreas, and gastrointestinal tract (Lande et al., 1976). Such aneurysms, which may affect the aorta, and the arteriovenous fistulae can often be demonstrated angiographically. Also, because the angiodysplastic

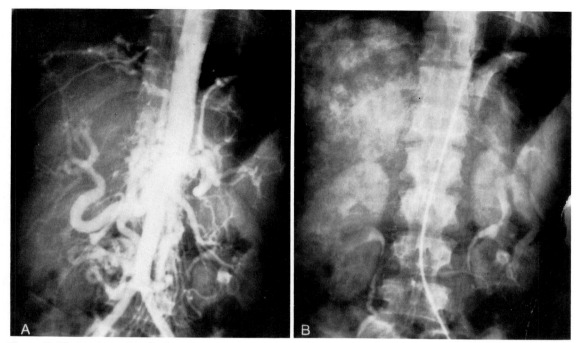

Figure 9–24. Angiographic findings in hereditary hemorrhagic telangiectasia (Rendu-Osler-Weber syndrome). *A,* Arterial phase. The diameter of the celiac axis approximates that of the aorta. There is early filling of hepatic veins and contrast pooling. *B,* Hepatographic phase. Irregular nodules are seen, rather than the normal homogeneous staining.

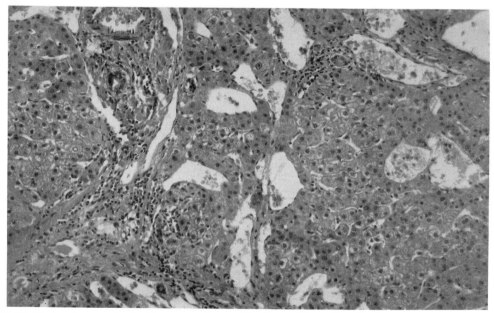

Figure 9–25. Photomicrograph of a biopsy specimen of the liver of the patient in Figure 9–24, showing dilatation of the sublobular portal tracts, central veins, and venous spaces. The findings shown here are characteristic of the pseudocirrhosis seen in this syndrome.

mucous membrane malformations exhibit varying degrees of arteriovenous shunting, these may be demonstrated as a cause of intestinal or other bleeding by selective arteriography. Early visualization of the hepatic veins and the right heart chambers is considered to be an important feature of hepatic angiodysplasia, distinguishing it from hepatic tumors that involve the portal venous system (Boijsen and Abrams, 1965). Telangiectatic liver cirrhosis also has a characteristic appearance (Lea Thomas and Carty, 1974) (Figs. 9–24 and 9–25).

Other conditions that may be associated with gastrointestinal bleeding are blue rubber bleb nevus syndrome and Maffucci's syndrome (Phillips and Yao, 1985).

Arterial anomalies, such as variations in size, position, and anatomical distribution, and congenital aneurysms occur, but they are much less frequent than those associated with the venous system and are generally not of clinical significance, although their demonstration may be desirable so that they can be avoided during operative exploration.

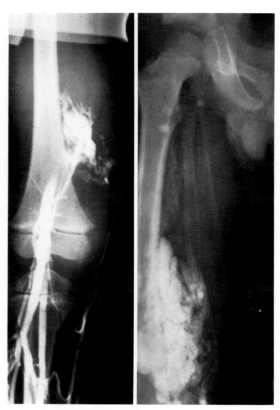

Figure 9–27. An extensive venous malformation of the thigh. The dilated spaces within the anomaly were filled by ascending phlebography, because a tourniquet was applied above the lesion to encourage retrograde venous filling from tributaries of the popliteal and femoral veins. An alternative way of showing this lesion would have been arteriophlebography.

Venous Malformations

Venous malformations or angiodysplasias are common. They form a spectrum from localized anomalies to diffuse phlebectasia involving the entire venous system of a limb, both superficial and deep. Arteriography must be carried out in doubtful cases to exclude arteriovenous fistulae (Lea Thomas and Andress, 1971). Venous investigations have already been mentioned and include ascending or descending phlebography of arms or legs, intraosseous phlebography, varicography (Lea Thomas and Posniak, 1985; Lea Thomas et al., 1986), arteriophlebography, and direct injections into the lesion (Figs. 9–26 to 9–32; see also Fig. 9–8).

Simple anomalies of veins are very common and include duplications, aplasia and hypoplasia (Fig. 9–33), ectasia, and anoma-

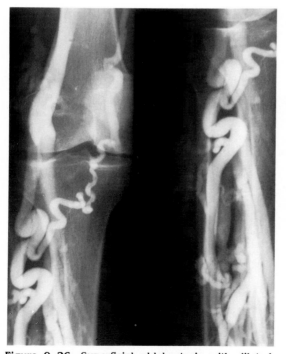

Figure 9–26. Superficial phlebectasia with dilated, valveless, tortuous, superficial veins in the calf on the short saphenous system. Phlebographically, these are indistinguishable from the more common adult varicose veins, as they were present since infancy (primary phlebectasia).

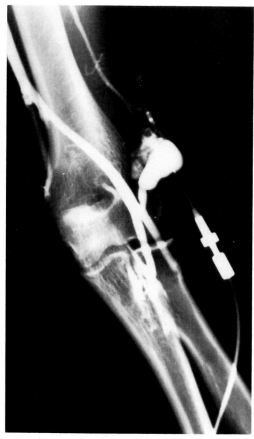

Figure 9–28. This simple venous malformation was shown by direct contrast injection. Its extent and connections with the venous system have been shown and enable localized excision to be carried out easily.

lous terminations. Venous aneurysms (Fig. 9–34) are very rare, usually occurring on the stem veins of the limbs (Cranley, 1975), but have been reported in many different regions (Anjaria et al., 1974; Jensen and Reingold, 1977). Congenital absence of valves (Leu, 1974) is also rare, and careful investigation must exclude past thrombosis in infancy or childhood.

Persistent Lateral Marginal Vein of Servelle

Because of the complicated embryology of the venous system, persistent developmental veins are relatively common. One of the most important is the lateral marginal vein of Servelle. This results from persistence of the primary embryological marginal vein and is usually observed in the legs (Fig. 9–35). The persistent vein can occur alone or, more usually, is associated with either the Servelle-Martorell syndrome (Vollmar and Voss, 1979) or the Klippel-Trenaunay syndrome. This persistent vein is often associated with hypoplasia or aplasia of some parts of the deep venous system of the extremity, and its presence should always alert one to this possibility and careful phlebography of the deep venous system should be carried out before surgical removal of the lateral vein or its tributaries is considered.

Klippel-Trenaunay Syndrome

The syndrome described by Klippel and Trenaunay (Klippel, 1900) consists of cutaneous capillary malformation confined to one limb, varicose veins of the same side dating from birth or infancy, and hypertrophy of bones and soft tissues of the affected limb without evidence of arteriovenous fistulae. Since the original description, there have been many more reports, and it is now known that not only one but even all four limbs may be involved (Servelle, 1964; Lindenauer, 1965; Lea Thomas and Macfie, 1974; Baskerville et al., 1985). Klippel-Trenaunay syndrome is the most common complex congenital venous malformation, and because it is readily recognized clinically the eponym can be conveniently retained. As already stated, deep vein aplasia or hypoplasia and a persistent valveless lateral channel are frequently associated. The termination of the lateral vein is variable and may be single or multiple and best shown by varicography. Common sites of termination are the profunda femoris vein, the common femoral vein, the internal iliac vein, and the lower inferior vena cava (Figs. 9–36 to 9–41).

Tissue enlargement of the affected limb is often considerable, and there is slight lengthening of the limb bones, rarely more than 2 cm, which can be assessed and followed up by scannography and computed tomography. The latter may be valuable in assessing the degree of soft tissue enlargement before and after the reducing operations that are sometimes required.

Maffucci Syndrome

Maffucci first reported multiple enchondromata associated with venous type vascular malformations (Maffucci, 1881). Phleboliths

Text continued on page 168

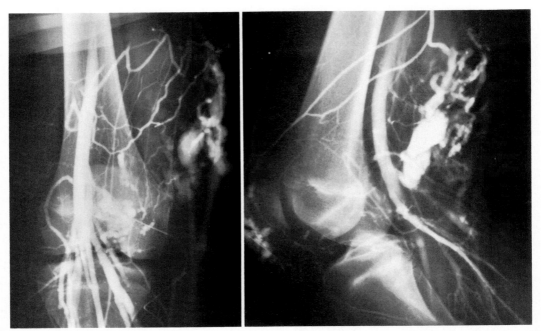

Figure 9–29. A venous anomaly of the lower thigh and popliteal region demonstrated by direct injection with a tourniquet above the lesion.

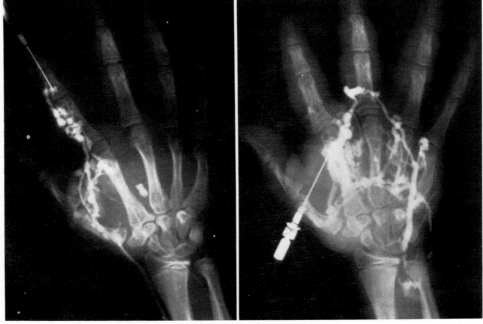

Figure 9–30. An attempt was made to demonstrate this extensive hand malformation by direct injections of specific parts of the lesion. A better method would have been arteriophlebography.

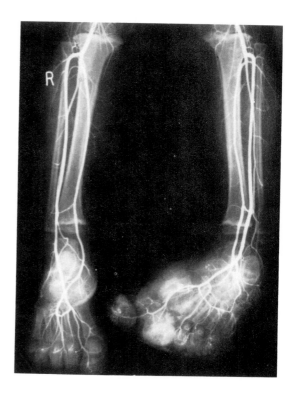

Figure 9–31. Arteriophlebograms (intermediate phase) showing a diffuse vascular abnormality of the left foot. Both legs were radiographed for comparison. Note that the calf arteries on both sides are of normal size, indicating that the malformation is primarily venous in type.

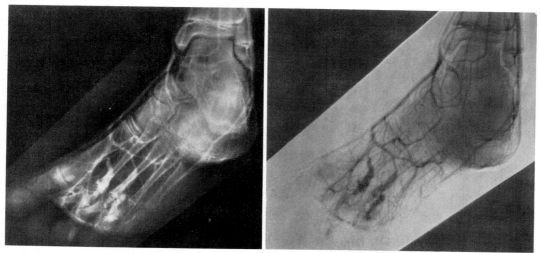

Figure 9–32. A venous anomaly of the forefoot is demonstrated by arteriophlebography. This lesion could not be demonstrated satisfactorily by direct phlebography. The tortuous, dilated veins in the forefoot are better seen in the photographic subtraction film (right panel).

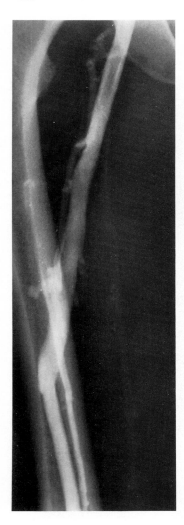

Figure 9–33. An ascending phlebogram shows hypoplasia of the femoral vein. The main venous drainage from the leg is through the profunda vein. The femoral vein is too regular to have resulted from past thrombosis, and there was no history of this.

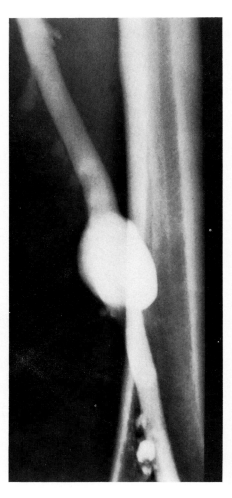

Figure 9–34. A congenital aneurysm of the superficial femoral vein in the adductor canal region. These lesions are very rare.

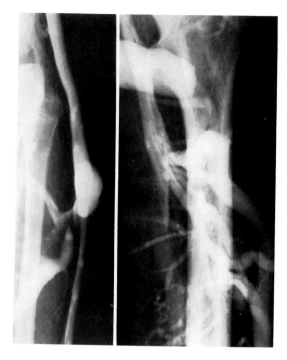

Figure 9–35. A persistent lateral marginal vein of Servelle demonstrated by varicography. The vein joins the profunda femoris vein.

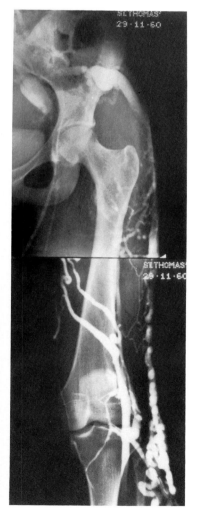

Figure 9–36. Ascending phlebogram in Klippel-Trenaunay syndrome showing the classical lateral valveless venous channel joining, in this case, the left internal iliac vein.

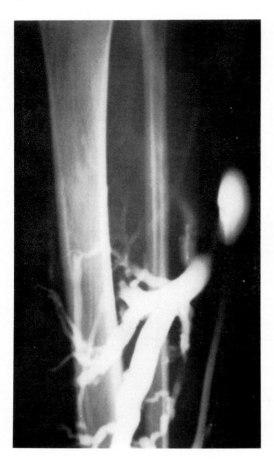

Figure 9–37. In this patient, the deep veins of the calf are absent and the drainage from the foot and lower calf are through a dilated persistent lateral vein (Klippel-Trenaunay syndrome).

Figure 9–38. In this patient with Klippel-Trenaunay syndrome, there is a large suprapubic vein (arrows) that joins the opposite common femoral vein. The iliac veins on the left side are aplastic, and the drainage from the left leg is through the suprapubic vein. Surgical interruption of this vein would result in edema of the left leg.

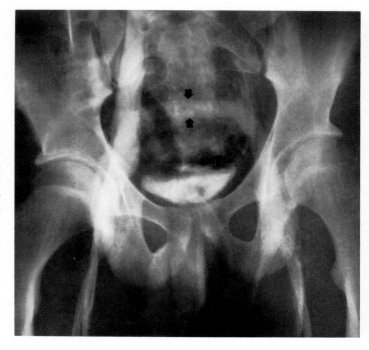

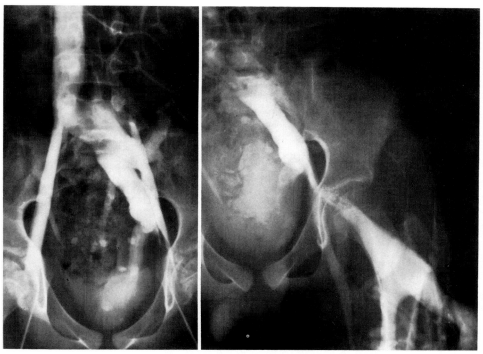

Figure 9–39. This is an example of an extensive venous malformation of the pelvis and left leg in Klippel-Trenaunay syndrome. The bilateral femoral venogram in the left panel shows a greatly enlarged left internal iliac vein. This does not indicate arteriovenous fistulae, but shows that there is an extensive malformation in the pelvis that drains through this vein. Phleboliths can be seen in the patient's pelvis, indicating extensive involvement, which was not possible to demonstrate phlebographically. There is a hypoplastic segment of the left external iliac vein (shown in the right panel), located just above the confluence of the normal common femoral vein and an abnormal draining vein from the leg.

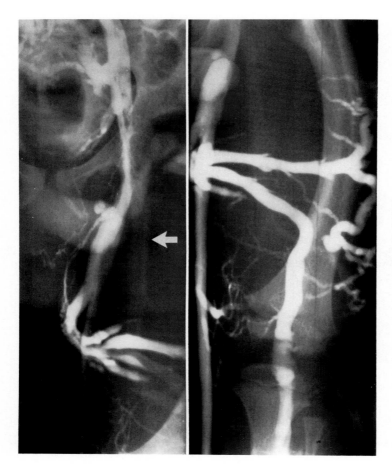

Figure 9–40. Abnormal draining veins in Klippel-Trenaunay syndrome. This varicogram shows abnormal veins draining into the superficial femoral vein, the lower part of which has faintly opacified (arrow).

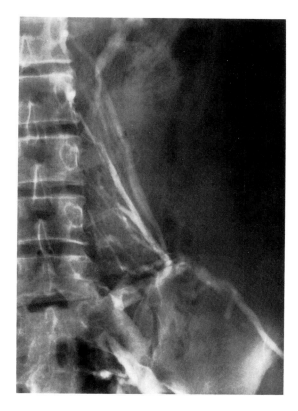

Figure 9–41. In Klippel-Trenaunay syndrome, several anomalous veins may drain into the inferior vena cava. In this case, there is also a connection with the left common iliac vein and distally (not shown) there was connection with the profunda femoris vein. Multiple connections of this sort are common and should be demonstrated phlebographically.

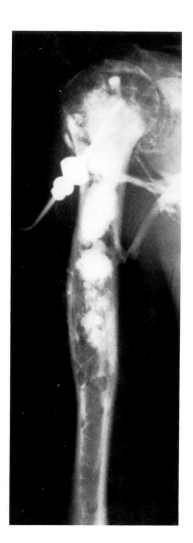

Figure 9–42. Extensive intraosseous involvement in a patient with diffuse combined lymphaticovenous malformation.

and the expansive bone lesions can be seen on plain films. Multiple organ involvement has been reported (Lewis and Ketcham, 1973; Kelikian, 1974).

Vascular Neurocutaneous Syndromes

The vascular neurocutaneous syndromes are a complicated, mixed group of conditions described under a number of eponymous designations, such as Sturge-Weber-Dimitri syndrome, Wyburn-Mason syndrome, and Brushfield-Wyatt syndrome, and as dermatospinal vascular anomalies (Vinken and Bruyn, 1972). There is much overlap between these various conditions, and radiological investigations depend on the clinical presentation of the patient. They are considered in Chapter Fifteen, Vascular Malformations of the Central Nervous System.

Lymphatic Malformations

As has already been indicated, congenital vascular malformations are frequently mixed with lymphatic anomalies coexisting with arterial, arteriovenous, and venous dysplasias.

Primarily lymphatic malformations include aplasia and hypoplasia of the lymph vessels and nodes (see Fig. 9–14), lymphangiectasia (see Fig. 9–15), and lymph cysts.

Primary lymphatic varices of the extremities are extremely rare (Bregt, 1952).

Localized lymphatic anomalies can be classified as simple, cavernous, or cystic (Schobinger, 1977). Investigation is by lymphography, combined with direct injection of cystic lymph spaces (see Fig. 9–13). In the rare cases with skeletal lymphaticovenous anomalies, intraosseous injection may be useful to show the extent of bone involvement (Fig. 9–42).

It seems likely that computed tomography and magnetic resonance imaging will play an increasing role in the investigation of these lesions because of their superior ability to outline tissue planes and define the extent of deep seated and impalpable lesions.

References

Anjaria, P. D., Vaidya, P. N., Vahia, V. N., and Dalvi, C. P.: Venous aneurysms (a case report). J. Postgrad. Med. 20:142, 1974.

Baskerville, P. A., Ackroyd, J. S., Lea Thomas, M., and Browse, N. L.: The Klippel-Trenaunay syndrome (clinical, radiological and haemodynamic features and management). Brit. J. Surg. 72:232, 1985.

Boijsen, E., and Abrams, H. L.: Roentgenologic diagnosis of primary carcinoma of the liver. Acta Radiol. 3:257, 1965.

Boyd, J. B., Mulliken, J. B., Kaban, L. B., et al.: Skeletal changes associated with vascular malformations. Plast. Reconstr. Surg. 74:789, 1984.

Bregt, H.: Lymphangiectasia pulmonum congenita. Archiv. f. Path. Anat. 321:517, 1952.

Burrows, P. E., Mulliken, J. B., Fellows, K. E., and Strand, R. D.: Childhood hemangiomas and vascular malformations: Angiographic differentiation. AJR 141:483, 1983.

Christenson, J. T., and Gunterberg, B.: Intramuscular haemangioma of the extremities. Is computerized tomography useful? Brit. J. Surg. 72:748, 1985.

Cranley, J. J.: Venous aneurysms. In Cranley, J. J.: Vascular Surgery Vol. II. Peripheral Venous Diseases. New York: Harper and Row, 1975, p. 272.

Dahl, E., and Tollefsen, I.: Congenital angiodysplasia with skeletal affection. VASA 9:67, 1980.

Erikson, U., and Hemmingsson, A.: Congenital vascular malformations of the hand. Acta Radiol. 14:754, 1973.

Grainger, R. G.: Osmolality of intravascular radiological contrast media. Brit. J. Radiol. 53:739, 1980.

Griffin, J. M., Vasconez, L. O., and Schatten, W. E.: Congenital arteriovenous malformations of the upper extremity. Plast. Reconstr. Surg. 62:49, 1978.

Jensen, J. L., and Reingold, I. M.: Venous aneurysms of the parotid gland. Arch. Otolaryngol. 103:493, 1977.

Kelikian, H.: Congenital Deformities of the Hand and Forearm. Philadelphia: W. B. Saunders Co., 1974, pp. 682–687.

Kinmonth, J. B.: Methods of lymphography. In Kinmonth, J. B.: The Lymphatics: Diseases, Investigation and Treatment. 2nd ed. London: Arnold, 1982, pp. 1–17.

Kinmonth, J. B., Young, A. E., Edwards, J. M., O'Donnell, T. F., and Lea Thomas, M.: Mixed vascular deformities of the lower limbs, with particular reference to lymphography and surgical treatment. Brit. J. Surg. 63:899, 1976.

Koblenzer, P. G.: In Goodman, R. M. (ed.): Genetic Disorders of Man. Boston: Little, Brown and Co., 1970, pp. 265–327.

Lande, A., Bedford, A., and Schechter, L. S.: The spectrum of angiographic findings in Osler-Weber-Rendu disease. Angiology 27:223, 1976.

Lea Thomas, M.: Phlebography of the Lower Limb. Edinburgh: Churchill Livingstone, 1982, pp. 153–179.

Lea Thomas, M., and Andress, M. R.: Angiography in venous dysplasias of the limbs. Am. J. Roentgenol. 113:722, 1971.

Lea Thomas, M., and Briggs, G. M.: Low osmolality contrast media for phlebography. International Angiology 3:73, 1984.

Lea Thomas, M., and Carty, H.: Hereditary haemorrhagic telangiectasia of the liver demonstrated angiographically. Acta Radiol. Diag. 15:433, 1974.

Lea Thomas, M., and Macfie, G. B.: Phlebography in the Klippel-Trenaunay syndrome. Acta Radiol. Diag. 15:43, 1974.

Lea Thomas, M., and Posniak, H. V.: Varicography. International Angiology 4:475, 1985.

Lea Thomas, M., Keeling, F. P., and Ackroyd, J. S.: Descending phlebography: A comparison of three methods and an assessment of the normal range of deep vein reflux. J. Cardiovasc. Surg. *27*:27, 1986.

Leu, H. J.: Familial congenital absence of valves in the deep veins. Human Genetik *22*:347, 1974.

Lewis, R. J., and Ketcham, A. S.: Maffucci's syndrome: Functional and neoplastic significance. J. Bone Joint Surg. *55A*:1465, 1973.

Lindenauer, S. M.: Klippel Trenaunay syndrome. Ann. Surg. *162*:303, 1965.

Maffucci, A.: Di un caso di encondroma ed angioma multiplo contribuzione al a genesi embrionale dei tumor. Movimento Med. Chir. (Naples) *3*:399, 1881.

Neiman, H. L., Mintzer, R. A., and Vogelzang, R. L.: Digital subtraction angiography. In Neiman, H. L., and Yao, J. S. T. (eds.): *Angiography of Vascular Disease.* New York: Churchill Livingstone, 1985, pp. 27–56.

O'Donnell, T. F., Jr: Congenital mixed vascular deformities of the lower limbs: The relevance of lymphatic abnormalities to their diagnosis and treatment. Ann. Surg. *185*:162, 1977.

Osler, W.: On a family form of recurring epistaxis associated with multiple telangiectases of the skin and mucous membranes. Bull. Johns Hopkins Hospital *12*:333, 1901.

Parkes Weber, F.: Angioma formation in connection with hypertrophy of limbs and hemihypertrophy. Br. J. Derm. *19*:231, 1907.

Parkes Weber, F.: Hemiangiectatic hypertrophy of limbs—congenital phlebectasiasis and so-called varicose veins. Br. J. Child Dis. *15*:13, 1918.

Phillips, J. F., and Yao, S. T. Y.: Congenital vascular malformations. In Neiman, H. L., and Yao, J. S. T. (eds.): *Angiography of Vascular Disease.* New York: Churchill Livingstone, 1985, pp. 393–419.

Reinhoff, W. R., Jr.: Congenital arteriovenous fistula: An embryological study, with the report of a case. Bull. Johns Hopkins Hosp. *35*:271, 1924.

Rendu, M.: Epistaxis répétées chez un sujet porteur de petits angiomes cutanés et muqueux. Bull. Soc. Méd. Hôp. des Paris *13*:731, 1896.

Robertson, D. J.: Congenital arteriovenous fistulae of the extremities. Ann. Roy. Coll. Surg. Engl. *18*:73, 1956.

Rose, R. S.: *Invasive Radiology: Risks in Patient Care.* Chicago: Year Book Medical Publishers, 1983, p. 5.

Schobinger, R. A.: Lymphatic dysplasias. In *Periphere Angiodysplasien.* Bern: Verlag Hans Huber, 1977, pp. 207–227.

Servelle, M.: Syndrome de Klippel Trenaunay. Press Med. *72*:3323, 1964.

Stewart, G., Hurst, P. A. E., Lea Thomas, M., and Burnand, K. G.: Immunology and haematology research. Monograph *2*:241, 1984.

Szilagyi, D. E., Smith, R. F., Elliott, J. P., and Hageman, J. H.: Congenital arteriovenous anomalies of the limbs. Arch. Surg. *111*:423, 1976.

Vinken, P. J., and Bruyn, G. W. (eds.): *The Phakomatoses. The Handbook of Clinical Neurology,* Vol. 14. New York: American Elsevier Publishing Co., 1972, p. 821.

Vollmar, J., and Voss, E.: Vena marginalis lateralis persistens—die vergessene—vene der angiologen. VASA *8*:192, 1979.

Weber, F. P.: Angioma-formation in connection with hypertrophy of limbs and hemihypertrophy. Brit. J. Derm. *19*:231, 1907.

Weber, F. P.: Haemangiectatic hypertrophy of limbs—congenital phlebectasiasis and so-called congenital varicose veins. Brit. J. Child. Dis. *15*:13, 1918.

Weber, F. P.: Haemorrhagic telangiectasias of the Osler type—"telangiectatic dysplasia." Brit. J. Dermatol. *48*:182, 1936.

Young, A. E.: Congenital mixed vascular deformities of the limbs and the associated lesion. Birth Defects, original article series *14*:289, 1978.

Ziedes des Plantes, B. G. Z.: Thesis: Klinik en ZN NV. Utrecht, 1934.

CHAPTER TEN

Capillary (Port-Wine) and Other Telangiectatic Stains

John B. Mulliken

One rapidly gets lost in a sea of eponyms which designate bizarre vascular syndromes . . .

W.B. Bean

NOMENCLATURE

Some birthmarks look as though the skin had been discolored by wine, hence the terms "claret" or "port" stain. Claret is synonymous with the unfortified dry red "Queen of Wines" from the Bordeaux district. The historical context accounts for the preferred use of the term port-wine rather than claret to portray vascular birthmarks in English literature.

During the late seventeenth century, the British Commonwealth retaliated to the protectionist policies of Louis XIV by placing a ban on French wines (Fletcher, 1978). Merchants elected to bypass Bordeaux and sail on to Portugal, "England's oldest ally." Reaching the city of Oporto, at the mouth of the Douro River, they would laden their ships with "Red Portugal," a sweet wine of the district, and then return to the thirsty British Isles. This fortified deep red wine, beloved by the English, became known as "Oporto" or "Port" (A New English Dictionary, 1909). From the early eighteenth century until the

Second World War, larger quantities of port were consumed in England than any other single wine (Fletcher, 1978). English novels and medical writings of this period used the term "port-wine stain" or "port-wine mark" to describe a vivid cutaneous vascular anomaly. Although claret has now reassumed its dominance on the English table and "port-wine stain" is a tautologism, the term remains hallowed in our medical lexicon. The Latin appellation for this vascular birthmark is *naevus flammeus*. Both these descriptive terms connote the superstition that the mother had a gravid craving for port or was, perhaps, frightened by fire during her pregnancy.

This birthmark is often incorrectly listed in textbooks as a "capillary hemangioma." Clinically and histologically, port-wine stains are not proliferative lesions, and thus they should not be called hemangiomas. Histologically, they are characterized by ectatic vessels within the upper dermis. The port-wine stain and various telangiectasias are best included under the broad heading of vascular malformation.

PORT-WINE STAINS

Port-wine stains are present at birth and have an equal sex distribution. They remain throughout life: there is no involution. Only 3 port-wine stains were found in a study of 1058 newborns, an incidence of 0.3% (Jacobs and Walton, 1976). The skin discoloration is usually, but not always, evident at birth. It may be hidden by the usual erythema of the neonatal skin, or may not be visible because of neonatal anemia.

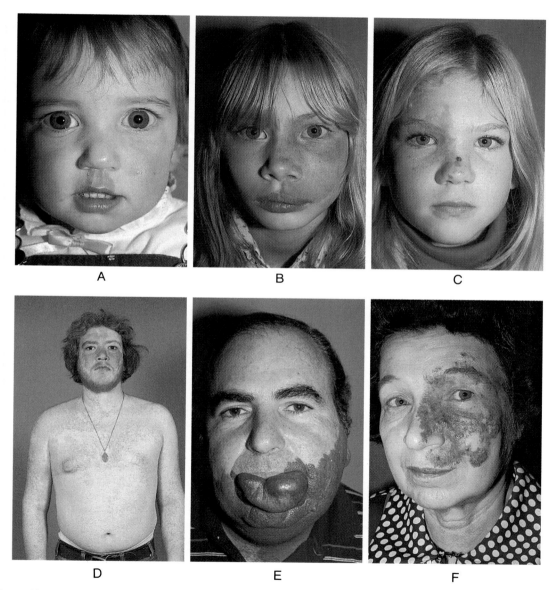

Figure 10–1. Patterns of port-wine stains. *A,* Tiny stain in central lip of a 15 month old child. *B,* Dermal stain in V1 dermatome (upper eyelid) and throughout V2 distribution with slight overgrowth of lip and maxilla. The brain CT and ophthalmologic studies are normal. *C,* "Pyogenic granuloma" in V1 port-stained area. This is a common occurrence; perhaps related to size and density of dermal vessels. *D,* Twenty-four year old male with diffuse staining of face, trunk, and all extremities. Note breast asymmetry; no evidence for CNS involvement. *E,* Forty-two year old male with V3 port-wine stain. Note dark color, soft tissue overgrowth, nodular areas, and venous ectasia of lower lip. *F,* Sixty year old woman with V2 stain. The "cobblestone" lesions (ectasia) make camouflage increasingly difficult.

In a study of 106 cases of facial port-wine stain by Enjolras and coworkers, they found that 45% were restricted to one of the three trigeminal sensory areas (Enjolras et al., 1985). Thus, 55% of facial port-wine stains were noted to overlap sensory dermatomes, cross the midline, or occur bilaterally (Fig. 10–1A to C). Diffuse scattered staining in geographic patterns may be present over the trunk and extremities, in association with or without a facial birthmark (Fig. 10–1D). The mucous membranes are often involved contiguously with facial port staining.

The port-wine stain is flat and sharply demarcated and grows proportionately with the child. The color ranges from pale pink to deep red—the hue deepens as the child cries, has a fever, or is in a warm environment. The pink color, characteristic of infancy, gradually darkens to a red shade during young adulthood and to a deep purple during middle age (Fig. 10–1E and F). In addition, with aging, the surface of the port stain becomes raised and studded with nodular lesions.

Curiously, pyogenic granulomata frequently develop within port-stained skin; this is particularly common with intraoral stains (Thoma, 1952; Swerlick and Cooper, 1983) (Fig. 10–1C). Perhaps increased dermal vascularity offers a fertile ground for the growth of pyogenic granulomata.

Associated Morphogenetic Deformities

The literature is replete with references to port-wine stains in association with other specific malformation syndromes. Most of these, however, are cases of mistaken identity and actually refer to the common macular neonatal stains of the glabella-frontal area that predictably fade in time.

Port-wine marks may be present in conjunction with other vascular anomalies. On the trunk or the extremities, there may be coexistent venous and lymphatic abnormalities (the Klippel-Trenaunay syndrome) (Fig. 10–2A). In this syndrome, the cutaneous stain can be pale and flat or a dark purple hue with scattered punctate nodules; these nodules are ectatic venolymphatic channels. Recurrent breakdown and bleeding are frequent occurrences in these nodular type stains. A port stain may also overlie a deep arteriovenous malformation anywhere on the body, as manifested by increased skin warmth, a bruit, and thrill (Figs. 10–2B and 10–3A). A port-wine stain on the posterior thorax may be the sign of an underlying arteriovenous malformation of the spinal cord (Cobb syndrome) (Cobb, 1915; Doppman et al., 1969; Jessen et al., 1977). However, less than one fourth of spinal vascular malformations have an associated cutaneous stain that may or may not be segmental. (See Chapter Fifteen for a detailed review of spinal vascular anomalies.) A vascular stain located over the lower lumbar midline is also a "red flag," signaling the possibility of underlying spinal dysraphism, lipomeningocele, tethered spinal cord, and diastematomyelia (Fig. 10–2C). In some cases, a tail-like skin appendage (acrochordon) is associated with these developmental lumbar anomalies. There may be subtle signs of neurogenic bladder dysfunction or lower extremity weakness (Bauer, 1986). In such a case, careful neurologic examination, spinal radiography, and bladder function studies are indicated (Fig. 10–3B).

A port-wine stain can accompany other developmental defects of the neural axis. Figure 10–2D illustrates a case of an infant with occipital dermal staining, abnormal tuft of hair, and underlying meningoencephalocele (Fig. 10–3C). A port-wine facial stain may also indicate a unilateral arteriovenous malformation of the retina and intracranial optic pathway, an entity known by the syndromic terms Bonnet-Dechaume-Blanc, in the French literature; and Wyburn-Mason, in the English literature (Théron et al., 1974). (See Chapter Fifteen for a discussion of this condition.) The Sturge-Weber syndrome is the most well-known vascular malformation complex associated with port-wine staining.

Sturge-Weber Syndrome

The Sturge-Weber complex constitutes vascular anomalies of the upper facial dermis, choroid, and ipsilateral leptomeninges. In 1879, Sturge presented a 6½ year old girl with a vascular stain on her right face, buphthalmos, and focal seizures on the left side (Sturge, 1879). He asserted to the audience of the Clinical Society of London that the girl should have a "port-wine mark" on the surface of the right brain. Several years

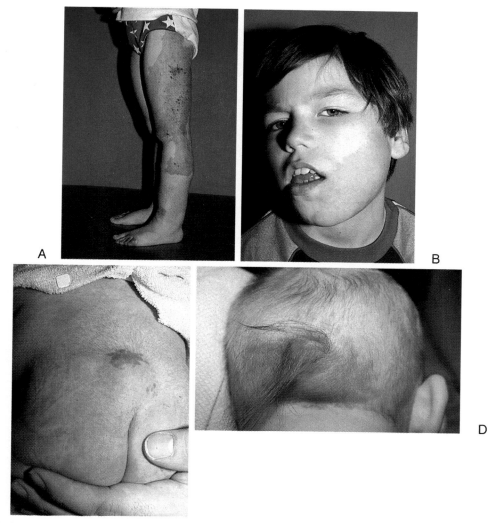

Figure 10–2. Port-wine stain is a "red flag" for possible underlying malformation. *A,* Port-wine stain is the emblem of the Klippel-Trenaunay syndrome (combined capillary, venous, lymphatic anomaly with osseous overgrowth). Note scattered purple punctate nodules. *B,* V3 stain of mandibular area with increased skin temperature and bruit (see Fig. 10–3*A*). *C,* Three week old child with stain of lumbosacral region and lipomatous mass. No evidence for lower motor neuron denervation (see Fig. 10–3*B*). *D,* Five month old child with occipital dermal stain and abnormal hair patch overlying meningoencephalocele (see Fig. 10–3*C*). (Courtesy of E. G. Fischer, M.D.)

later, an autopsy on a similar patient by Kalischer proved Sturge was correct (Kalischer, 1897). Cushing, apparently unaware of Sturge's report, operated on three children with "trigeminal nevi," who presented with spontaneous subdural hemorrhage (Cushing, 1906). Parkes Weber described this entity as a syndrome and published a roentgenogram showing typical intracranial calcifications (Parkes Weber, 1922, 1929).

The Sturge-Weber complex is often listed within the group of neuroectodermal dysplasias called the "phakomatoses." This latter term was introduced by van der Hoeve to emphasize the common "phakomata" (lenslike tumors) seen in the retina of patients with tuberous sclerosis, Recklinghausen's neurofibromatosis, and von Hippel–Lindau syndrome (van der Hoeve, 1932). There would seem to be no clinical pathological or heuristic value for labelling Sturge-Weber syndrome a "phakomatosis." It is not inher-

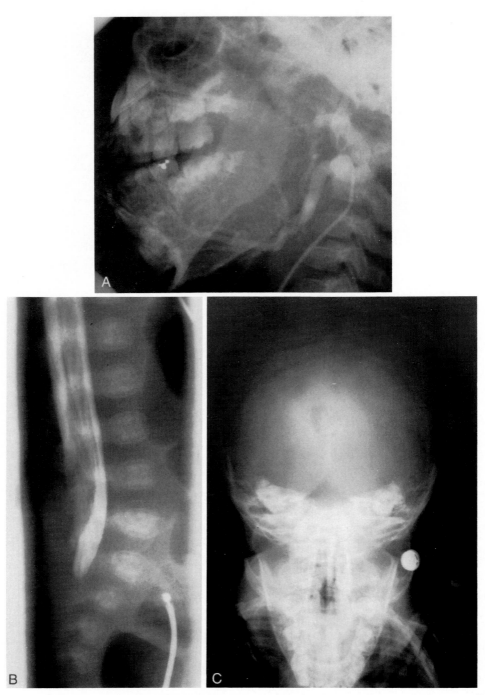

Figure 10–3. *A,* Selective arteriogram, arterial phase, demonstrates dilated, tortuous, internal maxillary and inferior alveolar arteries with arteriovenous shunting, confirming high-flow vascular malformations alongside mandible (see Fig. 10–2*B*). *B,* Myelogram of patient in Figure 10–2*C* demonstrates intraspinal mass and tethered cord attached at L5–S1 (rather than L1–L2) and spina bifida at L5–S1. Normal urodynamic evaluation following resection of lipomeningocele and untethering of cord. *C,* Tiny occipital cranial defect is seen on this Towne's projection of patient in Figure 10–2*D.*

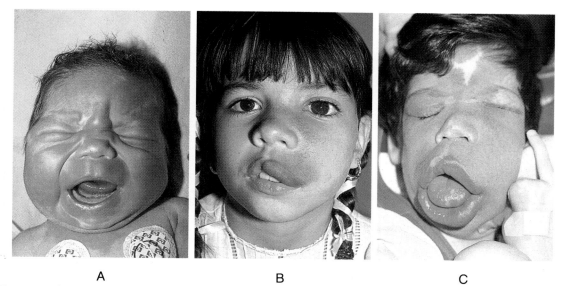

A   B   C

Figure 10–4. The spectrum of Sturge-Weber syndrome. *A,* Newborn with diffuse staining of face and neck. Abnormal choroidal vasculature seen on fundoscopy. CT study shown in Figure 10–6A and B. *B,* Ten year old girl with V1–V2 staining, normal intelligence, and normal CT scan. She has glaucoma OS (little improved by 4 operations), early cataract, 20/200 vision, and abnormal vessels of choroid and episclera. Note buphthalmos. *C,* Twelve year old boy with diffuse vascular anomaly of face, neck, and extremities. Note asymmetrical growth of facial bones, soft tissue hypertrophy, and macroglossia. He is mentally retarded. CT study is shown in Figure 10–6C.

ited, nor is it associated with the development of intracranial neoplasms. However, it is useful to consider this syndrome a maldevelopment of neural and other ectodermal structures. The facial connective tissue, ocular choroid, and leptomeninges, as well as pericytes, nerves, and smooth muscle cells lining vessels, are all mesectodermal derivatives of neuroectoderm. Enjolras and coworkers propose that the Sturge-Weber complex can be explained as an error of morphogenesis within a specific region of the cephalic neural crest, giving rise to abnormal vasculature in the upper facial dermis, choroid, and pia-arachnoid (Enjolras et al., 1985).

Although a strict definition of Sturge-Weber syndrome would include vascular anomalies of the brain, eye, and upper facial skin, the disorder presents in a spectrum of variable expressivity. The classic descriptions of Sturge-Weber type port-wine stain emphasize involvement of the upper eyelid and supraorbital area. Indeed, the study by Enjolras and colleagues documents that only those patients with a port-wine mark within the ophthalmic area alone or extending into the maxillary and mandibular regions are at high risk for having ocular and intracranial vascular anomalies (Enjolras et al., 1985) (Fig.

10–4A and B). Those infants with dermal staining of V2 and/or V3 trigeminal areas alone are not at increased risk. The port-wine stain in Sturge-Weber complex also frequently covers the entire face, neck, trunk, and extremities (Fig. 10–4C). The facial soft tissue in the area of the port stain is often hypertrophied, and frequently there is skeletal overgrowth in the region covered by the stain. Usually the skeletal enlargement involves the maxilla and particularly the alveolar ridge. Skeletal overgrowth may be noted at birth; it is progressive (Fig. 10–5). The ipsilateral mucous membranes are frequently hypertrophic and are prone to recurrent bleeding.

Cerebral angiography in patients with the fully expressed Sturge-Weber complex typically shows capillary and venous anomalies of the leptomeninges, even in the absence of calcification on skull roentgenograms (Poser and Taveras, 1957). Angiography may also demonstrate arterial thromboses, arteriovenous malformations, or anomalies of the veins and dural sinuses. The anomalous circulation is believed to be responsible for progressive degeneration and atrophy of the involved cerebral hemispheres (Lichtenstein, 1954).

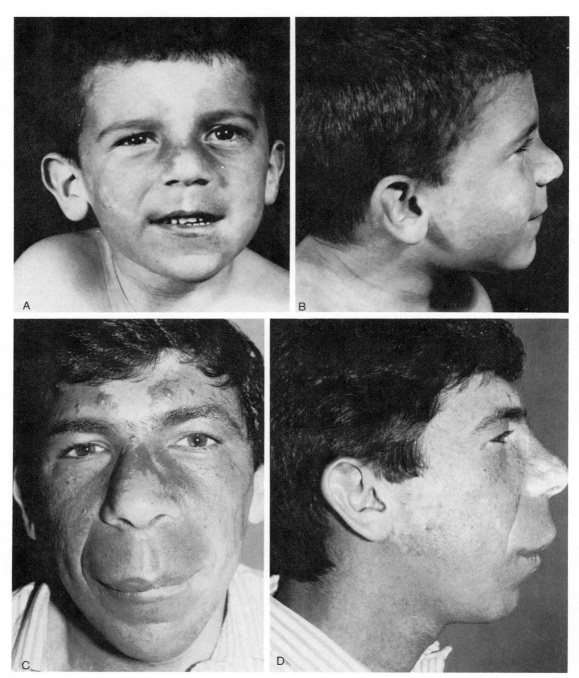

Figure 10–5. Skeletal and soft tissue growth abnormalities with Sturge-Weber syndrome. *A*, Six year old boy with bilateral V1–V2 dermal staining. *B*, Lateral photograph demonstrates normal facial proportions. *C*, The patient at age 24; note maxillary overgrowth and elongation of central face. Patient has glaucoma. *D*, Lateral photograph shows long lip and mid-facial hypertrophy; the upper gingiva, expanded with ectatic vasculature, often bleeds.

Gyriform calcifications can often be seen, usually in the temporal and occipital lobes. Krabbe demonstrated that the mineral deposition is in the outer layers of the cerebral cortex, rather than in the walls of the anomalous vessels (Krabbe, 1934). These "tramlike" calcifications are not pathognomonic of Sturge-Weber syndrome (Garwicz and Mor-

tensson, 1976). Computed tomography is the most sensitive technique for identifying cerebral calcification; this calcification may be seen in early infancy (Fig. 10–6A to D).

There are reported cases of patients with all the features of the syndrome, including intracerebral calcifications, but without facial port-wine stain (Peterman et al., 1958; Cros-

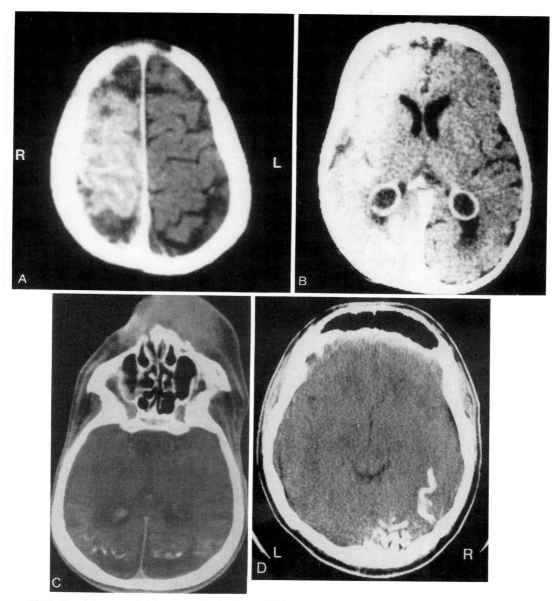

Figure 10–6. Cranial computed tomography in Sturge-Weber syndrome. A, Patient shown in Figure 10–4A, age 6 months; CT cut at level of lateral ventricles shows calcification in right cerebral cortex. There is also atrophy of opposite cerebrum. B, Lower CT slice of patient in Figure 10–4A, showing probable bilateral vascular anomaly of the choroid plexus at the ventricular trigone. C, Computed tomograph of patient in Figure 10–4C reveals bilateral cortical calcification in high parietal area. Note widened extracerebral space secondary to atrophy. D, Axial CT scan of patient in Figure 10–5 demonstrates serpentine calcifications in right occipital lobe.

ley and Binet, 1978). The neurological ramifications of the Sturge-Weber spectrum are discussed in Chapter Fifteen.

Associated Glaucoma

There is a 45% chance of a child having ipsilateral glaucoma if there is port-wine stain in the area supplied by both the ophthalmic (V1) and maxillary divisions (V2) of the trigeminal nerve (see Fig. 10–4B). Staining in either one of the upper divisions of the fifth cranial nerve is not associated with glaucoma (Stevenson et al., 1974). The diagnosis is based upon the presence of elevated intraocular pressure, increased corneal diameter, optic nerve cupping, and glaucomatous defects of the visual field. The presence of glaucoma is not strictly correlated with the finding of increased vascularity of the bulbar conjunctiva or the choroid or intracranial abnormalities.

Several pathogenetic mechanisms for this type of childhood glaucoma have been proposed, all relating to abnormal hemodynamics of the episclera and chamber angle. The ocular vascular anomaly may cause increased episcleral venous pressure, resulting in elevated intraocular pressure (Phelps, 1978). As in other types of congenital glaucoma, the Sturge-Weber cases may be secondary to a developmental anomaly of the filtration angle (Weiss, 1973). For open-angle cases of Sturge-Weber glaucoma, there is histologic evidence for degeneration of the trabecular meshwork of Schlemm's canal system, which could also account for the elevated pressure (Cibis et al., 1984).

An infant with a port-wine stain of the eyelid should be examined by an ophthalmologist every 6 months until age 2–3 years, and should continue to be seen yearly thereafter. It is critical that the diagnosis of glaucoma be made early, before irreversible ocular damage occurs. This is particularly important in the child with cortical degeneration of the ipsilateral occipital lobe resulting in contralateral hemianopsia. This type of glaucoma is often difficult to control by medical therapy. Surgical intervention is often

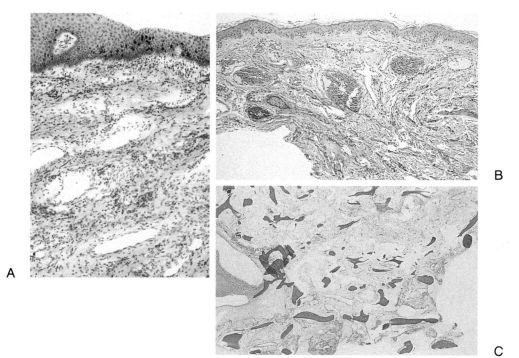

Figure 10–7. Histologic appearance of port-wine stains. A, Autoradiograph of mucosal biopsy of 10 year old with Sturge-Weber syndrome. There is tritiated thymidine uptake in the epidermis but no evidence for cellular replication in the abnormal dilated capillary-like vessels in upper dermis (H&E × 40). B, Biopsy of a 54 year old woman with facial port-wine stain. Note the large red blood cell–filled channels in upper dermis. Compare with Figure 10–7A (H&E × 25). (Courtesy of Seymour Rosen, M.D.) C, Biopsy of maxilla in a 3 month old child, with Sturge-Weber syndrome and skeletal overgrowth, shows thin-walled anastomosing network of vascular channels (venous-lymphatic) among thin spicules of lamellar and woven bone (H&E × 100).

necessary, may need to be repeated, and carries a risk of intraoperative bleeding.

Microscopic Findings in Port-Wine Stains

On histologic examination, a port-wine stain is characterized by ectatic capillary to venular sized channels within both papillary and upper reticular dermis. The vessel walls are thin and are lined by flat, mature appearing endothelium. Cell turnover is normal, i.e., undetectable, in these abnormal vessels (Fig. 10–7A). The detailed microscopic analyses of Barsky and colleagues show that a port-wine stain consists of an increased number of abnormally ectatic vessels in the dermis (Barsky et al., 1980). These investigators also point out that their findings could mean that a port-wine stain is a progressive dilatation of a cutaneous vascular plexus that was normal at one stage of development, with no true increase in vessel number. With aging, however, these channels undergo progressive dilatation; there is no evidence for an actual increase in the number of vessels (Fig. 10–7B). Studies in search of a possible morphogenetic defect to explain this curious dilatation are just beginning. Specialized staining techniques, including antibodies for Factor VIII, fibronectin, and collagenous basement membrane proteins, fail to show any differences from normal cutaneous tissue specimens (Finley et al., 1982). Using immunoperoxidase techniques, Smoller and Rosen demonstrate a significant decrease in perivascular nerve density in port-wine stains (Smoller and Rosen, 1986). They suggest that this deficit may be responsible for altered neural modulation of vascular tone and may lead to the progressive ectasia seen in port-wine stains.

Histologic examination of the enlarged maxilla, commonly seen in Sturge-Weber syndrome, reveals abnormal vascular channels within the marrow spaces (Fig. 10–7C).

Treatment of Port-Wine Stains

There is a long and colorful history of various ineffective methods to treat port-wine stains. Daniel Turner relates how, in a case of port stain of a maiden's hand, an old woman besmeared the lesion with "blood of an afterbirth"; this caused great pain, swelling, and inflammation. The girl's mother had reportedly been frightened by a fire during her pregnancy. Turner understood the challenge of treating this condition; his advice is worth remembering:

> To attempt the taking away discolourings of the skin such as redness from women's longing for claret, or having the same suddenly spilt upon them, is to little purpose; the stain going through the skin and the scar like to prove a greater blemish, if the part will admit of healing, than the discolouring itself. (Turner, 1714)

Scarification

In 1878, Mr. Balmanno Squire, surgeon to the British Hospital for Diseases of the Skin, promoted "linear scarification" for treating port-wine stains. A frozen scalpel was used to incise multiple parallel cuts, first in one direction, then in another (Squire, 1878). Later, Squire modified his scarification technique, using oblique cuts performed at 3 to 4 day intervals (Squire, 1879). The insertion of multiple acupuncture-like needles, attached to a source of electric current, was recommended by Beard in 1877 (Beard, 1877) and by Fox in 1882 (Fox, 1882). High-frequency fulguration, using spark-gap, was also tried (Morton, 1909). Radiation therapy, often protracted in port-wine stain cases, was used in several forms: radium salt (Wickham and Degrais, 1907), thorium X (Bowers, 1951), radioactive phosphorus, and grenz-rays. Unfortunately, radiation burns were not uncommon (Straatsma, 1930; Benedek, 1950); it is remarkable that only a few cases of late-developing basal cell carcinomas have been documented (Sagi, 1984). The Kromayer air-cooled ultraviolet lamp was also prescribed for port-wine nevi (Kromayer, 1910). MacCollum reported using the lamp to apply "blistering doses once each week for periods varying from four to nine months . . . with definite improvement or cure in 80 percent of this type" (MacCollum, 1935). A potentially less damaging form of scarification of the dermal capillaries is Jönsson's technique of rubbing the stain with ordinary sandpaper (Jönsson, 1947). Freezing with liquid nitrogen and carbon dioxide snow proved to be unsuccessful in obliterating port stains (Morel-Fatio, 1964; Goldwyn and Rosoff, 1969).

Tattooing

The first attempt to tattoo port-wine stains is credited to Pauli in 1835, who tried to cover a "congenital purple plaque" (Pauli, 1835). Tattooing was rediscovered in the late 1940's. Early reports failed to emphasize the transient nature of the coverage and the need for repeated treatments (Brown et al., 1946; Conway, 1948). With experience, other problems became obvious: variation in response to pigment deposition, color abnormality at the treated margin, and raised vascular papules secondary to needle trauma (Conway et al., 1967). Children, who probably need help the most, are at risk for scarring with tattooing. Even with more sophisticated color matching, the results have been inconsistent and disappointing (Thomson and Wright, 1971; Grabb et al., 1977). The tattooed skin has an unnatural, fixed, mask-like appearance, unalterable by stimuli that normally change facial color (Fig. 10–8A). Tattooing is no longer recommended.

Cosmetic Cover

Until better methods of treatment are devised, there is a place for cosmetic camouflage in the management of port-wine stains. The two most commonly used products are Covermark (Lydia O'Leary) and Dermablend (Flori Roberts). The base, or foundation, is an opaque, waterproof cream. The essential ingredient in the foundation is mineral oil; this helps to blend the preparation, and it gives the skin a soft, moist look. These commercial products offer a variety of foundation shades; usually two of these are mixed in order to match the patient's skin tone. In addition to the foundation cream, Lydia O'Leary offers a shading cream and a white primer, which further help to disguise the port-wine stain. The shading cream contains a red-brown base, which neutralizes the skin coloring and allows the patient to wear a thinner layer of foundation. The white primer cream is useful in concealing dark stains, especially in patients with a fair complexion. The foundation, with or without the shading or primer creams, also requires application of a setting powder to provide adherence of the make-up for 14–24 hours. The setting powder contains zinc oxide, talc, magnesium carbonate, and other iron oxides. These ingredients draw the mineral oil to the surface of the foundation layer, thus forming a barrier against water penetration. These products also have specially formulated creams for cleaning and make-up removal.

It requires an average of 20 minutes to apply the foundation, additional creams, and setting powder. Obviously, daily use of make-up for a port-wine stain demands the patient's full commitment. Cosmetics may be objectionable to those who need help the most—children. A mother is often willing to take the time to apply make-up each day, particularly for her little girl (Fig. 10–8B and C). Teenaged girls and young women are more likely to use make-up because, by that age, it is more socially acceptable (Fig. 10–8D and E). Very few boys, of any age, are about to use make-up. In one survey, only 28% of patients with port-wine stains were consistently using cosmetic cover, and the women were no more likely to do so than the men (Cosman, 1980).

Excision

With aging, the port-wine stain becomes hypertrophic, cobblestone-like in texture, and deep purple in color. Even thicker application of make-up will no longer hide the irregularly raised and pebbled skin. In selected patients, careful and artistic excision and thick split-thickness or full-thickness skin graft replacement, patterned to fit esthetic facial units, can give satisfactory results (Jonas, 1894; Snyderman and Wynn-Williams, 1966; Clodius, 1977, 1986). These grafts should be harvested from color-matched areas that normally evidence a blush response, e.g., posterior surface of the ear, retroauricular region, supraclavicular area, or scalp (Fig. 10–8F). For replacement of bearded areas, Clodius recommends that scalp skin from the mastoid region be used and that epilation be performed 10–14 days before grafting (Clodius and Smahel, 1979). Plucking causes the follicles to migrate upward into the dermis, thus increasing the hair density within the graft.

Potential problems with excision and grafting include: (1) scar hypertrophy at the juncture of the graft and normal skin, (2) unpredictable graft pigmentation, and (3) abnormal texture and skin quality of even the best full-thickness grafts. No matter what the quality of the grafted region, there is a border effect with normal skin that calls at-

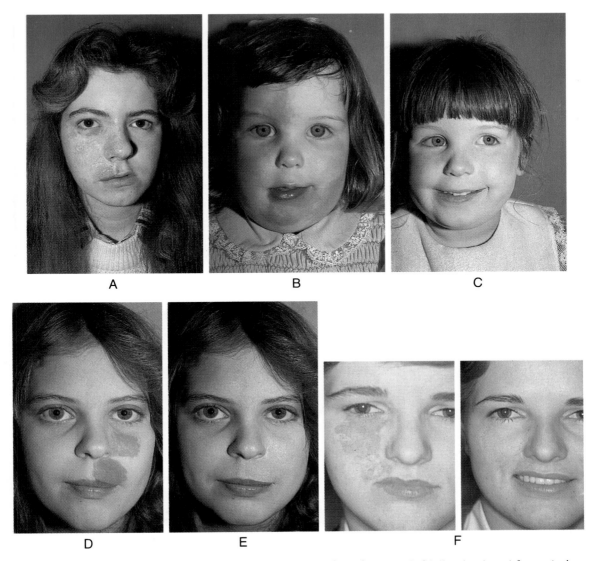

Figure 10–8. Treatment of port-wine stains. *A,* Young woman following repeated tattoo treatment for port-wine stain. Note variegated retention of pigment, giving talcum powder appearance. *B,* Two year old child with bilateral facial vascular stains. *C,* Child in *B* at age 4. Her mother applies the cosmetic cream daily. Now that she is older, her classmates ask, "Why do you wear make-up?" *D,* Dark, patchy port stains in a teenage girl. *E,* Patient in *D;* she takes 15 minutes to apply camouflage that lasts all day. Make-up is acceptable in this young woman's peer group. *F,* Excision of a localized port-wine stain of the cheek and replacement with full-thickness retroauricular skin graft. (Courtesy of J. E. Murray, M.D.)

tention to the reconstruction. Preliminary skin expansion is a new approach to excision of moderate-sized port-stained areas, allowing linear closure along facial unit borders (Argenta, 1983).

On a curiosity note, if a port-wine stain itself is transferred as a full-thickness skin graft, the abnormal vascular pattern persists (Johnson, 1960; Martin et al., 1985).

See Chapter Twenty for a discussion of laser therapy of port-wine stains.

NAEVUS FLAMMEUS NEONATORUM

("Angel's Kiss," "Stork Bite," "Salmon Patch," etc.)

The extremely common entity *naevus flammeus neonatorum* is often confused with the rather uncommon port-wine stain because it shares the same Latin term, *naevus flammeus.* Pratt found that 42% of white neonates and

31% of black neonates have a *naevus flammeus nuchae* (Pratt, 1967). A lower incidence of nuchal staining (23.4%) was noted in over 2000 normal Chinese and Malaysian infants (Tan, 1972). In a study of 1058 newborn infants, 40.3% had neonatal staining in the following distribution: 81% on the nape *(naevus flammeus nuchae)*, 45% on the eyelids, and 33% on the glabella (Jacobs and Walton, 1976). These stains are pink, macular, and irregularly outlined. They blanch completely with pressure and become suffused when the infant cries (Fig. 10–9A and B). These lesions are also known popularly as "stork bite," "salmon patch," or "angel's kiss." Dixey noted that these marks are "caused by an affectionate peck from the stork who delivers the child before taking final leave of its charge" (Dixey, 1955). To this, Bean affirmed that "this seems as good an explanation as any" (Bean, 1958).

The German dermatologist Unna ascribed nuchal and forehead stains to an intrauterine pressure phenomenon during birth (Unna, 1894). Unna's pressure theory has been discounted, because these lesions are also found in children delivered by cesarean section (Bettley, 1940). Schnyder, with thorough histologic examinations, could not demonstrate ectasia of the vessels in infants, but did find moderate ectasia of subpapillary vessels in older children with nuchal staining (Schnyder, 1955). These stains are sometimes found over the lower lumbar-sacral area, in addition to the nape of the neck. These observations have led some investigators to speculate that nuchal and lumbar stains represent persistence of embryological vascularity, in association with closure of the medullary tube.

Naevus flammeus neonatorum may be more of a physiological phenomenon than a true dermatopathological lesion. There is a remarkable tendency for these lesions to vanish within the first year of life, leaving no residual evidence. The nuchal patches seem to fade somewhat more slowly than the anterior facial stains (Smith and Manfield, 1962). Oster and Nielsen, in a study of more than 2000 Danish school children between the ages of 6 and 17 years, noted an incidence of persistent nuchal staining of 46.2% in females and 35% in males (Øster and Nielsen, 1970). In addition, they found an incidence of interscapular telangiectasia of 40% in girls and 32% in boys. They remarked that in girls, there was an increase in the incidence of

staining in the 12–13 year old group, with a subsequent decrease. The incidence seemed to be independent of age for boys. Hormones are known to modulate vascularity; endocrine changes may influence the dermal microcirculation in these anatomical regions. Nuchal staining can also remain into adulthood, becoming more obvious with blood pressure elevation, emotional episodes, or physical exertion. A persistent cervical stain is often referred to as "Unna's nevus" or "erythema nuchae" (Øster and Nielsen, 1970). There is evidence that Unna's nevus may have a familial tendency (Merlob and Reisner, 1985); this is also true for forehead stains (Fig. 10–9C).

Glabellar and nuchal staining is often listed as a phenotypic finding in a variety of malformation syndromes, including Beckwith-Wiedemann, trisomy 13–15, Brachmann–de Lange, Rubenstein-Taybi, SC-pseudothalidomide-Roberts, and others (Fig. 10–9D and E). A prominent V-shaped central forehead stain is also frequently seen with severe forms of craniosynostosis, particularly the cloverleaf (kleeblattschädel) skull deformity (Fig. 10–9F). However, because forehead staining is so commonly noted in normal infants, it is arguable that there is any pathological significance to its association with rare dysmorphologic syndromes.

HYPERKERATOTIC VASCULAR STAINS: CONGENITAL AND ACQUIRED

There are rare cases in which a vascular stain has a rough, warty surface. For many of these lesions, the term "angiokeratoma" has been generically applied. Imperial and Helwig have performed detailed histopathological studies of this group of cutaneous abnormalities. They prefer to restrict the designation "angiokeratoma" to the "acquired" vascular lesions, and to differentiate this category from the true telangiectatic malformation, also called "hypertrophic nevus flammeus" or "verrucous hemangioma" (Imperial and Helwig, 1967b). They also observe that in the congenital lesion, vascular ectasia involves both dermis and subcutaneous tissue, whereas in the "acquired" lesion, specified "angiokeratoma," the ectasia is seen only in the papillary dermis.

The hyperkeratotic vascular stains do not

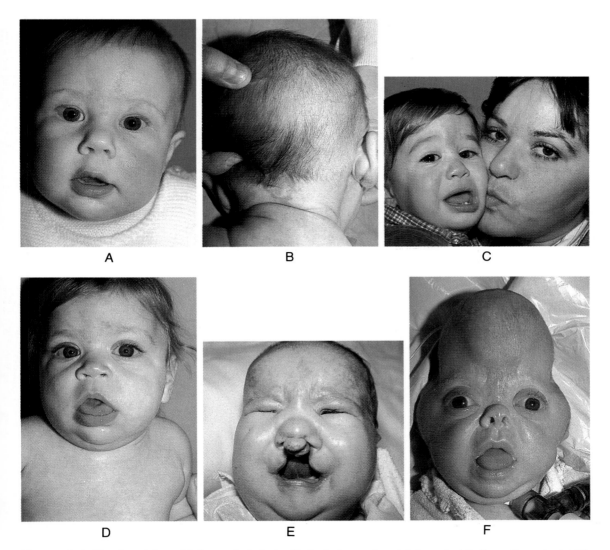

A   B   C

D   E   F

Figure 10–9. Macular stains of infancy. *A,* Infant with typical macular staining of glabella and upper eyelid regions. These usually fade within 1–2 years. *B,* Nuchal vascular patch ("stork bite"); these disappear slowly and may persist. *C,* Infant with forehead stain; also seen in his mother and other family members. Thus, not all salmon patches disappear. *D,* Beckwith-Wiedemann syndrome: omphalocoele, macroglossia, and macular forehead patch. *E,* Diffuse glabellar and eyelid stains in infant with trisomy-13 and bilateral complete cleft lip/palate. *F,* Central forehead dermal stain in infant with trilobar skull deformity (craniofacial synostosis).

demonstrate endothelial hyperplasia; therefore, the terms "verrucous hemangioma" and "angiokeratoma" are, in this sense, both misnomers. The more critical issue, however, is an overly rigid division between "acquired" versus "congenital" vascular anomalies. A vascular malformation may not become clinically apparent until adolescence or adulthood. The structural abnormality of the vessel walls may manifest itself in time. For this reason, the hyperkeratotic vascular stains are presented as true malformations, some congenital, and some apparently "acquired."

Capillary-Lymphatic Malformation
(Old Terms: "Hypertrophic Naevus Flammeus," "Verrucous Hemangioma")

Capillary-lymphatic malformations are usually obvious at birth. They may be light pink to bluish-red in color and are well demarcated. They are most commonly located on the lower extremities, but they are also seen on the chest, abdomen, and arms (Imperial and Helwig, 1967b). With trauma, altered hemodynamics, or possibly secondary infection, these lesions become more keratotic and wart-like. From both a clinical and histologic viewpoint, this lesion is a localized lymphatic malformation combined with abnormal dermal blood vessels. The color and consistency are determined by the amount of blood within the abnormal channels and by the verrucous changes (Fig. 10–10A and B). In the past, this lesion has been called "hypertrophic nevus flammeus," "verrucous hemangioma," "hemangio-lymphangioma," or "lymphangioma circumscriptum."

Histologically, these lesions demonstrate dilated, capillary to venular sized vessels in the dermis and subcutaneous tissue (Fig. 10–10C). The vessels are deficient in elastic fibers. Larger ectatic channels, some with proteinaceous material, are clearly abnormal lymphatic vessels. The epidermal hyperkeratosis and parakeratosis are reactive rather than primary features (Imperial and Helwig, 1967b). The clinical and pathological features of this lesion are consistent with those of a

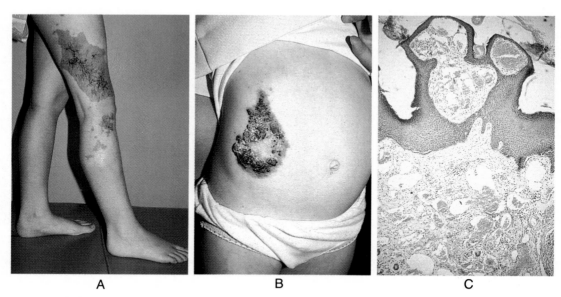

| A | B | C |

Figure 10–10. Patterns of hyperkeratotic vascular staining. *A, Klippel-Trenaunay syndrome* (combined capillary-lymphatic-venous malformation with skeletal overgrowth). In the past, this type of stain, with its warty excrescences, was called "hypertrophic naevus flammeus" or "verrucous hemangioma." The dermal component in this patient is a *capillary-lymphatic* anomaly. *B, Capillary-lymphatic malformation* of the abdomen. Note warty excrescences typical of dermal lymphatic anomaly. In the past, this lesion may have been labelled "angiokeratoma circumscriptum." *C,* Histologic section of excised lesion shown in *B.* Epidermis demonstrates papillomatosis and hyperkeratosis. Ectatic vessels invaginate the dermal papillae; organized thrombi are seen. Deeper sections show malformed, thick-walled, dilated veins and irregular channels in subcutaneous layer (H&E × 60).

true malformation of the dermal blood vessels and lymphatics. Therefore, the designation *capillary-lymphatic* malformation is accurate.

As for any cutaneous lymphatic malformation, this lesion must be widely excised, usually down to fascia. The defect may be closed in a linear fashion; more often, a split-thickness skin graft is needed for primary closure.

The "Angiokeratomas"

The term "angiokeratoma" refers to a group of skin lesions that present as dark-red to black papules measuring from 1 to 10 mm in size. These entities are usually remembered by their eponyms: *Mibelli, Fordyce,* and *Fabry.* There seems to be an anatomical predilection for the three angiokeratomas: (1) Mibelli's lesions on the hands or feet, (2) Fordyce's lesions on the scrotum, and (3) Fabry's lesions on the trunk or thighs. It is difficult to differentiate one angiokeratoma type from another by appearance; they are also indistinguishable by light microscopy. Braverman and Keh-Yen present elegant ultrastructural and three-dimensional reconstructions showing a close resemblance between the angiokeratomas of Fordyce and Fabry (Braverman and Keh-Yen, 1983). The lesions consist of dilated postcapillary venules within the dermal papillae, connected by very short channels. Multilaminated basement membrane material is noted within the thinnest walls of the saccular vessels that are adjacent to the epidermis. The Fordyce lesion is larger and contains no valves. The smaller Fabry angiokeratoma has valves, as well as vascular connections into the deep dermis, and characteristic intracellular inclusions (in endothelium, fibroblasts, and smooth muscle cells). Braverman and Keh-Yen conclude that the angiokeratomas of Fordyce and Fabry are abnormalities of pre-existing microvasculature and are not the result of proliferation of new vessels and random anastomoses.

There is evidence that the angiokeratomas may have an underlying genetic basis (Imperial and Helwig, 1967a), and in two types within this category, biochemical abnormalities have been detected, i.e., Fabry disease and fucosidosis.

Treatment of the angiokeratomas is usually symptomatic. Often these lesions bleed easily and weep, either spontaneously or following abrasion. The area should be kept clean and covered with petrolatum-based antibiotic ointment. Local electrocoagulation, cryotherapy, or laser treatment may be useful, particularly to control troublesome bleeding points (Flores et al., 1984).

Angiokeratoma of Mibelli

In 1889, Mibelli described warty, purplish spots over the bone prominences of the hands, elbows, knees, and feet in a 14 year old girl with a history of chilblain. For this dermatological entity, he coined the word "angiokeratoma" (Mibelli, 1889). The *Mibelli angiokeratoma* occurs in adolescence, first as telangiectasias that later coalesce to form tiny hemorrhagic keratotic papules (3–5 mm diameter) on the dorsal and volar surfaces of the hands and feet. It may also involve the ankles, knees, palms, and elbows. It is seen more commonly in females. The cause is unknown; however, the distribution and frequent association of angiokeratoma of Mibelli with acrocyanosis, chilblain, and frostbite suggest that cold-sensitivity is a precipitating factor. A pedigree reported by Smith and colleagues is evidence for a genetic basis for this disorder, transmitted with autosomal dominant inheritance (Smith et al., 1968). The disease is harmless, and treatment is necessary only for numerous and disfiguring lesions.

Imperial and Helwig have also described a "solitary angiokeratoma" type, histologically similar to the Mibelli lesions but occurring primarily in young adult males (Imperial and Helwig, 1967a). These patients relate a clinical history of less than 6 months, and usually present with a single lesion, most frequently located on the lower extremities. These authors believe that this type of angiokeratoma is a response of papillary vessels to trauma or chronic irritation.

Angiokeratoma of Fordyce

In 1896, Fordyce reported a case of a 60 year old man who developed warty vascular lesions of the scrotum, similar clinically and histologically to Mibelli's case but without the history of pernio (Fordyce, 1896). The designation *angiokeratoma of Fordyce* is restricted to red-purple lesions with minimal hyperkeratosis, seen most commonly in males over the age of 30 and located on the genitalia, lower abdomen, and thighs. Clinically and histologically similar lesions may also appear on the genital labia of older women. The lesions have a linear configuration, and on closer examination they are seen to be composed of tiny, red, soft, compressible papules (Fig. 10–11*A*). With advancing age of the patient, the lesions become larger, darker, more numerous, and keratotic in appearance. Although scrotal angiokeratomas tend to be asymptomatic, they can become pruritic and may bleed when traumatized. Some investigators believe that these lesions are venous ectasias secondary to venous obstruction, increased pressure, and thrombosis, caused by various genitourinary disorders such as varicocele, hernia, prostatitis, thrombophlebitis, or lymphogranuloma venereum (Evans, 1962; Imperial and Helwig, 1967c).

Angiokeratoma Circumscriptum

In 1915, Fabry described a localized hyperkeratotic-vascular skin disease, calling it *angiokeratoma circumscriptum* (Fabry, 1915). It consists of unilateral cutaneous purple papules and blood-filled cystic spaces located over the trunk, lower legs, and thighs. The lesions appear in infancy or early childhood and grow in proportion to the patient; they may enlarge to become several centimeters in diameter. Females are reportedly affected three times as frequently as males.

From descriptions in the literature, it is difficult to be certain whether "angiokeratoma circumscriptum" is, indeed, a truly acquired lesion, or a vascular malformation of the capillary-lymphatic category (see Fig. 10–10*B*).

Angiokeratoma Corporis Diffusum Universale (Fabry Disease)

This condition was described by Fabry and independently by Anderson in 1898 (Wallace, 1973). It is a rare, hereditary, sex-linked recessive disorder of sphingolipid metabolism (alpha-galactosidase A deficiency). The disorder is characterized biochemically by an abnormal glycolipid (ceramidetrihexoside) attached to sphingosine and deposited in cytoplasm of vascular endothelium and pericytes, renal epithelium, neural cells, corneal epithelium, and cardiac muscle fibers. The diagnosis can be confirmed by skin biopsy and appropriate histologic stains for glycolipid granules.

This disease presents in homozygous males during childhood or early adolescence, with intense burning pain in the fingers and toes. Vesicles usually appear over the hips, buttocks, and perineum (bathing trunk area) prior to puberty. The lesions can occur anywhere, but are rarely seen on the face (Fig. 10–11*B*). The lesions may emerge after trauma or application of heat. The cutaneous lesions are minute, blood-filled, hemispheric, purple or bluish-red papules, often with overlying keratosis (Fig. 10–11*C*). They do not disappear on pressure. In addition to the skin lesions, the condition manifests clinically by fevers, renal dysfunction, peripheral edema, and dyshidrosis. Most men with angiokeratoma of Fabry die in their early forties, as a result of renal failure or hypertensive cardiovascular disease. There is variable mild expressivity in the heterozygous female; only 20% develop skin lesions. The syndromology of this disorder is found in Gorlin, Pindborg, and Cohen's book (Gorlin et al., 1976). A comprehensive review, with emphasis on the metabolic basis, is given by Desnick and Sweeley (Desnick and Sweeley, 1987).

Fucosidosis

Fucosidosis is another enzymatic deficiency disorder that may present with diffuse angiokeratomas. This condition is inherited in an autosomal recessive manner, and is characterized by an absence or deficiency of the lysosomal enzyme alpha-L-fucosidase (Durand et al., 1966). Glycosaminoglycans and glycolipids accumulate in the tissues of affected homozygotic individuals, who evidence varying degrees of mental retardation, spasticity, and skeletal dysplasia (Smith et al., 1977; Hurwitz, 1981). Some affected individuals develop multiple angiokeratomas, located primarily on the trunk and upper legs and similar in appearance and distribution to the lesions of Fabry disease. Tissue specimens from patients with fucosidosis do not demonstrate the intracellular lipid inclusions of Fabry disease. The differential diagnosis between these two conditions is well presented by Smith and colleagues (Smith et al., 1977).

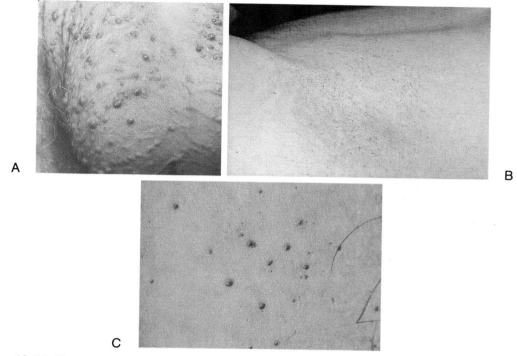

Figure 10–11. The eponymous "angiokeratomas." *A, Angiokeratoma of Fordyce,* scrotum, 50 year old male. (Courtesy of Harley A. Haynes, M.D.) *B,* Twenty-five year old male, *Fabry disease*: note diffuse telangiectatic lesions over flank and abdomen. (Courtesy of Harley A. Haynes, M.D.) *C, Fabry disease*: close-up photograph to show hemispheric papules in suprapubic area. (Courtesy of Harley A. Haynes, M.D.)

CUTIS MARMORATA TELANGIECTATICA CONGENITA

Some children exhibit a cutaneous marbling effect of the skin when they are placed in a low temperature environment. This mottling characteristically disappears when the child is warmed. This is merely an accentuated pattern of normal cutaneous vascularity, called *cutis marmorata* or *livedo reticularis* (Fig. 10–12*A*). This appearance is very similar to the veins visible in the skin of some delicate, fair-haired white women. This condition, once considered beautiful, is now regarded by some as a cosmetic embarrassment.

There are rare cases in which a newborn infant has a livid cutaneous marbling, even at normal temperatures, which becomes more pronounced with lower temperature or with crying. This is a pathological entity, first described by van Lohuizen in 1922 and now known by the ungainly term *cutis marmorata telangiectatica congenita* (CMTC) (van Lohuizen, 1922). The involved skin has a distinctive deep purple color and is depressed in a serpiginous reticulated pattern. The lesions occur in a localized, segmental, or generalized distribution. The trunk and extremities are more commonly involved than the face and scalp (Fig. 10–12*B*). Some cases of CMTC have associated deep venous anomalies, and this entity has been confused with "generalized phlebectasia." Neonatal ulceration of the depressed reticulated purple areas can occur. In some children, the involved limb and the subcutaneous tissue are hypoplastic (Moyer, 1966; Petrozzi et al., 1970). There are rare cases of CMTC in association with defective long bone growth (Fitzsimmons and Starks, 1970) and with congenital glaucoma and mental retardation (Petrozzi et al., 1970; South and Jacobs, 1978).

Biopsies of these lesions exhibit dilated capillaries and veins in the dermis and occasional thin-walled venous sinuses in the subcutaneous layer. Vascular occlusion is thought to be responsible for the observed local ulceration, scarring, and atrophy (Way et al., 1974). A possible clue to understanding CMTC is the case by Fitch and coworkers of a 16 week old fetus with lethal multiple pterygia syndrome and widespread cuta-

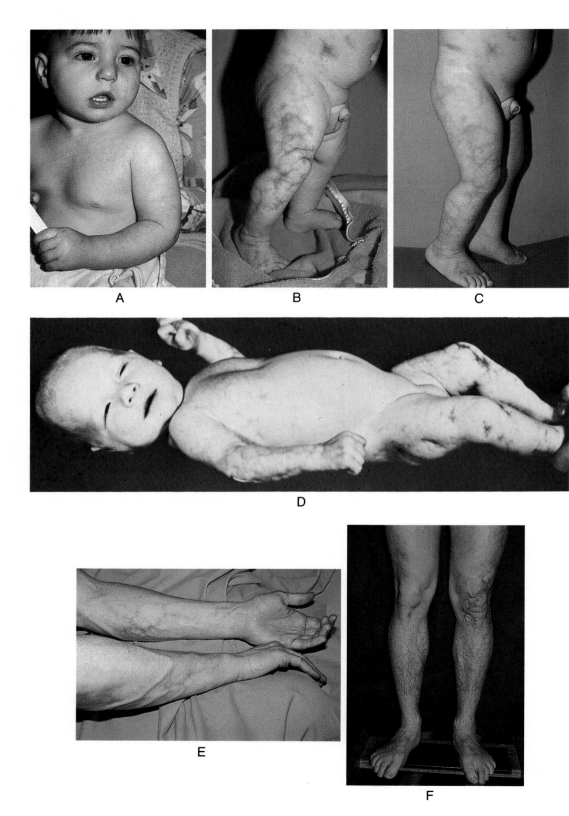

Figure 10–12 *See legend on opposite page*

neous vascular anomalies (Fitch et al., 1985). Histologically, the skin was found to contain a meshwork of abnormally dilated thin-walled vessels (capillary-venular sized) within dermis and subcutis. Elastic fibers were not found in these anomalous channels, and the blood vessels elsewhere in the body were normal.

Almost all affected infants with CMTC show steady improvement of their accentuated vascular pattern during the first year of life that continues into adolescence (Fig. 10–12C). This is probably the result of normal thickening and maturation of the skin. Nevertheless, the skin atrophy and deep vascular staining can persist into adulthood, along with diffuse ectasia of the veins in the involved extremities (Fig. 10–12D to F).

Most authors note that CMTC occurs sporadically, with an equal sex distribution (Way et al., 1974; South and Jacobs, 1978). There are reports suggesting that it may be an autosomal dominant disorder of low penetrance (Andreev and Pramatarov, 1979; Kurczynski, 1982).

RENDU-OSLER-WEBER SYNDROME (HEREDITARY HEMORRHAGIC TELANGIECTASIA)

The Rendu-Osler-Weber syndrome was first distinguished from hemophilia by Rendu in 1896 (Rendu, 1896). In 1901, Osler gave a complete clinical description and established the inherited nature of the disease (Osler, 1901). F. Parkes Weber presented another case in 1907 and invited Osler, newly appointed Regius Professor at Oxford, to examine the patient (Parkes Weber, 1907). In 1909, F. W. Hanes, a resident house officer at the Johns Hopkins Hospital, was the first investigator to describe the histopathology of the skin lesions. He accurately called the disease "hereditary hemorrhagic telangiectasia" (HHT) (Hanes, 1909). Nevertheless, the triple eponymous title "Rendu-Osler-Weber disease" tenaciously endures (Gibbs, 1986).

Inherited in an autosomal dominant pattern, the homozygous form of HHT is probably lethal. The incidence is 1–2 per 100,000 in the white European population and is considerably less in other races (Martini, 1978).

The characteristic lesions are discrete, spider-like, bright red maculopapules, usually 1–4 mm diameter and typically located on the face, tongue, lips, nasal and oral mucous membranes, conjunctiva, palmar aspect of the fingers, and nail beds (Fig. 10–13A). Lesions can occur on almost any mucosal surface, e.g., nasal septum, tongue, gastrointestinal tract, and bladder, and also in the bronchial and vaginal mucosa. They have also been found in liver, spleen, pancreas, kidney, and brain (Halpern et al., 1968; Chandler, 1965; Cooke, 1986). These telangiectatic lesions may appear in early childhood, but more commonly, they emerge after puberty, in the third to fourth decade. The lesions increase in number with advancing age. These vascular papules are prone to ulceration and bleeding. Hemorrhage may present as epistaxis or as painless hematemesis, hematuria, or melena. In women, hemorrhage from the gastrointestinal tract has been noted to worsen several days before menstruation, diminishing in the postmenopausal period and following ovariectomy (Heyde, 1954). Bleeding from telangiectasias in the brain or spinal cord can give neurologic symptoms. There is evidence for associated pulmonary arteriovenous fistulae and development of pulmonary hypertension (Sapru et al., 1969; Trell et al., 1972). With substantial shunting, the classic triad of cyanosis, clubbing of the fingers, and polycythemia appears. A familial history of HHT can be obtained in about 50–70% of patients with pulmonary arteriovenous fistulae.

Some patients with diffuse hepatic telangiectasis may have evidence of physiological effects of systemic arteriovenous fistulae, e.g., wide pulse pressure, rapid heart rate, and increased cardiac output (Graham et al., 1964; Trell et al., 1972). A peculiar type of liver cirrhosis or pseudocirrhosis has also been reported in this syndrome (Zelman,

---

Figure 10–12. Cutis marmorata telangiectatica. *A, Cutis marmorata* or *livedo reticularis:* an accentuation of normal vascular pattern of the arm and trunk, seen in fair-skinned children. *B, Cutis marmorata telangiectatica congenita (CMTC):* typical lesions of right leg and trunk in 5 month old child. Note depressed, serpiginous blue-purple craters. *C,* Improvement noted in same child, 1 year later. *D,* Infant with CMTC of trunk and extremities. *E,* Patient in *D,* now at age 24. Note dilated veins of forearm and persistent skin atrophy and pigmentation. *F,* Lower extremities of patient in *E:* venous ectasia and skin atrophy.

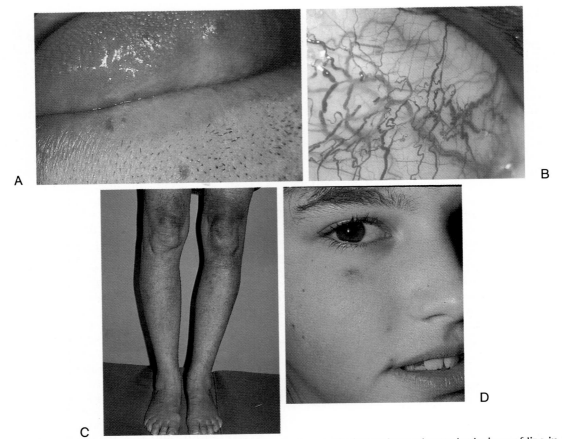

Figure 10–13. Telangiectasias. *A, Rendu-Osler-Weber syndrome.* Typical red maculopapular lesions of lips in a 55 year old male. (Courtesy of Harley A. Haynes, M.D.) *B, Ataxia-telangiectasia:* dilated, tortuous vessels in the bulbar conjunctiva of a 17 year old boy. (Reproduced by permission from Donaldson, D. D.: *Atlas of External Diseases of the Eye,* Vol II, St. Louis, 1968, The C. V. Mosby Co., p. 280.) *C, Generalized essential telangiectasia.* This healthy 60 year old woman noted gradual appearance of linear telangiectasia of lower extremities over the past 2 years. *D, Spider mark.* This common harmless lesion appeared in 11 year old girl.

1962; Feizi, 1972; Cooney et al., 1977; Martini, 1978). A study of four cases, which included the original cases described by Osler, showed specific local fibrovascular lesions in the livers of these patients, giving support to the concept that the fibrosis is, indeed, secondary to the vascular lesions (Daly and Schiller, 1976).

Aneurysms of large elastic arteries and the aorta have been repeatedly described in association with HHT (Schuster, 1937; Graham et al., 1964; Dondon et al., 1967; Borman and Schiller, 1969; Thomas, 1965; Trell et al., 1972). The common etiological factor is presumed to be an abnormality of the elastic and muscular components of the arterial wall.

The pathogenesis of HHT is still obscure. The architecture of the vascular abnormali-ties, their histologic appearance, and their hemodynamic significance have been convincingly reproduced by injection-corrosion casts of pulmonary telangiectases (Hales, 1956). These studies show that the structural abnormality is in the small arteries and arteriolar-precapillary sphincters that lack elastic fibers (Hales, 1956). The loss of the regulatory sphincteric mechanism and unrestricted flow could lead to formation of minute arteriovenous shunts. In time, the continuous hemodynamic load causes a secondary ectasia, elongation, and increased tortuosity of all parts of the vascular system. Other studies show remarkably few changes in the arterioles and suggest that the primary vascular abnormalities lie in the capillaries and small venules (Martini, 1978). Ultrastructural examination of the dilated vessels shows intact endothelium, continuous basal lamina but no elastic lamina, and inadequate smooth muscle elements (Jahnke, 1970). Thus, the pathogenesis may involve the new formation of structurally weak vessels that soon become dilated, elongated, and tortuous.

Studies of the mechanism of bleeding in HHT suggest that there is a local hemostatic abnormality. There is evidence that this may be related to increased plasminogen activator content, resulting in elevated fibrinolysis in the pericapillary tissues (Kwaan and Silverman, 1973). In 1952, Koch and colleagues reported that peroral treatment with ethinylestradiol diminished bleeding in this condition (Koch et al., 1952). Other investigators tried estrogen therapy to control epistaxis; the mechanism is thought to be induction of squamous metaplasia of the nasal septum (Flessa and Glueck, 1977). There is also ultrastructural evidence that estrogens might stabilize the brittle vascular walls in this syndrome (Menefee et al., 1975). However, a randomized double-blind trial with estrogen treatment, in 31 patients with HHT, showed no significant reduction in the frequency or intensity of bleeding (Vase, 1981).

Topical treatment of epistaxis is favored, e.g., pressure, packing, and microfibrillar collagen (Avitene). Laser coagulation is another therapeutic option (Shapshay and Oliver, 1984). If there is continued bleeding from a surgically accessible area, a split-thickness skin graft can be used to replace the involved septal mucosa (Saunders, 1960). This technique can be quite successful in diminishing epistaxis, although there is a tendency for crusting and fetor (Ulsø et al., 1983). In addition, telangiectasias can reappear within the skin graft (McCabe and Kelly, 1972; Ulsø et al., 1983).

ATAXIA-TELANGIECTASIA

Ataxia-telangiectasia (Louis-Bar syndrome) is transmitted by an autosomal recessive gene and is characterized by cerebellar ataxia, ocular and cutaneous telangiectasis, and frequent severe respiratory tract and sinus infections. Affected patients evidence severe immunologic deficiency with diminished levels of immunoglobulins A, G, and E; structural anomalies of the thymus and lymph nodes; and unusual susceptibility to lymphoma and T cell leukemia (Anmann et al.,

1969). Cultured fibroblasts from patients with this disorder show unusual sensitivity to x-rays and radiomimetic chemicals. It is postulated that the disease is causally related to defective repair of DNA.

Progressive cerebellar ataxia usually appears during the second or third year of life; the cutaneous and ocular abnormalities occur at 3–6 years of age. Symmetrical, bright red telangiectases are generally first noted in the nasal and temporal areas of the bulbar conjunctiva (Fig. 10–13B). Later, the cutaneous telangiectases appear on the eyelids, nasal bridge, cheeks, ears, neck, upper chest, and flexor surfaces of the forearms. Poorly controlled eye movements (oculomotor dyspraxia) often develop.

The course of the disease is progressive; as a rule, death usually occurs in the second decade of life from recurrent pulmonary infections and bronchiectasis, or from lymphoreticular malignancy. Kraemer has written a succinct review of the clinical and laboratory features of ataxia-telangiectasia (Kraemer, 1987).

GENERALIZED ESSENTIAL TELANGIECTASIA
("Angioma Serpiginosum")

In 1889, Hutchinson, in his own journal, described the case of a 15 year old girl who developed "A Peculiar Form of Serpiginous and Infective Naevoid Disease" (Hutchinson, 1889–1890). Radcliffe-Crocker proposed the term "angioma serpiginosum" for this entity in his 1893 textbook (Radcliffe-Crocker, 1893). The subject of considerable confusion in the literature, this condition has been mistaken for "angiokeratoma circumscriptum" and "nevus flammeus" (Stevenson, 1967).

Today, this skin disease is recognized as an acquired, idiopathic vascular ectasia and is best known as *generalized essential telangiectasia* (Becker, 1926; McGrae and Winkelmann, 1963; Rook et al., 1979). It occurs almost exclusively in females. The onset varies widely; lesions can appear before puberty, although middle adulthood is the usual age of presentation. Most reported cases are sporadic, although there may be a familial incidence (Marriott et al., 1975).

The primary lesions are pin-sized, red-purple vascular puncta, appearing in groups. The lesions extend frighteningly over several years, forming gyrate or serpiginous patterns or extensive sheets of telangiectases. Often there is a fiery red erythematous background (Fig. 10–13C). The telangiectasia occurs predominantly on the lower extremities, although any area of the body may be affected, except palms, soles, and mucous membranes. These patients show no evidence of systemic changes.

Histologic examination demonstrates thin-walled ectatic vessels in the upper corium with no signs of inflammation or hyperplasia (McGrae and Winkelmann, 1963).

Differential diagnosis is from other causes of telangiectasia, particularly Rendu-Osler-Weber syndrome. Generalized essential telangiectasia has a different distribution of lesions; presents in large, asymmetrical sheets; and usually does not hemorrhage. Late partial regression has been seen, but it is never complete. Successful treatment with oral tetracycline has been reported in one case (Shelley, 1971), but this is not confirmed. Whereas laser coagulation of facial telangiectasia is usually successful, the results following treatment of lower extremity telangiectasias have been unsatisfactory.

VASCULAR SPIDERS AND OTHER SIMILAR LESIONS

Acquired vascular marks called "spider nevus," "nevus araneus," or, incorrectly, "stellate hemangioma" have been comprehensively studied by Bean (Bean, 1958). These lesions most commonly occur over the dorsum of the hands and fingers, forearms, and face (Wenzl and Burgert, 1964). The spider mark consists of a central arteriole from which superficial vessels radiate (Fig. 10–13D). The blood flow is efferent, and therefore pressure with a tiny blunt instrument over the central vessel will cause blanching, and a centrifugal flush will occur when the pressure is released. Diascopy is another diagnostic maneuver: when a glass slide is pressed gently over the lesion, pulsations of the central vessel will be observed.

Spider marks typically appear on children in the preschool and school-aged group. Alderson found spider lesions in 47.5% of 1138 healthy English school children; the highest incidence occurred between 7 and 10 years, with no significant difference between boys and girls (Alderson, 1963). A study from the Mayo Clinic of normal children between the ages of 5 and 15 showed that 37% of boys and 48% of girls had at least one vascular spider (Wenzl and Burgert, 1964). They also noted that the incidence increased earlier and more rapidly in girls than in boys. Spontaneous disappearance of these marks does occur after puberty. Bean noted vascular spiders in 10–15% of normal adults (Bean, 1958).

Similar vascular lesions occur on the skin during pregnancy and have been called "hemangiomas of pregnancy" (Barter et al., 1963) or "granuloma gravidarum" when seen on the gingiva, palate, or septum. They usually appear during the second to fifth month of gestation and increase in size and number throughout the pregnancy. By the ninth month, 66% of pregnant white women have vascular spiders. The lesions may reach 5 mm in diameter. They usually disappear remarkably during the early puerperium. However, large lesions may persist, and vanished lesions often reappear in the same location with a subsequent pregnancy. Bean has beautifully documented the distribution of spider lesions in hepatic disease and pregnancy and has discussed the microanatomy. The lesion is an expansion of a normal dermal end artery, containing glomus cells, which then divides into radial vessels having the structure of veins (Bean, 1958).

There is gathering evidence that estrogen may account for the appearance of spider lesions in pregnancy, and that hormones somehow modulate the vasculature. This theory would account for the presence of spider marks in liver failure and the appearance of palmar erythema. The increased frequency of spider marks in pubertal females, more so than in males, also suggests a hormonal mechanism (Wenzl and Burgert, 1964).

Spider vascular lesions can be obliterated by punctate cautery or by argon laser directed at the central artery; however, the marks do tend to recur unless the abnormal vessels are completely obliterated.

References

A New English Dictionary on Historical Principles. Oxford: Clarendon Press, 1909, Vol. 7, p. 1138.

Alderson, M. R.: Spider naevi—their incidence in healthy school children. Arch. Dis. Child. *38*:286, 1963.

Andreev, V. C., and Pramatarov, K.: Cutis marmorata telangiectatica congenita in two sisters. Brit. J. Derm. *101*:345, 1979.

Anmann, A. J., Cain, W. A., Ishizaka, K., et al.: Immunoglobulin E deficiency in ataxia-telangiectasia. N. Engl. J. Med. *281*:469, 1969.

Argenta, L. C., Watanabe, M. J., and Grabb, W. C.: The use of tissue expansion in head and neck reconstruction. Ann. Plast. Surg. *11*:31, 1983.

Barsky, S. H., Rosen, S., Geer, D. E., and Noe, J.: The nature and evolution of port wine stains: A computer-assisted study. J. Invest. Dermatol. *74*:154, 1980.

Barter, R. H., Letterman, G. S., and Schurter, M.: Hemangiomas in pregnancy. Amer. J. Obstet. Gynec. *87*:625, 1963.

Bauer, S.: Pediatric neuro-urology. In Krane, R. J., and Siroky, M. B. (eds.): *Clinical Neuro-Urology*, 2nd ed. Boston: Little, Brown and Co., 1988.

Bean, W. B.: *Vascular Spiders and Related Lesions of the Skin*. Springfield, IL: Charles C Thomas Co., 1958, p. 372.

Beard, G. M.: Cases of naevi treated by electrolysis. N. Y. Med. J. *26*:616, 1877.

Becker, S. W.: Generalized telangiectasia: A clinical study with special consideration of etiology and pathology. Arch. Derm. *14*:387, 1926.

Benedek, T.: Facial hemiatrophy, sequel to the treatment of an extensive nevus flammeus (port-wine mark) with x-rays and radium. Milit. Surg. *106*:466, 1950.

Bettley, F. R.: Erythema nuchae. Brit. J. Derm. *52*:363, 1940.

Borman, J. B., and Schiller, M.: Osler's disease with multiple large vessel aneurysms. Angiology *20*:113, 1969.

Bowers, R. E.: Treatment of haemangiomatous naevi with thorium X. Brit. Med. J. *1*:121, 1951.

Braverman, I. M., and Keh-Yen, A.: Ultrastructural and three-dimensional reconstruction of several macular and papular telangiectases. J. Invest. Derm. *81*:489, 1983.

Brown, J. E., Cannon, B. and McDowell, A.: Permanent pigment injection of capillary hemangiomata. Plast. Reconstr. Surg. *1*:106, 1946.

Chandler, D.: Pulmonary and cerebral arteriovenous fistula with Osler's disease. Arch. Int. Med. *116*:277, 1965.

Cibis, G. W., Tripathi, R. C., and Tripathi, B. J.: Glaucoma in Sturge-Weber syndrome. Ophthalmology *91*:1061, 1984.

Clodius, L.: Excision and grafting of extensive facial haemangiomas. Brit. J. Plast. Surg. *30*:185, 1977.

Clodius, L.: Surgery for facial port-wine stain: Technique and results. Ann. Plast. Surg. *16*:457, 1986.

Clodius, L., and Smahel, J.: Resurfacing denuded areas of the beard with full-thickness scalp grafts. Brit. J. Plast. Surg. *32*:295, 1979.

Cobb, S.: Haemangioma of the spinal cord associated with skin naevi of the same metamere. Ann. Surg. *62*:641, 1915.

Conway, H.: Evolution of treatment of capillary hemangiomas of the face with further observation on the value of camouflage by permanent pigment injection (tattooing). Surgery *23*:389, 1948.

Conway, H., McKinney, P., and Climo, M.: Permanent camouflage of vascular nevi of the face by intradermal injection of insoluble pigments (tattooing): Experience through twenty years with 1022 cases. Plast. Reconstr. Surg. *40*:457, 1967.

Cooke, D. A. P.: Renal arteriovenous malformation demonstrated angiographically in hereditary haemorrhagic telangiectasia (Rendu-Osler-Weber disease). J. Roy. Soc. Med. *79*:744, 1986.

Cooney, T., Sweeney, E. C., Coll, R., and Greally, M.: 'Pseudocirrhosis' in hereditary haemorrhagic telangiectasia. J. Clin. Path. *30*:1134, 1977.

Cosman, B.: Clinical experience in the laser therapy of port-wine stains. Lasers Surg. Med. *1*:133, 1980.

Crosley, C. J., and Binet, E. F.: Sturge-Weber syndrome. Presentation as a focal seizure disorder without nevus flammeus. Clin. Pediatr. *17*:606, 1978.

Cushing, H.: Cases of spontaneous intracranial hemorrhage associated with trigeminal nevi. JAMA *47*:178, 1906.

Daly, J. J., and Schiller, A. L.: The liver in hereditary hemorrhagic telangiectasia (Osler-Weber-Rendu disease). Am. J. Med. *60*:723, 1976.

Desnick, R. J., and Sweeley, C. C.: Fabry's disease: alpha-Galactosidase-A deficiency (angiokeratoma corporis diffusum universale). In Fitzpatrick, T. B., Eisen, A. Z., Wolff, K., et al. (eds.): *Dermatology in General Medicine*, 3rd ed. New York: McGraw-Hill Book Co., 1987, p. 1739.

Dixey, J. R. B.: The "nape" nevus. Brit. Med. J. *1*:1032, 1955.

Dondon, J. R., Tanner, N. C., and Cowper, D. M.: Hepatic artery aneurysm hereditary haemorrhagic telangiectasia and peptic ulceration. Gut *8*:377, 1967.

Doppman, J. L., Wirth, F. P., DiChiro, G., and Ommaya, A. K.: Value of cutaneous angiomas in the arteriographic localization of spinal-cord arteriovenous malformations. N. Engl. J. Med. *281*:1440, 1969.

Durand, P., Borrone, C., and Della Cella, G.: A new mucopolysaccharide lipid-storage disease? Lancet *2*:1313, 1966.

Enjolras, O., Riché, M. C., and Merland, J. J.: Facial port-wine stains and Sturge-Weber syndrome. Pediatrics *76*:48, 1985.

Evans, H. W.: Angioma of the scrotum (Fordyce lesion). Arch. Intern. Med. *110*:520, 1962.

Fabry, J.: Über einen Fall von Angiokeratoma Circumscriptum am linken Oberschenkel. Derm. Zeit. *22*:1, 1915.

Feizi, O.: Hereditary hemorrhagic telangiectasia presenting with portal hypertension and cirrhosis of the liver. Gastroenterology *63*:660, 1972.

Finley, J. L., Clark, R. A. F., Covin, R. B., Blackman, R., Noe, J., and Rosen, S.: Immunofluorescent staining with antibodies to factor VIII, fibronectin, and collagenous basement membrane protein in normal human skin and port wine stains. Arch. Dermatol. *118*:971, 1982.

Fitch, N., Rochon, L., Srolovitz, H., and Hamilton, E.: Vascular abnormalities in a fetus with multiple pterygia. Amer. J. Med. Genet. *21*:755, 1985.

Fitzsimmons, J. S., and Starks, M.: Cutis marmorata telangiectatica congenita or congenital generalized phlebectasia. Arch. Dis. Child. *45*:724, 1970.

Flessa, H. C., and Glueck, H. I.: Hereditary hemorrhage telangiectasia (Osler-Weber-Rendu disease). Arch. Otolaryng. *103*:148, 1977.

Fletcher, J. S.: *Port: An Introduction to Its History and Delights*. London: Sotheby Publications by Philip Wilson Publishers, Ltd., 1978, p. 2.

Flores, J. T., Apfelberg, D. B., Maser, M. R., Lash, W., and White, D.: Angiokeratoma of Fordyce: Successful treatment with the argon laser. Plast. Reconstr. Surg. *74*:835, 1984.

Fordyce, J. A.: Angiokeratoma of the scrotum. J. Cutan. Genitourin. Dis. *14*:81, 1896.

Fox, G. H.: The treatment of wine-mark by electrolysis. Arch. Med. N.Y. *7*:166, 1882.

Garwicz, S., and Mortensson, W.: Intracranial calcification mimicking the Sturge-Weber syndrome. Pediatr. Radiol. 5:5, 1976.

Gibbs, D. D.: Rendu-Osler-Weber disease: A triple eponymous title lives on. J. Roy. Soc. Med. 79:742, 1986.

Goldwyn, R. M., and Rosoff, C. B.: Cryosurgery for large hemangiomas in adults. Plast. Reconstr. Surg. 43:605, 1969.

Gorlin, R. H., Pindborg, J. J., and Cohen, M. M., Jr.: Fabry syndrome. In Syndromes of the Head and Neck. New York: McGraw-Hill Book Co., 1976, pp. 295–299.

Grabb, W. C., MacCallum, M. S., and Tan, N. G.: Results from tattooing port-wine hemangiomas. Plast. Reconstr. Surg. 59:667, 1977.

Graham, W. P., III, Eisman, B., and Pryor, R.: Hepatic artery aneurysm with portal vein fistula in a patient with familial hereditary telangiectasia. Ann. Surg. 159:362, 1964.

Hales, M. R.: Multiple small arteriovenous fistulae of the lungs. Amer. J. Path. 32:927, 1956.

Halpern, M., Turner, A. F., and Citron, B. P.: Angiodysplasias of the abdominal viscera associated with hereditary hemorrhagic telangiectasia. Amer. J. Roent. 102:783, 1968.

Hanes, F. M.: Multiple hereditary telangiectases causing hemorrhage (hereditary hemorrhagic telangiectasia). Amer. J. Derm. Genito-Urinary Dis. 13:249, 1909.

Heyde, E. C.: Hereditary hemorrhagic telangiectasia: A report of pulmonary arteriovenous fistulae in mother and son: Medical (hormonal) and surgical therapy of this disease. Ann. Intern. Med. 41:1042, 1954.

Hurwitz, S.: Clinical Pediatric Dermatology. Philadelphia: W. B. Saunders Co., 1981, pp. 203–204.

Hutchinson, J.: A peculiar form of serpiginous and infective naevoid disease. Arch. Surg. (London) 1:Plate IX, 1889–1890.

Imperial, R., and Helwig, E. B.: Angiokeratoma. A clinicopathological study. Arch. Derm. 95:165, 1967a.

Imperial, R., and Helwig, E. B.: Verrucous hemangioma. A clinicopathologic study of 21 cases. Arch. Derm. 96:247, 1967b.

Imperial, R., and Helwig, E. B.: Angiokeratoma of the scrotum (Fordyce type). J. Urol. 98:379, 1967c.

Jacobs, A. H., and Walton, R. G.: The incidence of birthmarks in the neonate. Pediatrics 58:218, 1976.

Jahnke, V.: Ultrastructure of hereditary telangiectasia. Arch. Otolaryng. 91:262, 1970.

Jessen, R. T., Thompson, J., and Smith, E. G.: Cobb syndrome. Arch. Derm. 113:1587, 1977.

Johnson, H. A.: Transplantation's effect on capillary hemangiomas. Plast. Reconstr. Surg. 26:330, 1960.

Jonas, A. F.: Operative treatment for the cure of vascular nevi. Med. News Phila. 65:543, 1894.

Jönsson, G.: New method of treating capillary haemangiomas. Acta Chir. Scand. 95:275, 1947.

Kalischer, S.: Demonstration des Gehirns eines Kindes mit teleangiektasie der linksseitigen Gesichts-Kopfhaut und Hirnoberfläche. Berl. Klin. Wchnschs. 34:1059, 1897.

Kaplan, P., Hollenberg, R. D., and Fraser, F. C.: A spinal arteriovenous malformation with hereditary cutaneous hemangiomas. Amer. J. Dis. Child. 130:1329, 1976.

Koch, H. J., Escher, G. C., and Lewis, J. S.: Hormonal management of hereditary hemorrhagic telangiectasia. JAMA 149:1376, 1952.

Krabbe, K. H.: Facial and meningeal angiomatosis associated calcifications of brain cortex: A clinical and anatomicopathological contribution. Arch. Neurol. Psychiat. 32:737, 1934.

Kraemer, K. H.: Ataxia-telangiectasia. In Fitzpatrick, T. B., Eisen, A. Z., Wolff, K., et al. (eds.): Dermatology in General Medicine, 3rd ed. New York: McGraw-Hill Book Co., 1987, p. 1796.

Kromayer, von: Die Behandlung der roten Muttermale mit Licht und Radium nach Erfahrungen an 40 Fällen. Deutsche Med. Wochnschr. 36:299, 1910.

Kurczynski, T. W.: Hereditary cutis marmorata telangiectatica congenita. Pediatrics 70:52, 1982.

Kwaan, H. C., and Silverman, S.: Fibrinolytic activity in lesions of hereditary hemorrhagic telangiectasia. Arch. Derm. 107:571, 1973.

Lichtenstein, B. W.: Sturge-Weber-Dimitri syndrome: Cephalic form of neurocutaneous hemangiomatosis. A.M.A. Arch. Neurol. Psychiat. 71:291, 1954.

MacCollum, D. W.: Treatment of hemangiomas. Amer. J. Surg. 29:32, 1935.

Marriott, P. J., Munro, D. D., and Ryan, T.: Angioma serpiginosum—familial incidence. Brit. J. Derm. 93:701, 1975.

Martin, D. L., Chang, P. S., and McGrouther, D. A.: Full-thickness graft of haemangiomatous skin. Brit. J. Plast. Surg. 38:588, 1985.

Martini, G. A.: The liver in hereditary haemorrhagic telangiectasia: An inborn error of vascular structure with multiple manifestations: A reappraisal. Gut 19:531, 1978.

McCabe, W. P., and Kelly, A. P., Jr.: Management of epistaxis in Osler-Weber-Rendu disease. Recurrence of telangiectases within a nasal skin graft. Plast. Reconstr. Surg. 50:114, 1972.

McGrae, J. D., Jr., and Winkelmann, R. K.: Generalized essential telangiectasia: Report of a clinical and histochemical study of 13 patients with acquired cutaneous lesions. JAMA 185:909, 1963.

Menefee, M. G., Flessa, H. C., Glueck, H. I., and Hogg, S. P.: Hereditary hemorrhagic telangiectasia (Osler-Weber-Rendu disease): An electron microscopic study of the vascular lesions before and after therapy with hormones. Arch. Otolaryngol. 101:246, 1975.

Merlob, P., and Reisner, S. H.: Familial nevus flammeus of the forehead and Unna's nevus. Clin. Genet. 27:165, 1985.

Mibelli, V.: Di una nuova forma di cheratosi "angiocheratoma." Gior. Ital. d. Mal. Ven. 30:285, 1889.

Morel-Fatio, D.: Essai de traitement des angiomes plans par ponçage coloré de la peau congelée. Ann. Chir. Plastique 9:327, 1964.

Morton, E. R.: The treatment of naevi and other cutaneous lesions by electrolysis, cautery, and refrigeration. Lancet 2:1658, 1909.

Moyer, D. G.: Cutis marmorata telangiectatica congenita. Arch. Dermatol. 93:583, 1966.

Osler, W.: On a family form of recurring epistaxis associated with multiple telangiectases of skin and mucous membrane. Bull. Johns Hopkins Hosp. 12:333, 1901.

Øster, J., and Nielsen, A.: Nuchal naevi and interscapular telangiectasis. Acta Paediat. Scand. 59:416, 1970.

Parkes Weber, F.: Multiple hereditary developmental angiomata of the skin and mucous membranes associated with recurring haemorrhages. Lancet 2:160, 1907.

Parkes Weber, F.: Right-sided hemihypotrophy resulting from right-sided congenital spastic hemiplegia, with a morbid condition of the left side of the brain, revealed by radiograms. J. Neurol. Psychopath. 3:134, 1922.

Parkes Weber, F.: A note on the association of extensive haemangiomatous naevus of the skin with cerebral (meningeal) haemangioma, especially cases of facial vascular naevus with contralateral hemiplegia. Proc. Royal Soc. Med. (Sect. Neurol.) 22:431, 1929.

Pauli: Ueber das Fuermal und die einzig sichere Methode, diese Entstellung zu heilen. Siebold Archiv. f. Geburtshilfe, Frauenzimmer und Kinderrank 15:66, 1835.

Peterman, A. F., Hayles, A. G., Dockerty, M. B., and Love, J. G.: Encephalotrigeminal angiomatosis (Sturge-Weber disease). Clinical study of thirty-five cases. JAMA 167:2169, 1958.

Petrozzi, J. W., Rahn, E. K., Mofenson, H., and Greensher, J.: Cutis marmorata telangiectatica congenita. Arch. Dermatol. 101:74, 1970.

Phelps, C. D.: The pathogenesis of glaucoma in Sturge-Weber syndrome. Ophthalmology 85:276, 1978.

Poser, C. M., and Taveras, J. M.: Cerebral angiography in encephalotrigeminal angiomatosis. Radiology 68:327, 1957.

Pratt, A. G.: Birthmarks in infants. A.M.A. Arch. Derm. Syph. 67:302, 1967.

Radcliffe-Crocker, H.: Diseases of the Skin. Philadelphia: Blakiston Press, 1893, p. 646.

Rendu, M.: Epistaxis répétées chez un sujet porteur de petits angiomes cutanes et muqueux. Bull. Société Médicale des Hôpitaux de Paris 13:731, 1896.

Rook, A., Wilkinson, D. S., and Ebling, F. J. G.: Textbook of Dermatology, 3rd ed. Oxford: Blackwell Scientific Publications, 1979, p. 969.

Sagi, E., Aram, H., and Peled, I. J.: Basal cell carcinoma developing in a nevus flammeus. Cutis 33:311, 1984.

Sapru, R. P., Hutchison, D. C. S., and Hall, J. I.: Pulmonary hypertension in patients with pulmonary arteriovenous fistulae. Brit. Heart J. 31:559, 1969.

Saunders, W. H.: Septal dermoplasty for control of nosebleeds caused by hereditary hemorrhagic telangiectasia or septal perforations. Trans. Am. Acad. Ophthalmol. Otolaryngol. 64:500, 1960.

Schnyder, U. W.: Zur Klinik und Histologie der Angiome. Archiv. Derm. 200:483, 1955.

Schuster, H. N.: Familial haemorrhagic telangiectasia associated with multiple aneurysms of the splenic artery. J. Path. Bact. 44:29, 1937.

Shapshay, S. M., and Oliver, P.: Treatment of hereditary hemorrhagic telangiectasia by Nd-YAG laser photocoagulation. Laryngoscopy 94:1554, 1984.

Shelley, W. B.: Essential progressive telangiectasia. Successful treatment with tetracycline. JAMA 216:1343, 1971.

Smith, E. B., Graham, J. L., Ledman, J. A., and Snyder, R. D.: Fucosidosis. Cutis 19:195, 1977.

Smith, M. A., and Manfield, P. A.: The natural history of salmon patches in the first year of life. Brit. J. Dermatol. 74:31, 1962.

Smith, R. B. W., Prior, I. A. M., and Park, R. G.: Angiokeratoma of Mibelli: A family with nodular lesions of the leg. Aust. J. Dermatol. 9:329, 1968.

Smoller, B. R., and Rosen, S.: Port-wine stains: A disease of altered neural modulation of blood vessels? Arch. Dermat. 122:177, 1986.

Snyderman, R. K., and Wynn-Williams, D.: Complete replacement of port wine stains. N.Y. State Med. J. 66:1905, 1966.

South, D. A., and Jacobs, A. H.: Cutis marmorata telangiectatica congenita (congenital generalized phlebectasia). J. Pediatr. 93:944, 1978.

Squire, B.: Two cases of port-wine mark treated with a view to obliterating the mark without scar. Brit. Med. J. 1:865, 1878.

Squire, B.: An improvement in the treatment of port wine mark by linear scarification. Brit. Med. J. 2:732, 1879.

Stevenson, J. R., and Lincoln, C. S.: Angioma serpiginosum. Arch. Derm. 95:16, 1967.

Stevenson, R. F., Thomson, H. G., and Morin, J. D.: Unrecognized ocular problems associated with "port wine" stain of the face in children. Can. Med. Assoc. J. 111:953, 1974.

Straatsma, C. R.: Plastic repair of severe radium burns and angioma. N.Y. State Med. J. 30:9, 1930.

Sturge, W. A.: A case of partial epilepsy, apparently due to a lesion of one of the vaso-motor centres of the brain. Trans. Clinc. Soc. London 12:162, 1879.

Swerlick, R. A., and Cooper, P. H.: Pyogenic granuloma (lobular capillary hemangioma) within port-wine stains. J. Amer. Acad. Derm. 8:627, 1983.

Tan, K. L.: Nevus flammeus of the nape, glabella and eyelids. A clinical study of frequency, racial distribution, and association with congenital anomalies. Clin. Pediatr. 11:112, 1972.

Théron, J., Newton, T. H., and Hoyt, W. F.: Unilateral retinocephalic vascular malformations. Neuroradiology 7:185, 1974.

Thoma, K. H.: Sturge-Kalischer-Weber syndrome with pregnancy tumors. Oral Surg. Med. Oral Path. 5:1124, 1952.

Thomas, J. R.: Osler's disease with a dissecting aneurysm of the aorta. Arch. Int. Med. 116:448, 1965.

Thomson, H. G., and Wright, A.: Surgical tattooing of the port wine stain: Operative technique, results and critique. Plast. Reconstr. Surg. 48:113, 1971.

Trell, E., Johansson, B. W., Linell, F., and Ripa, J.: Familial pulmonary hypertension and multiple abnormalities of large systemic arteries in Osler's disease. Amer. J. Med. 53:50, 1972.

Turner, D.: De Morbis Cutaneis. A Treatise of Diseases Incident to the Skin. London: R. Bonwicke, W. Freeman, T. Goodwin, etc., 1714, p. 122.

Ulsø, C., Vase, P., and Stoksted, P.: Long-term results of dermatoplasty in the treatment of hereditary haemorrhagic telangiectasia. J. Laryngol. Otol. 97:223, 1983.

Unna, P. G.: Die Histopathologie der Hautkrankheiten. Berlin: Verlag von August Hirschwald, 1894, p. 920.

van der Hoeve, J.: The Doyne Memorial Lecture: Eye symptoms in phakomatoses. Trans. Ophth. Soc. U. K. 52:380, 1932.

van Lohuizen, C. H. J.: Über eine seltene angeborene Hautanomalie (cutis marmorata telangiectatica congenita). Acta Dermatovener. 3:202, 1922.

Vase, P.: Estrogen treatment of hereditary hemorrhagic telangiectasia. A double-blind controlled clinical trial. Acta Med. Scand. 209:393, 1981.

Wallace, H. J.: Anderson-Fabry disease. Brit. J. Derm. 88:1, 1973.

Way, B. H., Herrmann, J., Gilbert, E. F., Johnson, S. A. M., and Opitz, J. M.: Cutis marmorata telangiectatica congenita. J. Cutaneous Path. 1:10, 1974.

Weiss, D. I.: Dual origin of glaucoma in encephalotrigeminal haemangiomatosis. Trans. Ophthalmol. Soc. U.K. 93:477, 1973.

Wenzl, J. E., and Burgert, E. O.: The spider nevus in infancy and childhood. Pediatrics 33:227, 1964.

Wickham, L., and Degrais: The treatment of vascular naevi by radium. Brit. J. Dermat. 19:379, 1907.

Zelman, S.: Liver fibrosis in hereditary hemorrhagic telangiectasia. Arch. Path. 74:66, 1962.

CHAPTER ELEVEN

Venous and Arterial Malformations

A. E. Young

VENOUS MALFORMATIONS

Venous malformations may usefully be grouped as follows:
A. Defects of course, position, and number
B. Valvular anomalies
C. Aplasia, hypoplasia, and congenital obstruction of deep veins
D. Anomalous and ectatic veins, including
   1. True congenital varicose veins
   2. Phlebectasia
   3. Varicose dysplasia
E. Spongy venous malformations (called, in the past, "phlebangiomas"). These may be single or multiple, the latter encompassing Gorham's syndrome and the blue rubber bleb nevus syndrome.

Defects of Course, Position, and Number

The development of the venous system by the condensation of vessels from lacunae, with subsequent deletion of some vessels, frequently produces anomalies of course, position, and number of major, named veins as well as components of the tributary venous system. These variations are only rarely of clinical significance, and only those cases likely to present as a clinical problem are recorded here (Table 11–1).

Caval Veins

Anomalies of caval development are said to occur in 1–4% of the population and are usually asymptomatic (Fig. 11–1). They are not usually associated with a cutaneous birthmark, though they may be (Fig. 11–2), and most are only discovered at operation, at venographic examination, or postmortem. Caval anomalies include persistence of a left-sided superior vena cava or inferior vena cava with or without coexistence of right-sided vessels; the inferior vena cava (IVC) may be absent above the renal veins, with venous return via the azygos system. The inferior vena cava may be pre-ureteric, or there may be combined pre- and post-ureteric venae cavae. In addition, the left renal

Table 11–1. CLINICALLY SIGNIFICANT ANOMALIES OF MAJOR VEINS

Superior Vena Cava
Duplication
Left-sided
Anomalous systemic venous return

Inferior Vena Cava
Agenesis
Duplication
Left-sided
Pre-ureteric

Portal Vein
Agenesis
Duplication
Pre-duodenal
Congenital portosystemic connection

Peripheral Veins
Agenesis/hypoplasia
Duplication
Avalvulosis
Anomalous
Compression (femoral/iliac/axillary)

10% (Schobinger, 1977). These reduplicated segments go unnoticed until the limb is involved in venous thrombosis or until the anomalies are discovered during an operation.

Abnormalities of the course of the major veins in the root of the neck are uncommon, but when present they may predispose the patient to clot formation, so-called "effort thrombosis."

Valvular Anomalies

The most common vascular abnormality encountered in adults is varicosity of the superficial veins of the lower limb. It is usually a progressive and often familial condition, probably secondary to a primary congenital inadequacy of some or all of the valves in the affected veins. Although 30% of the working population have such varicosities, this condition is rarely noted before the late teens (Widmer, 1979). Another cause should be sought if varicose veins appear before puberty.

The number and distribution of venous valves vary considerably from person to person, and minor reductions in the total cannot be assessed. Thus there are, for example, functional valves in the iliac vessels in only 50% of the population. Total avalvulosis is described in which orthostatic dilatation of surface veins of the legs, together with mild edema, is noted in childhood (Plate et al., 1983). There may also be acrocyanosis of the hands and feet in this condition, and patients may suffer fainting spells as a result of the peripheral pooling of blood in the valveless veins. Dysplasia of the veins in Marfan's syndrome can cause similar problems. The condition of congenital avalvulosis is usually familial; Lodin and colleagues collected 30 cases over 10 years at the Karolinska Institute in Stockholm (Lodin et al., 1958), and Plate identified 15 patients from one Swedish family (Plate et al., 1983). However, sporadic cases are encountered and patients have been seen in the Department of Surgery at St. Thomas' Hospital, London, who have severe symptoms as a result of the avalvulosis. One patient, for example, presented with typical venous ulceration at the ankle and another had no physical evidence of anomalous veins but suffered venous claudication at 100 meters. Phlebography showed dilated, ectatic, valveless deep veins. These may involve just the lower limb or the lower and upper limbs (Fig. 11–3).

Aplasia, Hypoplasia, and Congenital Obstruction of Deep Veins

These anomalies are of particular importance because, though rare, they are usually symptomatic and are often associated with skeletal abnormalities, cutaneous varicosities, and capillary or dermal vascular malformations. The outward and visible signs present early, and it is of crucial importance that the physician treating these cutaneous problems be aware of the deeper abnormalities.

True atresia of the lower inferior vena cava or iliac veins is rare. There is, however, a common anomaly of the origin of the iliac vein encountered in about 20% of the population. This anomaly is found at the origin of the left common iliac vein at the point where it is crossed by the right common iliac artery. The anomalies take the form of longitudinal septa or "venous spurs" (May and DeWeese, 1979), or simple narrowing of the vein by the adjacent artery (McMurrick, 1906; DiDio, 1949; Cockett, 1965) (Fig. 11–4). These anomalies predispose the patient to a syndrome of swelling and aching of the leg, and some patients may experience venous claudication. There may or may not be varicosities of the legs. Indeed, although the patients may have definite symptoms, it is common for there to be no visible signs of the anomaly. The patients are prone to develop iliofemoral venous thromboses, and, indeed, in many cases the symptoms are largely due to the sequelae of the thrombosis rather than the anomaly itself. Because pelvic cross collaterals via the internal iliac system usually compensate for the primary partial obstruction in the iliac veins, symptoms may also develop when surgical dissection interferes with that collateral flow. Gynecological procedures involving the broad ligaments and uterine vessels are a particular cause of this interference of flow. Occasionally, pelvic cross collaterals are supplemented by transverse veins on the anterior abdominal wall. These may be mistaken as primarily ectatic veins. The abnormality of the common iliac vein has been described as the "iliac compres-

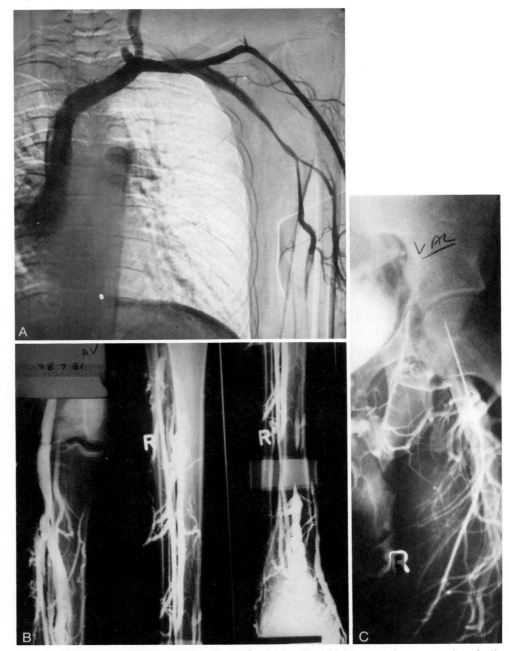

Figure 11–3. Congenital avalvulosis affecting the entire body. The phlebogram shows no valves in the upper limb veins *(A)*, nor in the lower limb *(B)*. C, A Valsalva maneuver following injection of contrast into the iliac veins fills the veins of the leg retrogradely.

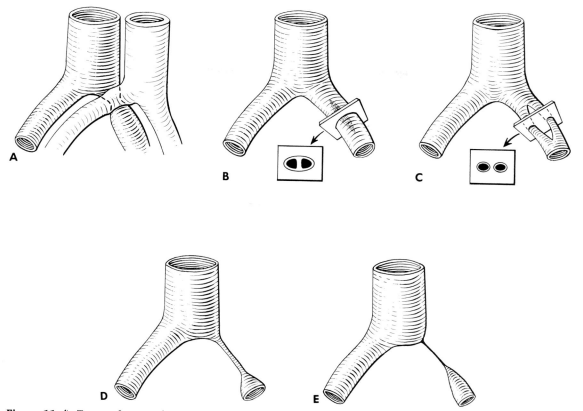

Figure 11–4. Types of congenital anomalies of the iliac veins. *A*, Compression by the overlying iliac artery. *B*, Partial occlusion by a septum. *C*, Double vein. *D*, Hypoplasia. *E*, True atresia.

sion syndrome," though compression of the iliac veins by the right common iliac artery is not always the cause (Cockett and Lea Thomas, 1965; Dodd and Cockett, 1979). Ninety-five per cent of cases occur on the left, as described, but in 5% of cases the abnormality is either bilateral or confined to the right side. The syndrome is never associated with skeletal anomalies or cutaneous markings, and for its diagnosis venography is needed, which may also include oblique and lateral views and intraosseous injection. Ideally, a raised femoral venous pressure should also be present. Isotope venography has been found to be a reliable way of demonstrating both the anatomical and the functional obstruction of the iliac veins (Buxton-Thomas et al., 1980). Complete atresias of the iliac vessels are occasionally encountered in association with the Klippel-Trenaunay syndrome. Iliac compression syndrome is further discussed in Chapter Nineteen.

Axillary vein compression is usually asymptomatic until thrombosis occurs. The compression is due to a fibrous or muscular band at the thoracic outlet or, more rarely, to the presence of an anomalous muscle in the axilla, the axillopectoral muscle (Sachatello, 1977).

Aplasias and hypoplasias of the femoral and/or popliteal veins are a more common association with the Klippel-Trenaunay complex and with the so-called "incomplete" variants of that syndrome, in which deep vein abnormalities are associated with hypertrophy of the limb but not with a cutaneous capillary stain or with visible varicose veins. There is argument about the incidence of deep vein anomalies in Klippel-Trenaunay syndrome. Servelle (Servelle and Babillot, 1980) maintains that it is almost invariable, but most other authors experience it in between 5 and 20% of patients (Baskerville et al., 1985). Servelle attributes the apparent hypoplasia to bands of fibrous tissue obstructing or encasing the vessels. There are examples of Klippel-Trenaunay syndrome with documented iliac vein atresia (Fig. 11–5).

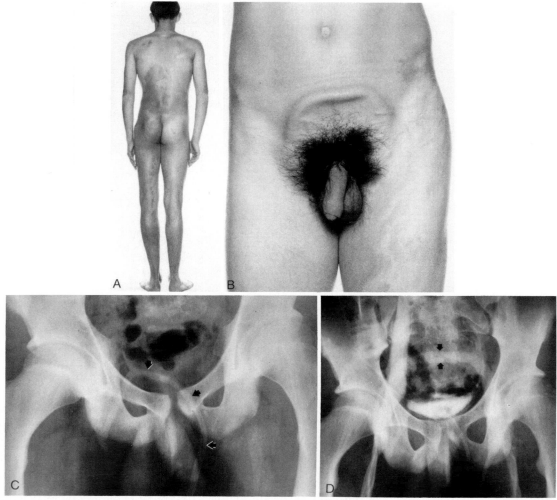

Figure 11–5. Klippel-Trenaunay syndrome with iliac vein atresia. *A,* The patient has a long leg with an extensive capillary malformation extending onto the trunk. *B,* A large cutaneous collateral vein crosses from the affected leg to the unaffected one. *C,* This is shown on direct puncture angiography to be an extension of the left long saphenous vein (arrows). *D,* Iliac phlebography shows the external iliac vein on the left crossing to the right via a large deep collateral (arrow).

Anomalous and Ectatic Veins

Anomalous Superficial Veins

Anomalous superficial veins are usually encountered as part of the Klippel-Trenaunay syndrome and are described in Chapter Fifteen. Occasionally the ectatic veins may, in the absence of overgrowth and a capillary malformation, be the only marker of the syndrome. Anomalously placed ectatic veins may sometimes be seen as part of a sporadic, unnamed genetic defect. We have, for instance, seen a girl with a hypoplastic lower leg with ectatic veins on it but without a capillary mark. The child also has epicanthal folds, sagittal alopecia, and arrested hydrocephalus (Fig. 11–6A). Often what appears to be an anomalous vein is merely a varicose or ectatic, but anatomically normal, vein (Fig. 11–6B).

Phlebectasia

Ectasia merely means dilatation (Greek "ek" = out + "teinein" = to stretch). The term *phlebectasia* thus indicates distension of veins and embraces both congenital and acquired lesions. Unfortunately, it is a hotch-potch of limited clinical use. Lea Thomas and Andress have stressed the importance of limiting the term both phlebologically and clinically to dilatation of venous trunks, in contrast to a localized anomaly of cavernous venous lakes (Lea Thomas and Andress, 1971). Congenitally ectatic veins may be solitary, localized, regional, or diffuse, and the various congenital types may be summarized as follows:

A. *Diffuse Phlebectasias*
  1. "Genuine diffuse phlebectasia"
  2. Cutis marmorata telangiectatica congenita (capillary/venular) (see Chapter Ten).
B. *Associated Phlebectasias*
  1. With deep vein aplasias/hypoplasias, as in Klippel-Trenaunay syndrome
  2. With overt arteriovenous malformations, as in Parkes Weber syndrome
  3. With venous valvular dysplasias, as in

commonly occurring banal or "idio-pathic" varicose veins
  4. In association with multiple spongy venous malformations ("phlebangio-matosis")

Diffuse Phlebectasia. Genuine diffuse phlebectasia ("of Bockenheimer") involves enlargements of all the veins, both large and small, superficial and deep, of part of the body (usually a limb) (Bockenheimer, 1907). Although the first description is attributed to Bockenheimer, Montfalcon noted in 1836 that Baron Alibert had seen, at the Hôpital de St. Louis, "the body of a man whose veins were all varicose—even the veins of the brain and the vena azygos" (Montfalcon, 1836). Diffuse phlebectasia is a rare condition and has to be carefully separated from the secondary varicosis noted with multiple congenital arteriovenous fistulae. Malan subdivides diffuse phlebectasias into two main types, regional and genuine diffuse (Malan and

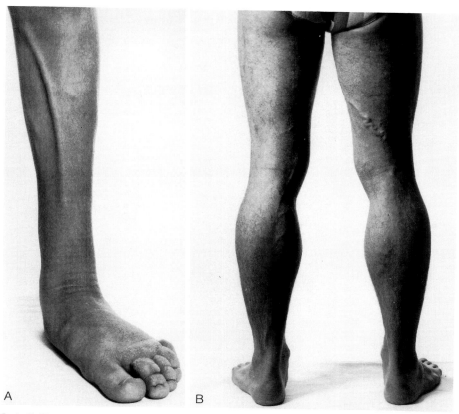

Figure 11–6. *A,* Solitary ectatic vein on a hypoplastic lower leg in a 7 year old girl with a dysmorphic face. *B,* An ectatic but anatomically normal vein had been present on the back of this man's thigh since infancy. The remainder of the venous system was normal; there was no long saphenous incompetence.

Puglionisi, 1964). He also notes a third type, in which there is associated deep vein hypoplasia. This last group, however, is best considered as part of the Klippel-Trenaunay syndrome. The true phlebectasias were first reviewed by Freund (1936). Diffuse phlebectasia has the following features:

1. Any limb can be affected, but the upper is more commonly affected than the lower.

2. The involved area shows enlargement of all veins into their finest ramifications, without preference for any specific anatomical distribution.

3. The ectasia may be saccular or tubular.

4. Dilatation of the veins is first noted in childhood but is slowly and inexorably progressive.

5. Histologic examination shows a primary maldevelopment of the vein wall with very little muscle and elastin in the media.

6. Thrombosis and phlebolith formation are common.

7. The affected limb may be longer or shorter than its fellow and the muscle wasted.

Pain, swelling, and ulceration have been observed. There may be an associated capillary malformation in the skin.

8. Surgical excision of the ectatic veins seems neither to help the symptoms nor halt the progression of the disease.

Varicose Dysplasia

Schobinger has described a syndrome of familial diffuse lower limb varicosis, noted at puberty and associated with mild limb hypertrophy and the presence of pigmented nevi in the skin of the affected leg (Schobinger, 1977). There may be ectatic deep veins, but there is no evidence to suggest arteriovenous shunting or malformation, apart from raised femoral vein oxygen tension. Of 4000 patients with "primary varicose veins" reviewed by Schobinger, 6% were considered to have "varicose dysplasia." The concept of varicose dysplasia suggests the existence of a continuum of malformation from banal primary varicosis to Klippel-Trenaunay syndrome.

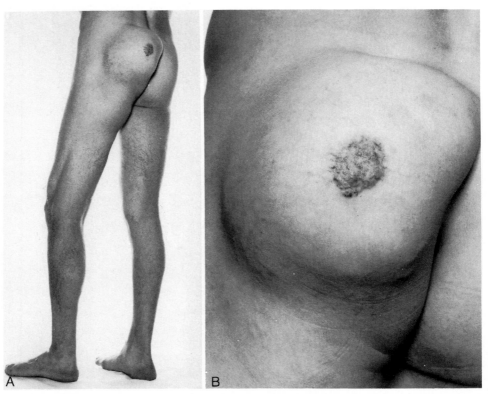

Figure 11–7. A, A large, circumscribed venous malformation. B, There is a small cutaneous capillary "marker" lesion. The patient remained asymptomatic until in late middle age, when he developed neurological symptoms in the leg from direct pressure of the malformation on sciatic nerve roots.

Spongy Venous Malformations ("Phlebangiomas")

Although spongy venous malformations may cause problems simply by their bulk, position, pressure on neighboring structures (Fig. 11–7), or hemorrhage, there are two specific situations that need to be considered when diffuse venous anomalies are associated with a major system disease: firstly, involvement of bone and, secondly, diffuse venous anomalies involving the gastrointestinal tract. The latter combination is popularly known as "blue rubber bleb nevus syndrome."

Localized Spongy Venous Malformations

Circumscribed knots of abnormal veins and/or venous spaces are frequently de-scribed as "phlebangiomas" and, where they are multiple, as "phlebangiomatosis." The terms are inaccurate, because the lesions are not true hemangiomas for, at cellular level, they are stable malformations.

There is a continuum of localized venous malformations from blue capillary spongy blebs through cavernous lesions (in which the venous lacunae are connected to the venous circulation by capillaries), through localized saccular anomalies (connected by veins to the venous circulation), to diffuse venous ectasias (Fig. 11–8). Furthermore, even apparently localized but multiple venous lesions tend to coexist with venous ectasias and deep vein anomalies. The localized lesions all have similar important characteristics:

1. A blue or purple color
2. Swelling when dependent or when the outflow is obstructed by a tourniquet

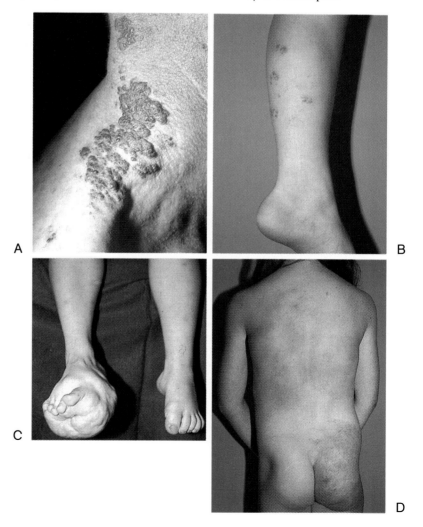

Figure 11–8. Spectrum of venous malformations. *A,* Multiple circumscribed venous anomalies in the skin of the neck. *B,* Localized venous blebs were scattered over the whole of this child's body (blue rubber bleb nevus syndrome). *C,* Large multiloculated saccular venous anomaly of the whole foot. *D,* Diffuse patches of cutaneous venous ectasia.

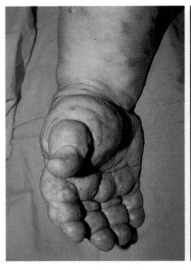 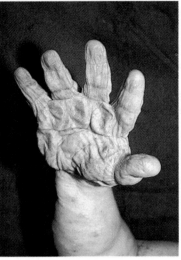

A   B

Figure 11–9. Diffuse saccular and ectatic venous malformation of the arm and hand. Its venous nature is confirmed by: *A.* Distension when dependent. *B.* Complete emptying when the hand is elevated.

3. Reduction in size and tissue tension when the lesion in elevated above the heart (Fig. 11–9)

4. Absence of clinical, radiological, or other evidence of arteriovenous fistulae

In addition, the neighboring veins may be enlarged. Calcified phleboliths may be present in the lesions. Hyperhidrosis over the lesion is common, and there may be recurrent attacks of thrombophlebitis in or near the lesions. Cruveilhier illustrated and described a typical case of multiple "phlebangiomas" in 1842 and noted the diverse size and character of the lesions (Cruveilhier, 1842). He also noted the common occurrence of phleboliths (Fig. 11–10). Spongy venous malformations are encountered not just in the skin but in all other tissues. The vast majority of deeply placed solitary venous anomalies cause no symptoms and are never discovered. They will, however, occasionally become symptomatic as a result of slow enlargement and pressure on surrounding structures, especially nerves (see Fig. 11–7). There is no good evidence, either histologic or clinical, that the enlargement of these lesions is malignant in a cellular sense; neither do they have malignant potential. Their "infiltration" of surrounding structures is present from the outset and is *not* malignant invasion. The enlargement is probably due to hemodynamic factors and simple stretching of the walls of the venous spaces. In addition to causing symptoms by pressure, these venous lesions may cause clinical problems by hemorrhage after trauma, by painful thrombosis, or by virtue of bulk. For example:

A. In the tongue. Small lesions are common,

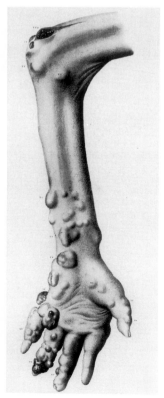

Figure 11–10. The first illustrated case of multiple "phlebangiomas" from Cruveilhier, 1842.

but large ones ("macroglossia angiomatosa") may interfere with speech and eating.

B. Orbital, causing exophthalmos.

C. Nasopharyngeal, causing bleeding.

D. Masseter/parotid, causing pain. Whereas arteriovenous malformations of the parotid are proportionately more common, venous anomalies are more often encountered in the masseter. Malan described 22 such cases (Malan, 1974).

E. Limb. When the lesions are diffuse and involve a limb, hypoplasia and shortening may occur.

F. Bone. Venous malformations may be associated with bone disease in several separate ways:

1. Disorders of growth: overgrowth and undergrowth.

2. By direct involvement of bone or by inclusion in bone of *solitary or multiple circumscribed lesions*. The latter may produce massive *osteolysis* (Gorham-Stout syndrome).

3. Association with dyschondroplasia (Maffucci's syndrome).

4. Association with other bone dysplasias.

In *1* and *2*, the bone abnormality may be caused by the venous lesion; in *3* and *4*, the lesion is merely concomitant.

Solitary vascular malformations in bone are very common, and Wallis notes that they are found in 10% of all autopsies (Wallis et al., 1964). If present in bone, they may be the site of pathological fractures, but the particular problem with solitary bone lesions is diagnosis. They occur most notably in the skull, vertebrae, scapulae, ribs, pelvis, and long bones and may be almost impossible to differentiate from benign tumors, cysts, and granulomas without biopsy. They represented 0.6% of primary bone tumors seen at the Mayo Clinic (Dahlin, 1957). Their radiological appearances have variously been described as "sunburst," "corduroy cloth," "honeycomb," and "soap bubbles" (Sherman and Wilner, 1961).

Multiple Intra-osseous Venous Malformations

These are much less common than solitary lesions and often behave differently, destroying rather than expanding bone. They are, however, frequently associated with cutaneous vascular malformations and are thus described in more detail here. The typical bone changes may be associated not only with venous malformations but also with lymphatic and capillary malformations and also may coexist with arteriovenous malformations elsewhere. The condition has been well reviewed under the misleading title of "diffuse skeletal hemangiomatosis" by Wallis and coworkers in 1964 (Wallis et al., 1964) and, more accurately, under "massive osteolysis" by Gorham and Stout (Gorham and Stout, 1955). The latter authors well deserve the eponymous syndrome for their very thorough reappraisal of all reported cases until 1955. The completeness of their attempts at marshalling all the pathological slides of all the reported cases was only handicapped by the destruction of the slides of four cases during the bombing of certain French and British pathology laboratories during the Second World War.

Gorham-Stout syndrome is sometimes described as "osteovascular dysplasia," "disappearing bone disease," "phantom bone disease," or "lithogenic phlebangiomatosis"; where it involves the upper limb, it has been called "hemangiomatosis braquial osteolitica of Martorell (and Trinquoste)" (Martorell, 1949). The venous anomalies involve bone and, usually, also nearby skin and soft tissues. The condition tends predominantly to affect the upper limb and shoulder girdle, though single bones and contiguous areas of adjacent bones may be involved (Fig. 11–11). Features that may be noted but that need not all be present are the following:

1. Progressive osteolysis with spotty lacunar patterns of resorption.

2. Pathological fractures.

3. Calcified phleboliths.

4. Coexistent shortening of the limb. Malan believes the shortening is due to destruction of the epiphyseal cartilage by the vascular malformation, but shortening of the limb has also been described as occurring with occult venous anomalies in the absence of radiological evidence of bone involvement. By contrast, the limb is enlarged in some patients.

The mechanism of the osteolysis is not clear. The radiographical changes are initially similar to those of chronic ischemia, and diminished blood flow at the epiphyses would account for the observed shortening. There may also be mechanical factors involved: for example, repeated alterations in

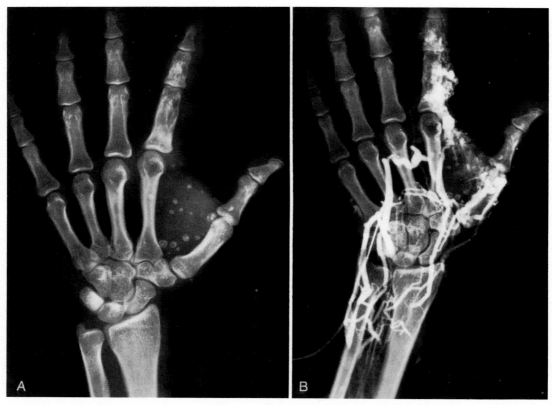

Figure 11–11. A localized spongy venous malformation of the hand. *A,* The plain film shows phleboliths and associated bone changes. *B,* The direct puncture venogram delineates the extent of the lesion.

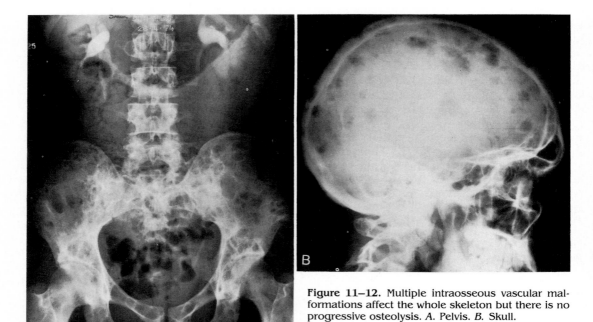

Figure 11–12. Multiple intraosseous vascular malformations affect the whole skeleton but there is no progressive osteolysis. *A.* Pelvis. *B.* Skull.

intravascular pressure caused by changes in posture. This may erode bone in a manner analogous to an aortic aneurysm eroding adjacent vertebrae. An increase in normal bone resorption seems unlikely, as biopsies do not show an increased number of osteoclasts. The histologic pattern is one of anomalous vascular channels with focal sclerosis. It may be of relevance to the proposed "hemodynamic" theory of bone resorption in

these patients that when the intraosseous anomalies are lymphatic (Fig. 11–12), progressive osteolysis does not usually occur. In venous intraosseous anomalies, resorption may be severe (Fig. 11–13).

The vascular channels in the bone may be capillary, venous, or lymphatic anomalies (Fig. 11–12). The dilated venous type is said to predominate in the vertebrae and skull. Capillary lesions are predominant in flat and

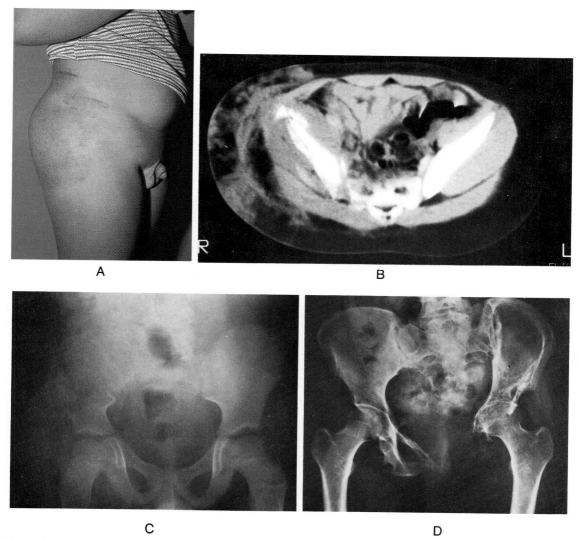

A   B

C   D

Figure 11–13. Four year old boy with history of gradual enlargement of a mass in the right hip region *(A–C)*. *A,* Faint vascular stain of skin overlying mass (combined capillary-venous anomaly). *B,* Computed tomographic scan at the same level showing extensive soft tissue mass and patchy osteolysis of the wing of the ileum. *C,* Plain pelvic radiograph demonstrates near total disappearance of the ileum and erosion of the adjacent sacrum. Irradiation reportedly can slow progression of this condition; this boy demonstrated such a response. *D,* This 35 year old Asian woman has had progressive pain and osteolytic destruction of the left side of the pelvis for 15 years. Biopsies show only venous vascular channels in bone (Gorham's syndrome). She has no visible vascular malformation in the overlying skin.

long bones. Both types may coexist. The early changes of osteolysis have a similar radiographical appearance to patchy osteoporosis. As the osteolysis progresses there is replacement by fibrous tissue, and if the process continues there is concentric bone resorption, giving a "sucked candy" appearance. Eventually the bone may disappear (Figs. 11–13 and 11–14). Pain may be severe in the area of bone resorption, and disability from bone loss may be considerable. There are anecdotal reports of beneficial effects from local radiotherapy.

The syndrome of primarily skeletal vascular anomalies with minimal visceral involvement is the typical variant encountered in children and young adults. When venous anomalies of the skeleton present in adults, they are usually part of a systemic or generalized vascular malformation syndrome (once known as "miliary angiomatosis"). The skeletal problems are then overshadowed by complications from pulmonary and pleural lesions (Wallis et al., 1964).

In one reported case with diffuse skeletal, cutaneous, hepatic, and CNS involvement, an increased urinary excretion of glycosaminoglycan (heparin sulfates) was discovered (Gordin et al., 1975). Bergoin and colleagues describe a case of lower limb osteolytic venous lesions associated with platelet and coagulation abnormalities (Bergoin et al., 1976). A few cases of osteolytic skeletal malformations in association with enchondromas in Maffucci's syndrome have been reported.

Another particularly aggressive variant of Gorham's syndrome is described by Haferkamp (1962), in which the vascular anomalies are widespread, the bone destruction rapid, and in which there is associated fatty infiltration of the liver and kidney. Hematologic assessment shows immature erythroid and myeloid cells (Haferkamp, 1962). The prognosis is poor in these diffuse forms of osteolysis.

Blue Rubber Bleb Nevus Syndrome

This syndrome, first described by Bean, is the association of multiple venous malformations in the skin and bleeding from similar vascular anomalies of the gastrointestinal tract (Bean, 1958). The skin lesions vary from the size of a pinhead to 1.5 cm in diameter. They are bluish, firm, dome shaped, and rubbery (Fig. 11–15). They are scattered over

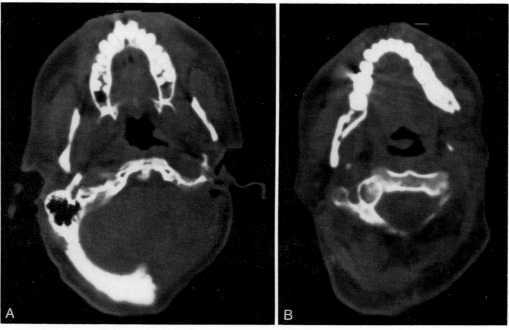

Figure 11–14. A 40 year old male presented with a 3 year history of neck pain. Computed tomography demonstrated "disappearing bone disease." The process has, to date, responded to radiation therapy. A, Bone loss in left occipital area. B, Erosion of posterior lateral elements of C1, C2, and mandibular ramus. (Radiographs courtesy of the patient.)

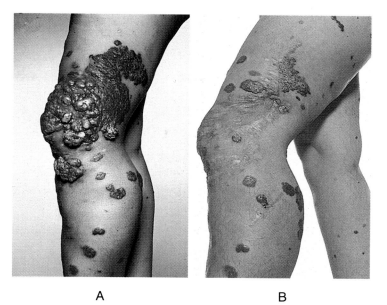

A   B

Figure 11–15. *A,* This boy has multiple spongy venous malformations involving the left leg, both superficially and deep, but he also has scattered lesions throughout his body. *B,* Affected areas about the knee, which bled repeatedly, were excised and split-thickness skin grafted.

the trunk and limbs, and similar lesions occur in the bowel, without any special association with one part of the bowel. In Bean's classic work *Vascular Spiders*, he noted, however, that the bluish nevi of the skin seen in this syndrome may occur in three main forms. Bean stated:

One is the large disfiguring cavernous hemangioma which may replace vital structures. . . . Another variety is the blood sac, looking like a blue rubber nipple covered with a milk white tissue of thin skin. These can be emptied of their contained blood. From the irregular mussed and rumpled state they resume their distended state by the gradual influx of blood. The third major variety of lesion is the irregular blue mark, sometimes with punctate, blackish spots merging with the adjacent normal skin in a series of color graduations through pale blue to white. Such lesions are elevated above the skin only if they are large. Small ones may or may not blanch on pressure. There is rarely complete fading, perhaps because of the complex range of coiled vascular spaces which trap blood when the structure is compressed (Bean, 1958).

The patients that Bean described had lesions in other sites (parotid, brain, liver, spleen, joints). Given this disparity of site and the variability in the characteristics of the lesions, it seems that Bean was describing merely a particular pattern of diffuse venous malformations complicated by gastrointestinal hemorrhage.

Other reports of multiple spongy venous malformations have similarly shown involvement of the liver, muscle, bones, lungs, kidneys, brain, nasal mucosa, spleen, gallbladder, adrenals, pleura, and peritoneum (Sakurane et al., 1967; Rice and Fischer, 1962; Waybright et al., 1978; Belsheim and Sullivan, 1980). It is not surprising, therefore, that hemoptysis, hematuria, epistaxis, and menorrhagia have been described in these patients, as well as the more common gastrointestinal hemorrhage and anemia. The lesions tend to enlarge with time and may be painful. Abnormal sweating is sometimes noticed adjacent to them. Histologically, sweat glands may be noted to be closely related to the dilated vascular spaces in the lesions. There are two reports of dominant inheritance. Berlyne traced the syndrome through five generations in one family (Berlyne and Berlyne, 1960), and Walshe found it in three generations in another (Walshe et al., 1966). Multiple cerebral venous malformations without cutaneous lesions have also been noted to be familial in some instances (Hayman et al., 1982). Nevertheless, in keeping with other vascular malformations, this condition generally occurs sporadically, with no family history. Waybright has noted that lingual or sublingual venous malformations may be markers of similar intracranial lesions (Waybright et al., 1981).

Diffuse venous anomalies are rare, and

whether the "blue rubber bleb nevus syndrome" truly exists as a separate disease is debatable. Nonetheless, the catchiness of its title will guarantee its survival, and familiarity with it serves to remind the clinician of the risks of deep-seated lesions in any patient with multiple cutaneous venous abnormalities. The problem of venous malformations involving the gastrointestinal tract is considered in Chapter Eighteen.

There are extremely rare cases of a cutaneous venous anomaly that clinically resembles blue rubber bleb nevus but that also demonstrates the remarkable capacity to perspire when stroked or pinched (Domonkos and Suarez, 1967). Like blue rubber bleb nevi, these lesions are painful on palpation. First reported by Beier in 1895 (Beier, 1895), this entity was called "hamartome angiomateux sudoripare secretant" by Vilanova in 1963 (Vilanova et al., 1963). The lesions of "sudoriparous angioma" are present at birth, dome shaped, and clustered, and measure 12–20 mm in diameter. Histologic examination shows thin-walled venular channels in the middle or deep corium with adjacent dilated eccrine structures. None of the reported cases demonstrated vascular lesions in the gastrointestinal tract.

An important differential diagnosis in localized nodular venous malformations is Kaposi's sarcoma.

Treatment of Venous Malformations

The great majority of venous malformations are asymptomatic, and treatment is fundamentally one of explanation, reassurance, and advice, where relevant, about the avoidance of trauma to the affected area. Venous malformations that cause discomfort, aching, or frank pain can be treated conservatively with elastic compression garments. Pain as a result of thrombosis in the lesion responds to analgesia and anti-inflammatory agents, but thrombosis in ectatic veins carries a risk of pulmonary embolism and may require treatment with anticoagulants.

Well-localized but troublesome cutaneous lesions are sometimes amenable to surgical excision, but deep extension of such lesions and lateral subcutaneous spread may cause hemorrhage at operation to be greater than expected. Deeply placed or very large lesions may best be treated by being thrombosed, by either percutaneous sclerosants, such as hyperosmolar saline, or pervascular embolization with agents such as Ethibloc (see Chapter Twenty-One). Such treatment should not be embarked upon in the asymptomatic patient and should be preceded by adequate investigation by angiography, CT scanning, and other imaging techniques. Venous malformations involving joints are particularly trou-

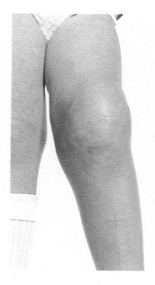

A

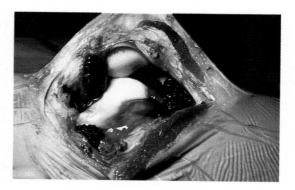

B

Figure 11–16. *A,* Painful, tense swelling of the knee caused by bleeding from a venous malformation. *B,* A venous malformation of the knee treated by synovectomy.

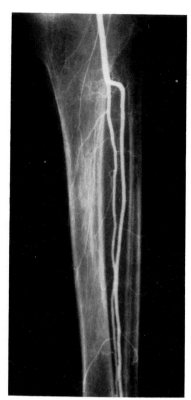

Figure 11–17. Atresia/agenesis of the posterior tibial artery.

blesome because of recurrent painful hemarthroses or thromboses and may thus require direct excision (Fig. 11–16).

ARTERIAL ABNORMALITIES

Arterial anomalies may be positional (supernumerary, absent, or of abnormal course) (Poynter, 1923) or structural (congenital hypoplasias, stenoses, aneurysms, and arteriectasias). They are almost invariably asymptomatic until late in life, when their presence may be revealed by coexistent acquired arterial disease (Fig. 11–17). They may be discovered incidentally.

Rob and Owen have described iliac artery hypoplasia (Rob and Owen, 1958), and Servelle has described agenesis of the femoral artery and vein (Servelle, 1952). True generalized arterial dilatation (arteriectasia) occurring primarily without evidence of arteriovenous fistulae or of atherosclerosis is an extreme rarity.

References

Baskerville, P., Ackroyd, J. S., Lea Thomas, M., and Browse, N. L.: The Klippel-Trenaunay syndrome. Brit. J. Surg. 72:232, 1985.

Bean, W. B.: *Vascular Spiders and Related Lesions of the Skin.* Springfield, IL: Chas. C Thomas, 1958, pp. 178–185.

Beier, E.: Ueber einen Fall von naevus subcutaneous (Virchow) mit hochgradiger Hyperplasie der Knäueldrüsen. Archiv. f. Derm. Syph. 31:337, 1895.

Belsheim, M. R., and Sullivan, S. N.: Blue rubber bleb nevus syndrome. Canadian J. Surg. 23:274, 1980.

Bergoin, M., Carcassonne, M., Legre, G., and Huguet, J. F.: Dysplasie veineuse congénitale du membre inférieur droit associée à un syndrome de Kasabach-Merritt chez une enfant de 14 ans. Chirurgie 102:68, 1976.

Berlyne, G. M., and Berlyne, N.: Anaemia due to "blue rubber bleb nevus" disease. Lancet 2:1275, 1960.

Bockenheimer, P.: Ueber die genuine diffuse Phlebektasie der oberen Extremität. Festschrift FGE Von Rindfleisch, Leipzig 38:311, 1907.

Buxton-Thomas, M. S., Tonge, C. M., and Croft, D. N.: A dynamic radioisotope technique for assessing venous abnormalities. Nuc. Med. Communic. 1:66, 1980.

Cockett, F. B., and Lea Thomas, M.: The iliac compression syndrome. Brit. J. Surg. 52:816, 1965.

Cruveilhier, J.: Atlas d'anatomie pathologique du corps humain. Vol. 2, Liv. 23, Pl. 3, 1842.

Dahlin, D. C.: *Bone Tumors.* General aspects and analysis of 2276 cases. Springfield, IL: Chas. C Thomas, 1957, pp. 84–89.

DiDio, L. J.: Estudio anatomico de particularidales normais e patologicas da superficie interna da vein iliaca. Arquivas de Cirurgia. Clin. E. Exp. 12:507, 1949.

Dodd, H., and Cockett, F. B.: Iliac compression syndrome. In *Pathology and Surgery of the Veins of the Lower Limb,* 2nd ed. Edinburgh: Churchill-Livingstone, 1979, p. 229.

Domonkos, A. N., and Suarez, L. S.: Sudoriparous angioma. Arch. Derm. 96:552, 1967.

Freund, D.: Diffuse genuine phlebectasia. Report of a case. Arch. Surg. 33:113, 1936.

Gordin, D., Edgren, J., Friman, C., and Holmström, T.: A case of disseminated hemangiomatosis with cutaneous, hepatic and skeletal manifestations and increased urinary excretion of glycosaminoglycans. Acta Med. Scand. 198:425, 1975.

Gorham, L. W., and Stout, A. P.: Massive osteolysis (acute spontaneous absorption of bone, phantom bone, disappearing bone). Its relation to hemangiomatosis. J. Bone Jt. Surg. 37A:985, 1955.

Haferkamp, O.: Über das Syndrome generalisierte maligne Haemangiomatosis mit Osteolysis. Krebforsch 64:418, 1962.

Hayman, L. A., Evans, R. A., Ferrell, R. E., et al.: Familial cavernous angiomas. Am. J. Med. Genet. 11:147, 1982.

Kimura, C. H., Shirotani, M., Hirooka, M., et al.: Membranous obliteration of the inferior vena cava in the hepatic portion. J. Cardiovasc. Surg. 4:87, 1963.

Lea Thomas, M., and Andress, M. R.: Angiography in venous dysplasias of the limbs. Am. J. Roentgenol. 113:722, 1971.

Lodin, A., Lindvall, N., and Gentele, H.: Congenital absence of venous valves as a cause of leg ulcers. Acta Chir. Scand. 116:256, 1958.

Malan, E.: Vascular malformations of the face. In *Vascular Malformations*. Milan: C. Erba, 1974, p. 150.

Malan, E., and Puglionisi, A.: Congenital angiodysplasias of the extremities. (Note I: Venous dysplasias). J. Cardiovasc. Surg. *5*:87, 1964.

Martorell, F.: Hemangiomatosis braquial osteolitica. Angiologia *1*:219, 1949.

May, R., and DeWeese, J. A.: In May, R. (ed.): *Surgery of the Veins of the Leg and Pelvis*. Stuttgart: Thieme, G., 1979, pp. 159–163.

McMurrick, J. P.: Congenital adhesions in the common iliac vein. Anat. Rec. *1*:78, 1906.

Montfalcon, M.: Dict. des Sciences Med., 1836.

Plate, G., Brudin, L., Eklof, B., et al.: Physiologic and therapeutic aspects in congenital vein valve aplasia of the lower limb. Ann. Surg. *198*:229, 1983.

Poynter, C. W. M.: *Congenital Anomalies of the Arteries and Veins of the Human Body*. Lincoln, NE: University Studies, 1923, p. 22.

Rice, J. S., and Fischer, D. S.: Blue rubber-bleb nevus syndrome. Arch. Derm. *86*:503, 1962.

Rob, C. G., and Owen, K.: Congenital hypoplasia of the iliac arteries. Postgrad. Med. J. *34*:391, 1958.

Sachatello, C. R.: The axillopectoral muscle (Langer's axillary arch): A cause of axillary vein obstruction. Surgery *81*:610, 1977.

Sakurane, H. F., Sugai, T., and Saito, T.: The association of blue rubber bleb nevus syndrome and Maffucci's syndrome. Arch. Derm. *95*:28, 1967.

Sarma, K. P.: Anomalous inferior vena cava—anatomical and clinical. Brit. J. Surg. *53*:600, 1966.

Schobinger, R. C.: *Periphere Angiodysplasien*. Bern: Hans Huber, 1977.

Servelle, M.: In *Pathologie Vasculaire Médicale et Chirurgicale*. Paris: Masson, 1952.

Servelle, M., and Babillot J.: Les malformations des veines profondes dans le syndrome des Klippel-Trenaunay. Phlébologie *33*:31, 1980.

Sherman, R. S., and Wilner, D.: The roentgen diagnosis of hemangioma of bone. Amer. J. Roentgenol. *86*:1146, 1961.

Smith, B. M., and Wolfe, W. G.: Venous disease in childhood. In Dean, R. H., and O'Neill, J. (eds.): *Vascular Disorders of Childhood*. Philadelphia: Lea and Febiger, 1983, pp. 120–141.

Vilanova, X., Pinol-Aguadé, J., and Castells, A.: Hamartome angiomateux sudoripare secretant. Dermatologica *127*:9, 1963.

Vollmar, J.: Malformations of leg and pelvic veins. In May, R. (ed.): *Surgery of the Veins of the Leg and Pelvis*, Stuttgart: Thieme, G., 1979.

Wallis, L. A., Asch, T., and Maisel, B. W.: Diffuse skeletal hemangiomatosis: Report of two cases and review of literature. Amer. J. Med. *37*:545, 1964.

Walshe, M. M., Evans, C. D., and Warin, R. P.: Blue rubber bleb naevus. Brit. Med. J. *2*:931, 1966.

Waybright, E. A., Selhorst, J. B., Chu, F., and Cogan, D. G.: Sublingual angiomas and blue rubber bleb nevus syndrome. Arch. Neurol. *38*:784, 1981.

Waybright, E. A., Selhorst, J. B., Rosenblum, W. I., and Suter, C. G.: Blue rubber bleb nevus syndrome with CNS involvement and thrombosis of a vein of Galen malformation. Ann. Neur. *3*:464, 1978.

Widmer, G., cited in May, R.: In preface to *Surgery of the Veins of the Leg and Pelvis*. Stuttgart: Thieme, G., 1979.

CHAPTER TWELVE

Lymphatic Malformations

A. E. Young

with a contribution by
G. Stewart

Purely lymphatic malformations are encountered in three formats. In the *first* and most common type, abnormalities of lymph vessels and nodes lead to inadequate clearance of lymph and are revealed as lymphedema. In the *second* format, solitary or multiple cystic lymphatic malformations present as deep or superficial lesions, posing a totally different set of management problems. The *third* category is disorders of the circulation of chyle. The first two clinical groups are briefly covered in this chapter; specific problems in the head and neck, arm, and lower limb are dealt with in Chapters Sixteen, Seventeen, and Nineteen, respectively. Detailed information about the chylous diseases may be found in the works of the late John Kinmonth (1976, 1982). Lymphatic abnormalities are often encountered in concert with venous and arteriovenous anomalies, and this association is reviewed in Chapter Fourteen.

MALFORMATIONS OF VESSELS AND NODES

The clinical appearance and course of these malformations are closely related to the morphological abnormalities that may be demonstrated by contrast lymphography, and the malformations are thus classified by lymphographic appearance. When on lymphographic examination nodes and/or lymphatic trunks are smaller or less numerous than normal, the generic descriptive term *hypoplasia* is used. When they are more numerous, broader, or ectatic, the generic term *hyperplasia* is employed.

Hypoplasia is the more common abnormality (Fig. 12–1). It usually involves only the lower limbs (Table 12–1), though the arms and face may be involved. It occurs more often in females and presents as edema of the lower limbs, most commonly in the teens and twenties (lymphedema praecox) or later (lymphedema tarda) (Fig. 12–2). Its investigation, diagnosis, and management are well described in Kinmonth's book *The Lymphatics* (Kinmonth, 1982). Although common, this form of lymphatic abnormality is not a problem in infancy, nor is it associated with a birthmark. Nevertheless, a small, separate peak of incidence is seen in neonates. This is a separately identifiable disease, historically referred to as *Milroy's disease* (Milroy, 1892). In such patients the lymphedema is congenital, as well as being inherited as an autosomal dominant trait (Esterly, 1965; Dale, 1984). The skin of the involved limbs of these patients may show a pink discoloration (as was noted in Milroy's original case in 1892), but this discoloration is not a true capillary malformation. The lymph nodes of these patients with congenital hypoplasia show fibrosis, and this may be the primary pathological finding even in patients with true familial

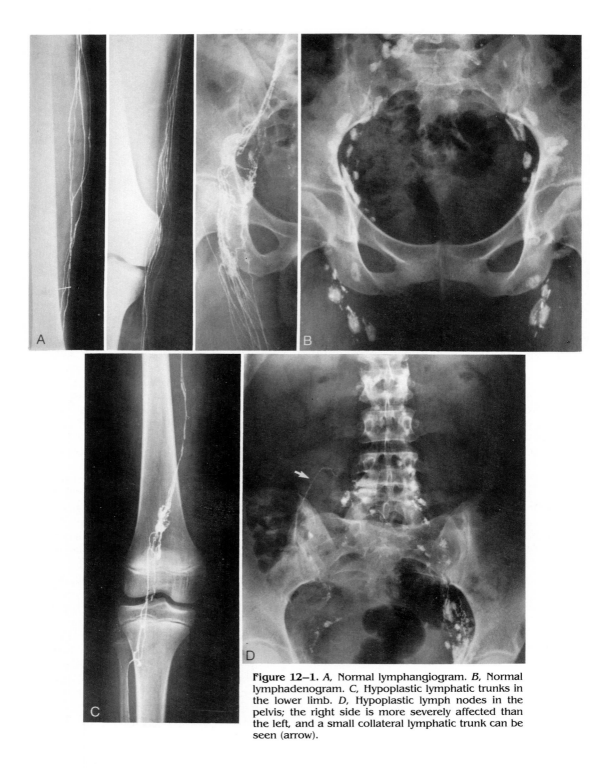

Figure 12–1. *A,* Normal lymphangiogram. *B,* Normal lymphadenogram. *C,* Hypoplastic lymphatic trunks in the lower limb. *D,* Hypoplastic lymph nodes in the pelvis; the right side is more severely affected than the left, and a small collateral lymphatic trunk can be seen (arrow).

Table 12–1. RELATIVE FREQUENCIES OF PRIMARY LYMPHATIC EDEMAS AND DEFECTS

	Patients
Lower limb lymphedema	1265
Upper limb lymphedema	109
Genital lymphedema	103
Facial lymphedema	45
Chylous defects	55
Localized lymphatic malformations ("lymphangiomas")	70
Combined vascular malformations with lymphatic abnormality	65
	1712

From Kinmonth, J. B.: The Lymphatics. 2nd ed. London: Edward Arnold, 1982, p. 84.

lymphedema (Kinmonth and Wolfe, 1980). Gabala recorded a family of 11 patients from five generations who had not only congenital lymphedema but also aplasia of the deep veins, superficial varices, and multiple arteriovenous fistulae in the thighs (Gabala et al., 1966). Lymphedema is often a concomitant finding of other extensive vascular malformations of the lower limbs, though almost all such cases are sporadic, not familial.

Hyperplasia

Patients who are found on lymphographic examination, to have dilated (ectatic) lymphatics fall into two groups: those with unilateral megalymphatics, and those with bilateral hyperplastic lymphatics.

Unilateral Megalymphatics

This condition is typically characterized by the following:

1. Unilateral lymphedema
2. Broad, valveless lymphatics, extending into the abdomen (Fig. 12–3)
3. Small, scattered, "spotty" lymph nodes (Fig. 12–4)
4. Proximal lymphatic abnormalities: for example, thoracic duct abnormalities and megalymphatics of the abdominal viscera (Fig. 12–5)
5. A cutaneous capillary malformation on the limb or adjacent trunk (Fig. 12–6)
6. Reflux of chyle into the limb or perineum, sometimes discharging through cutaneous vesicles (Fig. 12–7)

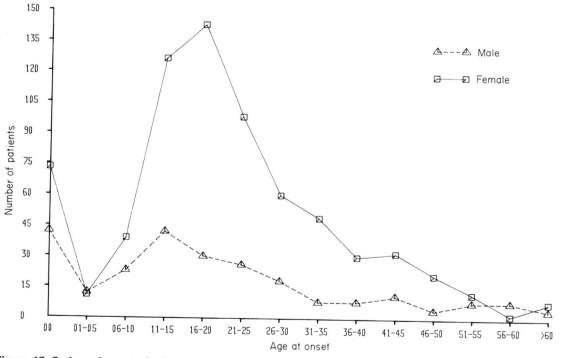

Figure 12–2. Age of onset of primary lymphedema in the lower limb in 948 patients studied at St. Thomas' Hospital, London, 1955–1980. There is a marked peak in the curve for females, coinciding with the years of onset of puberty and pregnancies. (From Kinmonth, J. B.: The Lymphatics, 2nd ed. London: Edward Arnold, 1982, p. 130.)

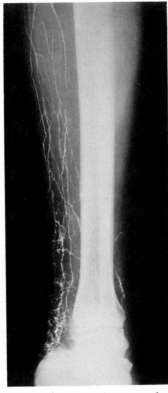

Figure 12–3. Unilateral valveless megalymphatics in lower limb.

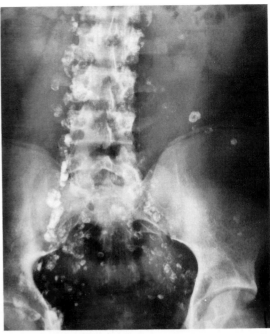

Figure 12–4. Typical fragmented pattern of lymph nodes in patients with unilateral megalymphatics.

7. No family history
8. Equal sex incidence

These patients may be in the spectrum of diffuse congenital arteriovenous fistulae, for in those patients similar lymphographic changes and clinical problems are encountered.

Bilateral Hyperplastic Lymphatics

Patients with bilateral hyperplastic lymphatics feature several or all of the following:

1. Bilateral lymphedema evident at birth or in childhood

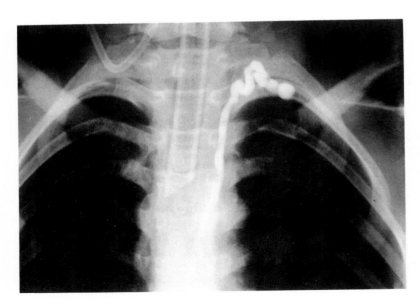

Figure 12–5. Ectatic thoracic duct in a patient with lower limb megalymphatics and chylometrorrhea.

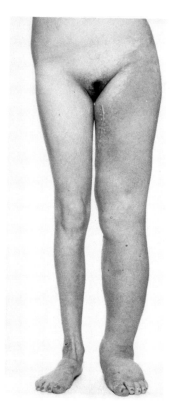

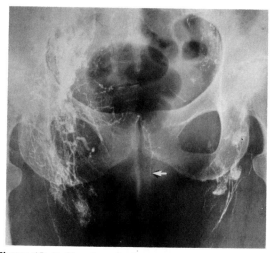

Figure 12–7. Megalymphatics with reflux of chyle into the vulva (arrow).

Figure 12–6. Extensive capillary malformation in the skin of a leg with unilateral megalymphatics and lymphedema. The leg is also longer than the unaffected fellow. All these features are compatible with diffuse arteriovenous fistulae, though none could be demonstrated in this patient.

2. Widespread dilatation of lymphatics in *both* limbs (Fig. 12–8)

3. Abnormally large lymph nodes (Fig. 12–9)

4. Symmetrical patchy redness on the sides of the feet, probably a capillary malformation (Fig. 12–10)

5. Familial incidence

6. Commonly, there are associated abnormalities, particularly distichiasis and cardiac anomalies (Robinow et al., 1970; Kinmonth, 1982) (Fig. 12–11)

These lymphographic abnormalities are also encountered in patients with multiple diffuse arteriovenous fistulae and are discussed in Chapter Thirteen.

Clinical Problems with Lymphedema

The difficulties that may be encountered in identifying lymphedema as the cause of leg swelling are discussed in Chapter Eight. Only with quite gross lymphedema is diagnosis easy for the clinician unfamiliar with the picture. Investigation by intradermal dye injection, isotopes, or direct injection lymphangiography may be necessary to establish the diagnosis confidently.

Conservative management with massage, skin care, and elastic support will suffice for most patients, though intermittent compression/massage by a special pneumatic legging or sleeve may be necessary to supplement this treatment. However, a return to normal contour is only rarely achieved. Probably no more than 10% of patients whose lymphedema is brought to specialist attention will need or benefit from ablative procedures to reduce the size of the limb, and in only a fraction of 1% is a reconstructive lymphatic procedure feasible, let alone successful.

Prognosis is predictable. Wolfe and Kinmonth studied 372 patients with lower limb lymphedema and showed that after the first year with lymphedema only 7% experienced further progression of disease and after five years only 1% still had progression. Nine per cent experienced edema of the opposite limb at a later date (Wolfe and Kinmonth, 1981).

There are rare instances of angiosarcoma arising in an area of congenital lymphedema (Taswell et al., 1962; Merrick et al., 1971; MacKenzie, 1971; Dubin et al., 1974; Chen and Gilbert, 1979). There are more cases of malignant degeneration in which severe lymphedema has followed radical mastectomy accompanied by axillary irradiation (Stewart

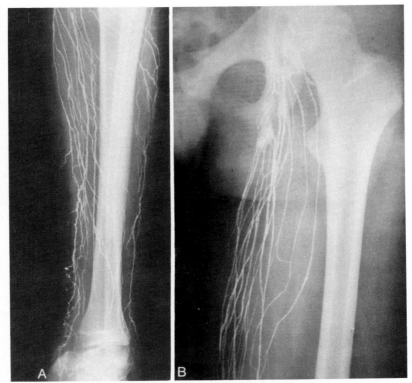

Figure 12–8. *A* and *B*, Hyperplastic lymphatics in the lower extremity.

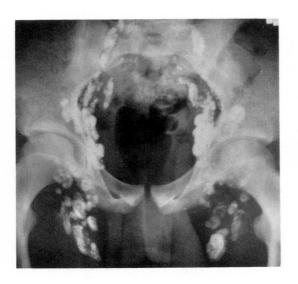

Figure 12–9. Abnormally large lymph nodes shown on a lymphadenogram of a patient with bilateral hyperplastic lymphatics.

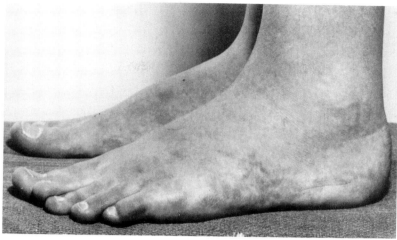

Figure 12–10. Patchy capillary malformations on the side of the feet in a patient with bilateral hyperplastic lymphatics.

and Treves, 1948; Enzinger and Weiss, 1983).

LYMPH CYSTS

Lymph cysts most commonly occur in the root of the neck, where they are usually called "cystic hygromas." These malformed lymphatic cysts contain a watery, sometimes lightly opaque fluid. The cysts may be single or multiple, interconnected or separate. They may communicate with adjacent lymphatics. Kinmonth describes one case in which a multiloculated cystic anomaly appeared as a developmental alternative to the thoracic duct. These cystic lymphatic malformations may be so large as to obstruct labor, but they tend to present more commonly as swellings at the root of the neck in infants. Occasionally

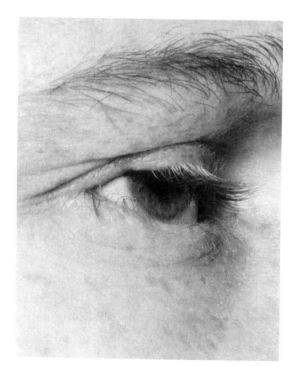

Figure 12–11. Distichiasis in a patient with bilateral hyperplastic lymphatics.

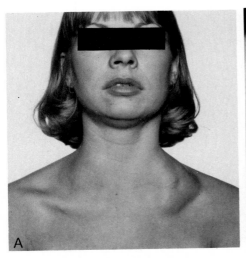
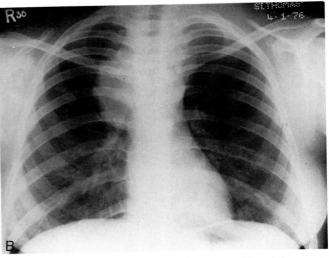

Figure 12–12. *A,* Cystic lymphatic anomaly at the root of the neck ("cystic hygroma") presented in adolescence. *B,* Chest radiograph of the same patient, showing extension into the upper mediastinum.

they present in adults, where they are a cosmetic embarrassment (Fig. 12–12) but rarely progress to become symptomatic (Broomhead, 1964).

Deep-seated lymph cysts in the trunk are recorded either in association with more extensive vascular malformations or alone. They are rare. They have been found throughout the length of the gastrointestinal tract (Colizza et al., 1981; Williams et al., 1981), in the liver and spleen (Rao et al., 1981), and in the mesentery and peritoneal cavity. In the gastrointestinal tract, the cysts can present at any age as a result of obstruction or ulceration and hemorrhage. Mesenteric cysts present as simple intra-abdominal masses requiring diagnosis, and very rarely they may be associated with the basal cell nevus syndrome (Gorlin's syndrome) (Case Records of M.G.H., 1986).

LOCALIZED MULTICYSTIC LYMPHATIC MALFORMATIONS ("LYMPHANGIOMAS")

"Lymphangioma" is an inaccurate term usually used to describe localized maldevelopments of the cutaneous, subcutaneous, or submucous lymphatic system. Despite the long usage of "lymphangioma," the term should be abandoned. Surface lymphatic abnormalities are encountered most commonly at the root of the limbs (Fig. 12–13), including the buttocks (Fig. 12–14) and shoulder

(Fig. 12–15), and are also seen in the neck and mouth (Fig. 12–16). They appear as persistent clusters of thin-walled vesicles, usually filled with clear, colorless fluid but occasionally discolored by the presence of fresh or altered blood or by surrounding capillar-

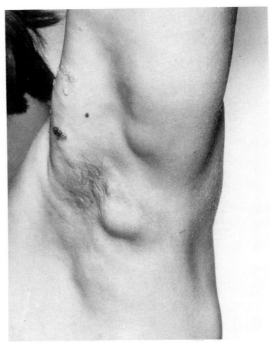

Figure 12–13. Localized lymphatic malformation at the root of the arm showing cutaneous cysts, some filled with clear fluid and some into which hemorrhage has occurred, and deep cysts.

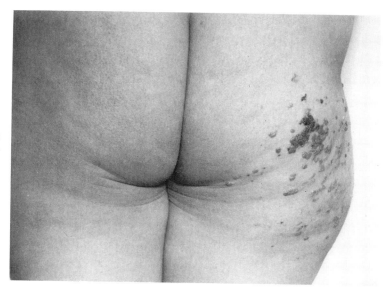

Figure 12–14. Localized lymphatic malformation of the buttock ("lymphangioma circumscriptum").

ies. Thus, a variety of clinical manifestations are seen (Fig. 12–17). Though they most commonly occur in the skin, there may be underlying thickened subcutaneous tissues that may contain palpable fluctuant cysts (as in Fig. 12–11). These may be very extensive, involving all soft tissues, viscera, and bones (Asch et al., 1974; Najman et al., 1967). Complications of these lymphatic lesions include troublesome, recurrent leakage of lymph and blood; recurrent cellulitis, causing pain and discomfort; and cosmetic disfigurement. Bacteria may readily enter via traumatized vesicles. Tissues affected by lymphatic anomalies are notorious for the speed at which infection can spread through them. At the first signs of inflammation, aggressive antibacterial therapy is mandatory. Such infections may well be life-threatening (Fig. 12–18).

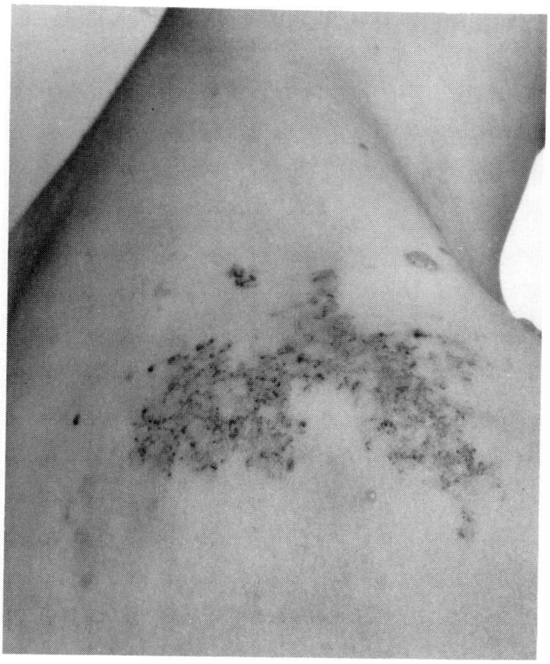

Figure 12–15. Localized lymphatic malformation on the shoulder.

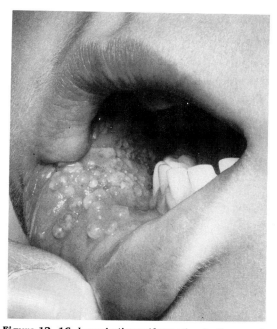

Figure 12–16. Lymphatic malformation in the mouth.

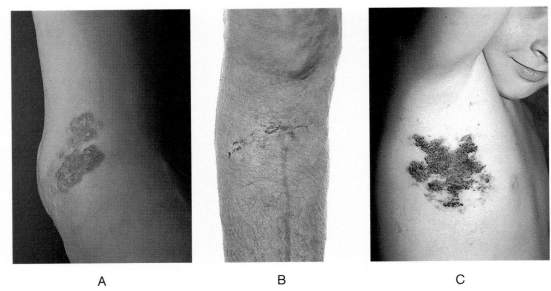

Figure 12–17. Various presentations of dermal lymphatic anomalies. *A*, Pink lymphatic vesicles, isolated near the lateral malleolus in a child. *B*, Patch of lymphatic blebs, leaking blood-stained lymph in a teenaged boy. *C*, These cutaneous vesicles gradually appeared following excision of an apparently simple cystic lymphatic malformation of the chest wall. The color is due to intralesional hemorrhage.

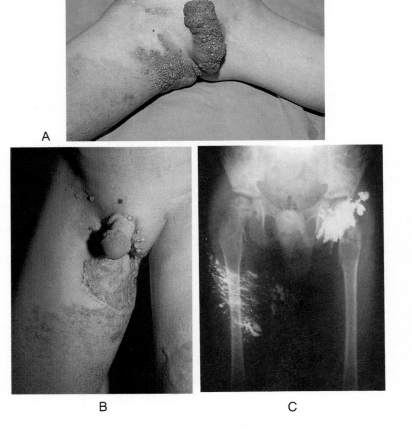

Figure 12–18. *A,* Four year old boy born with an extensive cutaneous visceral and skeletal lymphatic anomaly manifested externally by vesicles of the perineum and right thigh. *B,* Following full-thickness excision of the affected skin from the penile shaft and upper thigh and replacement with split-thickness skin grafts. *C,* Bilateral lymphangiogram shows pooling lipoidal globules in the subcutaneous tissues of the thighs. Both ilia and femoral heads show lytic lesions consistent with intraosseous lymphatic anomalies. At age 11, the patient presented with septic shock and died shortly thereafter despite antibiotic and supportive measures. Autopsy confirmed the presence of lymphatic anomalies within the liver, spleen, mesentery, retroperitoneum, and bones, as noted above.

Some lymphatic anomalies will undergo a degree of spontaneous improvement; Grabb noted complete disappearance in 44% of 94 patients and partial deflation in 29% (Grabb et al., 1980), while Broomhead has reported deflation in only 14% (Broomhead, 1964). However, these figures refer to children, and such malformations seen in adults do not regress. This subject is discussed further in Chapter Sixteen.

Malignant degeneration is a theoretical complication only. Girard and colleagues reported a case of lymphangiosarcoma arising at the site of a previous existing "lymphangioma circumscriptum," but they suggest that this may have been due to the substantial radiation therapy used in that case (Girard et al., 1970).

Although Wegner, in 1877 (Wegner, 1877), originally classified "lymphangiomata" into simplex, cavernous, and cystic forms, the first clinical report of the condition was probably that of Fox and Fox in 1879 (Fox and Fox, 1879). The term "lymphangioma circumscriptum" was first employed by Morris in 1889 (Morris, 1889). By 1893, Francis was able to collect 28 cases from the literature and described the main clinical and pathological features (Francis, 1893).

In 1970 Peachey, Lim, and Whimster reviewed 65 cases compiled from several centers and described the condition's clinical and histologic features (Peachey et al., 1970). They classified the lesions into two main groups, "localized lymphangioma circumscriptum" and "classical lymphangioma circumscriptum." The localized type was defined as a small lesion 1–2 cm in an area confined to the dermis and unlikely to recur. The "classical" type of lesion is much more common and is extensive in nature, often present at birth and commonly recurring after attempted excision. The difficulties experienced in surgical excision of these lesions led Kinmonth to suggest that they would be better termed "lymphangioma diffusum" rather than "lymphangioma circumscriptum."

Whimster described the histopathology of these lesions as a collection of subcutaneous lymphatic cisterns with a thick muscle coat that communicates through dilated lymphatic channels with the superficial vesicles (Whimster, 1976). He found no histologic evidence of communications between the cysts and the adjacent, normal lymphatics in 65 cases and

suggested that the subcutaneous cysts were sequestered segments of the primitive lymph system. The absence of connections between the subcutaneous lymphatics and the cysts has been confirmed by lymphography on many occasions (Edwards et al., 1972) (Fig. 12–19).

The muscular coat of the subcutaneous cysts may exhibit rhythmic contractions, as manifested by regular fluctuation of cyst pressure (Browse et al., 1986) (Fig. 12–20). Whimster has suggested that the skin vesicles are saccular outpouchings of the cysts secondary to the raised pressure that develops in the pulsating cisterns beneath them (Fig. 12–21). If this is true, it follows that excision of the skin vesicles without an adequate excision of the "feeding" cisterns will not effect a cure, because the cisterns will produce new outpouchings that will eventually appear on the skin as new vesicles (Jordan et al., 1977). This etiological theory also explains why many patients have subcutaneous vesicles over these areas many years later (Harkins and Sabiston, 1960). It also explains why skin grafts applied onto abnormal subcutaneous tissues after the removal of affected skin also develop vesicles.

Multiloculated lymphatic anomalies need not have cutaneous vesicles. The overlying skin can appear to be quite normal, or there

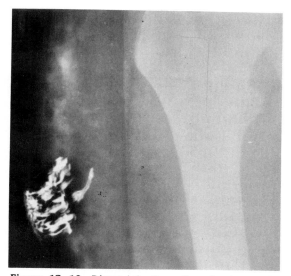

Figure 12–19. Direct injection of contrast material into the surface vesicles of the buttock malformation shown in Figure 12–14 indicates that there is no connection with the deep lymphatics in this case, as in all other cases of this lymphatic malformation.

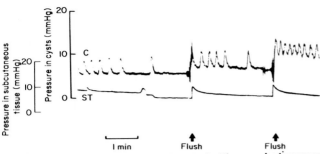

Figure 12–20. Pressure tracing from a cannula inserted into the cistern of a cutaneous lymphatic malformation. It demonstrates regular pulsations at the rate of about 4 per minute. The small fluctuations in the trace are those of respiration. The lower tracing is from a control cannula inserted into the subcutaneous fat adjacent to the lymphatic malformation. The minimal pressure difference between the malformation and the surrounding tissues suggests that the malformation maintains a small but constant tone, as well as contracting intermittently. (From Browse, N. L., Whimster, I. W., Stewart, G., et al.: The surgical management of lymphangioma circumscriptum. Brit. J. Surg. 73:585, 1986, by permission of the British Journal of Surgery.)

Figure 12–21. Diagram to illustrate the histologic findings of circumscribed lymphatic malformations ("lymphangioma circumscriptum"). The dermis in the subcutaneous area is packed with thick muscular walled deep cisterns that feed the superficial vesicles through short channels lined by lymphatic endothelium. The deep cisterns may extend well beyond the area of the superficial vesicles, and the channels feeding the vesicles are usually more complex than portrayed here. (From Browse, N. L., Whimster, I. W., Stewart, G., et al.: The surgical management of lymphangioma circumscriptum. Brit. J. Surg. 73:585, 1986, by permission of the British Journal of Surgery.)

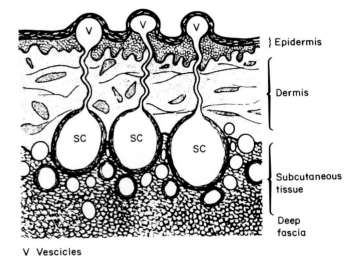

V Vescicles

SC Subcutaneous cisterns

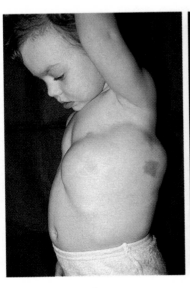
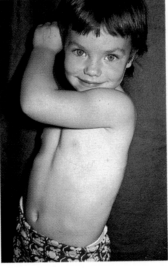

Figure 12–22. *A,* Four year old girl with a multiloculated lymphatic malformation of the chest wall with capillary stain in the skin. *B,* After resection of her lymphatic anomaly. (Procedure by J. B. Mulliken, M.D.)

A   B

may be an associated dermal capillary malformation (port-wine stain). These bulky lesions are amenable to surgical resection, with the proviso that, postoperatively, vesicles may bubble-up in the scar or the adjacent remaining lymphatic anomaly may expand (Fig. 12–22) (see also Fig. 12–17D).

Current evidence does not support the contention of Goetsch that lymphatic malformations have invasive or proliferative capacity (Goetsch, 1938). Vesicular extension from retained lymphatic cysts frequently occurs in the scar after subtotal excision. The question of potential for hyperplastic growth is not fully answered by a report of successful tissue culture of endothelium from a cystic lymphatic anomaly (Bowman et al., 1984). It is preferable to consider untouched lymphatic anomalies, like other vascular malformations, as stable, at a cellular level; hence the strict inaccuracy of the term "lymphangioma" (Mulliken and Glowacki, 1982).

References

Asch, M. J., Cohen, A. H., and Moore, T. C.: Hepatic and splenic lymphangiomatosis with skeletal involvement: Report of a case and review of the literature. Surgery 76(2):334, 1974.

Bowman, C. A., Witte, M. H., Witte, C. L., et al.: Cystic hygroma reconsidered: Hamartoma or neoplasm? Lymphology 17:15, 1984.

Broomhead, I. W.: Cystic hygroma of the neck. Brit. J. Plast. Surg. 17:225, 1964.

Browse, N. L., Whimster, I., Stewart, G., et al.: The surgical management of lymphangioma circumscriptum. Brit. J. Surg. 73:585, 1986.

Case Records of the Massachusetts General Hospital. Case 10–1986. N. Engl. J. Med. 314:700, 1986.

Chen, K. T. K., and Gilbert, E. F.: Angiosarcoma complicating lymphangiectasia. Arch. Path. Lab. Med. 103:86, 1979.

Colizza, S., Tiso, B., Bracci, R. G., et al.: Cystic lymphangioma of stomach and jejunum: Report of one case. J. Surg. Oncol. 17:619, 1981.

Dale, R.: Familial and genetic studies of primary lymphedema. M. S. Thesis, Univ. of London, 1984.

Dubin, H. V., Creehan, E. P., and Headington, J. T.: Lymphangiosarcoma and congenital lymphedema of the extremity. Arch. Dermatol. 110:608, 1974.

Edwards, J. M., Peachey, R. D. G., and Kinmonth, J. B.: Lymphangiography and surgery in lymphangioma of the skin. Brit. J. Surg. 59:36, 1972.

Enzinger, J. R., and Weiss, S. M.: Malignant vascular tumors. In Soft Tissue Tumors. St. Louis: C. V. Mosby, 1983, p. 422.

Esterly, J. R.: Congenital hereditary lymphedema. J. Med. Genet. 2:93, 1965.

Fox, T., and Fox, T. C.: On a case of lymphangiectodes, with an account of the histology of the growth. Trans. Path. Soc. London 30:470, 1879.

Francis, A. G.: Lymphangioma circumscriptum cutis. Brit. J. Dermatol. 5:33, 65, 1893.

Gabala, A., Klamut, H., Pietron, K., and Zdanowicz, H.: Congenital hereditary edema of the legs connected with developmental disturbances in the arterial and venous systems. Ann. Pediat. (Basel) 207:382, 1966.

Girard, C., Johnson, W. C., and Graham, J. H.: Cutaneous angiosarcoma. Cancer 26:868, 1970.

Goetsch, E.: Hygroma colli cysticum and hygroma axillae: Pathologic and clinical study and report of twelve cases. Arch. Surg. 36:394, 1938.

Grabb, W. C., Dingman, R. O., O'Neal, R. M., and Dempsey, P. D.: Facial hamartomas in children: Neurofibroma, lymphangioma, and hemangioma. Plast. Reconstr. Surg. 66:509, 1980.

Harkins, G. A., and Sabiston, D. C.: Lymphangioma in infancy and childhood. Surgery 47:811, 1960.

Jordan, P. R., Sanderson, K. V., and Wilson, J. S. P.: Surgical treatment of lymphangioma circumscriptum: A case report. Brit. J. Plast. Surg. 30:306, 1977.

Kinmonth, J. B.: Disorders of the circulation of chyle. J. Cardiovasc. Surg. 17:329, 1976.

Kinmonth, J. B.: The Lymphatics, 2nd ed. London: Edward Arnold, 1982.

Kinmonth, J. B., and Wolfe, J. H.: Fibrosis in the lymph nodes in primary lymphoedema. Ann. Roy. Coll. Surg. Engl. 62:344, 1980.

MacKenzie, D. H.: Lymphangiosarcoma arising in chronic congenital and idiopathic lymphedema. J. Clin. Path. 24:524, 1971.

Merrick, T. A., Erlandson, R. A., and Hajdu, S. I.: Lymphangiosarcoma of a congenitally lymphedematous arm. Arch. Path. 91:365, 1971.

Milroy, W. F.: An undescribed variety of hereditary edema. N. Y. Med. J. 5:505, 1892.

Morris, M.: Lymphangioma circumscriptum: In Unna, P., et al. (eds.): International Atlas of Rare Skin Diseases. London: H. K. Lewis, 1889, pp. 1–4.

Mulliken, J. B., and Glowacki, J.: Hemangiomas and vascular malformations in infants and children: A classification based on endothelial characteristics. Plast. Reconstr. Surg. 69:412, 1982.

Najman, E., Fabecic-Sabadi, V., and Temmer, B.: Lymphangioma in the inguinal region with cystic lymphangiomatosis of bone. J. Pediatrics 71:561, 1967.

Peachey, R. D. G., Lim, C-C, and Whimster, I. W.: Lymphangioma of the skin. Review of 65 cases. Brit. J. Derm. 83:519, 1970.

Rao, B. K., AuBuchon, J., Lieberman, L. M., and Polcyn, R. E.: Cystic lymphangiomatosis of the spleen: A radiologic-pathologic correlation. Radiology 141:781, 1981.

Robinow, M., Johnson, G. F., and Verhagen, A. D.: Distichiasis-lymphedema. Amer. J. Dis. Child. 119:343, 1970.

Steward, F. W., and Treves, N.: Lymphangiosarcoma in post mastectomy lymphedema. Cancer 1:64, 1948.

Taswell, H. F., Soule, E. H., and Coventry, M. B.: Lymphangiosarcoma arising in chronic lymphedematous extremities. J. Bone Joint Surg. 44A:277, 1962.

Wegner, G.: Ueber lymphangiome. Arch. Klin. Chir. 20:641, 1877.

Whimster, I. W.: The pathology of lymphangioma circumscriptum. Brit. J. Dermatol. 94:473, 1976.

Williams, S. M., Woltjen, J. A., and LeVeen, R. F.: Lymphangioma. One of the soft lesions of the colon. Amer. J. Gastroenterol. 75:70, 1981.

Wolfe, J. H. N., and Kinmonth, J. B.: The prognosis of primary lymphedema of the lower limbs. Arch. Surg. 116:1157, 1981.

CHAPTER THIRTEEN

Arteriovenous Malformations

A. E. Young

CLASSIFICATION

An arteriovenous fistula is an abnormal communication between an artery and a vein bypassing the normal capillary bed. The term "arteriovenous fistula" is best reserved for traumatic communications (including those deliberately made by surgeons). The congenital lesion is better described as an *arteriovenous malformation*. These communications between arteries and veins are always multiple and vary in diameter from several millimeters down to the size of the normal precapillary anastomosis. They can occur proximally between the major vessels and have been noted between, for example, the carotid artery and the jugular vein (Reinhoff, 1924) (Fig. 13–1), the subclavian vessels (O'Brien, 1965), the femoral vessels and the brachial vessels (Malan and Puglionisi, 1965), or at any level of the vascular tree as far distally as the capillaries. The length of the channels between the arteries and the veins can vary from millimeters to centimeters, and convoluted or cavernous abnormal vascular structures may be intercalated between the arterial and venous ends of the malformation.

The many possible permutations of these variables—position, size, length, and number—allow a very wide pattern of clinical appearance, but it is clinically useful to identify three major groups, based on structural criteria:

1. Truncal
2. Diffuse
3. Localized

In addition, any arteriovenous malformations may be hemodynamically "hyperactive" or "hypoactive."

Truncal fistulae arise from major arterial branches. They are usually localized, though many neighboring vessels may be involved. They are hemodynamically active and progressive. The connecting fistulae are anatomically demonstrable on arteriography and sometimes can be visualized at operation. Common examples are the so-called "cirsoid aneurysms" of the scalp (Fig. 13–2) and arteriovenous malformations in the hand (Fig. 13–3). Truncal fistulae are more common in the upper limb, head, and neck than in the lower limb and pelvis. Sometimes the connections are so short that the arteries and veins are adherent. By contrast, the interposed malformation may be quite bulky, like a tumor; hence the outdated term "arteriovenous angioma." It is important to note, however, that the bulk of these localized arteriovenous malformations is usually not the intercalated tissues but rather the enlarged inflow and outflow vessels.

Diffuse arteriovenous malformations are encountered particularly in the limbs, and, in contrast to truncal arteriovenous malformations, they are more frequently found in the lower limbs than in the upper limbs. The connections are small; millions may be present, and they may permeate the whole ex-

228

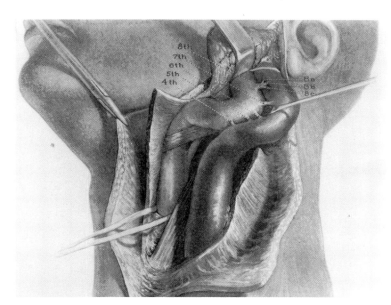

Figure 13–1. Congenital truncal arteriovenous fistulae between the carotid artery and jugular vein. (From Reinhoff, W. F., Jr.: Bull. Johns Hopkins Hosp. 35:271, 1924.)

tremity. In spite of these numbers, the connections may be less hemodynamically active than the truncal form. Though clinical features of heat and bruit may be demonstrable

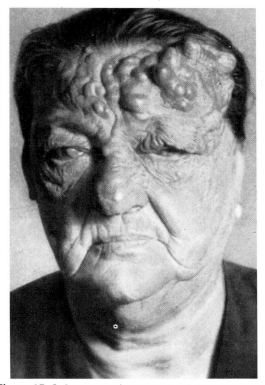

Figure 13–2. Large arteriovenous malformation of the forehead (cirsoid aneurysm). (Case of Prof. P. Niemeyer; from Olivecrona, H., and Ladenheim, J.: *Congenital Arteriovenous Aneurysms of the Carotid and Vertebral Arteries.* Berlin, Springer-Verlag, 1957, pp. 1–85.)

and angiography may show enlarged feeding arteries and rapid transit of contrast into enlarged draining veins, the fistulae themselves are not usually demonstrated angiographically. When these diffuse malformations are associated with limb hypertrophy and/or with superficial capillary malformations in the skin, they are encompassed by the term Parkes Weber syndrome.

Localized arteriovenous malformations are composed of a mass of abnormal intercalated tissues. These do not include the coiled arteries and veins associated with truncal arteriovenous malformations. These localized anomalies vary in hemodynamic activity. The majority are hemodynamically quiet, because of the high resistance and capacitance of the interstices of the lesion. Very inactive ones may be confused with venous lesions. Localized anomalies can occur in any organ: pulmonary, cerebral, hepatic, renal, and muscular ones being the most important, though all are less common than cutaneous ones.

All vascular malformations have in the past attracted a variety of clinical and pathological terms to describe them. These, though colorful and descriptive, are confusing and ought to be abandoned in favor of the simple but accurate phrase *arteriovenous malformation.*

HISTORY

Arteriovenous malformations have fascinated clinicians since the beginning of time, and it may have been an arteriovenous mal-

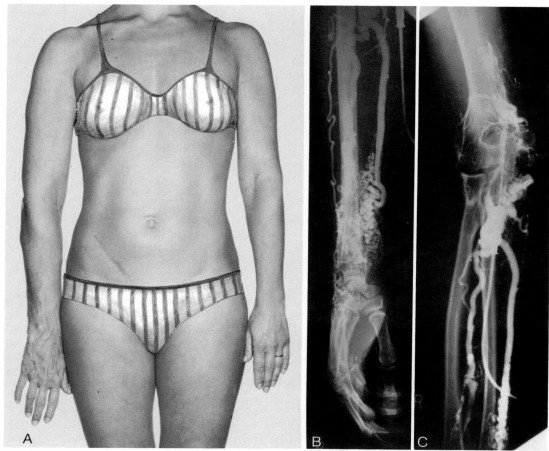

Figure 13–3. *A,* Diffuse arteriovenous malformation of the right forearm. Note the increased size and length of the limb. *B* and *C,* Arteriograms show extensive malformation in the wrist and at the elbow.

formation of the scalp that gave birth to the legend of Medusa (Fig. 13–4), the Gorgon whose hair was turned into a tangle of snakes by the goddess Athena because she had allowed herself to be seduced by Poseidon in one of Athena's temples (Homer; Smith, 1870). Anyone looking at Medusa's snakes was reputedly turned to stone, an experience familiar to a surgeon faced with the prospect of operating upon an extensive arteriovenous malformation!

However, the first properly recorded clinical case was described in the late sixteenth century by Guido (called Vidius), organizer of the medical faculty of the College de France and personal physician to King Francis I. The patient, one Allesandro Boscollo, a Florentine youth, had gross dilatation of his scalp veins from the forehead to the nape of the neck. The patient was referred to Gabriele Falloppio (Fallopius) in Padua, who

wisely declined to operate. From classical times through to the Renaissance, the notion of an aneurysm as a dilated artery was well understood, but without any accurate conception of the circulation the concept of an arteriovenous fistula and its effect on the circulation could not be grasped. Lancisi's *De Motu Cordis et Aneurysmatibus* (Lancisi, 1745) described the clinical and pathological features of true and false aneurysms at length, but it did not describe anything that is recognizable as an arteriovenous "aneurysm." In 1676, however, Sennertus of Wittenburg recorded an aneurysm that must have been an arteriovenous malformation, for it had "a thrill like boiling water" (quasi bullientes aquae). It was not only palpable but also audible, "as if the vital spirits were passing through a narrow orifice" (cited by Osler, 1915). However, the clinical association between this sort of lesion and an abnormal

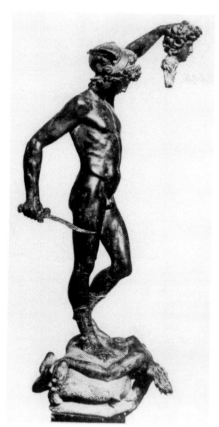

Figure 13–4. Perseus slew the Medusa by a technique that is not applicable to an arteriovenous malformation of the scalp. (Bronze statue by Benvenuto Cellini [1545], in Museo Nazionale, Florence.)

diately below the affected part. Both when the ligature was made tight and when it was removed they shrunk and remained of a small size while the finger was kept tight upon the artery at the point where the vein had been opened in bleeding. There was a general swelling and fullness at the affected part and in the course of the artery, which seemed to be larger and to beat stronger that what is natural all the way down the arm. There was likewise a pulsation in the dilated veins corresponding to the pulse in the artery; and there was a hissing sound and a tremulous jarring motion in the veins, which was very remarkable at the part which had been punctured, and became insensible at some distance both upwards and downwards.

Though such a case has never before entered my thought, I was so well convinced by the symptoms of its arising from a communication between the artery and the vein that I gave an opinion to that purpose and, therefore, advised her to do nothing while there should be no considerable alteration (Hunter, 1757).

John Bell published the first good clinical descriptions of a congenital arteriovenous malformation (Bell, 1815). Observations of congenital lesions were subsequently made by Bushe (1827), Adams (1858), Ghérini (1867), and Hewitt (1867). A postmortem anatomical demonstration was made by Warren in Boston in 1858 (Warren, 1858). In 1862, Krause described a 33 year old patient whose arm had been the site of an arteriovenous malformation all his life (Krause,

communication between an artery and a vein was not appreciated until William Hunter's description of a traumatic arteriovenous fistula in 1757 (Hunter, 1757). Although this lesion was traumatic (following an inadvertent arteriovenous injury with a lancet), the delineation is so clear and so classic for any active arteriovenous communication that it bears repetition, for not only did Hunter appreciate the significance of thrill but he also showed that occlusion of the fistula diminished the venous distension and eliminated the murmur (Fig. 13–5). Hunter wrote:

The veins in the bending of the arm, and especially the basilic, the vein that had been opened, were prodigiously enlarged at that place and came gradually to their natural size about two inches above and as much below the elbow. When emptied by pressure they filled again almost immediately; and this happened even when a ligature was applied tight about the forearm imme-

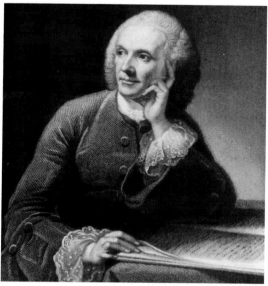

Figure 13–5. William Hunter, M.D., F.R.S. (1718–1783). Lithograph (1847) from the Robert Edge Pine painting in the Royal College of Surgeons of England.

1862). Krause noted the disparity in length and the progressive distal ischemia that led to amputation of the arm; injection studies of the amputated specimen demonstrated the connections between arteries and veins (Fig. 13–6).

The clinical assessment of arteriovenous communication was advanced in 1875 when Nicoladoni described the slowing of the pulse that followed occlusion of the subclavian artery proximal to a congenital arteriovenous fistula of the arm (Nicoladoni, 1875) (Fig. 13–7). He incorrectly ascribed the slowing to the pressure of a distended subclavian artery on the recurrent laryngeal nerve and thus the vagus. A similar observation was made by Branham in an acquired arteriovenous

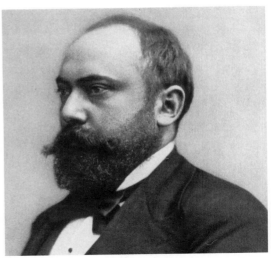

Figure 13–7. Carl Nicoladoni (1847–1902). In his short lifetime, this Austrian surgeon made remarkable contributions in a variety of fields: first to operate on esophageal diverticulum; described pollicization of the toe; wrote papers on tendon transfers, joint capsule innervation, and strangulated hernia; and did a fundamental study on torsion of the spine in scoliosis. He also described the reflex slowing of the pulse resulting from occlusion of congenital arteriovenous fistulae.

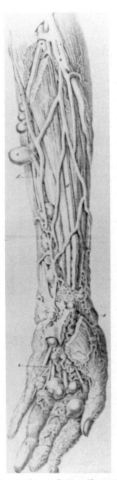

Figure 13–6. Engraving of the dissected amputation specimen from Krause's patient with an arteriovenous malformation of the arm. Krause accurately identified the enlarged feeding arteries and draining veins. (From Krause, W.: Arch. f. Klin. Chir. *ii*:142, 1862.)

fistula, and the physical sign based on this effect is now described, erroneously, as the Branham test (Branham, 1890).

The first scholarly collection of cases of arteriovenous malformation was made by William Halsted and his pupil Curle Callander. To Halsted is attributed the observation that "a congenital arteriovenous fistula without a nevus is very rare" (Reinhoff, 1924). Of Callander's 447 cases of arteriovenous communication from the literature, only 3 were congenital (Callander, 1920). The number of cases described in the nineteenth and early twentieth centuries was expanded by Osler (Osler, 1915), Rösler (Rösler, 1929), and Dean Lewis, whose review of 30 cases is the most detailed (Lewis, 1930). The first chapter of Emil Holman's classic work on abnormal arteriovenous communications also offers a good historical review of the subject (Holman, 1968).

The earliest clinical observations of cerebral arteriovenous malformations were reported by Steinheil in 1895 (Steinheil, 1895) and by Hoffmann in 1898 (Hoffmann, 1898). Cushing and Bailey's monograph of 1928 was the first thorough appraisal of these malformations (Cushing and Bailey, 1928), and its successor was the treatise of Olivecrona and

Ladenheim in 1957 (Olivecrona and Landenheim, 1957).

HEMODYNAMICS AND NATURAL HISTORY

There are normal communications ,between arteries and veins, bypassing the capillary bed, which are physiologically essential for temperature regulation, the distribution of flow to different organs, and adaptation to function. Their capacity is regulated by local autonomic and humoral controls. Congenital arteriovenous fistulae, by contrast, are probably free from such constraints. Whether they cause progressive hemodynamic and structural problems is due largely to their initial size, length, number, and position in the circulation. Thus, a single proximal arteriovenous fistula in a limb may cause a progressive, clinically dangerous increase in cardiac output without distal ischemia in the limb, whereas a multitude of small fistulae distally in the limb may not embarrass the heart but may cause distal ischemia, even to the point of gangrene. A knowledge of the hemodynamics of arteriovenous fistulae is crucial to understanding the clinical picture and to the planning of treatment. This knowledge of the pathophysiology and natural history of arteriovenous fistulae is largely based on the work of Holman, summarized in his book *Abnormal Arteriovenous Communications*, first published in 1936 and republished in 1968 (Purdy, 1964; Holman, 1968) (Fig. 13–8). Prior to that time, Reid had confirmed, experimentally, Halsted's contention that arteriovenous fistulae could produce cardiac enlargement (Reid, 1920). In 1913, Stewart had shown that the closing of an arteriovenous fistula was followed by reduction in cardiac size (Stewart, 1913), while both Gunderman and Nanu had described the changes in blood pressure that follow the closure (Gunderman, 1962; Nanu et al., 1922).

The fundamental circulatory changes that occur in association with an arteriovenous fistula are readily demonstrated by a patient with a Cimino-Brescia radiocephalic fistula formed for hemodialysis access. The pathological alterations are illustrated in Figure 13–9 and are described as follows:

1. There is shunting of blood from a high pressure area to a low pressure area, i.e.,

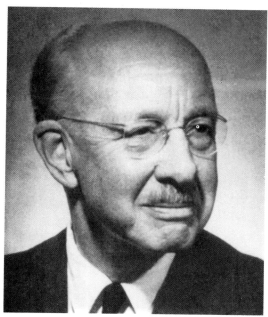

Figure 13–8. Emile Holman (1890–1977). Surgeon, graduated from Stanford and Oxford. He trained under Halsted at the Johns Hopkins Hospital and was stimulated to begin a life-long study of the pathophysiology of arteriovenous fistulae. After further work at the Peter Bent Brigham Hospital, under Cushing, he returned to Stanford, his alma mater.

from the arterial system to the venous system.

2. Two circuits are thus established; one of low resistance through the fistulae, and the other of high resistance through the normal peripheral capillary bed.

3. Because of the low resistance, flow in the afferent artery increases, causing dilatation, thickening, and tortuosity of the afferent artery. The same changes are seen in the efferent vein. The changes may be noted at great distances from the fistula. An arteriovenous malformation of the hand may, for instance, cause retrograde dilatation to the subclavian vessel. The dilatation is usually smooth and uniform.

4. If the potential for flow through the fistula is greater than that through the supplying artery, a "parasitic" circulation develops. This firstly involves flow into the fistula from that part of the afferent artery that is distal to the mouth of the fistula, i.e., there is a reversal of normal flow in that distal segment.

5. This distal arterial contribution may lower the arterial pressure in the distal artery and allow ischemia of the structures supplied by that artery to occur.

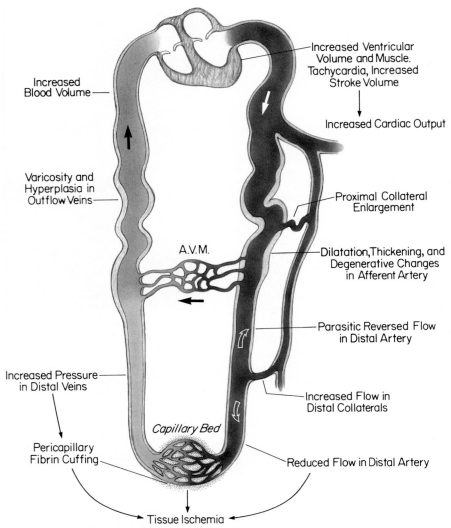

Increased Blood Volume

Increased Ventricular Volume and Muscle. Tachycardia, Increased Stroke Volume

Increased Cardiac Output

Varicosity and Hyperplasia in Outflow Veins

Proximal Collateral Enlargement

A.V.M.

Dilatation,Thickening, and Degenerative Changes in Afferent Artery

Parasitic Reversed Flow in Distal Artery

Increased Pressure in Distal Veins

Increased Flow in Distal Collaterals

Capillary Bed

Pericapillary Fibrin Cuffing

Reduced Flow in Distal Artery

Tissue Ischemia

Figure 13–9. Pathological effects of an arteriovenous fistula.

6. The lowering of arterial pressure as a result of loss of arterial blood through the fistula into the venous circulation may encourage the development of a collateral arterial circulation from adjacent arterial territories that are still at high pressure. This collateral flow is into the feeding artery both above and below the point at which the fistula is present.

7. The excess blood flowing into the venous circulation is usually accommodated by the veins between the fistula and the heart by an increase in diameter and velocity of flow. There is not necessarily an increase in pressure in these outflow veins. Hyperplastic structural alterations do, however, occur and

are usually described as "arterialization." There is thickening of the media by increased muscle fibers, fibrosis, and glycosaminoglycan accumulation.

8. The arterial blood flowing into the venous side causes turbulence, and this is responsible for the palpable thrill and audible bruit. The intensity of the thrill and bruit is, however, a composite of flow and geometry. The sharper the angle at which the fistula joins the vein, or the greater the disparity in sizes, the greater the turbulence. Thrill and bruit are not, therefore, a reliable indicator of the size of the flow through a shunt or set of shunts.

9. The pressure in veins peripheral to

the fistula is increased. This effect accentuates the peripheral arterial ischemia, which may already exist, and may precipitate edema, pain, and even ulceration and gangrene.

10. The inreased flow through the afferent arterial system may encourage degenerative changes in those vessels. At first these are pre-hypertrophic, and the walls may be thickened, especially the media: degenerative changes then occur, and frank atherosclerotic changes will eventually develop. The degenerative changes allow lengthening, and thus tortuosity, of the vessels near the fistula.

11. The potential drop in arterial pressure, caused by the presence of arteriovenous fistulae, is countered by an increase in blood volume and an increase in cardiac output, which may be associated with tachycardia, greater stroke volumes, ventricular dilatation, and, later, an increase in left atrial pressure and pulmonary arterial pressure.

Certain modifications of this model are needed to explain the changes seen in patients with congenital arteriovenous fistulae. We have already noted that these may be of two types, macrofistulous and microfistulous. Large solitary macrofistulae arising from large arteries, although rare, are a cause of major morbidity as a result of distal ischemia. At the opposite end of the scale, a limb permeated by millions of tiny tortuous arteriovenous fistulae occurring at an arteriolar level may display a greatly increased blood flow, but this need not be progressive or cause distal ischemia. Yao and coworkers noted that in such patients there may be an increased flow but no reduction in transit time (Yao et al., 1973). One such patient of ours has a 13 fold increase in flow through the affected leg, but the clinical condition has been stable for the 20 years that she has been under observation. Such multiple diffuse fistulae are more common in the lower limbs (Fig. 13–10) than in the head, neck, and trunk, and tend to be associated with skeletal overgrowth (Fig. 13–11). The macrofistulous lesions are most commonly seen in the head and neck and the upper limbs (Fig. 13–12).

Table 13–1 gives a listing of age at presentation with congenital arteriovenous fistulae.

It is generally accepted that when an arteriovenous malformation enlarges or extends, it does so by dilatation of existing channels and by the opening of collateral channels. Malan and Azzolini have, however, postulated that such progression occurs as a result of the "activation of dormant angioblasts" (Malan and Azzolini, 1968) that have, in the words of Medawar, escaped the "discipline of differentiation, persist into young adult life, later taking wing" (Medawar and Medawar, 1983). Convincing histologic proof of such angiogenesis in any form of vascular malformation is lacking. Fontaine's observation that puberty or pregnancy caused enlargement of arteriovenous malformations in

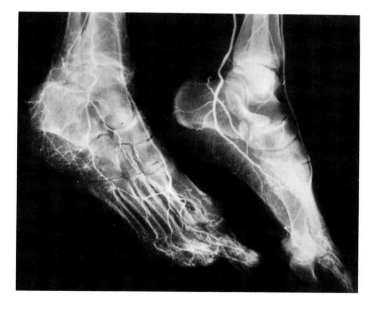

Figure 13–10. Translumbar arteriogram showing multiple diffuse arteriovenous malformations in the right foot. A synchronous arteriogram of the left foot shows the normal vasculature.

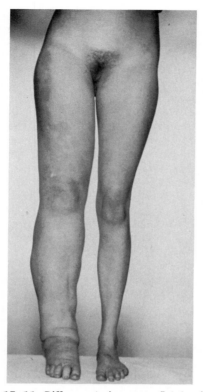

Figure 13–11. Diffuse arteriovenous fistulae involve the whole of the right lower limb of this pubertal girl. No enlarged veins were visible, but the limb was warmer, larger, and longer than its fellow; note the pelvic tilt. There is a pink capillary malformation involving the majority of the skin of the limb, especially the lateral side of the thigh. The measured blood flow per gram of tissue was 6 times greater than the unaffected side. Nicoladoni's sign was positive.

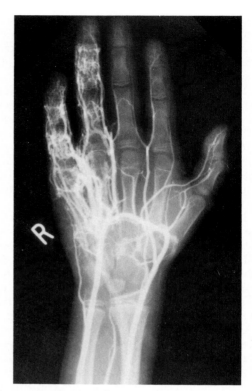

Figure 13–12. Macrofistulous arteriovenous malformation of the fourth and fifth fingers of the right hand.

25% of his female patients can be explained on hemodynamic grounds without invoking a concept of neoangiogenesis (Fontaine, 1967).

Most arteriovenous malformations are complex, drawing supply from several arter-

Table 13–1. AGE AT PRESENTATION WITH CONGENITAL ARTERIOVENOUS FISTULAE

Age (Yr)	Number Presenting
Birth	1
1	2
1–10	30
11–20	42
21–40	40
41–60	16
60+	7
	138

Combined series of Sako and Varco (1970), Szilagyi et al. (1976), and Young (1978).

ies and arterial territories at various levels and feeding into many different veins. Knowing this, the Holman model can be used to explain why proximal arterial "banding," or ligation, is such an ineffective treatment. The result of such proximal procedures is to lower the pressure in the distal artery without interfering with the fistula, which still has a lower resistance than the capillary bed. The shunt channels thus steal blood, and peripheral ischemia is worsened. The lowered peripheral arterial pressure stimulates further collateral development. If this is sufficient to restore the flow through the malformation, the treatment has failed in its primary objective. If it is inadequate, the worsened distal ischemia merely persists. Ligation of the artery above and below the arteriovenous fistula ("hunterian ligation") is rarely effective because other arterial afferents to the malformation usually exist and will enlarge to compensate. For "cure" the lesion must, in general, be excised or its central interstices blocked up with emboli. Both approaches will founder if the extent and pathological anatomy of blood supply to the lesion is not accurately mapped before treatment commences.

Symptomatic *cardiac decompensation* is rare in patients with congenital arteriovenous fistulae, though a few neonates with large, active arteriovenous malformations will develop potentially lethal cardiac failure within hours or days of birth (Flye et al., 1983). Few cardiac output studies have been performed on asymptomatic patients, but those that are reported show that even these patients have cardiac outputs of 2 or 3 times greater than normal (Natali et al., 1984). This merely confirms that the young and otherwise healthy heart can sustain an increased cardiac output for many years without clinically deteriorating, though enlargement of the cardiac diameter on a chest radiograph is a not uncommon finding.

Ulceration

The two major factors responsible for the ulceration that may complicate arteriovenous malformations are:

1. Pure arterial ischemia as a result of proximal steal through the malformation.

2. The effects on capillaries of the venous hypertension that occurs near the malformation. The effect is identical to that seen in acquired venous hypertension associated with varicose veins, deep vein thrombosis, deep vein obstruction, and valvular damage of deep veins. Indeed, the classic changes of "stasis dermatitis" may be the presenting feature of an arteriovenous malformation (Baer, 1969). The pathophysiology of these changes has been elucidated by Burnand (Burnand et al., 1982) and by Browse (Browse and Burnand, 1982). High venous pressure increases the permeability of dermal capillaries to fibrinogen, which leaks into the perivascular interstitial fluid where fibrin is produced (Burnand et al., 1982). This, in turn, forms a cuff around the capillaries, reducing diffusion of oxygen and nutrients from the capillary bed to the tissues (see Fig. 13–9). The affected skin can be shown by a transcutaneous PO_2 monitor to be hypoxic (Clyne et al., 1985), and positron emission studies show reduced oxygen extraction in the diseased ulcer bearing areas (Hopkins et al., 1986). By studying ulceration caused by a surgically fashioned arteriovenous fistula, Wood and coworkers have shown that the venous hypertension produced by the fistula can, per se, mimic the changes of banal "venous ulcers" (Wood et al., 1983). If there is concomitant arterial ischemia, the effect will clearly be worsened. Lymphatic abnormalities that often coexist with arteriovenous malformations may further exacerbate the process by reducing extraction of fibrinogen from the interstitial fluid. If venous hypertension is the dominant cause of ulceration, elastic compression may prevent recurrence of the ulceration when healing or grafting has been achieved, but where the underlying malformation has not been removed (Fig. 13–13).

TREATMENT

General Principles of Treatment of Arteriovenous Malformations

Of all the lesions described in this book, arteriovenous malformations are potentially the most difficult and frustrating to treat. Although many can be adequately managed by simple conservative measures, some will show an inexorable progression and require difficult and dangerous operations that will frequently fail. For this reason, it cannot be

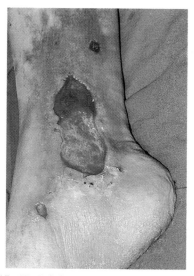

Figure 13–13. Painful chronic ankle ulcer in a patient with diffuse arteriovenous malformation of the lower left leg; note capillary stain. This was successfully treated by excision of the affected area and grafting, followed by life-long elastic compression.

said that the primary treatment of arteriovenous malformations is operative; however, as it is the form of treatment that is most difficult, proportionately more space will be given to it than to conservative forms of treatment. At present, the most promising avenue for the management of troublesome arteriovenous malformations is embolization, either alone or in conjunction with surgical excision.

Conservative Treatment

Symptoms of pain, heaviness, and tension in an area involved by an arteriovenous malformation are usually due to venous hypertension. Associated ulcers may also be due to this pathophysiology. The simplest way to counteract this venous hypertension is by the provision of elastic support. This is easily provided in the limbs. Many manufacturers now provide graduated compression elastic support stockings and sleeves capable of maintaining pressures of 30–40 mmHg. These graduated compression garments are preferable to elasticated tubular support, as these tend to be insufficiently tight at the periphery and have a tourniquet effect at the root of the limb.

Where a lesion is prone to ulceration and hemorrhage, extra compression in the form of an elasticated bandage with a foam rubber pad on the ulcer may be required. The elastic support has an additional virtue of minimizing the effect of trauma on superficial vessels.

Conservative management of ulcers associated with arteriovenous malformations may be effective and is described in Chapter Nineteen.

The use of radiotherapy and cryotherapy to eradicate superficial malformations has been very disappointing and can only be condemned.

Injection sclerotherapy may be used for small, cosmetically unacceptable varices in association with arteriovenous malformation but has not been found to be effective in treating the primary lesion.

Embolization

The treatment of arteriovenous malformations by the injection of emboli through a percutaneously introduced vascular catheter is finding an increasingly important role in the management of malformations for which conservative measures alone are insufficient.

Embolization may be used as the sole mode of treatment or as a preliminary maneuver to make the surgical procedure less vascular and easier. Its virtue is that not only can the major feeding vessels be occluded but also the central interstices of complex malformations may be filled up. Because the feeding vessels are not ligated, the procedures can be repeated if necessary. Embolization is technically difficult and requires an experienced interventional radiologist. The side effects are pain and tenderness in the embolized lesion, and the patient may have a transient fever and leukocytosis and clotting abnormalities. Reflux of embolic material into normal vessels occurs but is only problematic when it enters the cerebral or mesenteric circulation. Neurologic complications are the most feared. Ischemic necrosis of normal tissue, particularly skin, within the embolized territory is another worrisome possibility. Careful pre-embolization mapping of the vasculature and assessment of flow patterns by selective angiography, and the prevention of reflux from injected vessels by balloon catheters, together with skill and caution, minimize these complications. Embolization into the pulmonary circulation through the arteriovenous malformation is a theoretical, but not a practical, problem (Olcott et al., 1976). Embolization is normally achieved through a percutaneously introduced catheter, but direct access to vessels for embolization at the time of the operation may also be feasible. When surgical resection is used in combination with embolization, it is best to proceed with the operation 2–3 days after the embolization. Forty-eight hours is the time most commonly chosen, but there are no objective data to show what is the best interval, though data are accumulating that suggests that the hematological sequelae of embolization should have an important bearing on the timing and conduct of subsequent surgical intervention. In discussion at the Fifth International Workshop for Vascular Anomalies in Milan in 1984, Petrovici noted marked thrombocytopenia after embolization of four large head and neck malformations, reaching a maximum between 9 and 10 days after embolization; she suggested delaying extirpation until after this time. Hadjean, by contrast, prefers to operate 24 hours after

Ethibloc embolization and gives heparin to counteract problems of postoperative hemorrhage caused by consumptive coagulopathy. He has not, however, encountered similar problems after embolization of arteriovenous malformations.

Surgical Treatment

Malan divided the available surgical options into three groups (Malan and Puglionisi, 1965):

1. Radical resection aimed at elimination of the malformation itself
2. Hemodynamic surgical procedure necessitated by inability to perform radical removal or by failure of radical resection
3. Complementary operations

The surgeon embarking on intervention for an arteriovenous malformation should bear in mind that the operation will almost always be substantially more difficult, and probably less successful, than a procedure for the more frequently encountered traumatic arteriovenous lesion.

Resection

The attitude that arteriovenous malformations should be radically excised like cancer has, in the light of the high incidence of "recurrence" (re-expansion), much to recommend it. Unfortunately, experience shows that it is only very rarely that resection of an arteriovenous malformation in its entirety is feasible. Such lesions must be clinically and angiographically clearly localized and identified at the time of the procedure, even in these instances. Ablative operations may be associated with the following major problems:

1. Difficulty in delineating clearly the limits of the lesion. Even angiography may not clearly define the lesion because of rapid flow and multiple feeding vessels. Even when angiography has apparently defined the limits of the lesion, these may be difficult to identify at the time of operation. Furthermore, the venous run-off may be impressive and may give the lesion an appearance of greater size than it has in reality. Hypervascularity may be present throughout the affected and unaffected area, and difficulty in controlling blood loss may make distinction of the margins of the lesion impossible. The central question is *how* to identify the primarily malformed vessels and to determine which are the normal vessels that have become dilated collateral channels. Another important question is whether the resection must involve these secondarily involved vessels.

2. Absence of tissue planes. Where an arteriovenous malformation is buried in a single muscle group, block excision may be possible in a manner similar to the "compartmentectomy" used for soft tissue sarcomas. This is, however, a rare occurrence, and "infiltration" of tendons, nerves, and bones in the region of the malformation is the common finding. Arteriovenous malformations respect tissue planes less than do malignancies. Involvement of bones leads to particular difficulties with identification of fistulae and with hemostasis, and thus often necessitates amputation or excision of the bone (Lewis, 1930; Clay and Blalock, 1950; Nisbet, 1953).

3. Preservation of blood supply to distal or neighboring structures. As malformations are frequently closely related to major vessels, it may be necessary to excise arteries "en bloc" with the malformation. It is, however, possible in these circumstances to replace the artery with a prosthetic graft or a venous autograft. Where the malformation involves minor vessels, these can be removed "en bloc" with the malformation.

4. Hypervascularity. This, on its own, makes these operations difficult and dangerous. Hemostasis is difficult to achieve, and when operating in the limbs tourniquets may not be effective. Adjunctive preoperative embolization of the lesion can be used to reduce blood loss during operation. Even with preoperative embolization, however, proximal and distal vascular control is essential prior to excision and should be considered even if additional incisions are necessary to achieve it. Intraoperative embolization of the lesions through direct puncture of feeding vessels has been recommended, but there is not substantial experience of this in the literature as yet. Hypotensive anesthesia may also be of value to minimize excessive bleeding at operation (Rosales, 1983). In extreme cases, it may be necessary to place the patient on cardiopulmonary bypass, then establish hypothermia and temporary circulatory arrest during excision of the lesion (Mulliken et al., 1978). Natali recommended that facilities for autotransfusion be available when

extensive arteriovenous malformations are operated upon (Natali et al., 1984).

5. Hematological complications are infrequently encountered. However, coagulation problems may be precipitated by the large volumes of blood that are transfused. Preoperatively, there may be microthrombosis in adjacent vessels, leading tò platelet consumption; sometimes, disseminated intravascular coagulation may supervene.

6. Reconstruction after excision may be difficult. Skin grafts and local transposition flaps are often needed. Free tissue transfer of skin bone and muscle attached by microvascular anastomosis allows more aggressive approaches to some lesions that, at present, seem ineradicable or only, in the limbs, treatable by amputation.

Most arteriovenous malformations are not amenable to direct surgical excision, and those that seem to be frequently will re-expand after operation. In the pelvis, trunk, and head and neck, embolization may be the only feasible approach, but in the limb the appropriate treatment will often be amputation, though even this may fail if the whole limb is abnormal. There are, nonetheless, strong arguments against early amputation. Progression is often slow, and the indications for amputation should therefore be the same as for other forms of vascular disease, namely: intractable pain, intractable ulceration, gangrene, and loss of function, to which can be added the special problems of recurring hemorrhage or cardiac failure that less radical operations have failed to solve. A local palliative procedure is often justified even though it need not be expected to produce long-term cure. For example, such palliation may take the form of partial amputations of the hand, so as to remove painful ischemia tissue and leave a reasonable functioning limb, even though it is known that the extremity still contains abnormal arteriovenous connections. Partial removal of head and neck arteriovenous malformations may also be justified where more radical resections ;may carry an unacceptable risk of death. Flye, however, reports subsequent death from hemorrhage in two patients of three whose head and neck malformations were thus treated (Flye et al., 1983). Some writers have suggested that the application of normal tissues in the form of microvascular flaps may inhibit the expansion of the residual arteriovenous malformation (Hurwitz and Kerber,

1981). This, however, seems unlikely, and there is no firm evidence that this inhibition occurs. There is some dispute as to whether partial excisions of arteriovenous malformations are ever justified. Coursely and colleagues say that they should never be used (Coursely et al., 1956). Flanc, however, reports a case in which a child presenting at the age of 5 with an upper limb arteriovenous malformation was sustained to the age of 25 with partial resections and only then required a forequarter amputation (Flanc, 1968). We have had similar experiences in which the lesion was kept largely asymptomatic and the limb remained usable for many years (Fig. 13–14).

The presence of an arteriovenous malformation itself need not be a bad prognostic sign, and parents should not be threatened

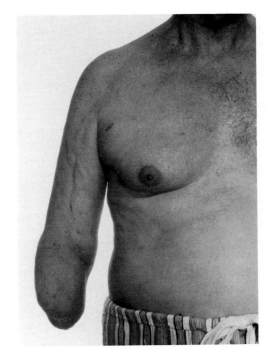

Figure 13–14. The whole of this man's right upper limb and shoulder was involved with multiple, hemodynamically active arteriovenous fistulae. The forearm was amputated in his twenties because of ischemia and ulceration. In spite of clear signs of substantial arteriovenous shunting in the residual limb and shoulder, he remained well until he died of myocardial ischemia àt the age of 56. Coronary angiography shortly before had shown the typical changes of atherosclerotic coronary artery disease, but the increased cardiac output consequent upon the multiple arteriovenous fistulae must have exacerbated the effects of this.

with the prospect of an eventual amputation when their child is diagnosed as having such a limb anomaly. The multiple diffuse fistulae, even those with very high flows and increased cardiac output, can remain stable over many years and may never need surgical intervention. In Robertson's series of 28 patients, amputation was never necessary for the management of diffuse arteriovenous fistulae (Robertson, 1965).

Hemodynamic Surgical Operation

When a lesion cannot be excised or when it has re-expanded after excision, there is clearly a temptation to interfere with the arterial supply to the lesion. Such a proposed operation may involve ligation of main arteries or tributary arteries. However, ligation of main arteries is almost never indicated, and ligation of tributary arteries is seldom called for.

Ligation of Main Arteries. Ligation of feeding vessels would, superficially, seem to be the best operation when one is faced with a daunting, extensive arteriovenous malformation, and many surgeons have opted for this simple answer. Unfortunately, not only does it usually fail to relieve the problem but also it will often worsen it. The reasons for this become clear when the pathophysiology of arteriovenous fistulae is considered, in particular the crucial role of collaterals. Proximal arterial ligation does not deprive an arteriovenous malformation of its arterial supply; it merely puts a greater demand on the collaterals, and these now supply the lesion at the cost of reduced supply to the normal peripheral vascular bed. In limb lesions, proximal ligation often precipitates the critical ischemia that precedes amputation. Therefore, peripheral ischemia worsens, not owing to the proximal ligation itself but to "steal" by the collaterals. Furthermore, it is unusual for an arteriovenous malformation to be supplied by only one major vessel, and for this reason even ligation of the artery both proximal and distal to a relatively circumscribed lesion also fails. "Banding," i.e., narrowing the vessel without occluding it, is also ineffective. The hazards of proximal ligation have been recognized for a century, but a more recent reason to deprecate such ligation is that by doing so the main access to the lesion for embolization through an arterial catheter is lost. This may be particularly critical in head and neck and in pelvic malformations, where the first maneuver in the definitive treatment of the lesion at a secondary referral center may have to be a reconstruction of the ligated vessel. At the Fourth International Workshop for Vascular Anomalies in Paris in 1982, Tricot reported on 13 patients with head and neck malformations in whom direct puncture beyond the ligated vessel was attempted for access for embolization, but with success in only one case. In five of eight patients, however, preliminary revascularization of the ligated external carotid allowed access. At the same meeting, Natali noted less success with revascularization after ligation of internal iliac arteries for pelvic and buttock malformations. Revascularization was attempted and failed in three patients, but embolization via collaterals was possible. It would have been preferable, in all these cases, if ligation had never been attempted. Even where major hemorrhages are occurring from an arteriovenous malformation, proximal ligation is an ineffective treatment.

Minor Vessel Ligation. Ligation of feeding vessels to arteriovenous malformations is not entirely "forbidden," as branch artery ligations are often effective in at least slowing enlargement of the lesion. Small arteries that angiography has shown to be primarily supplying the malformation may be ligated. These will usually be second or third order branches of a main trunk. These maneuvers, in contradistinction to proximal main vessel ligation, are not usually complicated by distal ischemia. The procedure is, however, of similar intent to embolization, and if small branch arteries feeding the lesion can be defined angiographically they are probably accessible for embolization. Embolization is a better method of occlusion, as it occludes not only the feeding vessels but also the interstices of the malformation. Several authors have reported on percutaneous placement of ligatures around arterial vessels to arteriovenous malformations, and other investigators have reported intraoperative embolization under direct vision (Malan and Puglionisi, 1965).

Carried to its limit, branch vessel ligation can be applied to the whole of the arterial tree in the region of a malformation, all the branches being ligated with the exception of the main feeding vessel. This is known as "de-afferentiation" (Malan and Puglionisi,

1965), or "skeletonization" (Cotton and Sykes, 1969)—an operation pioneered by Malan. It is, however, sometimes easier to excise the whole arterial segment and replace it with a prosthesis or venous autograft. When an assault on the vascular supply to a malformation is considered, angiography is the primary guide to planning and attention should be paid to achieving adequate films of the branches of all the major vessels in the area. In the limbs, temperature maps may help, as may a Doppler assessment.

Venous Ligation and Excision. In principle, venous ligation might help to reduce flow through an arteriovenous malformation, but in practice it is rarely helpful. It is more difficult to interrupt flow by ligation on the venous side because the venous drainage is so much less predictable, so multitudinous, and so difficult to map by venography accurately. In high flow vascular anomalies the operation may be counterproductive, causing painful enlargement of the malformation. Nevertheless, in some forms of minimally active arteriovenous fistulae with associated malformed veins, removal of these superficial varices may ease the symptoms without generating new ones.

However, Malan has recommended, that whenever possible excision of varices should be combined with a direct assault on the small arteries feeding the malformation (Malan and Puglionisi, 1965). In addition, the perforating veins should be ligated at a subfascial level. Our experience supports the generally proposed view that excision of varices should be performed under direct vision, through long incisions, rather than by use of a "stripper."

Complementary Operations

A direct attack on an arteriovenous malformation of an extremity is an uncommon operation. In our experience of limb malformations, only one in five malformations has been suitable for this approach, yet four out of five have required some form of complementary procedure. The average number of operations per patient has been five. The majority of the operations in the limbs have related to the excision and grafting of ulcers, the excision of abnormal veins, operations to control disparity in leg length, the excision of giant digits, and so forth.

Expected Results of Treatment

Results of surgical treatment of head and neck and upper limb malformations are described in Chapters Sixteen and Seventeen. In the lower limb, the most common site for arteriovenous malformations, best results are clearly to be expected in those with minimal symptoms of discomfort and fullness, as such people are satisfactorily treated with elastic support. Patients with malformations severe enough to require an operation will do best if their anomalies are small and closely localized, and where a confident "en bloc" resection can be performed with or without embolization. In 1965, Malan cited 43 limbs operated upon, with 77% benefiting from operation (Malan and Puglionisi, 1965). Other authors' experiences have been more disappointing. Szilagyi summarized his experience thus: "We intuitively thought that the only answer of a surgeon to the problem of disfiguring, often noisome and occasionally disabling blemishes and masses prone to cause bleeding, pain or other unpleasantness, was to attack them with vigor and with the determination of eradicating them" (Szilagyi et al., 1976). Szilagyi's results of this attempt at radical treatment were disappointing. Of the 82 patients considered in that series, only 18 were judged suitable for operation and improvement was produced in only 10. Two were the same following operation, and six were worse. Leonard and Vassos had a similar unsatisfactory experience: only 4 of 29 patients who came to operation for lower limb arteriovenous malformations were described as cured (Leonard and Vassos, 1951). These results compared with the excellent results from conservative treatment: Szilagyi's 1965 report, with a mean follow-up of 10 years, showed 12 patients improved on conservative treatments, 42 the same, and only 10 worse (Szilagyi et al., 1965). Leonard and Vassos' review of 1951 included 26 cases treated conservatively, with improvement in 21 (Leonard and Vassos, 1951). Most series show less than half the patients needing operation, and this has been our experience. Some series have shown higher operative rates; Flye, for example, reports 20 of 25 patients operated upon but with only short follow-up analysis (Flye et al., 1983).

Amputation

It is very difficult to quantify the risk of amputation in any particular patient with a limb malformation, as the amputation rates in the different reported series differ widely (Table 13–2). Even modern series such as Little's have cited amputation rates as high as 25% (Little, 1981). Once an arteriovenous malformation of the limb is serious enough to warrant a surgical procedure, it seems that between 10% and 30% will require amputation at some level. Figures from the Mayo Clinic series suggest that upper limb arteriovenous malformations are more likely to come to amputation than lower limb malformations (4 of 17 compared with 4 of 51) (Gomes and Bernatz, 1970).

Malformations Made Worse by Operation

An operation carries risks from hemorrhage and precipitation of hematological disease, as outlined previously. In addition, wounds made in the region of vascular malformations heal badly and the scars may become hypertrophic. Where lymphedema is a concomitant feature, it may be made worse. It has been suggested that an operation on an arteriovenous malformation may catalyze its subsequent expansion and that this growth

is not entirely attributable to altered collateral flow but to some other mechanism. It has been postulated that the physical trauma may break down septa between primarily arterial and primary venous lacunae in the malformations, thereby establishing new fistulae and tipping the hemodynamic balance in favor of progression. Though it is very speculative, one might wonder whether operation may release some humoral factor causing "angioneogenesis." Though there is no good objective evidence that this occurs, many surgeons have experienced a worsening of lesions after minimal interference or after trauma.

There is also the problem of accidental injury precipitating unstoppable deterioration of a previously quiescent lesion leading, eventually, to amputation. One of the first arteriovenous malformations recorded appears to have demonstrated this phenomenon (Letenneur, 1859). There is also the solitary but carefully reported case of Rudolph Matas, which he considered showed "metastases" developing in the chest wall and axillary scar 11 years after a forequarter amputation for an arteriovenous malformation (Matas, 1940).

The experience of major centers in managing arteriovenous malformations is summarized in the studies already quoted and additionally in Ward and Horton (1940), Adams (1951), Bertelesen and Dohn (1953), Lawton (1957), Cross (1958), Tice (1963), Cormier (1964), Sako and Varco (1970), Raskind and Weiss (1971), Dry (1972), and Knudson and Alden (1979).

Operation for arteriovenous malformations is almost never straightforward and is never to be lightly embarked upon. In this respect, little has changed from the time of Robert Liston who, in 1843, commenting on the successful removal of a vascular anomaly in the popliteal fossa, added: "The author may be allowed to premise that he would not willingly seek an intimate acquaintance with another such 'tumor mali moris' so situated and so connected, notwithstanding the completely favorable result of the operation in the case in question" (Liston, 1843).

Table 13–2. AMPUTATION RATES IN SERIES OF PATIENTS WITH CONGENITAL ARTERIOVENOUS FISTULAE

Investigator	Number of Patients	Amputation Rate (Per Cent)
Breschet (1833)	2	100
Pemberton (1928)	9	64
Lewis (1930)	30	43
Horton (1932)	23	9
Leonard (1951)	79	16
Robertson (1956)	28	18
Courseley (1956)	69	12
Malan (1965)	43	13
Sako (1970)	30	10
Young (1978)	26	8

References

Adams, H. D.: Congenital arteriovenous and cirsoid aneurysms. Surg. Gynec. Obstet. *92*:693, 1951.
Adams, J.: Singular case of hypertrophy of the right

lower extremity with superficial cutaneous naevus of the same side. Lancet 2:140, 1858.

Baer, R. L.: Multiple diffuse congenital arteriovenous aneurysms appearing as stasis dermatitis. Arch. Derm. 99:631, 1969.

Bell, J.: *The Principles of Surgery*. London: Longman, Hurst, Rees, et al., 1815, pp. 456–489.

Bertelsen, A., and Dohn, K.: Congenital arteriovenous communications of the extremities. Acta Chir. Scand. 105:448, 1953.

Branham, A. A.: Aneurysmal varix of the femoral artery and vein following a gunshot wound. Internat. J. Surg. 3:250, 1890.

Breschat, G.: Mémoire sur les anéurysmes. Mém. Acad. Roy. de Méd. Paris 3:101, 1833.

Browse, N. L., and Burnand, K. G.: The cause of venous ulceration. Lancet 2:243, 1982.

Burnand, K. G., Clemenson, G., Whimster, I., et al.: The effect of sustained venous hypertension on the skin capillaries of the canine hind limb. Brit. J. Surg. 69:41, 1982.

Burnand, K. G., Whimster, I., Naidod, A., and Browse, N. L.: Pericapillary fibrin in the ulcer bearing skin of the leg. Brit. Med. J. 285:1071, 1982.

Bushe, G.: A case, after the excision of an anastomosing aneurism from the right temple, ligature of the external carotid became necessary to restrain haemorrhage. Lancet 2:413, 1827–1828.

Callander, C. L.: Study of arteriovenous fistula with analysis of 447 cases. Ann. Surg. 71:428, 1920.

Clay, R. C., and Blalock, A.: Congenital arteriovenous fistulas in the mandible. Surg. Gynec. Obstet. 90:543, 1950.

Clyne, C. A. C., Ramsden, W. H., Chant, A. D. B., and Webster, J. H. H.: Oxygen tension on the skin of the gaiter area of the limbs with venous disease. Brit. J. Surg. 7:644, 1985.

Cormier, J. M.: Surgical treatment of arteriovenous aneurysms and fistulas of the lower extremity. Presse Med. 72:2601, 2717, 1964.

Cotton, L. T., and Sykes, B. J.: The treatment of diffuse congenital arteriovenous fistulae of the leg. Proc. Roy. Soc. Med. 62:245, 1969.

Coursley, G., Ivins, J. C., and Nelson, W. B.: Congenital arteriovenous fistulas in the extremities: An analysis of 69 cases. Angiology 7:201, 1956.

Cross, F. S., Glover, D. M., Simeone, F. A., and Oldenburg, F. A.: Congenital arteriovenous aneurysms. Ann. Surg. 148:649, 1958.

Cushing, H., and Bailey, P.: *Tumors Arising from the Blood Vessels of the Brain*. Springfield, IL, Charles C Thomas, 1928.

Dry, L. R., Conn, J. H., Chavez, C. M., and Hardy, J. D.: Arteriovenous fistula: An analysis of 58 cases. Amer. Surg. 38:154, 1972.

Flanc, C.: Congenital arterio-venous fistulas of the extremities. Austr. N Z J. Surg. 37:222, 1968.

Flye, M. W., Jordan, B. P., and Schwartz, M. Z.: Management of congenital arteriovenous malformations. Surgery 94:740, 1983.

Fontaine, R.: Les anéurysmes cirsoïdes dans le cadre des fistules artéro-veineuses. Lyon Chir. 63:3332, 4495, 1967.

Ghérini (of Milan): Varice anéurysmatique congénitale. Gaz. de Hop. de Paris, 27 Juin, 1867, p. 303.

Gomes, M. M. R., and Bernatz, P. E.: Arteriovenous fistulas. A review and ten year experience at the Mayo Clinic. Mayo Clin. Proc. 45:81, 1970.

Gunderman, W., Cited by Allen, E. V., Barker, N. W., and Hines, E. A.: In *Peripheral Vascular Diseases*, 3rd ed. Philadelphia: W. B. Saunders Co., 1962, p. 476.

Hewitt, P.: A case of congenital aneurysmal varix. Lancet 1:146, 1867.

Hoffmann, J.: Krankenvorstellung. Münch. Med. Woschr., 30 August, p. 1159, 1898.

Holman, E.: *Abnormal Arteriovenous Communications*, 2nd ed. Springfield, IL: Charles C Thomas, 1968.

Homer: *Odyssey*. XI, 633.

Hopkins, N. F. G., Spinks, T. J., Rhodes, C. G., et al.: Positron emission tomography in venous ulceration and liposclerosis: Study of regional tissue function. Brit. Med. J. 286:333, 1986.

Horton, B. T.: Hemihypertrophy of extremities associated with congenital arteriovenous fistula. JAMA 98:378, 1932.

Hunter, W.: The history of an aneurysm of the aorta with some remarks on aneurysms in general. Med. Obs. Soc. Phys. (London) 1:323, 1757.

Hurwitz, D. J., and Kerber, C. W.: Hemodynamic considerations in the treatment of arteriovenous malformations of the face and scalp. Plast. Reconstr. Surg. 67:421, 1981.

Knudson, R. P., and Alden, E. R.: Symptomatic arteriovenous malformations in infants less than 6 months of age. Pediatrics 64:238, 1979.

Krause, W.: Traumatische angiectasie der linken armes. Arch. f. Klin. Chir. ii:142, 1862.

Lancisi, G. M.: *De Motu Cordis et Aneurysmatibus (1745)*, Text and Translation. New York: MacMillan, 1952.

Lawton, R. C., Tidrick, R. T., and Brintnall, E. S.: A clinicopathological study of multiple congenital arteriovenous fistulae of the lower extremities. Angiology 8:161, 1957.

Leonard, F. C., and Vassos, G. A.: Congenital arteriovenous fistulization of lower limb. N. Engl. J. Med. 245:885, 1951.

Letenneur (de Nantes): Etat cirsoïde des artères de l'avant-bras, compliqué de phlébectasie artérielle. Gaz. de Hop., 15 Mars, 1859, p. 122.

Lewis, D.: Congenital arteriovenous fistulae. Lancet 2:621, 680, 1930.

Liston, R.: Case of erectile tumour in the popliteal space. Med. Chir. Trans. 26:120, 1843.

Little, J. M.: Vascular malformations. Aust. N Z J. Surg. 51:219, 1981.

Malan, E., and Azzolini, A.: Congenital arteriovenous malformations of the face and scalp. J. Cardiovasc. Surg. 9:109, 1968.

Malan, E., and Puglionisi, A.: Congenital angiodysplasia of the extremities. (Note II. Arterial, arterial and venous, and haemolymphatic dysplasias.) J. Cardiovasc. Surg. 6:255, 1965.

Matas, R.: Congenital arteriovenous angioma of the arm. Metastases eleven years after amputation. Ann. Surg. 111:1021, 1940.

Medawar, P. B., and Medawar, J. S.: *Aristotle to Zoos*. Cambridge, MA: Harvard University Press, Preface, p. v, 1983.

Mulliken, J. B., Murray, J. E., Castaneda, A. R., et al.: Management of a vascular malformation of the face using total circulatory arrest. Surg. Gynec. Obstet. 146:168, 1978.

Nanu, I., Alexandrescu-Dersca, C., and Lazeanu, E.: Les troubles cardiaques consécutifs aux anéurysmes artérioveineux. Arch. Mal Coeur *15*:829, 1922.

Natali, J., Jue-Denis, P., Kieffer, E., et al.: Arteriovenous fistulae of the internal iliac vessels. J. Cardiovasc. Surg. *25*:165, 1984.

Nicoladoni, C.: Phlebarteriectasie der rechten oberen extremität. Arch. Klin. Chir. *18*:252, 1875.

Nisbet, N. W.: Congenital arteriovenous fistula in the extremities. Brit. J. Surg. *41*:658, 1953.

O'Brien, S. F.: A large solitary congenital arteriovenous fistula presenting as lymphoedema. Brit. J. Surg. *52*:358, 1965.

Olcott, C., Newton, T. H., Stoney, R. J., and Ehrenfeld, W. K.: Intra-arterial embolization in the management of arteriovenous malformations. Surgery *79*:3, 1976.

Olivecrona, H., and Ladenheim, J.: *Congenital Arteriovenous Aneurysms of the Carotid and Vertebral Arteries.* Berlin: Springer Verlag, 1957, pp. 1–85.

Osler, W.: Remarks on arteriovenous aneurysm. Lancet *1*:949, 1915.

Pemberton, J., and Saint, J. H.: Congenital arteriovenous communications. Surg. Gynec. Obstet. *46*:470, 1928.

Purdy, A.: Contributions by Emile Holman to surgical literature. J. Cardiovasc. Surg. *5*:187, 1964.

Raskind, R., and Weiss, S. R.: Arteriovenous malformations. Follow-up of 68 cases. Vasc. Surg. *5*:30, 1971.

Reid, M. R.: The effect of arteriovenous fistula upon the heart and blood vessels: An experimental and clinical study. Bull. Johns Hopkins Hosp. *31*:43, 1920.

Reinhoff, W. F., Jr.: Congenital arteriovenous fistula. An embryological study with the report of a case. Bull. Johns Hopkins Hosp. *35*:271, 1924.

Robertson, D. J.: Congenital arteriovenous fistulae of the extremities. Ann. Roy. Coll. Surg. Engl. *18*:73, 1956.

Rosales, J. K.: Hypotensive anesthesia in the surgery of hemangiomas. In Williams, H. B. (ed.): *Symposium on Vascular Malformations and Melanocystic Lesions.* St. Louis: C. V. Mosby, 1983, pp. 52–57.

Rösler, H.: Über herzvergrösserlung bei angeborener arteriovenöser kommunikation. Klin. Woch. *8*:1621, 1929.

Sako, Y., and Varco, R.: Arteriovenous fistula: Results of management of congenital and acquired forms, blood flow measurements, and observations on proximal arterial degeneration. Surgery *67*:40, 1970.

Smith, W. (ed.): *A Dictionary of Greek and Roman Biography and Mythology.* London: J. Murray, Vol. 2, 1870, p. 285.

Steinheil, S. O.: Über einen fall von varix aneurysmaticus im bereich der gehirngefasse. Wurzburg: F. Froome, 1895.

Stewart, F. T.: Arteriovenous aneurism treated by angeiorrhaphy. Ann. Surg. *57*:574, 1913.

Szilagyi, D. E., Elliott, J. P., DeRusso, F. J., and Smith, R. F.: Peripheral congenital arteriovenous fistulas. Surgery *57*:61, 1965.

Szilagyi, D. E., Smith, R. F., Elliott, J. P., and Hageman, J. H.: Congenital arteriovenous malformations of the limbs. Arch. Surg. *111*:423, 1976.

Tice, D. A., Clauss, R. H., Keirle, A. M., and Reed, G. E.: Congenital arteriovenous fistulae of the extremities. Observations concerning treatment. Arch. Surg. *86*:460, 1963.

Ward, C. E., and Horton, B. T.: Congenital arteriovenous fistulas in children. J. Pediatr. *16*:746, 1940.

Warren, J. M.: Extracts from the records of the Boston Society for Medical Improvement—unusual case of varicose aneurysm. Amputation. Boston Med. Surg. J. *57*:528, 1858.

Wood, M. L., Reilly, G. D., and Smith, G. T.: Ulceration of the hand secondary to a radial arteriovenous fistulae: A model for varicose ulceration. Brit. Med. J. *287*:1167, 1983.

Yao, S. T., Needham, T. N., Lewis, J. B., and Hobbs, J. T.: Limb blood flow in congenital arteriovenous fistula. Surgery *73*:80, 1973.

Young, A. E.: Mixed vascular malformations. MChir Thesis, University of Cambridge, 1978.

CHAPTER FOURTEEN

Combined Vascular Malformations

A. E. Young

with contributions by
J. Ackroyd
P. Baskerville

*Monstrosities belong to the class of things
contrary to Nature, not any and every kind of
Nature, but Nature in her usual operations;
nothing can happen contrary to Nature
considered as eternal and necessary.*
Aristotle, De genera. Animale II, i, 732 b1–25

The development of the embryonic vascular system is closely integrated, abnormalities of one part influencing the growth and morphogenesis of another. It is not surprising, therefore, that close study of vascular malformations, especially those involving large areas, should show abnormalities in more than one of the components: the veins, arteries, lymphatics, and capillaries (Fig. 14–1). These overlaps are so common that Kinmonth suggested grouping certain vascular malformations together as "mixed vascular deformities" (Kinmonth et al., 1976). The word "deformities" was used because of the frequent association of tissue hyperplasia and skeletal overgrowth in these patients. We prefer, however, the term *combined vascular malformations,* as it is more comprehensive.

There are seven specific situations in which combined anomalies in different systems are of clinical importance:

1. Klippel-Trenaunay syndrome
2. Parkes Weber syndrome
3. Combined venous-lymphatic malformations
4. Maffucci's syndrome
5. Multiple dysplasia syndromes
6. Weber's diffuse phlebarteriectasis
7. The vascular neurocutaneous syndromes

KLIPPEL-TRENAUNAY AND PARKES WEBER SYNDROMES

In the galaxy of congenital vascular malformations, Klippel-Trenaunay syndrome and Parkes Weber syndrome are perhaps the

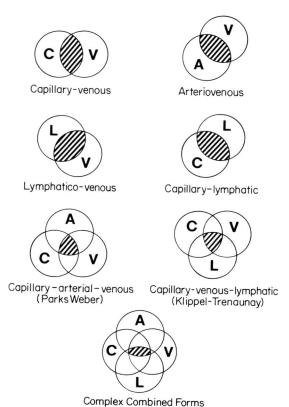

Capillary-venous

Arteriovenous

Lymphatico-venous

Capillary-lymphatic

Capillary-arterial-venous
(Parks Weber)

Capillary-venous-lymphatic
(Klippel-Trenaunay)

Complex Combined Forms

Figure 14–1. Schematic drawing of types of combined vascular malformations. The overlapping circles in these diagrams show the progressive complexity of abnormality that is possible when more than one component of the vascular system is malformed.

most common gross abnormalities encountered. They are characterized by impressive physical findings that rarely fail to fascinate and puzzle the physician. The symptomatology, pathology, and complications are described in this chapter. In 95% of cases the lower limb is the site of the malformations, and the practical management of these conditions is thus described in Chapter Nineteen.

The dominant features of Klippel-Trenaunay and Parkes Weber syndrome are three:

1. Cutaneous capillary malformations on a limb with
2. Congenital varicose veins with
3. Limb hypertrophy (gigantism)

Klippel-Trenaunay and Parkes Weber syndromes are, however, *not* the same, though they may present clinically as similar-looking malformations. Klippel-Trenaunay syndrome is predominantly a venous lesion of good prognosis, whereas Parkes Weber syndrome is characterized by the presence of an arteriovenous malformation and the prognosis is less sanguine. In both syndromes, there are frequent concomitant lymphatic abnormalities.

Historical Background

Throughout the nineteenth century medical literature, there appeared sporadic case reports of gigantism of the limbs associated with vascular lesions of the skin. A few of these case reports are published in English, and these are usually brief (Simpson, 1855; Adams, 1858; Hawthorne, 1902). By contrast, many reports from Europe are sufficiently full and accurate for us to be sure that the descriptions are of patients with congenital vascular malformations, e.g., those of Beck (1837), Friedberg (1867), Chaissaignac (1858), and Bryk (1879). Few of the cases were illustrated, but Friedberg's patient, described in 23 pages of text in Virchow's Archiv of 1867, provides an elegant exception (Fig. 14–2). Since the deformities of these patients sometimes verge on the grotesque, it is strange that none appear to have been described or illustrated in the medical literature before the nineteenth century. However, it is conceivable that the giant leg bearing a varicose vein that appears on a votive relief from the Asklepeion in Athens may indeed represent a venous ectasia on a leg hypertrophied in fact as well as in the sculptor's fancy (Fig. 14–3).

The first attempt at collecting these isolated case reports was made by Trélat and Monod in 1869 (Fig. 14–4). Under the title "De L'hypertrophie Unilatérale Partielle ou Totale du Corps," they collated the reports of 12 patients with limb hypertrophy (Trélat and Monod, 1869). Of these, all but three had some form of associated vascular lesion. Trélat and Monod defined no sub-groups; however, they did note the regular presence of varicose veins and, in some patients, an increased temperature of the limb and an enlargement in the size of the limb arteries. They noted three particular features of these varices: "La limitation de ces varices a un seul membre. L'absence de toutes les causes ordinaires de ces dilatations veineuses, la jeune âge du subjet."

Although Trélat and Monod had all but recognized a true syndrome, it was not until

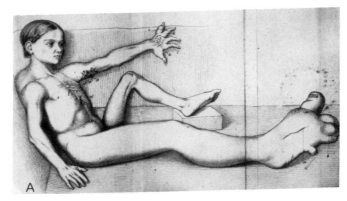

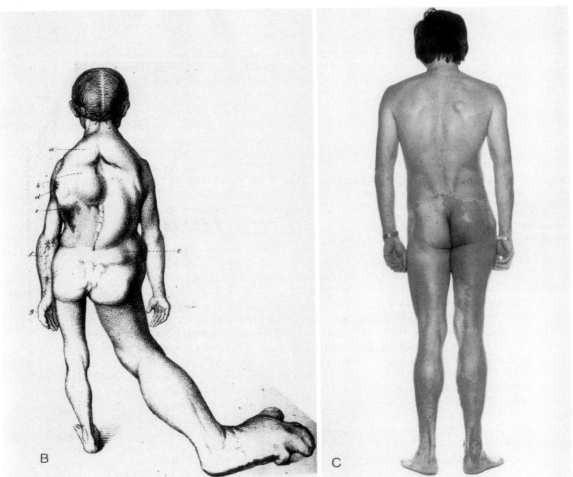

Figure 14—2. Friedberg's case of 1867. *A,* Side view showing the giant limb and scattered vascular malformations on the trunk and arms. *B,* He described a lipoma on the scapula labelled "b." (*A* and *B* from Friedberg, H.: Virchow's Archiv f. Path. Anat. *40:*353, 1867.) *C,* A current patient with Klippel-Trenaunay syndrome and a lipoma at a similar site; this is not an uncommon finding.

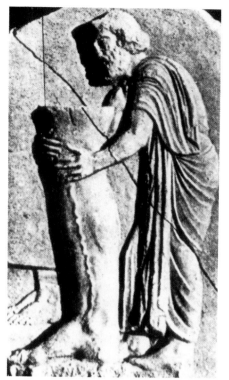

Figure 14–3. Votive relief from the Asklepeion in Athens showing a giant limb and varix.

the paper of Klippel and Trenaunay in 1900 that the association of hypertrophy and a vascular abnormality was recognized as "a syndrome" (Klippel and Trenaunay, 1900a)

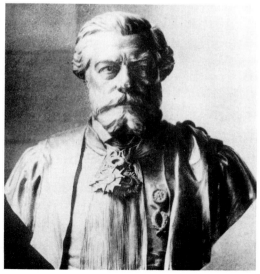

Figure 14–4. Ulysse Trélat (1828–1890), Professor of Surgery, Hôpital Necker, Paris. Illustration courtesy of the Wellcome Institute Library, London.

(Fig. 14–5). Their first account described a single case of limb hypertrophy associated with a vascular malformation. They quickly followed this case report of their classic paper "Du noevus variqueux ostéohypertrophique" (Klippel and Trenaunay, 1900b). This is a thorough and articulate review of 51 cases reported in the European (predominantly French) literature. On the basis of this analysis, they delineated a syndrome comprising three features:

1. A vascular nevus (birthmark) extending the full length of the lower limb with metameric distribution ("Un *noevus* étendu à tout le membre inférieur, à distribution métamérique")

2. Varices on the affected side dating from birth or infancy ("Des *varices* précoces exclusivement limitées au côté malade et datant de l'enfance, sinon de la naissance")

3. Hypertrophy of all the tissues of the affected side, particularly the skeleton, which is enlarged in all dimensions—length, breadth, and thickness ("Une *hypertrophie* portant sur l'ensemble des tissus du côté malade, mais en particulier du côté du squelette, qui se montre augmenté en toutes ses dimensions, longueur, largeur, epaisseur")

They stated clearly, for the first time, that these were not "lesions groupées par accident ou par coincidence mais comme resultat d'une seule et même maladie." There was, however, no suggestion that the vascular abnormality might *cause* the hypertrophy. The syndrome to which they gave the unwieldy title "noevus variqueux ostéohypertrophique" (described by Vollmar as "ein linguistiches Ungetum"—a linguistic monstrosity) has subsequently been known as Klippel-Trenaunay syndrome (Vollmar, 1974).

Seven years after Klippel and Trenaunay's papers, Frederick Parkes Weber* (Fig. 14–6), apparently in ignorance of Klippel and Trenaunay's work, presented a paper describing a syndrome that he named "haemangiectatic hypertrophy" (Parkes Weber, 1907). He subsequently expanded this work in two further papers in 1908 and 1918 (Parkes

---

*Frederick Parkes Weber was a dermatologist whose name is associated with six syndromes: 1. Rendu-Osler-Weber syndrome; 2. Parkes Weber syndrome. 3. Sturge-Weber syndrome. 4. Weber-Cockayne syndrome (epidermolysis bullosa of the feet); 5. Weber-Christian disease (relapsing, febrile, nodular, non-suppurative panniculitis); and 6. Weber-Hellenschmied syndrome (telangiectasia macularis eruptica perstans).

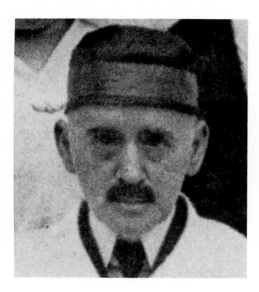

Figure 14–5. Maurice Klippel (1858–1942), French neurologist whose name is associated with three syndromes: Klippel-Trenaunay, Klippel-Feil, and Klippel-Feldstein. This illustration from the Revue Illustrée des Hôpitaux 1923, page 26, is the only known illustration of Dr. Klippel. Nothing is known of his compatriot Trenaunay.

Weber, 1908, 1918). Parkes Weber reviewed a historical and personal series of patients in whom three features coexisted:

1. "Phlebarteriectasis' (enlargement of the arteries and veins of the limb)
2. Capillary or venous malformations
3. Gigantism of the affected limb

On superficial examination of these separate reports the triads of signs seem similar,

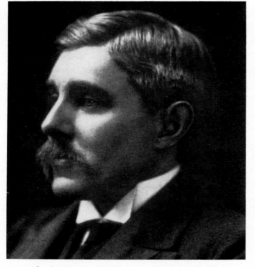

Figure 14–6. Frederick Parkes Weber (1863–1962). This Austrian dermatologist spent his working life in London. His name is attached to six syndromes, of which three contain vascular birthmarks: Parkes Weber, Sturge-Weber, and Rendu-Osler-Weber. (Photograph courtesy of Wellcome Institute for the History of Medicine.)

but there are important differences, namely the presence in the Parkes Weber syndrome of multiple arteriovenous fistulae. In his 1918 paper, Parkes Weber speaks of the phlebarteriectasis thus: "Sometimes the communication between the arterial channels and the venous channels may be so free that a definite kind of thrill or pulsation rhythmical with the heart's contraction is transmitted to the veins *as in cases of arteriovenous anastomosis of traumatic origin.*" He clearly understood this to be a feature of the syndrome he described. By contrast, Klippel and Trenaunay (who must have been familiar with the signs of fistulation) did not include any of the signs of arteriovenous shunting in their description and, in fact, stated, "Les altérations des veines et l'angiome semblent constitués les seules lésions du système vasculaire," and added that, in their case, the pulses were normal. There are thus two distinct syndromes associated with limb hypertrophy and capillary (dermal) vascular malformation. One is *Klippel-Trenaunay syndrome,* in which the vascular lesion is predominantly venous. The other is *Parkes Weber syndrome,* in which arteriovenous fistulae are the major vascular lesions. It is necessary to stress the importance of making this distinction because many authors, in the past and still, have confused the two syndromes or lumped them together as "Klippel-Trenaunay-Weber syndrome" or depersonalized them as the "osteoangiohypertrophic syndrome." (It is interesting to note that Parkes Weber himself does not seem to have objected to this conjunction [Parkes Weber, 1946].)

Modern techniques for measuring blood flow and arteriovenous shunt size show that patients with Klippel-Trenaunay syndrome do, indeed, have slightly increased blood flow and may have an increase in shunting through physiological arteriovenous connections, but this is always trivial and never clinically important (Baskerville et al., 1985). Investigations of the lymphatic system in patients with Klippel-Trenaunay syndrome and Parkes Weber syndrome show different patterns of abnormality (Young, 1978b).

Authors of any respectably sized series of these patients have invariably concluded that not only are the two syndromes usually clinically separable, but also this separation has valuable prognostic and therapeutic implications (Lindenauer, 1971). Although Klippel-Trenaunay and Parkes Weber syndromes were described as lower limb anomalies, equivalent lesions are seen in the upper limbs, separately or in conjunction with lower limb lesions, and by common usage are allowed the same titles. Vollmar published a full and closely argued paper showing the justification for separating the two syndromes (Vollmar, 1974).

Occasionally, there are patients who demonstrate features of both syndromes, but there is overlap between all varieties of vascular malformation such that obsessionally pure classification becomes impossible. This is, however, not a reason to abandon clinically useful subdivisions. Bourde attempted to deal with this problem by identifying five different levels of Klippel-Trenaunay syndrome, in which genuine Klippel-Trenaunay syndrome is considered to fade into Parkes Weber syndrome (Bourde, 1974). The classifications of Coget and Merlen (1980) and of Schobinger (1977) are far more useful.

The terms "Klippel-Trenaunay-Weber syndrome" and "osteoangiohypertrophic syndrome" should be abandoned. The features that separate the two syndromes are shown in Table 14–1. A useful, simple classification for Klippel-Trenaunay syndrome (KTS) has been proposed by Schobinger (Schobinger, 1977):

Type I   KTS without deep vein anomalies and without detectable arteriovenous fistulae.

Type II   KTS with detectable arteriovenous fistulae (i.e., Parkes Weber syndrome).

Table 14–1. COMPARISON BETWEEN KLIPPEL-TRENAUNAY SYNDROME AND PARKES WEBER SYNDROME

	Klippel-Trenaunay Syndrome	Parkes Weber Syndrome
Cutaneous vascular malformation	Almost invariably tends to be dark. May be verrucous.	Frequent. Usually a pink capillary malformation.
Arteriovenous fistulae	Not significant	Invariable
Deep vein	Common	Absent
Lateral venous anomaly	Common	Absent
Gigantism	Usually disproportionte, with soft tissue thickening predominating. Often giant toes present.	Usually proportionate
Lengthening of limb	Usually minor	Often major
Associated lesions (see Table 14–2)	Common	Rare
Lymphatics	Often hypoplastic	Usually hyperplastic
Prognosis	Good. Stable after childhood.	May be progressive deterioration

Type III   KTS with abnormalities of the deep veins but without detectable arteriovenous fistulae.

Lymphatic anomalies are also seen in patients with the Klippel-Trenaunay anomaly. Therefore, the possible extent of this syndrome can only be encompassed by the designation "combined capillary-venous-lymphatic malformation" (see Fig. 14–1).

KLIPPEL-TRENAUNAY SYNDROME

Clinical Features

Males and females are equally affected. In 95% of patients, the lower limb is involved. In 5%, the upper limb alone is affected. In 15%, both upper and lower limbs are involved. Eighty-five per cent of cases are unilateral, and occasionally the lower limb on one side and the arm on the opposite side are involved. In a few cases, the whole trunk is also involved in the malformation. Very occasionally the varices, capillary malformation, and hypertrophy may appear in different limbs, a condition noted by Klippel and Trenaunay in their original paper and described as crossed dissociation ("forme croisée-dissociée") (Figs. 14–7 and 14–8). In all cases, the malformation is present at birth but will usually be asymptomatic at that time. Nevertheless, 75% of the patients who become symptomatic will present before the age of 10, though some may not come to specialist medical attention until late middle age. In the Mayo Clinic series of 40 patients, all were white (Gloviczki et al., 1983). In the St. Thomas' Hospital (London) series of 50 patients, some blacks and Asian Indians were seen (Baskerville et al., 1985). Almost all reported cases have been sporadic, without any familial tendency to vascular abnormalities. A few exceptions have been reported. Lian and Alhomme recorded congenital varicose veins in three generations of one family (Lian and Alhomme, 1945), and Lindenauer noted them in a brother and sister (Lindenauer, 1965). There has been no recorded evidence of particular problems occurring during gestation, or of exposure of known teratogens.

Symptoms

The patients usually present because of varicose veins or because of anxiety about the nevus; bleeding from the varices, rectum, or bladder; ulceration of the skin; a long leg and scoliosis; edema; or the associated skeletal anomalies.

Signs

The Capillary Malformation

The capillary malformation is flat, minimally raised, or can be studded with vascular nodules (Fig. 14–9). It is usually widespread but, as Klippel and Trenaunay originally required, need not spread down the whole limb. In color, it ranges from pink to deep purple, though it is usually bluish and often contains small included venous "flares" and small ectatic veins, or frank localized venous lesions or vesicular lymphatic lesions. The

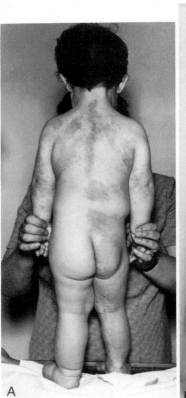
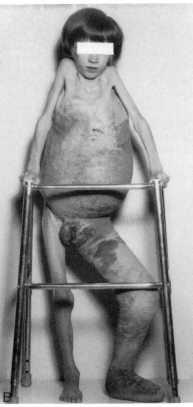

Figure 14–7. *A,* Klippel-Trenaunay syndrome of the right lower extremity and the left upper extremity. There are distended veins and skeletal overgrowth in both limbs. *B,* A 10 year old girl with severe Klippel-Trenaunay syndrome involving not only the limb with a length discrepancy of 11.8 cm but also extensive vascular malformations of the trunk. She died at the age of 11. (Illustration courtesy of Dr. L. H. Hollier, Mayo Clinic; Ann. Surg. *197:*353–362, 1983.)

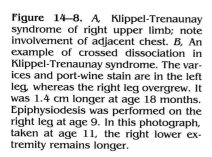

Figure 14–8. *A*, Klippel-Trenaunay syndrome of right upper limb; note involvement of adjacent chest. *B*, An example of crossed dissociation in Klippel-Trenaunay syndrome. The varices and port-wine stain are in the left leg, whereas the right leg overgrew. It was 1.4 cm longer at age 18 months. Epiphysiodesis was performed on the right leg at age 9. In this photograph, taken at age 11, the right lower extremity remains longer.

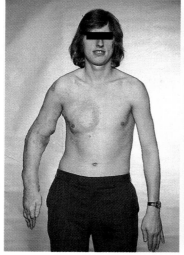 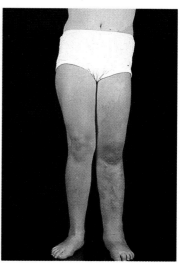

A　　　　　　　　　B

dermal vascular malformation does not blanch significantly on pressure. The shape of the capillary nevus resembles a map of Scotland in shape, but was originally described as "metameric." In fact, it is not truly metameric. None of the 25 cases whose nevi were carefully studied by the author could be matched to any cutaneous sensory nerve distribution or other known metameric distribution (Young, 1978a) (Fig. 14–10). In

17% of the St. Thomas' Hospital series (Baskerville et al., 1985), the capillary malformation affected the whole of one side of the body. As the patient ages, the skin over the malformation thickens and some capillaries may thrombose, leading to slow fading of the capillary malformation. We have never seen complete disappearance of the malformation, but pink ones may fade to be of no cosmetic significance. In contrast, the marks may be-

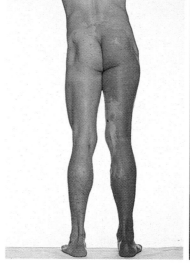 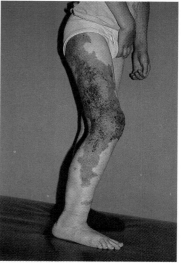

Figure 14–9. Cutaneous capillary malformations in Klippel-Trenaunay syndrome can be flat and pale *(A)* or dark purple, raised, and verrucous *(B)*.

A　　　　　　　　　B

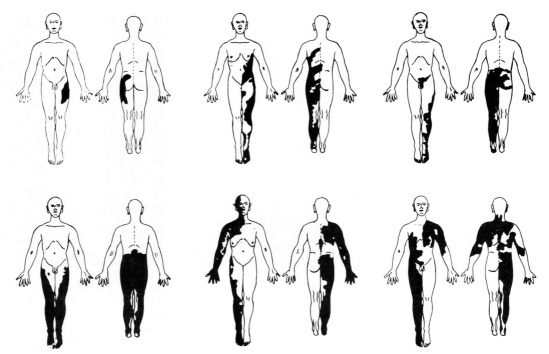

Figure 14–10. Examples of the distribution of the capillary malformation seen in patients with Klippel-Trenaunay syndrome.

come more prominent during puberty and pregnancy. Some patients do not have the capillary malformation, and in black patients it may be all but invisible.

Many authors have noted that profuse sweating may occur in the area involved by the capillary malformation and have even noted an abnormally high chloride content in the sweat. The affected areas may also feel warmer than normal. We have noticed subcutaneous lipomas in several patients, and the first illustrated case of what is probably Klippel-Trenaunay syndrome (Friedberg's) also showed a lipoma (see Figs. 14–2B and C). The nails may be deformed and ridged. The capillary nevus may also contain small lymphatic anomalies with vesicles that leak lymph.

Limb Hypertrophy

Klippel and Trenaunay defined the syndrome as requiring enlargement of the limb in all dimensions as a *sine qua non*. In the St. Thomas' Hospital series, however, the limb was noted to be longer than its fellow in only 72% of cases and thicker in only 58%. The increase in thickness is classically due to an increased thickness in bone, together with

hypertrophy of muscle and all other soft tissues. In our experience, however, there is usually very little increase in bone diameter, though it may be denser. The greater girth of the limb is more often due to muscle hypertrophy, thickened skin, and excessive fat, together with bulky abnormal vascular tissue. There is sometimes concomitant lymphedema, which may not be typical in appearance (Fig. 14–11). The enlargement of the limb in Klippel-Trenaunay patients may be in proportion but is often disproportionate in parts of the limb, especially the toes and feet (Fig. 14–12). Such gigantism is noted at birth, but the more common, milder degrees of hypertrophy and elongation may not be noted until late infancy or adolescence, if at all. The disparity in length does not progress in a predictable way.

A few patients with otherwise classic Klippel-Trenaunay syndrome may have a short and/or hypotrophic limb (see Fig. 14–8B).

Varicosities

The most common abnormality is a lateral venous anomaly (Fig. 14–13). This starts from a plexus of veins on the dorsum and lateral side of the foot and extends a variable

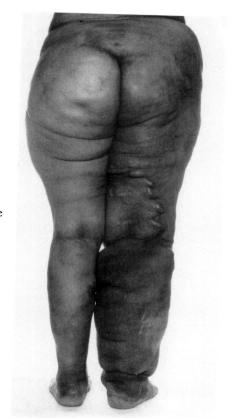

Figure 14–11. Asian-Indian woman with Klippel-Trenaunay syndrome of the right leg and associated lymphedema, present since birth.

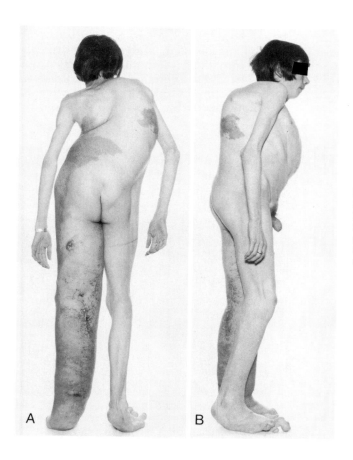

A   B

Figure 14–12. A and B, Klippel-Trenaunay syndrome of the left leg with gross associated lymphatic and skeletal abnormalities; in particular, the commonly associated feature of giant toes in this patient is found on the opposite side, suggesting that the vascular anomaly was not itself the cause.

Lateral venous anomaly

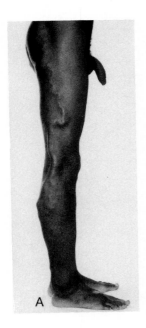

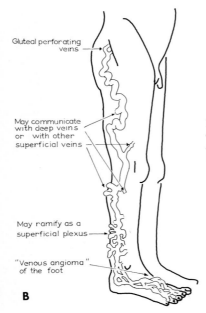

Gluteal perforating veins

May communicate with deep veins or with other superficial veins

May ramify as a superficial plexus

"Venous angioma" of the foot

A   B

Figure 14–13. *A,* Klippel-Trenaunay syndrome with a full length lateral venous anomaly. *B,* Diagram to show the typical features of lateral venous anomalies.

distance up the leg. In the St. Thomas' Hospital series, it was noted in 70% of cases and was found on phlebography to terminate in the popliteal vein in 11%; the superficial femoral vein in 17%; the profunda femoris vein in 19%; the external iliac vein in 6%; and, in 33% of cases, it extended the full length of the leg and penetrated the lateral aspect of the buttock, entering the internal iliac system via the gluteal veins (Fig. 14–14). The vein may or may not be valveless. It is usually thick-walled and may be deeply placed under the skin, such that it is not externally visible (though it may be palpated). Particularly in the lower part of the leg, it may be embedded in a dense fibrous plexus

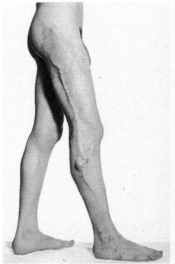

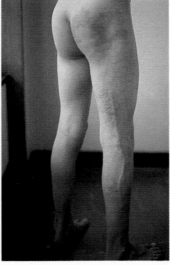

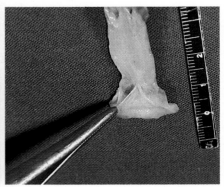

A   B   C

Figure 14–14. Other forms of the lateral venous anomaly (*A* and *B*); these veins can contain valves (*C*).

of anomalous veins. There are usually incompetent perforating veins, especially in the full length "lumbar foot" lateral anomaly (Myers and Janes, 1955). Perforating veins can occur along the full length of the anomaly. The long and short saphenous systems may also be varicose, either secondarily to the lateral anomaly, with associated incompetent communicating veins, or primarily. Myers and Janes have described four variants of the venous abnormalities (Myers and Janes, 1955):

1. The lateral venous anomaly that they describe as a "lumbar foot pattern" (see Fig. 14–13)

2. The "long saphenous pattern" with multiple perforating veins (Fig. 14–15)

3. The "long saphenous pattern" in which gluteal veins communicate via posterior thigh veins with the short saphenous system (see Fig. 14–11)

4. The "short saphenous pattern" associated with lateral ankle and foot perforating veins (Fig. 14–16).

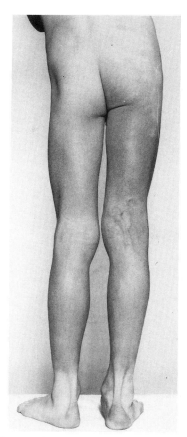

Figure 14–16. Klippel-Trenaunay syndrome with short saphenous pattern varices.

The multiple patches of stellate venous flare frequently seen in the skin adjacent to the venous anomaly may be primarily ectatic veins occurring in the area of the capillary malformation, or may be the result of reflux of venous blood secondary to hypertension in the main abnormal vein.

In the St. Thomas' Hospital series, 22% of patients had bled from their varices, either spontaneously or secondary to trauma. Eczema, verrucosity of the skin, or the frank changes of lipodermatitis secondary to venous hypertension and progressing to ulceration are rare; none of our patients had a "varicose ulcer" at any time, though two patients of the Mayo Clinic series had such ulceration (Gloviczki et al., 1983), and Servelle records it as occurring in 10% of a large series of congenital venous anomalies in the lower limb (Servelle, 1985). However, episodes of both superficial and deep thrombophlebitis are common and may be associated with pain and with pulmonary embolism. Phleboliths may be seen as monuments to

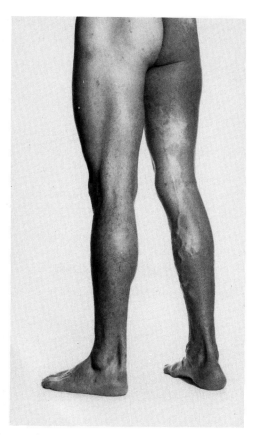

Figure 14–15. Klippel-Trenaunay syndrome with long saphenous pattern varices.

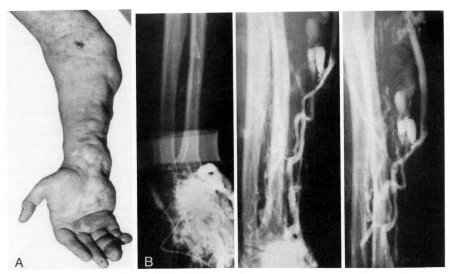

Figure 14–17. *A,* Klippel-Trenaunay syndrome of the arm. *B,* Direct puncture venogram of arm showing nest of abnormal veins at the wrist connecting with abnormal and ectatic forearm veins.

past thromboses. We have not seen any co-agulopathy or other hematological abnor-mality in patients with Klippel-Trenaunay syndrome confined to one or more limbs. However, it may be encountered where the abnormality involves the trunk with a large mass of abnormal malformed vascular tissue, in which case platelet and fibrinogen deple-tion can occur. Although clinically significant hematological changes are rare, low-grade, localized consumption coagulopathy is prob-ably common.

At the Children's Hospital in Boston, three cases of refractory septicemia have been seen in young patients with extensive Klippel-Trenaunay anomalies. Localized signs of in-fection were noted in the proximal thigh and buttock. Gram-negative organisms were cul-tured from the blood of these patients, thus raising the question whether bacterial seed-ing of the malformed vascular spaces, per-haps the lymphatic component, can originate in the lower gastrointestinal tract. Prolonged intravenous antibiotic therapy was necessary to prevent recurrent sepsis.

Varicosities in the rare cases of Klippel-Trenaunay syndrome seen in the upper limbs do not appear to show any specific pattern, and we are not aware of any instances of deep vein aplasia or hypoplasia associated with the superficial varicosities (Fig. 14–17).

Associated Abnormalities

Klippel-Trenaunay syndrome, like an ice-berg, has a visible, often impressive element,

but also has an invisible and sometimes dan-gerous deep component. The "submerged" parts of the syndrome include
1. Deep vein abnormalities
2. Lymphatic abnormalities
3. Associated abnormalities in other sys-tems
4. Venous thrombosis and pulmonary em-bolism

Deep Vein Abnormalities

Most of the papers on the topic of deep vein abnormalities are in the French litera-ture. The largest experience is that of Ser-velle, who claims that the deep veins are abnormal in all instances of Klippel-Trenau-nay syndrome of the lower limb (1957, 1965, 1980, 1985). In his report reviewing a per-sonal series of 614 patients operated upon between 1944 and 1978, 51% were consid-ered to have popliteal vein abnormalities, usually occlusion by a fibrous band (Fig. 14–18), but occasionally in the form of agenesis or atresia; 16% had femoral vein obstruction, manifested by long external compression, but atresias were also found; 3% had iliac vein malformations; and 1% had inferior vena cava malformations. In the iliac and caval segments, atresias and agenesis were more common than external bands. Lindenauer found deep vein anomalies in 13 of 14 pa-tients with Klippel-Trenaunay syndrome, but other investigators found the abnormality in far fewer cases—on average 1 in 5 (Linden-auer, 1965). This has also been our experi-

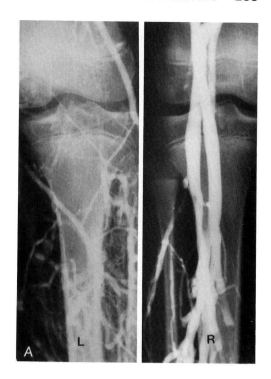

Figure 14–18. *A,* This patient with Klippel-Trenaunay syndrome of the left leg has only minimal visible varices on the surface, but venography shows an absent or obstructed popliteal vein with extensive collaterals. The right popliteal vein is normal. *B,* Servelle suggests that this clinical pattern is associated with anatomical obstruction to the deep venous drainage, as shown in his diagram. (From Servelle, M.: *Oedemes Chroniques des Membres.* Paris, Masson, 1962.)

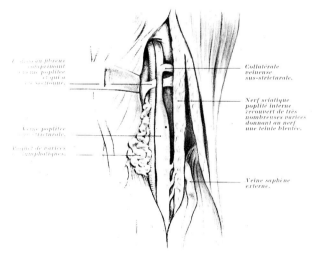

ence. However, a confident assessment of the deep veins does require a surgical exploration, and hardly any such explorations have been performed, except by Servelle. Phlebographic appraisal is confused by the well-recognized difficulties in displaying the deep trunks because of dilution of contrast, difficulties with tourniquets, occlusion of large superficial veins, and dilution in capacious venous abnormalities. Extensive bandaging of the legs and/or direct injection into the deep veins may be necessary to demonstrate their anatomy. Other measures, such as venous phase arteriography, retrograde venography, or intraosseus venography, may be needed to display the deep system properly. We have seen a clear example of the fallibility of venography in this syndrome. A patient with "atretic" deep veins died, and, at postmortem, the deep veins were found to be entirely normal. Hemodynamic studies are also often normal in patients with phlebographically abnormal deep veins (see later discussion). Vermeulen and Wiffels found that the popliteal stenoses seen on static phlebography disappeared on dynamic phlebography (Vermeulen and Wiffels, 1970).

A collateral venous circulation around deep vein obstruction occurs via lateral venous anomalies, by the vein accompanying the sciatic nerve, by veins anastomosing with the profunda femoris vein, by the long and short saphenous veins, by venae comitantes of the femoral artery, and by other abnormal veins (Servelle, 1985).

We have been surprised by the paucity of symptoms and clinical complications encountered in patients with quite gross phlebographic deep vein abnormalities (Fig. 14–18). The pattern of swelling, aching, lipodermatitis, and ulceration is rarely seen, and in the St. Thomas' Hospital series none of the patients with Klippel-Trenaunay syndrome had a "venous ulcer."

Hemodynamics of Klippel-Trenaunay Syndrome

Hemodynamics of the Venous System. Ackroyd and coworkers (1984) investigated the calf pump function in patients with Klippel-Trenaunay syndrome using a modification of the foot volumetric techniques as first described by Thulesius and Norgren (Thulesius et al., 1973). The ability of the calf muscles to pump blood up the leg away from the foot was assessed by measuring water displacement in a foot bath. The technique also allowed measurement of any reflux down the deep veins of the leg. Twenty-seven of 32 abnormal limbs studied in this fashion showed a normal or greater than normal reduction in foot volume during exercise (Fig. 14–19). Of the five patients with an abnormally small reduction of foot volume, suggesting an inefficient calf pump or obstruction, only one had atretic deep veins on phlebography. Thus, in spite of a high incidence of phlebographic deep venous abnormalities, calf pump function in almost all these patients remained normal. The major abnormality lay in the refilling rate of the foot: most limbs had an abnormally rapid refilling rate, which suggests reflux down the deep veins or through perforating veins (Fig. 14–19). In spite of this chronic reflux, it seems that the calf pump still manages to compensate, because the incidence of skin changes and ulceration normally associated with venous hypertension is remarkably low in the patients studied.

Arteriovenous Hemodynamics. Although the diagnosis of Klippel-Trenaunay syndrome should specifically exclude the pres-

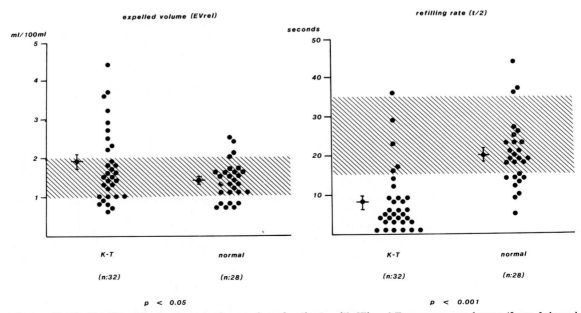

Figure 14–19. Results of foot volumetry in a series of patients with Klippel-Trenaunay syndrome (from Ackroyd et al., 1984). The normal legs are compared with the involved limbs. Values for the normal population are shown hatched.

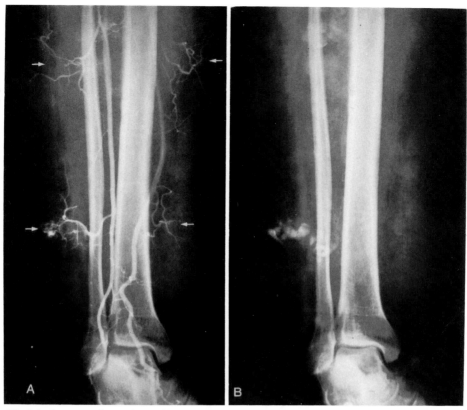

Figure 14–20. Arteriogram of a patient with apparently typical Klippel-Trenaunay syndrome; however, angiography shows discrete arteriovenous malformations in the calf (arrows). *A,* The arterial phase. *B,* The later venous pooling in the malformations.

ence of an arteriovenous fistula, we have already noted that some authors continue to classify cases as Klippel-Trenaunay syndrome when they have an obvious arteriovenous fistula, which is an abnormality characteristic of the Parkes Weber syndrome. It would seem that some clinicians equate an enlarged limb with the presence of arteriovenous fistulae and fail to use any objective tests to confirm or exclude their presence. However, if a limb contains active arteriovenous fistulae, hypertrophy of bone or soft tissue will be progressive in nature. In patients with Klippel-Trenaunay syndrome, hypertrophy rarely continues after the age of 12 years. Therefore, before one makes a diagnosis of Klippel-Trenaunay syndrome, arteriovenous fistulae should be excluded by clinical and physiological investigations (Fig. 14–20).

A study of calf blood flow in patients with Klippel-Trenaunay syndrome using strain gauge phlethysmography has shown that although their flow lies within normal limits in all limbs, flow in the abnormal limb is greater than in the normal limb (Ackroyd et al., 1984) (Fig. 14–21). Furthermore, in the absence of arteriovenous fistulae, the increase in flow appears to be associated with the presence of a nevus (Baskerville et al., 1985) and probably simply reflects increased flow through the skin and subdermal venules. Ackroyd found that when the limb opposite to that bearing the Klippel-Trenaunay syndrome also bore a capillary nevus, the flow in that limb, though less than the flow in the limb with the Klippel-Trenaunay abnormality, was nonetheless greater than in a normal limb.

Lymphatic Abnormalities

In a prospective study of the lymphatic system of 26 patients with Klippel-Trenaunay syndrome undertaken in 1975, 6 (23%) had clinically apparent lymphedema and 6 had cutaneous lymphatic vesicles (Kinmonth, 1982). Lymphography of the 26 patients, including those with and without clinically apparent lymphatic disease, showed that 72%

ml/100 ml/min   n:22

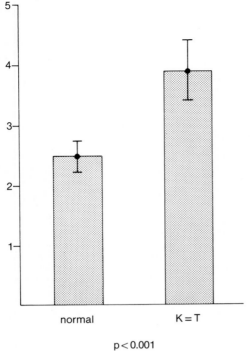

Figure 14–21. Calf blood flows in 22 patients with Klippel-Trenaunay syndrome.

p < 0.001

had abnormalities of the lymphatic system demonstrable by venography. St. Thomas' Hospital is, nonetheless, a referral center for lymphatic problems and it is likely to have had a slight preponderance of lymphatic disease in the series of patients with Klippel-Trenaunay syndrome. Nonetheless, the fact remains that patients without any clinical evidence of lymphatic abnormality can regularly be shown to have a lymphographic abnormality. This is typically in the form of reduction of the number of lymph trunks and nodes (Fig. 14–22). Lymphatic hypoplasia is not the result of chronic sepsis and is probably a primary intrauterine developmental defect.

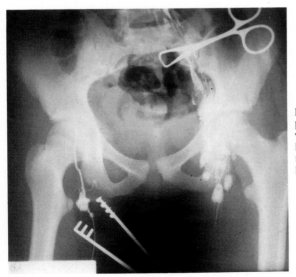

Figure 14–22. Lymphangiogram of the right leg of a patient with Klippel-Trenaunay syndrome. No lymphatic vessels could be found in the foot, and an intranodal injection was made into the single lymph node identifiable in the groin. There is only one efferent groin lymphatic. The left side is normal.

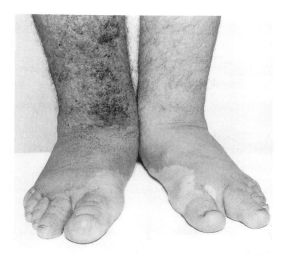

Figure 14–23. Bilateral Klippel-Trenaunay syndrome with hemorrhagic lymphatic vesicles covering the right shin. Troublesome leakage was experienced from these vesicles. The problem was resolved by excision of the affected area and coverage with a split skin graft.

Servelle and colleagues consider that the lymphatic abnormalities in Klippel-Trenaunay syndrome patients with deep vein malformations are due to entrapment of juxta-venous lymphatic vessels by the fibrous bands that also obstruct the veins (Servelle et al., 1957; Servelle and Babilliot, 1980). These authors also note an instance of chylous reflux into the limb. Although only Servelle has exposed the lymphatics surgically in patients with Klippel-Trenaunay syndrome, Müller and Schmidt (1969), Pokrovosky and coworkers (1971), Biasi and colleagues (1973), and Hamatake (1974) have also noted lymphographic evidence of "hypoplasia."

The lymphatic vesicles seen on the skin may be isolated lymphatic abnormalities ("lymphangioma circumscriptum") out of contact with the deep system, or they may represent dermal backflow from an obstructed deep lymphatic system (Fig. 14–23). Very rarely they may leak chyle, reflecting chylous reflux into the limb. Where Klippel-Trenaunay syndrome involves the trunk as well as the limb, intestinal lymphangiectasis may occur with associated protein-losing enteropathy.

Associated Abnormalities in Other Systems

A great variety of abnormalities have been recorded in other systems and are annotated in Table 14–2. These concomitant abnormalities usually occur in, or adjacent to, the limb involved by the Klippel-Trenaunay syndrome (Fig. 14–24) but can occur at a distance, suggesting a more generalized meso-dermal and/or ectodermal dysplasia or that the tissue at these different sites has been subject to a common teratogenic influence. The concomitant abnormality seen in a limb need not be interpreted as a secondary result of the vascular malformation. Importantly, however, the neurological problems encountered in some patients with Klippel-Trenaunay syndrome, in whom the malformation involves the spine and the brain, are entirely secondary to the direct effects of the abnormal vascular tissue on the central nervous system. There is no primary neuronal defect. We have seen no evidence of mental retardation in association with Klippel-Trenaunay syndrome.

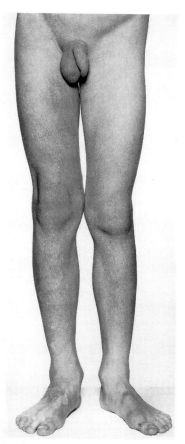

Figure 14–24. Klippel-Trenaunay syndrome of the right leg with left cryptorchidism. This was noted in 4 of 15 males with this anomaly (Young, 1978).

Table 14–2. KLIPPEL-TRENAUNAY SYNDROME ASSOCIATIONS

The following lesions have been recorded in association with Klippel-Trenaunay syndrome:

Vascular Malformations
Of spinal cord (Djindjian, 1977)
Of bladder (Kuffer, 1968; Servelle, 1976)
Of colon and rectum (Ghahremani, 1976; Servelle, 1976)
Of retroperitoneum (Kuffer, 1968)
Of penis, vulva, and vagina
Of buccal mucosa (Brooksaler, 1966)
Sturge Weber syndrome (Harper, 1971)
Pulmonary vein varicosis (Malan, 1964; Owens, 1973; Kessler, 1983)

Skeletal Malformations
Disproportionate gigantism, especially of toes
Dwarfism of limb
Facial, pelvic asymmetry
Jaw anomalies (mandibular cyst, dentigerous cyst, malocclusion, premature eruption of teeth (Kontras, 1974; Sciubba, 1977)
Spine anomalies (kyphosis, scoliosis, vertebral segmentation defects, spina bifida occulta)
Hand and foot anomalies (syndactyly, polydactyly, clinodactyly, metatarsal agenesis, phalangeal agenesis, talipes calcaneovarus and equinovarus) (Young, 1978; Gloviczki, 1983)
Hip anomalies (congenital dislocation, coxa vara, pelvic non-fusion, congenital dislocation of shoulder) (Young, 1978)
Atresia of auditory canal (Gloviczki, 1983)
Rudimentary rib
Fibrous dysplasia
Chondroma, osteoma, fibroma
Melorheostosis (Young, 1978; Kessler, 1983)

Lymphatic Malformations
Hypoplasia of vessels and nodes
Intestinal lymphangiectasis causing protein-losing enteropathy
Localized lymphatic anomalies (Belovic, 1974; Young, 1978)

Skin Malformations
Café-au-lait spots
von Recklinghausen's disease
Lipomas
Hypertrichosis
Alopecia
Sebaceous and salivary gland hypertrophy (Klippel, 1900b)

Other Malformations
Lipodystrophies (Smith, 1982)
Mucosal ulceration (Brooksaler, 1966)
Congenital glaucoma, heterochromia (Kontras, 1974; Smith, 1982)
Choanal atresia (Feldmuller, 1976)
Atrial septal defect
Indirect inguinal hernia
Cryptorchidism, hydrocele, testicular hypoplasia
Gynecomastia
Wilms tumors/nephroblastomas (Mankad, 1974; Ehrich, 1979)
Temporal lobe astrocytoma (Howitz, 1979)
Tuberous sclerosis (Troost, 1975)
Ehlers-Danlos syndrome (Poulet, 1979; Alberti, 1976)
von Hippel–Lindau syndrome (Hartog Jager, 1949)
Muscle atrophy (Bereston, 1965; Korting, 1969)

Venous Thrombosis and Pulmonary Embolism

Venous thrombosis is common in patients with Klippel-Trenaunay syndrome. This, and the risks of pulmonary embolism, are documented in Chapter Nineteen.

PARKES WEBER SYNDROME

Parkes Weber syndrome is substantially less common than Klippel-Trenaunay syndrome. When present, it most commonly affects the lower limb but is more likely to be found in the upper limb than Klippel-Trenaunay syndrome. Of Robertson's 28 patients, 7 had upper limbs involved and 23 had lower limb involvement (Robertson, 1956). Twenty of the 28 patients had cutaneous vascular malformations of varying types, though in our experience the dermal lesion is usually more diffuse and pinker than that seen in Klippel-Trenaunay syndrome (Fig. 14–25 and 14–26).

Almost all patients with Parkes Weber syndrome present in childhood, and it is usually possible to judge before the age of 10 which patients will have a bad prognosis. Robertson identified a positive bradycardiac reaction in childhood (Nicoladoni-Branham sign) as indicating a bad prognosis. Of six of his patients with that sign, three came to amputation and three had signs of cardiac enlargement when reviewed. This has also been our experience. Patients with clinically obvious arteriovenous malformations (the large, hot leg) in infancy are also more likely to develop clinically important leg disparity in limb length, and about 15% of cases will require operations for epiphyseal arrest. Other complications encountered are ulceration and severe lymphedema. We have seen one patient with associated chylous reflux into the limb and a spinal vascular malformation, a combination of all these complications in the one patient leading to amputation in childhood. Direct surgical attack on the arteriovenous fistulae is usually not possible,

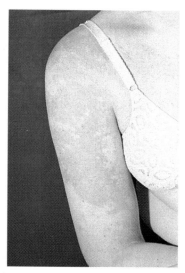

Figure 14–25. A pink capillary cutaneous malformation associated with multiple arteriovenous fistulae of the arm.

as they are diffuse and permeate the whole limb.

COMBINED VENOUS-LYMPHATIC MALFORMATIONS

It has already been noted that in many cases of Klippel-Trenaunay syndrome and Parkes Weber syndrome there are concomitant anomalies of the lymphatic system. There is, in addition, another small group of patients in whom multiple circumscribed venous, capillary, and lymphatic malformations are the dominant feature. Malan describes these merely as "complex mixed forms" or "hemolymphangiomas" (Malan and Puglionisi, 1964), and Schobinger's classification concurs (Schobinger, 1977). Such patients have multiple cutaneous and deeply placed lesions of varying types, some capillary, some nodular and venous, some vesicular and predominantly lymphatic. There may be associated proportionate or disproportionate gigantism and abnormality of venous and lymphatic trunks. The dominant clinical problem is hemorrhage and lymphatic ooze, often with secondary infection. Even when only a limb seems to be involved, there may be gastrointestinal, urinary, and other deeply placed lesions (Figs. 14–27 to 14–29; see also Fig. 14–7B). In our experience, the management of these patients is difficult and the prognosis poor. Multiple operations may be indicated to control the bleeding and lymphatic leakage. Radiotherapy, sclerosant therapy, or cryotherapy are unhelpful.

MAFFUCCI'S SYNDROME

Maffucci's syndrome is the coexistence of a vascular malformation and dyschondroplasia (Ollier's disease). The first case was described by Maffucci in 1881 (Maffucci, 1881) (Fig. 14–30). He described a woman, presenting at the age of 40, who from the age of 3 had had enlarging, scattered cartilaginous tumors, particularly of the upper limbs and predominantly involving the hands. These were associated with blue vascular lesions, many containing phleboliths. One of the lesions on the left scapula appeared to have undergone sarcomatous change. The left arm and the tumor were amputated, but the patient died of pyemia. Maffucci delineated all the features of the syndrome, including the risks of sarcomatous degeneration, and the eponym is rightly his, though the name of Kast who, with von Recklinghausen, described a case in 1889 is sometimes added (Kast and von Recklinghausen, 1889). Streudel illustrated a case in 1892 (Streudel, 1892)

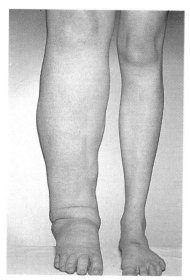

Figure 14–26. A young woman with Parkes Weber syndrome of the right leg. Arteriovenous fistulae could be demonstrated only in this extremity, whereas the capillary malformation involved the whole of the right side of the body.

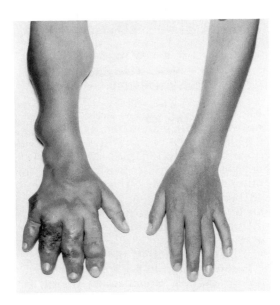

Figure 14—27. Multiple nodular venous-lymphatic malformations of the right arm.

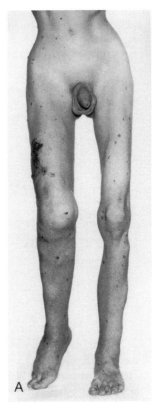

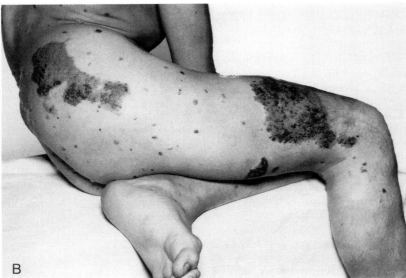

Figure 14—28. *A* and *B,* Extensive combined (capillary, arteriovenous, venous, and lymphatic) malformation of the leg. This patient suffered in addition from joint contractures, hematuria, and rectal bleeding. Control of lymphatic leakage and bleeding presented major clinical problems. The child died at the age of 13.

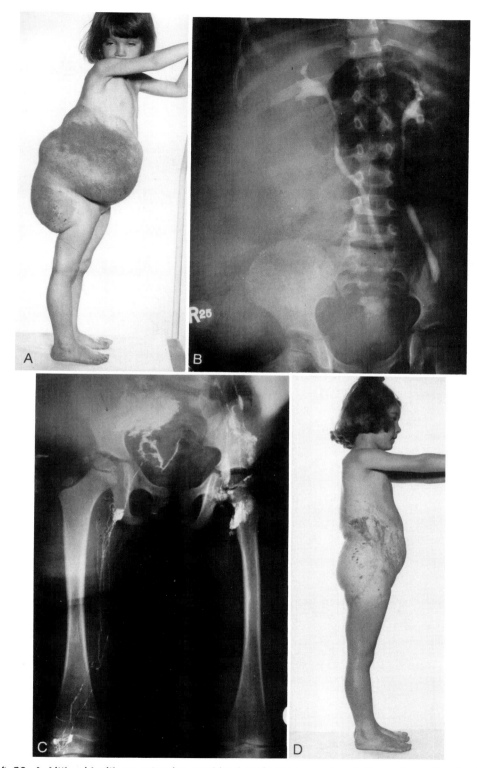

Figure 14–29. *A,* Little girl with an extensive combined capillary-venous-lymphatic malformation involving the whole loin (Kippel-Trenaunay syndrome). *B,* Intravenous urography shows the deep extension of the lesion with displacement of the ureter. *C,* The lymphangiogram shows communication with the pelvic lymphatic system and cysts. *D,* Following multiple excisions, a good cosmetic and functional result was achieved.

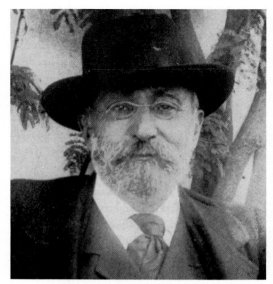

Figure 14–30. Angelo Maffucci (1847–1903). Photograph taken while he was director of the Instituto di Anatomica Patologica at Pisa. (Reproduced from Costa, 1965, by permission of Tipografia Il Sedicesimo, Florence.)

and also noted the phleboliths (Fig. 14–31). The 18 cases described up to 1942 were very carefully reviewed by Carlton and colleagues, who proposed Maffucci's name for the syndrome (Carlton et al., 1942). Carlton's description of such a patient cannot be bettered (Fig. 14–32):

In a typical case, the child, generally male, is apparently normal at birth. During the years before puberty, any time from the first to the 12th year, a hard nodule 1–2 cm. in diameter appears, most commonly on a finger or toe. This is soon followed by others, involving the extremities and limbs. The distribution may be unilateral or extremely asymmetrical. Dilated veins and soft bluish tumours occur in the affected limbs and elsewhere. Fractures of one or more bones may follow a trivial injury and union is slow and unsatisfactory. It may be noticed that development is uneven on the two sides. One or more of the long bones have short shafts, irregularly expanded ends and cartilaginous tumours, especially near the epiphyseal line. One whole side of the child may remain dwarfed and deformed. The curved uneven bones bring about secondary deformities, such as genu valgum, pes planus etc. Though the condition is very asymmetrical, careful examination generally reveals that it is rarely absolutely unilateral. Throughout the period of development the deformities increase. In severe cases the hands and feet become almost unrecognizable and are transformed into huge masses of tumour growth, in which only the protrusion of a nail reveals the

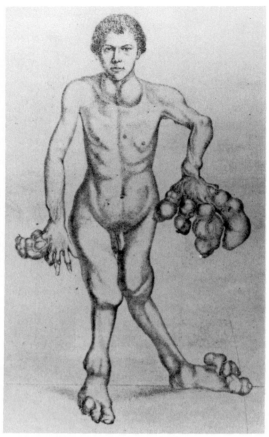

Figure 14–31. The first illustrated case of Maffucci's syndrome from Streudel, 1892.

presence of a digit. The vertebrae, ribs, scapulae and pelvis may all be the site of tumours. The skull, carpus and tarsus, though not exempt, are rarely involved. In the early twenties, as growth

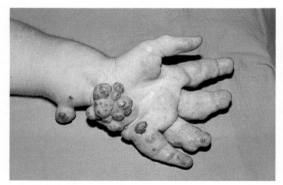

Figure 14–32. Twenty-five year old woman of short stature and the signs of Maffucci's syndrome; note protruding vascular anomalies and skeletal deformations.

draws to an end, the disease becomes stationary but injury may cause excerbation of cartilage growth at any age, or even the appearance of further nodules. Malignant changes have been observed in a certain number of cases. Affected persons are generally of low stature and poor muscular development. Intelligence is average and the internal organs appear normal. There is no pain.

Many more cases have now been described: in 1973, Lewis and Ketcham enumerated 84 further patients (Lewis and Ketcham, 1973). The types of vascular malformation encountered have also multiplied. The most common associated lesions are complex venous anomalies (Fig. 14–33). These are often large, subcutaneous, and associated with major veins. The veins themselves may be ectatic. Deep cavernous venous lesions may be present and may also appear in the gastrointestinal tract; one case was complicated by major bleeding (Sakurane et al., 1967). Rarely, there are associated lymphatic lesions (Fig. 14–34).

The syndrome has been noted in all races and equally affects women and men. No familial tendency has been discovered, and there are affected women who have borne

Table 14–3. DISTRIBUTION OF SKELETAL LESIONS IN 102 CASES OF MAFFUCCI'S SYNDROME

	Number
Hand	88
Foot	62
Tibia and fibula	60
Femur	54
Radius and ulna	42
Humerus	43
Ribs	32
Scapula	26
Pelvis	23
Vertebrae	11
Skull	8
Clavicle	4
Sternum	3

Data from Lewis, R. J., and Ketcham, A. S.: J. Bone Jt. Surg. 55A:1465, 1973; Tilsley, D. A., and Burden, P. W.: Brit. J. Derm. 105:331, 1981.

normal children. Twenty-five per cent of patients have symptoms at birth or in the first year, and 78% have had their symptoms develop before puberty. Table 14–3 shows the skeletal involvement in 100 cases described by Lewis and Ketcham (1973), with one of ours and one of Tilsley and Burden's (1981) (Fig. 14–34). Twenty per cent of pa-

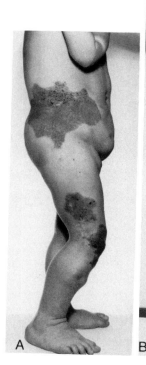
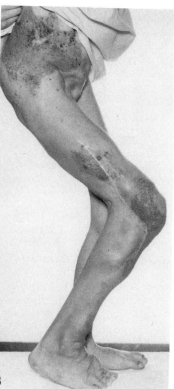

Figure 14–33. Photographs taken at the age of 2 *(A)* and 8 *(B)* to show the progressive and destructive deformity produced by a combined vascular and skeletal anomaly. This girl also had lymphedema. The vascular component of the syndrome resembles Klippel-Trenaunay syndrome and is not typical of Maffucci's syndrome.

A   B

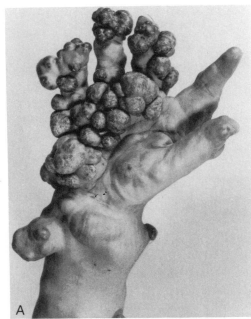

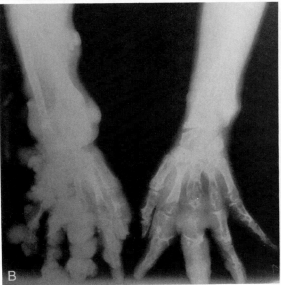

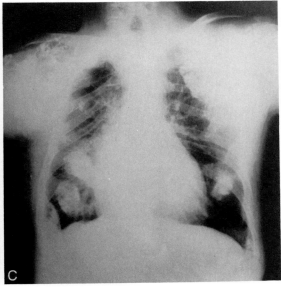

Figure 14–34. *A,* The appearance of the hand in a 24 year old male with Maffucci's syndrome. *B,* Radiograph of the hand showing extensive enchondromatosis and phleboliths in the vascular malformations. *C,* Similar changes are seen in the chest wall and shoulder girdle. (Courtesy of Dr. D. A. Tilsley; Brit. J. Derm. *105:*331, 1981.)

tients have been found to suffer malignant change, usually chondrosarcomas but also malignancy of mesodermal structures (Table 14–4). The chondrosarcomas may be multiple and can even occur in patients only mildly affected (Banna and Parwani, 1969).

Jaffe estimated the risk of neoplasia in dyschondroplasia to be 50% (Jaffe, 1958). Although this proportion does not seem to be reached in Maffucci's syndrome, Rubin suggested that chondrosarcomas grow more rapidly in Maffucci's syndrome, possibly be-

cause of the rich blood supply associated with the concurrent vascular malformations (Rubin, 1964). Other malignancies have been noted, including angiosarcoma, lymphangiosarcoma, glioma, fibroadenoma, and ovarian teratoma (Cremer, 1981; Cheng, 1981).

Lewis and Ketcham attempted to assess the degree to which patients were affected by the syndrome (Lewis and Ketcham, 1973). They found that 40% were only minimally affected, but almost all required a surgical procedure. Many patients required multiple

Table 14–4. MALIGNANCIES IN 105 CASES OF MAFFUCCI'S SYNDROME

Malignant

Chondrosarcoma	16
Hemangiosarcoma	1
Lymphangiosarcoma	1
Fibrosarcoma	1
Glioma	2
Ovarian tumor	2
Carcinoma of pancreas	1
	24

Benign

Pituitary chromophobe adenoma	1
Uterine polyp	1
Uterine fibroid	1
Adrenal cortical adenoma	2
Thecoma of ovary	1
Multiple fibromas	1
	7

From Lewis, R. J., and Ketcham, A. S.: Maffucci's syndrome. Functional and neoplastic significance. J. Bone Jt. Surg. *55A*:1465, 1973.

cosmetic, diagnostic, ablative, and reconstructive operations.

Because of the risk of malignancy, these patients require close follow-up examination; regular radiographic assessment; and biopsy of any lesions that enlarge rapidly, cause symptoms, or are suspicious on radiology. Radiotherapy is of no therapeutic value.

MULTIPLE DYSPLASIA SYNDROMES

Many combined vascular anomalies reflect extensive and disparate abnormalities of mesodermal and ectodermal development. Several constellations of soft tissue and skeletal anomalies have been identified at the extreme end of this spectrum. In 1960, Riley and Smith reported on a family who all demonstrated macrocephaly, pseudopapilledema, and multiple subcutaneous nodular vascular malformations (Riley and Smith, 1960). There was no hydrocephalus. In 1971, Bannayan described a case in which macrocephaly occurred in conjunction with multiple subcutaneous lipomas and vascular malformations together with lymphedema (Bannayan, 1971). Other similar cases were discovered by Higginbottom and Schultz (1982), who noted an increased risk for developing intracranial neoplasm, and by Stephan and coworkers, who noted an association with Klippel-Trenaunay syndrome (Stephan et al., 1975). Most of these cases

demonstrated autosomal dominant inheritance.

In 1983, Wiedemann published details of four boys with partial gigantism of the hands and/or feet, hemihypertrophy, and macrocephaly and/or other skull anomalies, together with subcutaneous nodular vascular malformations (Wiedemann et al., 1983). He proposed the term *Proteus syndrome,* after the polymorphic Greek god Proteus (Fig. 14–35).

Another closely related dysmorphic complex is the *epidermal nevus syndrome* (Solomon et al., 1968). In addition to patchy or linear epidermal defects, over two thirds of these patients have associated vascular anomalies of the skin and central nervous system and skeletal malformations, e.g., digital gigantism, craniofacial bone overgrowth, hemihypertrophy, and vertebral defects (Fig. 14–36). Epidermal nevi are also occasionally seen in lymphatic anomalies of the face; these patients also may evidence skeletal overgrowth.

Thus, there is broad overlapping of these various syndromes, none of which is particularly pure in its expression. The concomitance of vascular and musculoskeletal malformations suggests that these entities are part of a continuum with Klippel-Trenaunay and Maffucci's syndromes.

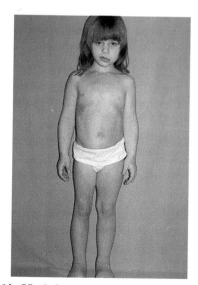

Figure 14–35. A 6 year old girl with selective asymmetrical skeletal overgrowth and diffuse vascular staining—categorized as "Proteus syndrome." There is bone and soft tissue overgrowth of her left face, hands, and feet. There is no visceromegaly by physical examination or computed tomographic study.

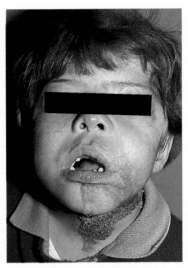

Figure 14–36. Epidermal nevus syndrome in a 5 year old boy. Note the cervicofacial verrucous nevus with capillary staining of the left face and underlying soft tissue and skeletal overgrowth. The patient had a transient ischemic attack, and angiographic study showed multiple stenoses of the intracranial vasculature with hypertrophy of collaterals ("moya-moya" changes). At age 7, he presented with a giant cell tumor of the left maxilla.

WEBER'S DIFFUSE PHLEBARTERIECTASIS

In 1869, Karl Otto Weber described a rare anomaly in which all the arteries and veins of a limb progressively dilate and lengthen. Sonntag, in 1919, furthered the concept of what was described as "genuine diffuse phlebarteriectasis" (Sonntag, 1919). However, there is considerable doubt as to whether this condition is, indeed, genuine and whether the few cases described are not merely reflecting diffuse arteriovenous connections that may be difficult to demonstrate. Malan describes two cases that could fit the declared picture of diffuse phlebarteriectasis (Malan and Puglionisi, 1964). Both were investigated by arteriography without demonstration of the usual radiographic features of arteriovenous fistulation. In one patient, venous oxygen tension measurements were claimed to exclude arteriovenous malformations, but this test may be normal in known cases of diffuse arteriovenous malformation. The case for "Weber's phlebarteriectasis" remains unsubstantiated until appropriate cases have been properly investigated with blood flow measurements, isotope shunt volume assess-

ments, and histologic examination, though there is no *a priori* reason why a primary ectatic defect of arteries and veins should not exist.

VASCULAR NEUROCUTANEOUS SYNDROMES

Vascular cutaneous birthmarks may be linked with neurological disease in two quite separate ways: *Firstly,* the cutaneous malformation may be merely the marker of other vascular malformations in or adjacent to the central nervous system that, by pressure of bulk or by "steal" of blood or by venous hypertension or thrombosis, may generate secondary neurological symptoms. Sturge-Weber syndrome, the association of a dense capillary malformation on the face and intracranial vascular malformation causing seizures, is the most common example of this. In Cobb syndrome, the vascular malformation is in the lumbar skin or vertebrae and underlying spinal meninges—neurological damage being produced by the bulk of the malformation. *Secondly,* the cutaneous mark may simply coexist with a primary neurological lesion, there being no demonstrable causal connection between the vascular and the neurological defects. An example is "ataxia-telangiectasia" (Louis-Bar syndrome), in which cutaneous telangiectasiae are associated with progressive cerebellar ataxia.

In van Bogaert–Divry syndrome, cutis marmorata is associated with non-calcified cerebral vascular malformations, mental retardation, and spasticity. Several other neurological syndromes that have associated vascular malformations are identified in the glossary. For further information on these anomalies, the reader is referred to specialist neurological texts.

References

Ackroyd, J. C., Baskerville, P. A., Young, A. E., and Browse, N. L.: The Pathophysiology of the Klippel-Trenaunay Syndrome. 5th International Workshop for Vascular Anomalies, Milan, 1984.

Adams, J.: Singular case of hypertrophy of the right lower extremity with superficial cutaneous naevus of the same side. Lancet 2:140, 1858.

Alberti, E.: Ischaemic infarct of the brain stem combined with bisymptomatic Klippel-Trenaunay-Weber syndrome and cutis laxa. J. Neurol. Neurosurg. Psychiat. *39*:581, 1976.

Banna, M., and Parwani, G. S.: Multiple sarcomas in Maffucci's syndrome. Brit. J. Radiol. 42:304, 1969.

Bannayan, G. A.: Lipomatosis, angiomatosis, and macrencephalia. A previously undescribed congenital syndrome. Arch. Pathol. 92:1, 1971.

Baskerville, P. A., Ackroyd, J. S., and Browse, N. L.: The etiology of the Klippel-Trenaunay syndrome. Ann Surg. 202:624, 1985.

Baskerville, P. A., Ackroyd, J. S., Lea Thomas, M., and Browse, N. L.: The Klippel-Trenaunay syndrome. Brit. J. Surg. 72:232, 1985.

Beck, G.: Hypertrophie congéniale d'un membre. Archiv. Gén. Med. Tome I:99, 1837.

Belovic, B., Nethercott, J., and Donsky, H. J.: An unusual variant of Klippel-Trenaunay-Weber syndrome. Canad. Med. Assoc. J. 111:439, 1974.

Bereston, E. S., and Roberts, D: Congenital hypertrophy of the extremities. Southern Med. J. 58:302, 1965.

Biasi, G., Sala, A., and Biglioli, R.: La linfografia nelle angiodisplasie degli arti. Angiologia: Minerva Chir. 28:918, 1973.

Bourde, C.: Classification des syndromes de Klippel-Trenaunay et de Parkes Weber d'après données angiographiques. Ann. Radiol. (Paris) 17:153, 1974.

Brooksaler, F.: The angioosteohypertrophy syndrome. Klippel-Trenaunay-Weber syndrome. Am. J. Dis. Child 112:161, 1966.

Bryk, A.: Ulceröses Lymphangiom der Füsse. Arch. Klin. Chir. 24:273, 1879.

Carlton, A., Elkington, J. StC., Greenfield, J. G., and Robb-Smith, A. H. T.: Maffucci's syndrome. Quart. J. Med. 11:203, 1942.

Chaissaignac, M.: Hypertrophie congéniale des deux membres droits. Taches sanguines multiples, varices, etc. Gaz. Des. Hôp. 8 May 1858, p. 215.

Cheng, F. C.: Maffucci's syndrome with fibroadenomas of the breasts. J. Roy. Coll. Surg. Edinburgh 26:181, 1981.

Coget, J. M., and Merlen, J. J.: Klippel-Trenaunay, syndrome ou maladie? Phlébologie 33:37, 1980.

Costa, A: Ricordo di Angelo Maffucci (1847–1903). Archivio "De Vecchi" 45:1, 1965.

Cremer, H., Gullotta, F., and Wolf, L.: Maffucci-Kast syndrome. J. Cancer Res. Clin. Oncol. 101:231, 1981.

Djindjian, M., Djindjian, R., Hurth, M., et al.: Spinal cord arteriovenous malformations and the Klippel-Trenaunay-Weber syndrome. Surg. Neurol. 8:229, 1977.

Ehrich, J. H. H., Ostertag, H., Flatz, S., and Kamran, D.: Bilateral Wilms tumour in Klippel-Trenaunay syndrome. Arch. Dis. Child 54:405, 1979.

Feldmuller, V. M., and Becker, B.: Angiographische Befunde einer mit choanalatresie Kombinierten Gemischten Angiodysplasie (Klippel-Trenaunay-Weber syndrome). Fortschr. Rontgenstr. 124:76, 1976.

Friedberg, H.: Riesenwuchs des rechten Beines. Virchow's Archiv f. Path. Anat. 40:353, 1867.

Ghahremani, G. G., Kangarloo, H., Volberg, F., and Meyers, M. A.: Diffuse cavernous hemangioma of the colon in the Klippel-Trenaunay syndrome. Radiology 118:673, 1976.

Gloviczki, P., Hollier, L. H., Telander, R. L., et al.: Surgical implications of Klippel-Trenaunay syndrome. Ann. Surg. 197:353, 1983.

Hamatake, Y.: Clinical studies of congenital angiodysplasias in limbs. Fukuoka Acta Med. 65:833, 1974.

Harper, P. S.: Sturge Weber syndrome with Klippel-Trenaunay-Weber syndrome. Birth Defects 7:314, 1971.

den Hartog Jager, W. A.: About two new forms in the group of phacomatoses. Folia. Psychiat. 52:356, 1949.

Hawthorne, C. O.: Rep. Soc. Stud. Dis. Child ii:114, 1902.

Higginbottom, M. C., and Schultz, P.: The Bannayan syndrome: An autosomal dominant disorder consisting of macrocephaly, lipomas, hemangiomas, and risk for intracranial tumors. Pediatrics 69:632, 1982.

Howitz, P., Howitz, J., and Gjerris, F.: A variant of Klippel-Trenaunay-Weber syndrome with temporal lobe astrocytoma. Acta Paediatr. Scand. 68:119, 1979.

Jaffe, H. L.: *Tumors and Tumorous Conditions of the Bones and Joints.* Philadelphia: Lea and Febiger, 1958.

Kast, A., and von Recklinghausen, F. D.: Ein Fall von Echondrom mit ungewöhnlicher Multiplication. Archiv Pathol. Anat. 118:1, 1889.

Kessler, H. B., Recht, M. P., and Dalinka, M. K.: Vascular anomalies in association with osteodystrophies— a spectrum. Skeletal Radiol. 10:95, 1983.

Kinmonth, J. B.: *The Lymphatics,* 2nd ed. London: Edward Arnold, 1982.

Kinmonth, J. B., Young, A. E., Edwards, J. M., et al.: Mixed vascular deformities of the lower limbs with particular reference to lymphography and surgical treatment. Brit. J. Surg. 63:899, 1976.

Klippel, M., and Trenaunay, P.: Noevus variqueux ostéohypertrophique. J. des Praticiens February 3, 1900a.

Klippel, M., and Trenaunay, P.: Du noevus variqueux ostéohypertrophique. Arch. Gén. Méd. Tome III:641, 1900b.

Kontras, S. B.: The Klippel-Trenaunay-Weber syndrome. Birth Defects 10:177, 1974.

Korting, G. W., and Dolcher, G.: Unusual Klippel Trenaunay and Parkes Weber syndrome with homolateral muscle atrophy. Med. Welt. 46:2543, 1969.

Kuffer, F. R., Starzynski, T. E., Girolam, A., et al.: Klippel-Trenaunay syndrome, visceral angiomatosis and thrombocytopenia. J. Ped. Surg. 3:65, 1968.

Lewis, R. J., and Ketcham, A. S.: Maffucci's syndrome: Functional and neoplastic significance. J. Bone Jt. Surg. 55A:1465, 1973.

Lian, C., and Alhomme, P.: Les varices congénitales par dysembryoplasie (syndrome de Klippel-Trenaunay). Arch. Mal. Coeur 38:176, 1945.

Lindenauer, S. M.: Klippel-Trenaunay syndrome. Ann. Surg. 162:303, 1965.

Lindenauer, S. M.: Congenital arteriovenous fistula and the Klippel-Trenaunay syndrome. Ann Surg. 174:248, 1971.

Maffucci, A.: Di un caso di encondroma ed angioma multiplo contribuzione al a genesi embrionale dei tumor. Movimento Med. Chir. 3:399, 1881.

Malan, E., and Puglionisi, A.: Congenital angiodysplasias of the extremities (Note I: venous dysplasias). J. Cardiovasc. Surg. 5:87, 1964.

Mankad, V. N., Gray, G. F., Jr., and Miller, D. R.: Bilateral nephroblastomatosis and Klippel-Trenaunay syndrome. Cancer 33:1462, 1974.

Müller, J. H. A., and Schmidt, K. H.: Angiographische befunde beim Klippel-Trenaunay-Weber syndrome. Fortschr. Roentgenstr. 110:540, 1969.

Myers, T. T., and Janes, J. M.: Comprehensive surgical management of cavernous hemangioma of the lower extremity with special reference to stripping. Surgery 37:184, 1955.

Owens, D. W., Garcia, E., Pierce, R. R., and Castrow, F. F.: Klippel-Trenaunay syndrome with pulmonary vein varicosity. Arch. Dermatol. 108:111, 1973.

Parkes Weber, F.: Angioma formation in connection with hypertrophy of limbs and hemi-hypertrophy. Brit. J. Derm. *19*:231, 1907.

Parkes Weber, F.: Haemangiectatic hypertrophies of the foot and lower extremity. Med. Press (London) *136*:261, 1908.

Parkes Weber, F.: Haemangiectatic hypertrophy of the limbs—congenital phlebarteriectasis and so-called congenital varicose veins. Brit. J. Child Dis. *15*:13, 1918.

Parkes Weber, F.: *Further Rare Diseases and Debatable Subjects.* London: Staples Press, 1946, p. 55.

Pokrovosky, A. V., Moskalenko, J. D., and Tkhor, S. N.: The state of the lymph system in congenital arterial and venous diseases of the lower extremities. Vestn. Khir. *107(9)*:74, 1971.

Poulet, J., and Ruff, F.: Les dysplasies veineuses congénitales des membres. Presse Med. 77:163, 1969.

Riley, H. D., and Smith, W. R.: Macrocephaly, pseudopapilledema and multiple hemangiomata. Pediatrics 26:293, 1960.

Robertson, D. J.: Congenital arteriovenous fistulae of the extremities. Ann. Roy. Coll. Surg. Engl. *18*:73, 1956.

Rubin, P.: *Dynamic Classification of Bone Dysplasias.* Chicago: Year Book Medical Publishers, 1964, p. 218.

Sakurane, H. F., Sugai, T., and Saito, T.: The association of blue rubber bleb nevus and Maffucci syndrome. Arch. Derm. 95:28, 1967.

Schobinger, R. C.: *Periphere Angiodysplasien.* Bern: Hans Huber, 1977.

Sciubba, J. J., and Brown, A. M.: Oral-facial manifestations of Klippel-Trenaunay-Weber syndrome: Report of two cases. Oral Surg. 43:227, 1977.

Servelle, M.: Agénésie d'une des veines principales du membre inférieur. Coeur et Med. Int. 4:53, 1965.

Servelle, M.: Klippel and Trenaunay's syndrome. Ann. Surg. 201:365, 1985.

Servelle, M. and Babilliot, J.: Les malformations des veines profondes dans le syndrome de Klippel et Trenaunay. Phlébologie *33*:31, 1980.

Servelle, M., Albeaux-Fernet, M., Laborde, S., Chabot, J., and Rougeulle, J.: Lésions des vaisseaux lymphatiques dans les malformations congénitales des veines profondes. Presse Méd. 65:531, 1957.

Servelle, M., Bastin, R., Loygue, J., et al.: Hematuria and rectal bleeding in the child with Klippel and Trenaunay syndrome. Ann. Surg. 183:418, 1976.

Servelle, M., Zolotas, E., Soulié, J. et al.: Syndrome de Klippel et Trenaunay: Malformations des veines il-

iaques, fémorale et poplitée. Arch. Mal. Coeur 58:1187, 1965.

Simpson, B.: Monthly J. Med. (Edinburgh) *20*:173, 1855.

Smith, D. W.: *Recognizable Patterns of Human Malformation*, 3rd ed. Philadelphia: W. B. Saunders Co., 1982.

Solomon, L. M., Fretzin, O. F., and Dewald, R. L.: The epidermal nevus syndrome. Arch. Derm. 97:273, 1968.

Sonntag, E.: Ueber genuine Diffuse Phlebektasie am Bein. München. Med. Wochschr. 66:155, 1919.

Stephan, M. J., Hall, B. D., Smith, D. W., and Cohen, M. M.: Macrocephaly in association with unusual cutaneous angiomatosis. J. Pediatr. 87:353, 1975.

Steudel: Multiple Enchondrome der Knochen in Verbindung mit Venosen Angiomem der Weichteile. Beitr. Z. Klin. Chir. 8:503, 1892.

Thulesius, O., Norgren, L., and Gjöres, J. E.: Footvolumetry, a new method for objective assessment of edema and venous function. VASA 2:325, 1973.

Tilsley, D. A., and Burden, P. W.: A case of Maffucci's syndrome. Brit. J. Derm. *105*:331, 1981.

Trélat, U., and Monod, A.: De l'hypertrophie unilatérale partielle ou totale du corps. Arch. Gén. de Méd. *13*:536, 1869.

Troost, B. T., Savino, P. J., and Lozito, J. C.: Tuberous sclerosis and Klippel-Trenaunay-Weber syndrome. J. Neurol. Neurosurg. Psychiat. 38:500, 1975.

Vermeulen, F. E. E., and Wiffels, C. C. S. M.: In Van Der Molen, H. R. (ed.): *Progres Cliniques et Therapeutiques dan la Domaine de la Phlebologie.* Apeldorn: Stenvert and Zoon, 1970, p. 317.

Vollmar, J.: Zur Geschichte und Terminologie der Syndrome nach F. P. Weber und Klippel-Trenaunay. VASA *3*:231, 1974.

Weber, K. O., Quoted by Sonntag, E.: München. Med. Wochschr. 66:155, 1919.

Wiedemann, H. R., Burgio, G. R., Aldenhoff, P., Kunze, J., Kaufmann, H. J., and Schirg, E.: The proteus syndrome: Partial gigantism of the hand and/or feet, nevi, hemihypertrophy, subcutaneous tumors, macrocephaly, or other skull anomalies and possible accelerated growth and visceral affections. Eur. J. Pediatr. *140*:5, 1983.

Young, A. E.: Congenital mixed vascular deformities of the limbs and their associated defects. Birth Defects; Original Article Series *14*:289, 1978a.

Young, A. E.: Mixed vascular deformities. M. Chir. Thesis, Univ. Cambridge, 1978b.

PART FOUR

Problems and Solutions

CHAPTER FIFTEEN

Vascular Malformations of the Central Nervous System

Michael J. Aminoff

Several different types of congenital vascular malformations occur in the central nervous system. Saccular aneurysms probably relate to congenital maldevelopment of the wall of a cerebral artery, but these are beyond the scope of this chapter. *Capillary telangiectasias* are usually found within the substance of the brain, especially the pons or basal ganglia, and consist of an unencapsulated mass of pathologically enlarged capillaries. They are generally an incidental finding at postmortem examination, but occasionally bleed in life. *Complex ("cavernous") malformations* consist of a compact, tangled web of sponge-like vascular spaces without intervening neural parenchyma. *Simple venous malformations* sometimes look like a collection of engorged veins, but many of these lesions probably represent arteriovenous malformations with an inconspicuous arterial component because only rarely can they be distinguished from the latter either angiographically or pathologically. Other true venous malformations consist of a collection of small veins converging on to a dilated venous trunk. *Arteriovenous malformations (AVMs)* are the most important anomalies occurring in the nervous system, and attention here will be directed primarily at them. They consist of an abnormal arteriovenous communication without intervening capillaries.

Intracranial Vascular Malformations

Vascular malformations may occur in relation to either the brain or the dura, and they are best considered with this in mind. Malformations located primarily in the scalp, orbit, or calvaria are addressed in Chapter Sixteen. In this review of the intracerebral malformations, discussion will be directed primarily to those of major clinical relevance, that is, to arteriovenous malformations in particular.

CEREBRAL ARTERIOVENOUS MALFORMATIONS

Regional maldevelopment of the brain may be associated with the AVM and underlie any clinical disturbance, but neurological symptoms and signs commonly relate to intracranial or subarachnoid hemorrhage from one of the vessels involved in the malformation, or from a coexisting arterial aneurysm. They may also relate to cerebral ischemia that is due to diversion of blood to the AVM from the normal cerebral circulation ("steal"), or to venous stagnation because the cerebral venous pressure has been increased by the AVM. Enlarged anomalous vessels may compress or distort adjacent cerebral tissue or cause obstructive hydrocephalus by interfering with the normal circulation of cerebrospinal fluid, whereas a communicating hydrocephalus may relate to previous hemorrhage.

Progressive gliosis of surrounding brain tissue as a result of mechanical and ischemic factors may also play a role in symptom production.

In approximately 10% of cases of cerebral AVM there is an associated arterial aneurysm (Stein, 1979), whereas 1.4% of patients with intracranial aneurysms have coexistent AVMs (Perret and Nishioka, 1966). The association may relate to multiple disorders of vascular development or may be purely coincidental. Alternatively, the aneurysms may arise from hemodynamic stresses resulting, in turn, from the presence of the AVMs. Thus, there is often a close relationship between the site of the aneurysm and the source of blood to the AVM. Hayashi and colleagues (1981) reported a case in which three aneurysms were found arising from an enlarged anterior cerebral artery feeding an AVM, and although two of the aneurysms were not treated surgically, they disappeared almost completely following excision of the AVM.

Clinical Features of Supratentorial AVMs

Symptoms

Most cerebral AVMs are supratentorial and usually lie in the rolandic area, where they are supplied by the middle cerebral artery. Patients may present at any age with intracranial hemorrhage, seizures, headache, or a focal neurological deficit, but a higher incidence of hemorrhage is likely among referrals to a neurosurgical unit. A male preponderance of cases is found in some series.

Between 50 and 70% of AVMs bleed at some point in their natural history, and small AVMs seem more likely to bleed than large ones (Henderson and Gomez, 1967; Waltimo, 1973; Luessenhop, 1976). There is no obvious correlation between liability to bleed and site of the AVM, or the age and sex of the patient. The peak age for hemorrhage is between 15 and 20 years, and about three quarters of all cerebral AVMs (supratentorial and infratentorial) that will bleed have done so by the age of 40 (Perret and Nishioka, 1966). The hemorrhage is usually subarachnoid, but it may be partly or wholly intracerebral. Therefore, the typical clinical presentation is with severe headache, neck stiffness, photophobia, and a depressed level of consciousness, accompanied—in about 50% of

cases—by a focal neurological deficit. About 10% of patients die from the initial hemorrhage, and among the survivors the rebleeding rate from supratentorial lesions is between 20 and 25% (Perret and Nishioka, 1966). The second hemorrhage has a mortality rate of between 10 and 15%. There is general agreement that the risks of hemorrhage are greater in patients with an AVM that has already bled than in other patients (Perret and Nishioka, 1966; Drake, 1979; Graf et al., 1983).

Seizures may accompany or follow an intracranial hemorrhage, but in between 20 and 40% of patients they are the initial symptom of the AVM. The prevalence of seizures ranges between 28% (Perret and Nishioka, 1966) and 50% (Houdart and Le Besnerais, 1963) in different series of patients with supratentorial AVMs. Seizures are especially likely with frontal or parietal AVMs, may be either focal or generalized, and are usually controlled pharmacologically without difficulty. In patients with seizures as the sole presenting feature of an AVM, Forster and colleagues (1972) reported a 25% chance of a hemorrhage occurring in the next 15 years, giving a bleeding rate of approximately 1.6% per year. Similarly, based on the data of the cooperative study, Drake (1979) calculated that the incidence of hemorrhage was approximately 1% per year in patients presenting with unruptured AVMs. More recently, Graf and colleagues (1983) calculated an average yearly risk for first hemorrhage of between 2% and 3%, and the cumulative risk of a first hemorrhage among 66 patients with an unruptured AVM when first seen was 2% at the end of the first year, and 39% over 20 years.

Headache unrelated to hemorrhage is sometimes particularly troublesome, especially when the external carotid arteries are involved in the AVM. It may simulate classical migraine, but visual or other prodromata then show a consistent lateralization to one side, and "auras" accompany or follow the headache rather than preceding it. The headache itself may also be lateralized, generally to the side of the underlying lesion. More commonly, the headaches are non-specific, with nothing about them to suggest an underlying structural lesion.

Other neurological symptoms or focal neurological deficits may also lead to medical consultation. Bruit or pulsatile tinnitus is rarely a presenting symptom except of lesions that are dural, at least in part. Although intellectual deterioration has been described (Olivecrona and Riives, 1948; Mackenzie, 1953; Paterson and McKissock, 1956), and dementia may certainly result from the communicating hydrocephalus that sometimes follows a bleed, Waltimo and Putkonen (1974) found no psychometric evidence that AVMs had any general influence on intellectual function.

In patients presenting during infancy, symptoms generally relate to congestive cardiac failure as a result of the abnormal arteriovenous shunt or to obstructive hydrocephalus, whereas in older children the presenting symptoms are similar to those in adults, with hemorrhage and seizures being the most typical (Kelly et al., 1978).

Physical Signs

The presence of a systolic bruit over the eye or head may suggest the presence of an AVM, and any focal neurological signs will help to localize it. Although a bruit may also be found with other vascular anomalies or with meningiomas, it is a very useful sign. It is found in between 15 and 40% of patients with AVMs, and is especially common if branches of the external carotid arteries are involved in the malformation. It is best heard over the ipsilateral eye or mastoid region. Large, pulsatile vessels may be present over the scalp and neck, and other vascular anomalies may be found in the skin and retina. Arteriovenous shunts of large volume may also be associated with tachycardia, cardiomegaly, and even cardiac failure, especially in infants and children, and particularly when the vein of Galen is involved.

Clinical Features of Infratentorial AVMs

Between 5 and 30% of intracranial AVMs are situated in the posterior fossa in different series. Hemorrhage from a cerebellar AVM may cause meningeal irritation and an acute cerebellar syndrome, sometimes associated with a sixth cranial nerve palsy and minor pyramidal signs (Logue and Monckton, 1954). In other instances, such AVMs may lead to an obstructive hydrocephalus or to a brainstem syndrome.

Subarachnoid or intracranial hemorrhage or an acute obstructive hydrocephalus (Logue and Monckton, 1954) may be a clinical manifestation of brainstem AVMs, but focal neurological deficits may also develop and follow a progressive or relapsing course. There may be a combination of cranial nerve (often oculomotor), pyramidal, and cerebellar signs, sometimes accompanied by sensory disturbances. A steadily progressive neurological deficit may be attributed to a neoplasm, and a stepwise progression may lead to an erroneous diagnosis of multiple sclerosis despite the clinical evidence of a lesion at only a single site in the nervous system.

Investigations

An electroencephalogram is often performed in patients presenting with seizures or non-specific neurological symptoms, and it may show consistently focal or lateralized abnormalities that suggest the presence of an underlying structural lesion without indicating its nature. Plain radiographs of the skull are usually normal. Abnormal intracranial calcification is sometimes seen, but this also occurs with tumors or aneurysms (Rumbaugh and Potts, 1966). There may be displacement of a calcified pineal or choroid plexus, especially if an intracerebral hematoma is present, but similar findings are encountered with any space-occupying lesion. It is sometimes possible to recognize enlarged vessels feeding or draining an AVM, particularly if meningeal vessels are involved.

The computed tomography (CT) scan (Figs. 15–1 to 15–3) is usually the first diagnostic study now performed in patients presenting with hemorrhage. It is a reliable indicator of recent intracranial hemorrhage, may permit the source of bleeding to be localized, and facilitates the early diagnosis of AVMs. These typically appear as nonhomogeneous areas of mixed density with irregular—often tubular—calcifications, with serpiginous areas of enhancement after infusion of contrast material. Cerebral atrophy may be evident on the affected side, and large malformations or an intracerebral hematoma may also distort the normal intracranial anatomy. Diagnostic changes and/or focal abnormalities are present in the CT scans of most patients with intracranial AVMs (Kendall and Claveria, 1976). Hematomas from AVMs are often situated in the cortex or adjacent white matter and thus can usually be distinguished from hypertensive hematomas, which are usually deeply placed.

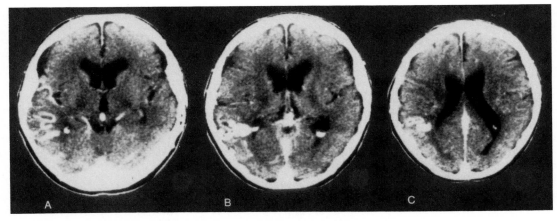

Figure 15–1. *A, B,* and *C,* Post-contrast CT scans at different levels, showing a right temporoparietal arteriovenous malformation in a 44 year old woman presenting with seizures. Serpiginous contrast enhancing shadows are present in the right temporoparietal region. The vein of Galen is prominent, probably representing the site of drainage. The ventricles are mildly enlarged, but not displaced.

Magnetic resonance imaging (MRI) may also reveal the presence of cerebral AVMs (Kucharczyk et al., 1985; Lee et al., 1985). The typical appearance is of a latticework of signal-void spaces highly contrasted against surrounding cerebral tissue on both T1- and T2-weighted sequences, intermixed with which are regions of various signal intensities corresponding to hematomas in different stages of evolution and to regions containing calcium as well as hemosiderin. The serpiginous shape of vessels may be distinctive.

Angiography (Figs. 15–2 and 15–4) is the definitive investigation, because it permits the nature and extent of the lesion to be established and its blood supply and venous drain-

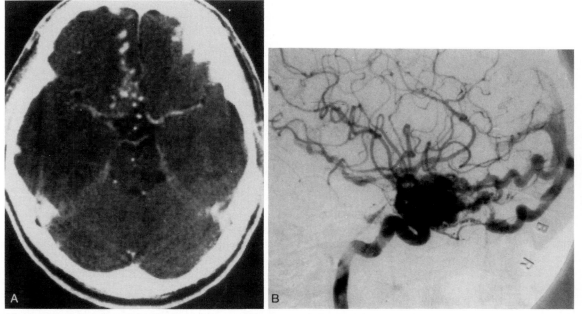

Figure 15–2. Inferior right frontal lobe arteriovenous malformation in a 35 year old man presenting with generalized seizures. *A,* Post-contrast CT scan through the circle of Willis. Multiple rounded and serpiginous contrast-enhanced structures are noted in the inferior right frontal lobe, and have the appearance of vascular channels. *B,* Right internal carotid arteriogram, showing an arteriovenous malformation in the posterior inferior aspect of the right frontal lobe. Prominent draining veins (well shown on the CT scan) extend anteriorly.

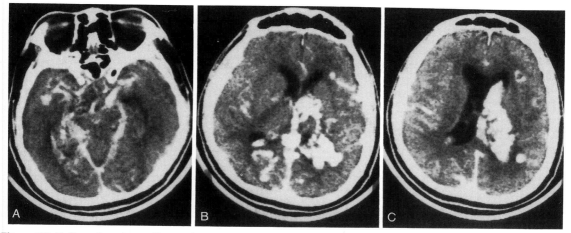

Figure 15–3. Deep basal ganglia arteriovenous malformation in a 53 year old man presenting with sudden onset of occipital headache and loss of consciousness. *A, B,* and *C,* Post-contrast CT scans. Multiple enlarged serpiginous contrast-enhanced vessels are seen in the most inferior cut *(A).* More superior sections show bilateral rounded enhancing lesions projecting into the left lateral ventricle. The ventricular system is moderately enlarged.

age to be determined. It generally includes bilateral opacification of both the internal and external carotid arteries and the vertebral arteries in order to ensure that all vessels supplying the AVM are visualized. It is often

not appreciated that 15% of cerebral AVMs receive some of their blood supply from ipsilateral or contralateral meningeal arteries (Newton and Cronqvist, 1969). The typical angiographic appearance of an AVM is of

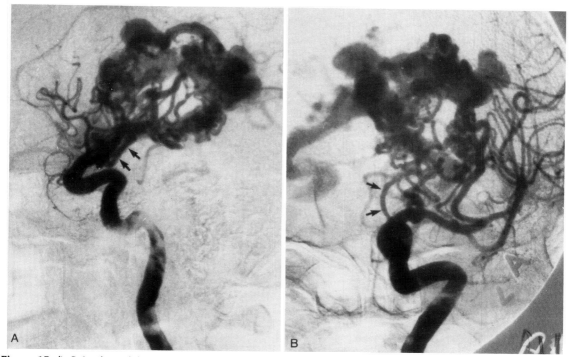

Figure 15–4. Selective left internal carotid arteriogram, lateral *(A)* and frontal *(B)* projections; same patient as in Figure 15–3. The lenticulostriate and anterior choroidal (arrows) arteries are enlarged, supplying a deep arteriovenous malformation that drains into the deep venous system bilaterally. In addition, a left vertebral angiogram (not shown) showed feeders to the malformation from posteromedial and posterolateral choroidal arteries.

distended tortuous afferent and efferent vessels connecting with a tangled vascular mass, through which the circulation time is rapid, with arteriovenous shunting. Other vessels or structures are not displaced unless an intracerebral hematoma is present, when an avascular mass is related to the malformation. Distinction of a small AVM from a highly vascularized malignant glioma may be difficult (Goree and Dukes, 1963). Angiography occasionally fails to demonstrate an AVM despite suggestive CT findings, usually because of partial or complete thrombotic occlusion of feeding vessels, and it may then be hard to distinguish the lesion from a partially calcified, avascular low-grade glioma (Kramer and Wing, 1977; Wharen et al., 1982). Other suggested causes of an angiographically occult AVM include small size, compression by adjacent clot, and destruction at the time of hemorrhage. The incidence of angiographically occult AVMs was 11% in one series (Leblanc et al., 1979).

Static or dynamic scintigraphy has been used to detect AVMs, but the results depend in part on technical and anatomical factors (Landman and Ross, 1973; Waltimo et al., 1973; Gates et al., 1978; Petersen et al., 1983). Such an approach is relatively inexpensive and does not require use of iodinated contrast agents, but it fails to provide as much information as the CT scan. Regional cerebral blood flow studies show that blood flow is increased on the side of an AVM, especially when the lesion is superficial (Menon and Weir, 1979), but despite the development of a non-invasive technique the method has little diagnostic relevance.

Treatment

Surgery

Treatment is essentially operative, but the precise indications for operation are not clear, owing in part to incomplete knowledge of the natural history of untreated AVMs. Comparison of the results within and among published series is difficult because of differences in case selection, duration of follow-up, technical facilities, and operative expertise.

Once hemorrhage has occurred, surgical treatment to prevent further bleeding is clearly warranted if the AVM is surgically accessible and if the patient otherwise has a reasonable life expectancy. The mortality and rebleeding rates following an initial hemorrhage have already been indicated. Because rebleeding may not occur for some years and because there is a definite operative morbidity, Forster and colleagues (1972) have stressed that the benefits of surgical therapy only become apparent statistically after a follow-up period approaching 10 years. Surgical treatment is also necessary when there is increased intracranial pressure or cardiac decompensation, and it can sometimes prevent further progression of a focal neurological deficit.

In most instances, however, surgery is unnecessary for unruptured cerebral AVMs (Aminoff, 1987). Pharmacological maneuvers or partial obliteration of the AVM by nonoperative means will help most of the nonhemorrhagic manifestations of unruptured malformations. Nevertheless, because these measures do not influence the risk of an intracranial bleed with its associated morbidity and mortality, some surgeons advocate operation for AVMs that have not bled, especially if they are favorably situated for excision with minimal risk of producing a functional deficit (Wilson et al., 1979; Heros and Tu, 1986). However, surgery itself is not without risk, and even if the most favorable morbidity and mortality rates for surgical treatment are used, there does not appear to be any clear advantage to surgical excision over conservative management for unruptured AVMs over a 20 year period (Aminoff, 1987).

The aim of surgical treatment is total excision of the AVM if feasible. Moderate hypothermia may reduce the extent of any cerebral edema resulting from operative exposure of a deeply situated lesion. If the AVM is massive or situated in a critical or totally inaccessible region of the brain, occlusion of one or more of its feeders may help in reducing ischemia of adjacent cerebral tissue, but this is not curative.

At operation, a wedge-shaped mass of tortuous, engorged, pulsating vessels is often found on the surface of the hemisphere, with its apex directed inward. Besides any major feeders visualized at angiography, other small arterial branches may be seen supplying the abnormal mass. Venous structures may be seen pulsating and engorged with red arterial blood. In other instances, however, AVMs are so small that it is hard to identify them, especially in the presence of a related hematoma.

There are differences in operative morbidity and mortality rates in different published series, and these differences presumably relate to different criteria by which patients are selected for surgery, and to differences in preoperative clinical state, location and anatomical features of AVMs, and surgical expertise. Thus, Aminoff (1987) noted from a number of published series that the overall operative mortality rate varied between 1% and 11%, and the morbidity rate varied between 5% and 28%. There was some evidence that the operative risks were lower for AVMs that were angiographically small.

Brainstem AVMs are frequently considered to be inoperable because they lie within the substance of the brain. However, Drake (1975) was able to remove the lesion successfully in four patients with multiple bleeds from AVMs involving the brainstem and cerebellopontine angle; operation in one other patient had a fatal outcome from subsequent intraventricular bleeding. In most of these cases, the AVM lay superficially on the brainstem and could be dissected free in an extrapial plane.

Embolization

Embolization with particles via the afferent blood supply using an intravascular catheter technique is a simple, relatively safe adjunct to more definitive surgical treatment. Its main use is to reduce the size of the AVM before its surgical removal. Embolization is facilitated if the main feeders to the AVM are large compared with vessels supplying adjacent cerebral tissue. The manner in which a feeder comes off its parent artery is also important, since embolization is more difficult if this is at an acute or right angle. Moreover, emboli are more likely to stray if distal branches of a long, tortuous artery supply the AVM rather than proximal branches of a relatively straight vessel (Wolpert and Stein, 1979). Complications may result from stray emboli, but Wolpert and Stein (1979) reported permanent complications in only 1 patient among a series of 34 patients subjected to 59 embolization procedures.

AVMs that are surgically inaccessible or involve a critical area of the brain are sometimes treated solely by embolization with solid particles. Unfortunately, small feeding vessels are likely to remain patent and will then enlarge unless the fistulous portion of the malformation is removed. Partial embolic obliteration of an AVM is an unsatisfactory solution, since the incidence of hemorrhage remains high (Luessenhop and Presper, 1975). Nevertheless, progressive neurological deterioration may stabilize or reverse if the deficit is of relatively short duration and has not resulted from a hemorrhage (Luessenhop and Presper, 1975; Kusske and Kelly, 1974). Unfortunately, this has not been the experience of all investigators, and Wolpert and coworkers (1982) found, for example, that neither the incidence and progression of neurological deficits nor the frequency of seizures was affected by embolization procedures.

Serbinenko (1974) developed a technique for the temporary or permanent occlusion of major vessels using balloon catheters. Temporary occlusion of specific vessels can suggest the likely outcome of obliterating or embolizing vessels to an AVM. Such an approach may therefore be of particular importance in planning treatment of malformations located in critical areas of the brain. The procedure also permits angiographic study of any blood supply to the malformation from neighboring vessels. Permanent occlusion of the vessels feeding a malformation is finally achieved using a detachable balloon that is positioned in the desired site and then inflated with quickly solidifying contrast material. The results of this approach (Romodanov et al., 1979; Serbinenko, 1979) have been questioned on several grounds by Debrun and colleagues (1982), including the lack of subtracted films, of angiography in the capillary-venous phase, of opacification of the other cerebral vessels after vascular occlusion, and of follow-up review.

Another approach is the use of a Silastic or latex calibrated-leak balloon that is directed to one of the main feeders of the AVM so that the nidus of the malformation can be embolized with bucrylate (isobutyl-2-cyanoacrylate). This substance rapidly solidifies inside the AVM, thereby obliterating it. However, it must be delivered into the feeder at its point of entry into the AVM, with no injection of adjacent normal cortical vessels. There are a number of technical complications, including rupture of the balloon, gluing of the catheter in place, and passage of the injected material through the AVM and into its draining venous structures. Intraoperative embolization with bucrylate is an alternative procedure (Cromwell and Harris, 1980), in which a feeder is exposed and cannulated directly.

Debrun and colleagues (1982) reported their experience of embolization with bucrylate in 46 patients with cerebral AVMs. Among 22 patients with non-resectable AVMs selected for treatment with the Silastic calibrated-leak balloon, embolization was successfully achieved in 16, but complete obliteration of the AVM occurred in only 2. Complications included subarachnoid hemorrhage in 5 patients (with 1 death), owing to bursting of the balloon with dissection of the feeding vessel, and a transient or permanent mild neurological deficit in 7. Among 13 patients treated by intraoperative embolization, the AVM was completely obliterated in 4. The other 9 patients had only partial obliteration, but 5 patients then underwent total resection. Three of the 13 patients were left with a mild neurological deficit, and 2 had transient deficits. Finally, of 11 patients treated using a new latex calibrated-leak balloon, the AVMs were completely obliterated in 2 and were only partially obliterated in the others. There were no mortalities, but the catheter was glued in place in 2 instances, and hemianopia occurred in another.

Other studies using a similar technique have been published, for example, that of Bank and coworkers (1981). The long term result in patients whose AVM was completely obliterated by these procedures is unknown, but an optimistic outlook seems reasonable. Moreover, with increasing experience and technical refinements, the number of patients successfully treated by such approaches will almost certainly increase.

Irradiation

One study suggests that Bragg-peak proton beam therapy is useful for treating intracranial AVMs that, because of location, size, or operative risk, are not suited to other forms of treatment (Kjellberg et al., 1983). The aim was to induce subendothelial deposition of collagen and hyaline substance in order to narrow the lumens of small vessels and thicken the walls of the malformation over the following months. The procedure was performed under local anesthesia in a single session lasting for up to 2 hours. However, no protection from hemorrhage was conferred during the first year, and over that time there were two deaths among 75 consecutive patients from bleeding. Fatal or disabling hemorrhages did not occur subsequently, and in many instances seizures, headaches, and progressive neurological deficits were helped or arrested. Further studies to evaluate the place of this therapeutic approach therefore seem warranted.

Gamma ray and x-ray treatment of AVMs has been in use for some years. For example, Steiner is reported by Drake (1983) as having been very successful in obliterating small AVMs by using a stereotactically focused gamma unit. Thus, in a group of 67 cases, 84% of the AVMs had disappeared on follow-up angiography 2 years after treatment. With regard to conventional x-ray treatment, Johnson (1975) reported that small, deeply situated AVMs disappeared on angiograms obtained 2 or more years after treatment in all of 9 cases, in contrast to large surface AVMs, which remained apparently unaffected by the treatment in all of 11 cases.

The available evidence is incomplete, but it would seem that radiation therapy is not helpful for AVMs larger than 5 cm in diameter. Whether it has a role in the management of AVMs treated incompletely by operation or embolization is not known.

COMPLEX ("CAVERNOUS") MALFORMATIONS

Intracranial "cavernous" malformations are relatively rare and usually occur within the cerebral parenchyma. The surrounding tissues may be scarred, and they often contain calcifications. Most malformations occur singly, but occasionally two or more are located in different parts of the brain. There may be coexisting vascular anomalies elsewhere in the body, especially the skin. A familial incidence has been reported (Clark, 1970), but there is no sex predominance and presentation may be at any age (Voigt and Yasargil, 1976). "Cavernous" vascular malformations may never give rise to symptoms, being discovered incidentally at autopsy, or may be responsible for a variety of neurological complaints.

Giombini and Morello (1978) reviewed some of the literature on these lesions and reported another 14 cases. The first symptom was intracranial (subarachnoid or intracerebral) bleeding in 23% of cases, seizures in 38%, headache in 28%, and focal neurological disturbances in 12%. Since complex ("cavernous") malformations are usually located in the hemispheres, often close to the cortex, their early epileptogenic potential is easily understood. In many of the cases reviewed, there were focal neurological signs that helped to localize the lesion, accompanied in some patients by papilledema. However, such clinical features do not permit the distinction of these complex vascular malformations from other mass lesions.

Voigt and Yasargil (1976) reported 1 new case and reviewed 163 previously published ones. In 126 cases (76.8%) the malformations were supratentorial, in 34 (20.7%) they were infratentorial, in 4 (2.5%) they were multiple and in various locations, and in 4 (2.5%) they were intraventricular. Macroscopic calcifications were observed in 18 cases (11.0%). Among 31 cases in which cerebral angiography was undertaken, normal findings or an avascular mass was encountered in 20. In the remainder, the angiographic findings were mixed and non-specific.

Numaguchi and colleagues (1977) also reviewed the angiographic findings in a series of previously published cases. Unlike most cases of AVM, no large feeding arteries were observed. Angiography was either normal, or suggested a mass effect with arterial displacement in 10 of 17 cases. In the patient reported by Voigt and Yasargil (1976), repeated angiograms were normal, but the fifth study revealed an avascular mass in the right temporal lobe. These authors suggested that the angiographic findings depended upon the timing of the study in relation to any hemorrhage. Other authors have reported that a large, draining vein and/or early venous filling around an avascular mass are features of these anomalies (Bogren et al., 1970; Roberson et al., 1974), and neovasculature and a "blush" is sometimes present (Jonutis et al., 1971).

The findings in two other large series of patients with "cavernous" malformations have been published (Simard et al., 1986; Tagle et al., 1986), and they generally confirm the observations in these earlier series. The CT findings are sometimes strongly suggestive of "cavernous" malformations, the typical appearance consisting of well defined collections of multiple, rounded densities showing mild contrast enhancement and no significant mass effect (Bartlett and Kishore, 1977).

A rare variant of these cavernous malformations is the so-called "hemangioma calcificans," in which there is gross intracranial calcification. An example was reported by DiTullio and Stern (1979) of a woman who presented with mental status changes, a past history of absence attacks, and a skull radiograph showing several areas of mottled intracranial calcification. These lesions appeared avascular on cerebral angiography, but microscopic examination of two specimens removed at operation permitted a diagnosis of hemangioma calcificans to be made.

In view of the tendency of these lesions to bleed, Voigt and Yasargil (1973) proposed the removal of all readily accessible solitary "cavernous" vascular malformations. Because they are clearly demarcated from adjacent cerebral tissue, most accessible lesions can be removed with relative ease.

There have been occasional reports of this type of vascular anomaly situated extra-axially in the middle cranial fossa, and these have been distinguished from similar lesions situated elsewhere in the intracranial cavity by Mori and coworkers (1980). They tend to occur in middle-aged women and usually lead to such symptoms as diplopia, ptosis, exophthalmos, and visual field defects that may be exacerbated by pregnancy. Calcification occurs rarely in such anomalies. The appearance on a CT scan is indistinguishable from that of a meningioma, a high density mass with homogeneous enhancement being found. The angiographic appearance may also simulate that of a meningioma, since an extra-axial mass with persisting tumor stain that is opacified by either the external or the internal circulation is found. Total surgical removal may be difficult because of profuse bleeding and adherence to the cavernous sinus (Mori et al., 1980).

The rare occurrence of a "cavernous" vascular anomaly as a cryptic lesion of the pituitary gland has also been described (Sansone et al., 1980).

SIMPLE VENOUS MALFORMATIONS

These simple, low flow malformations consist of venous structures, separated by normal neural parenchyma, that converge on a dilated venous trunk. No arterial component can be identified either angiographically or at autopsy in these malformations. In the earlier literature, a number of arteriovenous malformations were incorrectly classified as venous in type because a small arterial component was overlooked on inspection at operation or autopsy.

A review of the more recently published cases with adequate angiographic documentation indicates that in most patients with true venous malformations, the diagnosis is made between the ages of 20 and 40 years. There is an approximately equal sex incidence. The malformation is usually found incidentally following investigations performed for some unrelated disorder (Saito and Kobayashi, 1981). Very occasionally, the anomaly is responsible for the presenting complaint, such as with intracranial hemorrhage. In fact, hemorrhage from these malformations occurs only in rare instances (Constans et al., 1968; Maehara and Tasaka, 1978; Moritake et al., 1980; Scotti et al., 1975), and consequently its relative morbidity and mortality as compared with intracranial hemorrhage from other sources are unknown. Similarly, the natural history of venous malformation remains poorly defined at the present time, although most seem to follow a benign course and surgical treatment of these lesions seems rarely to be indicated (Martin et al., 1984). It has, however, been suggested that venous malformations in the cerebellar hemispheres are more prone to bleeding than similar malformations in other locations (Rothfus et al., 1984).

Venous malformations are usually demonstrated initially by CT scan (Fig. 15–5). In non-contrast scans, they appear as high density nodular lesions without calcification, edema, or mass effect. With contrast, they appear as linear densities that probably represent the dilated major venous trunk (Maehara and Tasaka, 1978; Fierstien et al., 1979; Michels et al., 1977). With the use of thin slices and coronal cuts, both the malformation and its pattern of venous drainage may be identified on CT, and with dynamic CT studies the specificity of the technique in diagnosing venous malformations may be increased (Valavanis et al., 1983). Magnetic resonance imaging also reveals a characteristic abnormality, with an enlarged transcerebral draining vein frequently associated with an area of increased parenchymal signal on T2-weighted images, and occasionally with

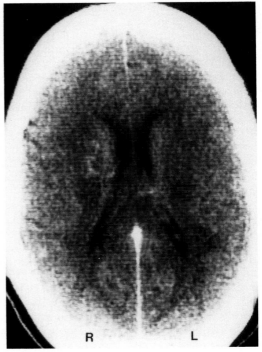

Figure 15–5. CT scan with contrast, showing abnormal serpiginous density in right paraventricular region in a 43 year old woman with parkinsonism.

reduced parenchymatous signal on T1-weighted images (Augustyn et al., 1985).

At angiography, the characteristic finding is of small, radially arranged vessels that converge on a distended vein that in turn is connected with the deep venous system or empties into a dural sinus (Fig. 15–6). In rare instances, these malformations show a blush during the capillary phase of the study (Preissig et al., 1976; Wendling et al., 1976).

Surgical treatment of venous malformations is usually not indicated unless intracerebral hemorrhage has occurred and the responsible lesion is accessible and not located in a critical region.

INTRACRANIAL DURAL VASCULAR ANOMALIES

Abnormal arteriovenous shunts may be fed by meningeal branches of the carotid (internal and external) and/or vertebral arteries and drain through dural veins and sinuses. These durally situated shunts may have a developmental basis, and, in keeping with

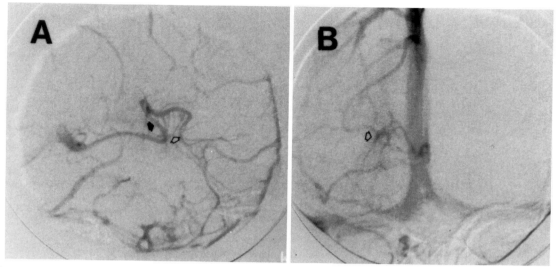

Figure 15–6. Right internal carotid arteriogram. *A,* Lateral projection, showing complex of abnormal veins (open arrow) draining into the thalamostriate vein (black arrow). *B,* Anteroposterior projection, showing the complex of abnormal veins (open arrow) adjacent to the wall of the lateral ventricle. Same patient as in Figure 15–5.

this, angiography sometimes shows the feeding arteries to divide into branches that communicate with the sinus at several different sites along its length (Aminoff and Kendall, 1973). However, similar lesions may develop in adult life, often following trauma, presumably because of the intimate relationship of certain meningeal arteries to venous structures (Wilson and Cronic, 1964; Newton and Hoyt, 1970), or after dural sinus thrombosis (Houser et al., 1979). Subsequent dilatation of pre-existing anastomotic channels from other arterial sources may then lead to the angiographic appearance of an AVM. Pathological examination of resected specimens often fails to indicate the congenital or acquired nature of the abnormality (Aminoff, 1973), although some lesions have the histopathological features of cavernous malformations (McCormick and Boulter, 1966). Accordingly, reference here will be made to vascular anomalies rather than to malformations to avoid general etiological implications.

The clinical features of these anomalies are similar to those of cerebral AVMs, but headache and tinnitus are common presenting symptoms, and a bruit is found more often than with cerebral lesions. Seizures and focal neurological deficits occur less often than with cerebral AVMs, but hemorrhage has a similar incidence (Aminoff, 1973). The definition of these lesions depends upon angiography. They may not be detected on CT

scans because of their close relationship to overlying bone, but reported findings include hydrocephalus, hemorrhage, and abnormal enhancement of dilated veins. In three cases, Miyasaka and coworkers (1980) reported vermiform or patchy enhancement after intravenous contrast infusion, local mass effects, and dilatation of the major draining route; hydrocephalus was present in two cases, and prominent vascular grooving of the skull inner table was seen in one. Most of these changes were attributed to the raised venous sinus pressure caused by the anomalous shunt.

Dural vascular anomalies are best considered further in relation to their venous drainage. They can be classified into an anterior-inferior group (involving the cavernous, intercavernous, sphenoparietal, superior and inferior petrosal sinuses, and basilar plexus) and a superior-posterior group (involving the superior and inferior sagittal, straight, transverse, sigmoid, and occipital sinuses).

Anterior-Inferior Group

The clinical features of a shunt between meningeal arteries and the cavernous sinus, or a venous structure draining into it, were reviewed in a series of 11 patients by Newton and Hoyt (1970). There is a female preponderance among the reported cases, and patients usually present in middle or later life. The initial complaint is often pain about the orbit, frontal, or temporal region on one side of the head. Diplopia from a sixth cranial nerve palsy is another common early symptom. Other patients present with a red eye, unilateral tinnitus, or mild protrusion of the eye. Typical findings on the affected side include mild proptosis, dilated conjunctival veins, increased intraocular pressure, and sometimes a transient sixth cranial nerve palsy; there may also be an orbital bruit. Unlike a direct carotid-cavernous fistula, there are no ocular pulsations, and marked proptosis with chemosis and swelling of the lid is uncommon. Spontaneous thrombosis of the venous component of the anomaly may obliterate the fistulous communication, sometimes shortly after angiography (Newton and Hoyt, 1970). Failing vision or intolerable symptoms may lead to the attempted occlusion of feeders, and embolization may enable this to be achieved without a direct operative approach (Aminoff, 1973; Hilal and Michelsen, 1975).

As already indicated, the cause of these lesions is unclear. Congenital anomalies may be responsible in some cases, but rupture of the thin-walled dural arteries traversing the cavernous sinus—either spontaneously, following mild trauma, or for other reasons— may be the cause in others. Trauma was directly implicated in all three cases described by Hayes (1963), and in some of the cases reported by others. Symptoms sometimes commence in the postpartum period (Newton and Hoyt, 1970; Taniguchi et al., 1971), perhaps because of straining during labor or the circulatory changes accompanying pregnancy.

The dural shunt is usually of low volume and is supplied by meningeal branches of the external and/or internal carotid arteries, sometimes from the contralateral side. The most common feeders from the external circulation are terminal meningeal branches of the internal maxillary artery, whereas the meningohypophyseal trunk is the most common source from the internal carotid artery. The vertebral artery may occasionally give rise to a major feeder through one of its meningeal branches (Laine et al., 1963; Edwards and Connolly, 1977). Drainage is usually anteriorly into the ophthalmic veins, especially the superior ophthalmic vein, and there may also be some drainage posteriorly

through the petrosal sinuses or the venous plexus of the clivus.

Newton and Hoyt (1970) subdivided these anomalies into those draining directly into the cavernous sinus, and those involving a more distant dural sinus or a venous structure that communicates with the cavernous sinus. Most of their cases were of the former type. Taniguchi and coworkers (1971) reported a further 11 patients in whom angiography revealed abnormal arteriovenous communications about the cavernous sinus. Their clinical features were similar to those reported by Newton and Hoyt (1970). The precise source of feeders to the shunts was not clear from the paper by Taniguchi and associates, but venous drainage was primarily through the inferior petrosal sinus, ophthalmic veins, and/or the superficial sylvian veins.

Post-traumatic or apparently spontaneous abnormal dural arteriovenous shunts between the middle meningeal artery and the superior petrosal or sphenoparietal sinuses have also been described (Fincher, 1951; Pakarinen, 1965; Markham, 1961). Tinnitus, sometimes pulsatile, is the main complaint and may be the sole symptom. On examination a bruit may be audible in the region about the ear, but there are usually no other abnormalities. Simple ligation of the external carotid artery sometimes relieves symptoms, but resection of the fistula may be necessary.

Superior-Posterior Group

Shunts involving the transverse-sigmoid sinus are the most common anomalies of the superior-posterior group (Fig. 15–7). Their clinical features have been reviewed in detail elsewhere (Houser et al., 1979; Aminoff, 1973; Obrador et al., 1975; Kuhner et al., 1976). There is a female preponderance of cases, and most patients present when they are older than 40 years. Symptoms and signs may relate to the shunt itself, or to hemorrhage, intracranial hypertension, or cerebral ischemia. Increased intracranial pressure may result from elevated venous pressure in involved sinuses or to associated venous sinus thrombosis (Aminoff and Kendall, 1973); hydrocephalus may also relate to previous subarachnoid bleeding or aneurysmal dilatation of the vein of Galen. Cerebral ischemia may relate to "steal" of blood by the anomalous

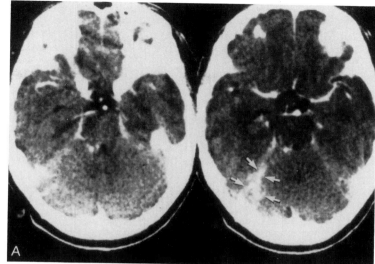

Figure 15–7. Supratentorial dural arteriovenous malformation in a 48 year old woman presenting with headaches. *A,* Post-contrast CT scan. Irregular enhancement is noted in the region of the right posterior tentorium (arrows). *B,* Selective right exernal carotid arteriogram. The middle meningeal branches are moderately enlarged, supplying a dural arteriovenous malformation draining into the torcular region and sigmoid sinus.

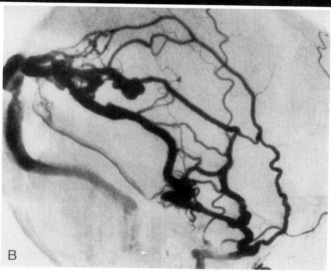

shunt, or to focal venous stagnation (Houser et al., 1979). The most common presenting complaint is of tinnitus, but headache, visual failure, subarachnoid hemorrhage, seizures, and various neurological deficits may also occur. Examination frequently reveals a bruit that is best heard in the mastoid region or behind the ear and that may be the sole abnormality, but papilledema and other neurological signs are also sometimes found. The vascular anomaly is occasionally asymptomatic, being found incidentally at angiography (Aminoff and Kendall, 1973) or at autopsy (McCormick and Boulter, 1966). It often has multiple feeders, and these commonly arise from the ipsilateral and/or contralateral occipital artery, middle meningeal artery, tentorial branches of the internal carotid artery, and meningeal branches of the vertebral artery.

Abnormal dural arteriovenous shunts to the superior sagittal sinus may follow head injury (Dennery and Ignacio, 1967) or may occur without any history of previous trauma (Aminoff, 1973; Newton et al., 1968; Ramamurthi and Balasubramanian, 1966; Kunc and Bret, 1969). Anomalies involving the vein of Galen, the torcular, or the superficial cerebral or cerebellar veins are also well described (Aminoff, 1973; Newton et al., 1968; Kunc and Bret, 1969; Ciminello and Sachs, 1962). These anomalies may have multiple feeders from the carotid (external and/or internal) and vertebral circulations. The usual clinical presentation is with papille-dema, headache, subarachnoid hemorrhage, or tinnitus.

Venous sinus thrombosis sometimes occurs spontaneously (Houser et al., 1979; Handa et al., 1975), and leads to clearing of symptoms (Magidson and Weinberg, 1976). If treatment is necessary, ligation of individual feeding vessels may occasionally relieve symptoms, although it is often unrewarding. Benefit may also follow embolization of feeders (Hilal and Michelsen, 1975; Lamas et al., 1977). Surgical extirpation of the anomaly, with occlusion of all feeders, is the most satisfactory treatment of patients with disabling symptoms or a history of hemorrhage (Sundt and Piepgras, 1983). An alternative approach to the treatment of lesions involving the transverse and sigmoid sinuses is to isolate these sinuses surgically from all dural attachments; apparent benefit (partial or complete relief of pulsatile tinnitus) has been reported by Hugosson and Bergstrom (1974) with this technique.

MALFORMATIONS INVOLVING THE VEIN OF GALEN

The clinical features of the rare AVMs involving the vein of Galen depend on the age of presentation. Neonates generally develop congestive cardiac failure that often has a fatal outcome, and other congenital anomalies may also be present (Gold et al., 1964). In infants, the typical presentation is with hydrocephalus (as a result of aqueductal compression by the dilated vein of Galen), convulsions, or distended tortuous scalp veins, sometimes followed by psychomotor retardation, cardiomegaly, and the development of diverse neurological signs, usually including a cranial bruit. Headache, subarachnoid hemorrhage, or seizures are common presentations in older children, and focal neurological deficits subsequently develop, but a cranial bruit is rare. Radiographs of the skull may suggest increased intracranial pressure in infants and young children, whereas the wall of the vein of Galen may be outlined by calcification in older teenagers and adults (Thomson, 1959). Bilateral carotid and vertebral angiography indicates the nature of the lesion and is required to define all the involved vessels. There is marked enlargement of feeding vessels and draining sinuses and a midline collection of contrast material (Fig. 15–8). The definitive treatment is surgical, but medical management to support cardiac function and control seizures is important.

STURGE-WEBER SYNDROME

In the Sturge-Weber syndrome, which has an equal sex incidence and occurs sporadi-

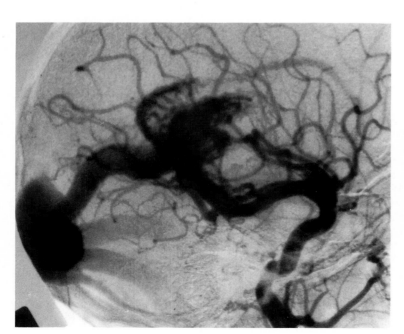

Figure 15–8. Right internal carotid arteriogram in a 6 year old boy with ease of fatigue, cardiomegaly, and facial venous distension. There is a large arteriovenous communication involving the vein of Galen, with drainage into a globular-shaped torcula via a markedly dilated straight sinus.

cally, a congenital, usually unilateral, capillary dermal malformation of the upper part of the face is associated with leptomeningeal vascular anomalies and often also with a choroidal lesion. The cutaneous stain may be associated with overgrowth of connective tissue and is often very disfiguring, except in black patients. Focal or generalized seizures are common presenting features of neurological involvement and often commence during infancy. Intracranial hemorrhage is uncommon. In addition to the cutaneous lesion, examination classically reveals mental subnormality; a contralateral homonymous hemianopia, hemiparesis, and hemisensory disturbance; and contralateral limbs that are often small and poorly developed. There is no cranial bruit. Ipsilateral buphthalmos or glaucoma may be found.

Skull radiographs usually reveal gyriform ("tramline") intracranial calcification, especially in the parieto-occipital region, after the first 2 years of life as a result of mineral deposition in the cortex beneath the leptomeningeal lesion. The overlying skull vault may be thickened and have an enlarged diploic space (Nellhaus et al., 1967). Electroencephalographic abnormalities include a depression of normal background rhythms over the affected hemisphere, and the occurrence on that side of irregular slow activity and sharp transients (Brenner and Sharbrough, 1976).

Many authorities regard the intracranial lesion as inoperable, but occipital lobectomy is sometimes performed with the aim of alleviating or preventing the seizure disorder and limiting intellectual decline (Alexander, 1972). Medical treatment consists of pharmacological management of seizures. The patient should be referred to an ophthalmologist if choroidal vascular abnormalities are present or if there is increased intraocular pressure.

WYBURN-MASON SYNDROME

The rare association of a mesencephalic AVM with an ipsilateral retinal vascular anomaly and, sometimes, with a facial port-wine stain is referred to as the Wyburn-Mason (1943a) or Bonnet-Dechaume-Blanc (1937) syndrome. In rare instances, a dural lesion may coexist with the cerebral AVM (Tamaki et al., 1971).

The cerebral lesion is unilateral; frequently involves the optic pathway, sometimes in its entirety from the retina to the occipital cortex; and is supplied from the carotid and/or vertebral circulations. It most often involves the optic chiasm, hypothalamus, basal ganglia, and midbrain. It may lead to seizures, headaches, a bruit, hemorrhage, and focal neurological deficits, but occasionally it is asymptomatic. Homonymous field defects, pyramidal and other focal signs, and/or mental retardation may be found on examination.

Among 25 cases (including 3 new ones) reviewed by Théron and coworkers (1974), a cutaneous vascular stain involving the ipsilateral face or eyelids was present in 6 patients, and facial asymmetry was sometimes evident as well. Ten patients had a vascular malformation involving the jaws, nose, or mouth, manifest in some by recurrent bleeding. The ipsilateral retinal AVM was always unilateral and was easily recognized ophthalmoscopically, and clusters of peripherally situated microaneurysms were sometimes present as well. Other ophthalmological findings often included a mild non-pulsatile proptosis, dilatation of conjunctival vessels, and a decrease in visual acuity. Retrobulbar involvement by the malformation was frequent, and dilated vascular channels were often apparent within the optic nerve at angiography. Rare cases without retinal involvement have been described (Brown et al., 1973).

The extent of the cerebral and facial malformation cannot be predicted on clinical grounds. Patients commonly present with monocular amblyopia, and this leads to discovery of the retinal lesion, but without further investigations the coexisting lesions are likely to be missed.

HEREDITARY HEMORRHAGIC TELANGIECTASIA

Hereditary hemorrhagic telangiectasia, an autosomal dominant, familial disorder, also known as Rendu-Osler-Weber syndrome, is characterized by the occurrence of repeated hemorrhages from multiple cutaneous, mucosal, and visceral telangiectasias. In addition, various vascular anomalies, including telangiectasias, complex (cavernous) malformations, AVMs, and aneurysms, may occur in the brain or spinal cord (Roman et al., 1978).

The most common neurological manifestations include cerebral abscess, hypoxia, and embolic phenomena as complications of the pulmonary arteriovenous fistulae that occur in this disorder. Other neurological manifestations consist of seizures, progressive hydrocephalus, and/or focal neurological deficits that may result from minor hemorrhages.

Intradural and Extradural Spinal Vascular Anomalies

Spinal vascular anomalies may occur in association with intracranial AVMs and with intracranial (Brion et al., 1952; Doppman and Di Chiro, 1965) or spinal (Herdt et al., 1971; Caroscio et al., 1980) arterial aneurysms. They may also occur in the Rendu-Osler-Weber syndrome and with other vascular or lymphatic anomalies (Aminoff, 1976), and are the underlying cause in many cases of subacute necrotic myelopathy (Antoni, 1962). Most symptomatic spinal vascular anomalies are AVMs, and their clinical and radiological features depend upon their location. Their topographical classification has generally been based on their relationship to the different compartments of the spinal canal, i.e., on whether they are intradural, extradural, or vertebral. Studies have shown, however, that in many of those previously considered to be situated intradurally the actual arteriovenous shunt lies on the dura (Kendall and Logue, 1977; Symon et al., 1984; Oldfield et al., 1983). Accordingly, intra- and extradural spinal AVMs will be considered together, especially since their clinical and myelographic features are similar.

The majority of spinal AVMs (80%) are situated below the second or third thoracic cord segment, are found two or three times more frequently in males than in females, and are not diagnosed before middle age. They are usually extramedullary, commonly lying behind the cord, where they are supplied by just one or two feeders that either do not supply the cord at all or contribute only to the posterior spinal circulation. In contrast, cervical AVMs have an approximately equal sex incidence and, perhaps because of their tendency to bleed, are usually diagnosed at an earlier age. They are commonly anterior to the cord, are often partly intramedullary, may have multiple feeders, and frequently are supplied at least in part by vessels supplying the cord as well.

CLINICAL FEATURES

Spinal AVMs present either with hemorrhage or, more commonly, with a myeloradiculopathy. Numerous case reports have been published, and are reviewed by Wyburn-Mason (1943b), Aminoff (1976), and others.

Non-traumatic spinal subarachnoid hemorrhage is uncommon, but when it does occur it is usually from an AVM. Other reported but rarer causes are telangiectasias, mycotic or other aneurysms of a spinal artery, coarctation of the aorta, tumors (such as ependymomas, neurofibromas, and meningeal sarcomas), blood dyscrasias, vasculitides, and various infective states (Aminoff, 1976). About 10–15% of patients with spinal AVMs experience a hemorrhage, and this is especially likely from cervical malformations (Aminoff, 1976).

The hemorrhage is heralded by a sudden, severe back pain, initially at the level of the bleed but rapidly becoming more widespread, when it may be accompanied by root pain, especially in the legs. Signs of meningeal irritation then develop, and if blood passes intracranially there may also be headache, a depressed level of consciousness, papilledema, cranial nerve palsies, and other more widespread signs. Unless a spinal source for the bleeding is indicated by signs of hematomyelia or cord compression, diagnosis may be delayed because the hemorrhage is presumed to have originated intracranially. However, the presence of a cutaneous vascular stain on the trunk or a spinal bruit favors a spinal lesion, and should specifically be searched for.

The overall mortality rate of subarachnoid hemorrhage from spinal AVMs is at least 15% (Aminoff, 1976). About half of the survivors will have a second bleed, and this occurs within a year in about 40% of cases with recurrent hemorrhage. Half of the subsequent survivors will have further hemorrhages unless the AVM is treated. Unfortunately, cervical AVMs are more likely to bleed than more caudally placed lesions, and their adequate treatment is often precluded by their anatomical features. If there is a coexisting arterial aneurysm, however, this may be a more likely source of bleeding (Herdt et al., 1971; Caroscio et al., 1980) than the AVM itself.

Extradural hemorrhage sometimes accounts for a cord disturbance when it has an acute onset. Back pain, usually accompanied by girdle or extremity pain, is conspicuous initially; the CSF findings are usually of no diagnostic help because of the extradural location of the blood, but there may be manometric evidence of a total or partial block in the subarachnoid space.

Most patients present with a myeloradiculopathy rather than with hemorrhage. Symptoms and signs develop either gradually (80% of cases) or acutely (20%) and resemble those of cord compression from any cause. Among 60 patients reported by Aminoff and Logue (1974a), pain was the most common initial symptom, occurring either alone or in combination with other symptoms in 42%; it was radicular in 23%, confined to the back in 12%, and remote and non-specific in the limbs in 7%. Other initial symptoms consisted of sensory disturbances in 33%, leg weakness in 32%, a disturbance of sphincter or sexual function in 10%, and subarachnoid hemorrhage in 5%. Progression of symptoms was usually steady but was occasionally episodic, with intervening periods of partial remission. By the time of diagnosis, 65% of the patients complained of leg weakness, sensory symptoms, pain, and disturbed micturition.

Certain features of the history are suggestive of an underlying AVM in patients with a myeloradiculopathy of uncertain cause. In 19 of the 60 cases reported by Aminoff and Logue (1974a), for example, there were symptoms of neurogenic intermittent claudication. Pain in the legs or back or in both sites was precipitated or enhanced by exercise and was relieved by rest. Leg pain usually had a radicular distribution, unlike that of peripheral vascular disease, and other symptoms sometimes accompanied it. A few patients developed motor or sensory disturbances, without associated pain, on exercise. The exercise tolerance varied in different patients, but it tended to diminish with time. In 14 of the 60 patients, postural factors (such as bending forward) provoked pain or other symptoms, and in a few patients symptoms were related to pregnancy, increased body temperature, or trauma. The exacerbation of symptoms by the menstrual cycle, breath-holding, or straining at stool is also well described (Aminoff, 1976), and recur-

rent, transient postprandial paresis of the legs has been reported (Oliver et al., 1973).

A combined upper and lower motor neuron deficit is commonly found in the legs on examination, accompanied by sensory impairment that may be extensive or radicular. A purely motor deficit is sometimes found, however, and may consist solely of an upper or lower motor neuron disturbance. The presence of cutaneous vascular stains, especially if related segmentally to the level of the spinal lesion, may be of diagnostic relevance, and should be searched for (Cobb syndrome). Their recognition is facilitated if the skin is inspected while patients perform the Valsalva maneuver. Although segmentally related cutaneous lesions were not present in any of the 60 patients reported by Aminoff and Logue (1974a), their incidence was 12% (Djindjian et al., 1970) and 21% (Doppman et al., 1969), respectively, in two other series. A spinal bruit is sometimes audible in the region overlying a spinal AVM (Hook and Lidvall, 1958; Matthews, 1959), and careful auscultation over the spine is therefore important in patients with subarachnoid hemorrhage, myelopathy, or a radiculopathy of uncertain cause. An AVM cannot, however, be excluded by the absence of a bruit.

Of the 60 patients evaluated by the author, 33 eventually became totally unable to walk, or required two sticks or crutches to get about; 10 patients were disabled to this extent within 6 months, and 28 within 3 years, of the onset of any leg weakness or disturbance in walking (Aminoff and Logue, 1974b). Once an AVM has become symptomatic, this major disability is likely to result unless effective treatment is instituted.

DIAGNOSTIC INVESTIGATIONS

Plain radiographs of the spine are usually unhelpful diagnostically, although widening of the interpeduncular distance or other radiological evidence of an intraspinal space-occupying lesion is sometimes seen. Signs of an associated vertebral vascular anomaly are occasionally found.

Examination of the cerebrospinal fluid is helpful if subarachnoid hemorrhage is suspected, but the findings are otherwise of little diagnostic relevance. The protein concentration is frequently increased in the absence of obstruction of the subarachnoid space, and there may be an accompanying pleocytosis; an increased cell content is sometimes the sole abnormality.

Positive contrast myelography is the most important screening procedure (Fig. 15–9). The length of the cord is visualized in both prone and supine positions, using a large volume of contrast material. Tortuous filling defects as a result of vascular impressions in the column of contrast material, without any obstruction in the subarachnoid space, are characteristic of an AVM. The defects may be localized or extensive and in the thoracic region may only be shown on supine films. Such typical abnormalities were found in at least 80% of cases by several authors (Aminoff and Logue, 1974a; Lombardi and Migliavacca, 1959; Svien and Baker, 1961) but

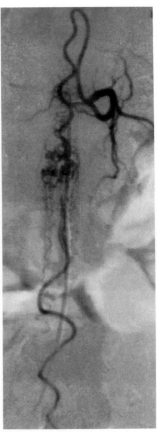

Figure 15–10. Selective spinal arteriogram in a 24 year old woman with a 2 week history of low back pain, with weakness and numbness in the right leg. There is an arteriovenous malformation at the level of the conus supplied by a spinal branch of the left L1 intercostal artery, and drained by a single large descending vein.

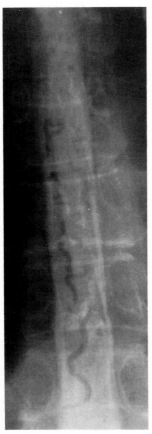

Figure 15–9. Metrizamide myelogram in a 35 year old woman with progressive paraparesis and sensory disturbance in the legs, accompanied by mild bladder and bowel dysfunction. Serpiginous filling defects are seen in the column of contrast material, indicating the presence of a vascular malformation in the midthoracic region.

were less commonly seen by others. For example, Djindjian and coworkers (1970) reported them in only about half of their patients; many of their remaining patients had other myelographic abnormalities, but these were less characteristic. The myelographic appearances of true vascular tumors with prominent draining veins may resemble those of an AVM. Tortuous, redundant lumbar nerve roots can be distinguished by examining the spine in slight flexion to straighten them (Kendall, 1976).

If myelography suggests that a vascular anomaly is present, selective spinal angiography (Fig. 15–10) is undertaken to confirm that this is the case; to determine its level, extent, and position in relation to the spinal cord; and to identify all of its feeders. In addition, the normal blood supply to the adjacent spinal cord, and especially the regional supply to the anterior spinal artery, must be determined so that it can be safeguarded at operation. Contrast material is injected into the orifices of the segmental arteries arising from the aorta so that the vessels entering the spinal canal can be visualized. The clinical or myelographic findings will determine which vessels are injected first, and in this regard the presence of a cutaneous vascular lesion may be particularly helpful in suggesting the likely level and side of feeders. Further details are given by Kendall (1976).

Because epidural AVMs may drain into the coronal venous plexus on the surface of the cord (Kendall and Logue, 1977), their myelographic appearances may be indistinguishable from those of intradural AVMs unless epidural hemorrhage has occurred, when an obstructive lesion will be evident. However, angiography generally permits the epidural site of the arteriovenous shunt to be recognized, because it usually lies lateral to the cord and outside the plain of the dura. In most instances, no more than one or two feeding vessels are involved in the lesion.

Di Chiro and Wener (1973) described three types of angiographic appearance of spinal AVMs. The most common appearance, Type 1, is of an AVM fed by only one or two vessels that do not supply the cord at all. Most of the malformation consists of long, tortuous vessels on the back of the cord, and blood flow through it is slow. The Type 2 malformations are characterized by a more compact coil of vessels but are otherwise similar to the preceding variety. Type 3 malformations, which occur mainly in children and young adults, are supplied by several vessels that may also supply the cord, and blood flow through them is rapid; their fistulous portion may lie in front of or behind the cord and is often intramedullary, at least in part. The angiographic appearances relate in part to the level of the lesion (Aminoff, 1976). Cervical AVMs are often of the Type 3 variety, whereas more caudal malformations are usually of Type 1 or 2.

Spinal AVMs can sometimes be visualized with contrast-enhanced CT scans (Di Chiro et al., 1977), but the value of this technique as a screening procedure for AVMs is unclear. For the present, myelography and angiography are the investigative methods of choice. Similarly, magnetic resonance imaging may permit the detection of intramedullary or extramedullary spinal AVMs, or the presence of localized hematoma, but the sensitivity of this technique compared with myelography for the detection of these lesions is not clear at the present time.

PATHOLOGY AND PATHOPHYSIOLOGY

At autopsy or operation, abnormal distended intradural vessels are found overlying part of the cord. Microscopically, they have defects in the elastica and media and hypertrophied walls of irregular thickness; some may be occluded by thrombus. Fine vessels may run between them and the cord, particularly when the AVM is placed anteriorly. The cord itself may be swollen as a result of hemorrhage, edema, or an intramedullary lesion, or atrophic from ischemic necrosis. Leptomeningeal thickening and adhesions are common. Within the cord, there is a proliferation of small vessels, with thickened hyalinized walls, especially posteriorly and laterally, and variable degeneration of neurons and axons, demyelination of nerve fibers, and glial proliferation. Thrombotic vascular occlusion may be prominent in some cases and absent in others. The cord itself may be infarcted, show hematomyelic changes, or contain an intramedullary component of the malformation.

The development of an acute neurological deficit may relate to extradural, intramedullary (Odom et al., 1957), or subarachnoid hemorrhage (Hensen and Croft, 1956), or to intravascular thrombosis (Wyburn-Mason, 1943b). However, the basis of symptoms that develop gradually and progressively is unclear. There is no evidence to support the early notion that the cord is compressed by the AVM. Short-circuiting of blood through the AVM could conceivably lead to cord ischemia by depriving the normal intraspinal circulation of part of its blood supply, but it is unlikely that such "steal" is responsible for the production of symptoms in most cases. If cervical AVMs are excluded, the arteries feeding an AVM usually do not arise from a vessel supplying the cord, individual arteries to the AVM and cord are usually not derived from the same segmental stem, and the circulation through the AVM and cord are generally quite separate (Aminoff et al., 1974).

Aminoff and colleagues (1974) suggested that neurological dysfunction related to increased pressure in the interconnected plexus of coronal veins that drains both the AVM and the intramedullary circulation. As the pressure in these veins increases, the arteriovenous pressure gradient across the spinal cord declines, thereby reducing intramedullary blood flow and leading to ischemic hypoxia. A mechanism of this sort would account for the relationship of symptoms to mechanical factors such as posture.

TREATMENT

There is no satisfactory medical treatment for spinal AVMs. Surgical treatment is generally reserved for AVMs that are symptomatic, but the prospects for complete recovery are generally greater in patients with no incapacity than in those with marked disability. Operative treatment is clearly indicated once subarachnoid hemorrhage has occurred and for rapidly progressive symptoms or incapacity influencing the normal pattern of daily life. The advisability of surgical exploration for patients with mild symptoms and no significant disability is harder to assess, and factors such as the age and general condition of the patient, the available technical facilities, and the angiographic character of the lesion will assume greater importance. Treatment of epidural hemorrhage is by urgent evacuation of the hematoma at laminectomy.

Surgical treatment poses no particular problem for the majority of malformations, as they are extramedullary, lie behind the cord, and are fed by vessels not supplying the anterior spinal circulation. If the AVM is actually extradural in location, the incidence of neurological complications should be low because the vessels on the surface of the cord can be left undisturbed (Logue, 1979). The aim is to abolish the blood supply of the AVM by ligation of feeders, and this is combined with excision of the fistulous portion to reduce any possibility of its revascularization. Technical details are given elsewhere (Aminoff, 1976; Symen et al., 1984; Oldfield et al., 1983; Logue, 1979). A previously progressive downhill course is generally halted by surgical excision, and pain is usually relieved. Definite improvement in gait occurs in at least 60% of cases, and disturbances of sensory and sphincter function may also improve. Thus, of the seven chairbound patients operated on by Logue (1979), two were subsequently enabled to walk without support, one could get about with a cane and two could walk with crutches, and only two remained unable to walk at all.

Malformations lying in front of or within the cord are harder to treat because of their inaccessibility, and they are commonly supplied by the anterior spinal artery or its feeding vessels, occlusion of which may further impair the cord circulation. Cervical AVMs are usually of this type, but the occasional thoracolumbar malformation is supplied either by the anterior spinal artery or by the artery of Adamkiewicz. Therapeutic occlusion of the artery of Adamkiewicz may then be well tolerated (Di Chiro and Wener, 1973; Newton and Adams, 1968), but it is hard to predict the outcome of such a procedure. Controlled embolization to occlude the feeding branches but preserve the main arterial supply to the cord may be a useful therapeutic approach in these circumstances (Djindjian, 1975).

Percutaneous embolization of feeding vessels is a simple, safe technique for the treatment of spinal AVMs. Progressive neurological improvement was reported by Doppman and coworkers (1971) in three of five patients in whom embolization was successful, but Djindjian (1976) found that among his ten patients with retromedullary vascular anomalies, embolization with Gelfoam was definitely ineffective in seven and probably ineffective in another two patients.

The technique of embolization is of importance when direct operative treatment is especially hazardous, not warranted, or not feasible. For example, in paraplegic patients with gross sphincteric dysfunction, embolization may still reduce pain and lessen the risk of subarachnoid hemorrhage even though the neurological deficit is irreversible. The procedure, however, is not innocuous. The AVM may enlarge or rupture if the embolus passes through to block its draining veins. Moreover, occlusion of vessels other than the intended ones may lead to an enhanced or additional deficit. Thus, although selective embolization of certain intramedullary malformations supplied through the anterior spinal circulation is sometimes feasible

(Djindjian, 1975), a severe neurological deficit may result if the main vessels to the cord itself are occluded inadvertently.

An exciting new therapeutic approach consists of the intra-arterial injection of a material that will form an intravascular cast within the AVM so that all of the feeding vessels are occluded. Whether such a technique has any practical relevance in the management of spinal lesions remains to be established, but the results in one preliminary study, using intra-arterial cyanoacrylate, were encouraging (Kerber et al., 1978).

References

Alexander, G. L.: Sturge-Weber syndrome. In Vinken, P. J., and Bruyn, G. W. (eds.): *Handbook of Clinical Neurology*. Amsterdam: North-Holland, 1972, Vol. 14, p. 223.

Aminoff, M. J.: Vascular anomalies in the intracranial dura mater. Brain *96*:601, 1973.

Aminoff, M. J.: *Spinal Angiomas*. Oxford: Blackwell, 1976.

Aminoff, M. J.: Treatment of unruptured cerebral arteriovenous malformations. Neurology *37*:815, 1987.

Aminoff, M. J., and Kendall, B. E.: Asymptomatic dural vascular anomalies. Brit. J. Radiol. *46*:662, 1973.

Aminoff, M. J., and Logue, V.: Clinical features of spinal vascular malformations. Brain *97*:197, 1974a.

Aminoff, M. J., and Logue, V.: The prognosis of patients with spinal vascular malformations. Brain *97*:211, 1974b.

Aminoff, M. J., Barnard, R. O., and Logue, V.: The pathophysiology of spinal vascular malformations. J. Neurol. Sci. *23*:255, 1974.

Antoni, N.: Spinal vascular malformations (angiomas) and myelomalacia. Neurology *12*:795, 1962.

Augustyn, G. T., Scott, J. A., Olson, E., Gilmor, R. L., and Edwards, M. K.: Cerebral venous angiomas: MR imaging. Radiology *156*:391, 1985.

Bank, W. O., Kerber, C. W., and Cromwell, L. D.: Treatment of intracerebral arteriovenous malformations with isobutyl 2-cyanoacrylate: Initial clinical experience. Radiology *139*:609, 1981.

Bartlett, J. E., and Kishore, P. R. S.: Intracranial cavernous angioma. AJR *128*:653, 1977.

Bogren H., Svalander, C., and Wickbom, I.: Angiography in intracranial cavernous hemangiomas. Acta Radiol. (Diagn.) *10*:81, 1970.

Bonnet, P., Dechaume, J., and Blanc, E.: L'anévrysme cirsoïde de la retiné (Anévrysme racemeux), ses relations avec l'anévrysme cirsoïde de la face et avec l'anévrysme cirsoïde du cerveau. J. Med. Lyon *18*:165, 1937.

Brenner, R. P., and Sharbrough, F. W.: Electroencephalographic evaluation in Sturge-Weber syndrome. Neurology *26*:629, 1976.

Brion, S., Netsky, M. G., and Zimmerman, H. M.: Vascular malformations of the spinal cord. Arch. Neurol. Psychiatry *68*:339, 1952.

Brown, D. G., Hilal, S. K., and Tenner, M. S.: Wyburn-Mason syndrome. Report of two cases without retinal involvement. Arch. Neurol. *28*:67, 1973.

Caroscio, J. T., Brannan, T., Budabin, M., Huang, Y. P., and Yahr, M. D.: Subarachnoid hemorrhage secondary to spinal arteriovenous malformation and aneurysm. Arch. Neurol. *37*:101, 1980.

Ciminello, V. J., and Sachs, E.: Arteriovenous malformations of the posterior fossa. J. Neurosurg. *19*:602, 1962.

Clark, J. V.: Familial occurrence of cavernous angiomata of the brain. J. Neurol. Neurosurg. Psychiatry *33*:871, 1970.

Constans, J. P., Dilenge, D., and Vedrenne, C.: Angiomes veineux cerebraux. Neurochirurgie *14*:641, 1968.

Cromwell, L. D., and Harris, A. B.: Treatment of cerebral arteriovenous malformations. A combined neurosurgical and neuroradiological approach. J. Neurosurg. *52*:705, 1980.

Debrun, G., Vinuela, F., Fox, A., and Drake, C. G.: Embolization of cerebral arteriovenous malformations with bucrylate. Experience in 46 cases. J. Neurosurg. *56*:615, 1982.

Dennery, J. M., and Ignacio, B. S.: Post-traumatic arteriovenous fistula between the external carotid arteries and the superior longitudinal sinus: Report of a case. Can. J. Surg. *10*:333, 1967.

Di Chiro, G., and Wener, L.: Angiography of the spinal cord. A review of contemporary techniques and applications. J. Neurosurg. *39*:1, 1973.

Di Chiro, G., Doppman, J. L., and Wener, L.: Computed tomography of spinal cord arteriovenous malformations. Radiology *123*:351, 1977.

DiTullio, M. V., and Stern, W. E.: Hemangioma calcificans. Case report of an intraparenchymatous calcified vascular hematoma with epileptogenic potential. J. Neurosurg. *50*:110, 1979.

Djindjian, M.: Les malformations artério-veineuses de la möelle epinière et leur traitement. These pour le doctorat en médicine, Université de Paris VI, 1976.

Djindjian, R.: Embolization of angiomas of the spinal cord. Surg. Neurol. *4*:411, 1975.

Djindjian, R., Hurth, M., and Houdart, R.: *L'Angiographie de la Moelle Epiniere*. Paris: Masson, 1970.

Doppman, J. L., and Di Chiro, G.: Subtraction-angiography of spinal cord vascular malformations. Report of a case. J. Neurosurg. *23*:440, 1965.

Doppman, J. L., Di Chiro, G., and Ommaya, G.: Percutaneous embolization of spinal cord arteriovenous malformations. J. Neurosurg. *34*:48, 1971.

Doppman, J. L., Wirth, F. P., Di Chiro, G., and Ommaya, A. K.: Value of cutaneous angiomas in the arteriographic localization of spinal-cord arteriovenous malformations. N. Engl. J. Med. *281*:1440, 1969.

Drake, C. G.: Surgical removal of arteriovenous malformations from the brain stem and cerebellopontine angle. J. Neurosurg. *43*:661, 1975.

Drake, C. G.: Cerebral arteriovenous malformations: Considerations for and experience with surgical treatment in 166 cases. Clin. Neurosurg. *26*:145, 1979.

Drake, C. G.: Arteriovenous malformations of the brain. The options for management. N. Engl. J. Med. *309*:308, 1983.

Edwards, M. S., and Connolly, E. S.: Cavernous sinus syndrome produced by communication between the external carotid artery and cavernous sinus. J. Neurosurg. *46*:92, 1977.

Fierstien, S. B., Pribram, H. W., and Hieshima, G.: Angiography and computed tomography in the evaluation of cerebral venous malformations. Neuroradiology *17*:137, 1979.

Fincher, E. F.: Arteriovenous fistula between the middle meningeal artery and the greater petrosal sinus. Case report. Ann. Surg. *133*:886, 1951.

Forster, D. M. C., Steiner, L., and Hakanson, S.: Arteriovenous malformations of the brain. A long-term clinical study. J. Neurosurg. *37*:562, 1972.

Gates, G. F., Fishman, L. S., and Segall, H. D.: Scintigraphic detection of congenital intracranial vascular malformations. J. Nucl. Med. *19*:235, 1978.

Giombini, S., and Morello, G.: Cavernous angiomas of the brain. Account of fourteen personal cases and review of the literature. Acta Neurochir. *40*:61, 1978.

Gold, A. P., Ransohoff, J., and Carter, S.: Vein of Galen malformation. Acta Neurol. Scand. *40*(Suppl. 11):1, 1964.

Goree, J. A., and Dukes, H. T.: The angiographic differential diagnosis between the vascularized malignant glioma and the intracranial arteriovenous malformation. Am. J. Roentgenol. Radium Ther. Nucl. Med. *90*:512, 1963.

Graf, C. J., Perret, G. E., and Torner, J. C.: Bleeding from cerebral arteriovenous malformations as part of their natural history. J. Neurosurg. *58*:331, 1983.

Handa, J., Yoneda, S., and Handa, H.: Venous sinus occlusion with a dural arteriovenous malformation of the posterior fossa. Surg. Neurol. *4*:433, 1975.

Hayashi, S., Arimoto, T., Itakura, T., Fujii, T., Nishiguchi, T., and Komai, N.: The association of intracranial aneurysms and arteriovenous malformation of the brain. Case report. J. Neurosurg. *55*:971, 1981.

Hayes, G. J.: External carotid-cavernous sinus fistulas. J. Neurosurg. *20*:692, 1963.

Henderson, W. R., and Gomez, R. de R. L.: Natural history of cerebral angiomas. Br. Med. J. *4*:571, 1967.

Henson, R. A., and Croft, P. B.: Spontaneous spinal subarachnoid haemorrhage. Quart. J. Med. *25*:53, 1956.

Herdt, J. R., Di Chiro, G., and Doppman, J. L.: Combined arterial and arteriovenous aneurysms of the spinal cord. Radiology *99*:589, 1971.

Heros, R. C., and Tu, Y. K.: Unruptured arteriovenous malformations: A dilemma in surgical decision making. Clin. Neurosurg. *33*:187, 1986.

Hilal, S. K., and Michelsen, J. W.: Therapeutic percutaneous embolization for extra-axial vascular lesions of the head, neck, and spine. J. Neurosurg. *43*:275, 1975.

Hook, O., and Lidvall, H.: Arteriovenous aneurysms of the spinal cord. A report of two cases investigated by vertebral angiography. J. Neurosurg. *15*:84, 1958.

Houdart, R., and Le Besnerais, Y.: Les anevrysmes arterio-veineux des hemispheres cerebraux. Paris: Masson, 1963.

Houser, O. W., Campbell, J. K., Campbell, R. J., and Sundt, T. M.: Arteriovenous malformation affecting the transverse dural venous sinus—an acquired lesion. Mayo Clin. Proc. *54*:651, 1979.

Hugosson, R., and Bergstrom, K.: Surgical treatment of dural arteriovenous malformation in the region of the sigmoid sinus. J. Neurol. Neurosurg. Psychiatry *37*:97, 1974.

Johnson, R. T.: Radiotherapy of cerebral angiomas: With a note on some problems in diagnosis. In Pia, H. W., Gleave, J. R. W., Grote, E., and Zierski, J. (eds.): *Cerebral Angiomas: Advances in Diagnosis and Therapy*. New York: Springer-Verlag, 1975, p. 256.

Jonutis, A. J., Sondheimer, F. K., Klein, H. Z., and Wise, B. L.: Intracerebral cavernous hemangioma with an-

giographically demonstrated pathologic vasculature. Neuroradiology *3*:57, 1971.

Kelly, J. L., Mellinger, J. F., and Sundt, T. M.: Intracranial arteriovenous malformations in childhood. Ann. Neurol. *3*:338, 1978.

Kendall, B. E.: Radiological investigations. In Aminoff, M. J.: *Spinal Angiomas*. Oxford: Blackwell, 1976, p. 97.

Kendall, B. E., and Claveria, L. E.: The use of computed axial tomography (CAT) for the diagnosis and management of intracranial angiomas. Neuroradiology *12*:141, 1976.

Kendall, B. E., and Logue, V.: Spinal epidural angiomatous malformations draining into intrathecal veins. Neuroradiology *13*:181, 1977.

Kerber, C. W., Cromwell, L. D., and Sheptak, P. E.: Intraarterial cyanoacrylate: An adjunct in the treatment of spinal/paraspinal arteriovenous malformations. AJR *130*:99, 1978.

Kjellberg, R. N., Hanamura, T., Davis, K. R., Lyons, S. L., and Adams, R. D.: Bragg-peak proton-beam therapy for arteriovenous malformations of the brain. N. Engl. J. Med. *309*:269, 1983.

Kramer, R. A., and Wing, S. D.: Computed tomography of angiographically occult cerebral vascular malformations. Radiology *123*:649, 1977.

Kucharczyk, W., Lemme-Pleghos, L., Uske, A., Brant-Zawadzki, M., Dooms, G., and Norman, D.: Intracranial vascular malformations: MR and CT imaging. Radiology *156*:383, 1985.

Kuhner, A., Krastel, A., and Stoll, W.: Arteriovenous malformations of the transverse dural sinus. J. Neurosurg. *45*:12, 1976.

Kunc, Z., and Bret, J.: Congenital arterio-sinusal fistulae. Acta Neurochir. *20*:85, 1969.

Kusske, J. A., and Kelly, W. A.: Embolization and reduction of the "steal" syndrome in cerebral arteriovenous malformations. J. Neurosurg. *40*:313, 1974.

Laine, E., Galibert, P., Lopez, C., Delahousse, J., Delandtsheer, J. M., and Christiaens, J. L.: Anévrysmes arterio-veineux intra-duraux (developpes dans l'épaisseur de la dure-mère) de la fosse postérieure. Neurochirurgie *9*:147, 1963.

Lamas, E., Lobato, R. D., Esparza, J., and Escudero, L.: Dural posterior fossa AVM producing raised sagittal sinus pressure. Case report. J. Neurosurg. *46*:804, 1977.

Landman, S., and Ross, P.: Radionuclides in the diagnosis of arteriovenous malformations of the brain. Radiology *108*:635, 1973.

Leblanc, R., Ethier, R., and Little, J. R.: Computerized tomography findings in arteriovenous malformations of the brain. J. Neurosurg. *51*:765, 1979.

Lee, B. C. P., Herzberg, L., Zimmerman, R. D., and Deck, M. D. F.: MR imaging of cerebral vascular malformations. AJNR *6*:863, 1985.

Logue, V.: Angiomas of the spinal cord: Review of the pathogenesis, clinical features, and results of surgery. J. Neurol. Neurosurg. Psychiatry *42*:1, 1979.

Logue, V., and Monckton, G.: Posterior fossa angiomas. A clinical presentation of nine cases. Brain *77*:252, 1954.

Lombardi, G., and Migliavacca, F.: Angiomas of the spinal cord. Br. J. Radiol. *32*:810, 1959.

Luessenhop, A. J.: Operative treatment of arteriovenous malformations of the brain. In Morley, T. P. (ed.): *Current Controversies in Neurosurgery*. Philadelphia: W. B. Saunders Co., 1976, p. 203.

Luessenhop, A. J., and Presper, J. H.: Surgical embolization of cerebral arteriovenous malformations through internal carotid and vertebral arteries. Long-term results. J. Neurosurg. *42*:443, 1975.

Mackenzie, I.: The clinical presentation of the cerebral angioma. A review of 50 cases. Brain *78*:184, 1953.

Maehara, T., and Tasaka, A.: Cerebral venous angioma: Computerized tomography and angiographic diagnosis. Neuroradiology *16*:296, 1978.

Magidson, M. A., and Weinberg, P. E.: Spontaneous closure of a dural arteriovenous malformation. Surg. Neurol. *6*:107, 1976.

Markham, J. W.: Arteriovenous fistula of the middle meningeal artery and the greater petrosal sinus. J. Neurosurg. *18*:847, 1961.

Martin, N. A., Wilson, C. B., and Stein, B. M.: Venous and cavernous malformations. In Wilson, C. B., and Stein, B. M. (eds.): *Current Neurosurgical Practice: Intracranial Arteriovenous Malformations.* Baltimore: Williams and Wilkins, 1984.

Matthews, W. B.: The spinal bruit. Lancet *2*:1117, 1959.

McCormick, W. F., and Boulter, T. R.: Vascular malformations ("angiomas") of the dura mater. Report of two cases. J. Neurosurg. *25*:390, 1966.

Menon, D., and Weir, B.: Evaluation of cerebral blood flow in arteriovenous malformations by the Xenon 133 inhalation method. Can. J. Neurol. Sci. *6*:411, 1979.

Michels, L. G., Bentson, J. R., and Winter, J.: Computed tomography of cerebral venous angiomas. J. Comput. Assist. Tomogr. *1*:149, 1977.

Miyasaka, K., Takei, H., Nomura, M., Sugimoto, S., Aida, T., Abe, H., and Tsuru, M.: Computerized tomography findings in dural arteriovenous malformations. Report of three cases. J. Neurosurg. *53*:698, 1980.

Mori, K., Handa, H., and Mori, K.: Cavernomas in the middle fossa. Surg. Neurol. *14*:21, 1980.

Moritake, K., Handa, H., Mori, K., Ishikawa, M., Morimoto, K., and Takebe, Y.: Venous angiomas of the brain. Surg. Neurol. *14*:95, 1980.

Nellhaus, G., Haberland, C., and Hill, B. J.: Sturge-Weber disease with bilateral intracranial calcifications at birth and unusual pathologic findings. Acta Neurol. Scand. *43*:314, 1967.

Newton, T. H., and Adams, J. E.: Angiographic demonstration and nonsurgical embolization of spinal cord angioma. Radiology, *91*:873, 1968.

Newton, T. H., and Cronqvist, S.: Involvement of dural arteries in intracranial arteriovenous malformations. Radiology *93*:1071, 1969.

Newton, T. H., and Hoyt, W. F.: Dural arteriovenous shunts in the region of the cavernous sinus. Neuroradiology *1*:71, 1970.

Newton, T. H., Weidner, W., and Greitz, T.: Dural arteriovenous malformation in the posterior fossa. Radiology *90*:27, 1968.

Numaguchi, Y., Fukui, M., Miyake, E., Kishikawa, T., Ikeda, J., and Matsuura, K.: Angiographic manifestations of intracerebral cavernous hemangioma. Neuroradiology *14*:113, 1977.

Obrador, S., Soto, M., and Silvela, J.: Clinical syndromes of arteriovenous malformations of the transverse-sigmoid sinus. J. Neurol. Neurosurg. Psychiatry *38*:436, 1975.

Odom, G. L., Woodhall, B., and Margolis, G.: Spontaneous hematomyelia and angiomas of the spinal cord. J. Neurosurg. *14*:192, 1957.

Oldfield, E. H., Di Chiro, G., Quindlen, E. A., Rieth, K.

G., and Doppman, J. L.: Successful treatment of a group of spinal cord arteriovenous malformations by interruption of dural fistula. J. Neurosurg. *59*:1019, 1983.

Olivecrona, H., and Riives, J.: Arteriovenous aneurysms of the brain. Their diagnosis and treatment. Arch. Neurol. Psychiatry *59*:567, 1948.

Oliver, A. D., Wilson, C. B., and Boldrey, E. B.: Transient postprandial paresis associated with arteriovenous malformations of the spinal cord. Report of two cases. J. Neurosurg. *39*:652, 1973.

Pakarinen, S.: Arteriovenous fistula between the middle meningeal artery and the sphenoparietal sinus. A case report. J. Neurosurg. *23*:438, 1965.

Paterson, J. H., and McKissock, W.: A clinical survey of intracranial angiomas with special reference to their mode of progression and surgical treatment: A report of 110 cases. Brain *79*:233, 1956.

Perret, G., and Nishioka, H.: Report on the cooperative study of intracranial aneurysms and subarachnoid hemorrhage. Section VI. Arteriovenous malformations. J. Neurosurg. *25*:467, 1966.

Petersen J., Andersen, E. B., Dige-Petersen, H., Ahlgren, P., and Mortensen, E. L.: Intravenous radionuclide angioscintigraphy and computer tomography in cerebral arteriovenous malformations. Acta Neurol. Scand., Suppl. *94*:49, 1983.

Preissig, R. S., Preissig, S. H., and Goree, J. A.: Angiographic demonstration of a cerebral venous angioma. Case report. J. Neurosurg. *44*:628, 1976.

Ramamurthi, B., and Balasubramanian, V.: Arteriovenous malformations with a purely external carotid contribution. Report of two cases. J. Neurosurg. *25*:643, 1966.

Roberson, G. H., Kase, C. S., and Wolpow, E. R.: Telangiectases and cavernous angiomas of the brainstem: "Cryptic" vascular malformations. Report of a case. Neuroradiology *8*:83, 1974.

Roman, G., Fisher, M., Perl, D. P., and Poser, C. M.: Neurological manifestations of hereditary hemorrhagic telangiectasia (Rendu-Osler-Weber disease): Report of 2 cases and review of the literature. Ann. Neurol. *4*:130, 1978.

Romodanov, A. P., Zozulia, Y. A., and Shcheglov, V. I.: Balloon catheter occlusion of the feeding vessels of arteriovenous malformations of the brain. Zentralbl. Neurochir. *40*:21, 1979.

Rothfus, W. E., Albright, A. L., Casey, K. F., Latchaw, R. E., and Roppolo, H. M. N.: Cerebellar venous angioma: "Benign" entity? A.J.N.R. *5*:61, 1984.

Rumbaugh, C. L., and Potts, D. G.: Skull changes associated with intracranial arteriovenous malformations. Am. J. Roentgenol. Radium Ther. Nucl. Med. *98*:525, 1966.

Saito, Y., and Kobayashi, N.: Cerebral venous angiomas. Clinical evaluation and possible etiology. Radiology *139*:87, 1981.

Sansone, M. E., Liwnicz, B. H., and Mandybur, T. I.: Giant pituitary cavernous hemangioma. Case report. J. Neurosurg. *53*:124, 1980.

Scotti, L. N., Goldman, R. L., Rao, G. R., and Heinz, E. R.: Cerebral venous angioma. Neuroradiology *9*:125, 1975.

Serbinenko, F. A.: Balloon catheterization and occlusion of major cerebral vessels. J. Neurosurg. *41*:125, 1974.

Serbinenko, F. A.: Six hundred endovascular neurosurgical procedures in vascular pathology. A ten-year experience. Acta Neurochir. Suppl. *28*:310, 1979.

Simard, J. M., Garcia-Bengochea, F., Ballinger, W. E., Jr., Mickle, J. P., and Quisling, R. G.: Cavernous angioma: A review of 126 collected and 12 new clinical cases. Neurosurgery *18*:162, 1986.

Stein, B.: Arteriovenous malformations of the brain and spinal cord. In Hoff, J. (ed.): Neurosurgery volume in *Goldsmith's Practice of Surgery.* Hagerstown, MD: Harper and Row, 1979, Ch. 17, p. 1.

Sundt, T. M., and Piepgras, D. G.: The surgical approach to arteriovenous malformations of the lateral and sigmoid dural sinuses. J. Neurosurg. *59*:32, 1983.

Svien, H. J., and Baker, H. L.: Roentgenographic and surgical aspects of vascular anomalies of the spinal cord. Surg. Gynecol. Obstet. *112*:729, 1961.

Symon, L., Kuyama, H., and Kendall, B.: Dural arteriovenous malformations of the spine: Clinical features and surgical results in 55 cases. J. Neurosurg. *60*:238, 1984.

Tagle, P., Huete, I., Mendez, J., and Del Villar, S.: Intracranial cavernous angioma: Presentation and management. J. Neurosurg. *64*:720, 1986.

Tamaki, N., Fujita, K., and Yamashita, H.: Multiple arteriovenous malformations involving the scalp, dura, retina, cerebrum, and posterior fossa. Case report. J. Neurosurg. *34*:95, 1971.

Taniguchi, R. M., Goree, J. A., and Odom, G. L.: Spontaneous carotid-cavernous shunts presenting diagnostic problems. J. Neurosurg. *35*:384, 1971.

Théron, J., Newton, T. H., and Hoyt, W. F.: Unilateral retinocephalic vascular malformations. Neuroradiology *7*:185, 1974.

Thomson, J. L. G.: Aneurysm of the vein of Galen. Br. J. Radiol. *32*:680, 1959.

Valavanis, A., Wellauer, J., and Yasargil, M. G.: The radiological diagnosis of cerebral venous angioma: Cerebral angiography and computed tomography. Neuroradiology *24*:193, 1983.

Voigt, K., and Yasargil, M. G.: Cerebral cavernous haemangiomas or cavernomas. Neurochirurgia *19*:59, 1976.

Waltimo, O.: The relationship of size, density and localization of intracranial arteriovenous malformations to the type of initial symptom. J. Neurol. Sci. *19*:13, 1973.

Waltimo, O., Eistola, P., and Vuolio, M.: Brain scanning in detection of intracranial arteriovenous malformations. Acta Neurol. Scand., *49*:434, 1973.

Waltimo, O., and Putkonen, A-R.: Intellectual performance of patients with intracranial arteriovenous malformations. Brain *97*:511, 1974.

Wendling, L. R., Moore, J. S., Kieffer, S. A., Goldberg, H. I., and Latchaw, R. E.: Intracerebral venous angioma. Radiology *119*:141, 1976.

Wharen, R. E., Scheithauer, B. W., and Laws, E. R.: Thrombosed arteriovenous malformations of the brain. An important entity in the differential diagnosis of intractable focal seizure disorders. J. Neurosurg. *57*:520, 1982.

Wilson, C. B., and Cronic, F.: Traumatic arteriovenous fistulas involving middle meningeal vessels. JAMA *188*:953, 1964.

Wilson, C. B., Sang, U. H., and Domingue, J.: Microsurgical treatment of intracranial vascular malformations. J. Neurosurg. *51*:446, 1979.

Wolpert, S. M., and Stein, B. M.: Factors governing the course of emboli in the therapeutic embolization of cerebral arteriovenous malformations. Radiology *131*:125, 1979.

Wolpert, S. M., Barnett, F. J., and Prager, R. J.: Benefits of embolization without surgery for cerebral arteriovenous malformations. AJR *138*:99, 1982.

Wyburn-Mason, R.: Arteriovenous aneurysm of midbrain and retina, facial naevi and mental changes. Brain *66*:163, 1943a.

Wyburn-Mason, R.: *The Vascular Abnormalities and Tumours of the Spinal Cord and its Membranes.* London: Kimpton, 1943b.

CHAPTER SIXTEEN

Vascular Malformations of the Head and Neck

John B. Mulliken

INTRODUCTION

Mont Reid reflected that it is a wonder, not that vascular abnormalities occur, but that they do not happen more often, considering the common bed of vascular development and complex morphologic changes necessary before the final pattern is reached (Reid, 1925). Indeed, perhaps the intricate vascular anatomy of the head and neck predisposes this region to aberrations. This very same anatomy certainly complicates the management of vascular anomalies in this location.

The road to understanding cervicofacial vascular anomalies has been cluttered by fanciful names, such as "cirsoid aneurysm," "cystic hygroma," and "pulsatile nevus," as well as various eponymous designations. As emphasized in this text, the first diagnostic step is to determine whether a vascular birthmark is a malformation or a hemangioma. The second step in the algorithm is to decide whether it is a "low flow" or a "high flow" malformation. The low flow anomalies are anatomically subdivided into (1) capillary, (2) lymphatic, and (3) venous categories. The high flow lesions constitute a different anatomical class, the arteriovenous malformations, which may contain microscopic or macroscopic shunts. A vascular malformation consists of a single (predominant) vessel type, or there are combined anomalies with more than one channel type and complex interconnections.

CAPILLARY MALFORMATIONS

The simple capillary malformations are examined in detail in Chapter Ten. Dermal capillary or venular ectasia can also overlie a venous, venous-lymphatic, or arteriovenous vascular malformation. Less commonly, a port-wine stain is noted in association with a lymphatic anomaly. In these conjoined capillary lesions, it is the underlying major channel component (venous, lymphatic, or arterial) that determines the natural history and consequent management of the vascular malformation.

LYMPHATIC MALFORMATIONS

Terminology

Redenbacker is credited with the first description of a cervicofacial lymphatic malformation in 1828; he called it "ranula congenita" (Redenbacker, 1828). Wernher introduced the term "cystic hygroma," and in his 1843 monograph, he accurately described the gross pathology, noted the propensity for the head and neck region, and distinguished these lesions from branchial cleft cysts and thyroglossal duct anomalies (Wernher, 1843). Virchow considered these lesions to be tumors, capable of independent growth and proliferation (Virchow, 1863). Virchow's student Wegner dutifully proposed a histomorphologic classification for lymphatic anomalies that was closely patterned after his professor's schema for "angiomas" (Wegner, 1877). Wegner's classification remains popular today as "lymphangioma": "simplex," "cavernous," and "cystoides." The additional designation "lymphangioma circumscriptum" was introduced by Morris in 1889 to describe a localized lymphatic anomaly with vesicular skin lesions (Morris, 1889).

There is a pervasive notion that these anomalies have the potential for neoplastic growth and "recurrence" after excision. This misconception is fostered by the terms "lymphangioma" and "cystic hygroma." In a strict sense, the suffix "-oma" implies a potential for growth by cellular mitosis and invasion. Since the papers by Arnold (1865) and Koes ter (1872), the majority of authors admit that these lesions are abnormalities of lymphatic development; yet the discussion continues over whether they have proliferative capacity (Dowd, 1913; Harkins and Sabiston, 1960; Bill and Sumner, 1965; Broomhead, 1964; Baksakis, 1979).

The lymphatic anomalies have engendered other semantic problems. For example, the infelicitous hybrid terms "lymphangiohemangioma" or "hemangiolymphangioma" have been incorrectly applied to lesions that upon histologic examination have admixed lymphatic and blood-filled spaces. Instead, these lesions should be envisioned as combined vascular anomalies containing both lymphatic and venous channels. A more precise and useful designation for these lesions is either *lymphatic-venous* or *venous-lymphatic malformation*, depending on the predominant clinical presentation.

Pathogenesis

Normal Development of the Lymphatic System

In 1877, Wegner proposed three ways by which these anomalies could originate: (1) by the obliteration of efferent lymph vessels, secondary to compression, inflammation, or embryonic occlusion; (2) by the proliferation of lymphatic endothelium to form new lymph clefts; or (3) by the formation of granulation tissue into which lymphatics penetrate (Wegner, 1877). By the early nineteenth century, a lively debate in embryology was taking place on the Eastern coast of the United States that would give insight into the etiology of lym-

phatic anomalies. Working in Mall's laboratory at the Johns Hopkins Hospital and using fresh pig embryos, Florence Sabin observed that lymphatic vessels grow out into surrounding mesenchyme from lymph sacs that derive from veins (Sabin, 1902, 1904, 1905, 1909). F. H. Lewis confirmed Sabin's observations, using serially sectioned rabbit embryos; he also noted that the lymphatic sacs separated from parent veins and later made new connections (Lewis, 1905). The Sabin-Lewis studies are the basis for the *centrifugal theory* of lymphatic development. This view was challenged by the contemporaneous *centripetal theory* of Huntington and McClure. Studying cat embryos in the Princeton University Anatomy Laboratory, they concluded that lymphatic channels form from clefts in the primitive mesenchyme and then secondarily communicate with the venous system (Huntington and McClure, 1906–1907). Their theory presupposed that vascular endothelium arises independently from local mesenchyme to form the peripheral lymphatic system (Huntington and McClure, 1910; McClure, 1915). This theory was later supported by Kampmeier (Kampmeier, 1960). The investigations by van der Putte, who sectioned 40 human embryos (ages 35–65 days), confirm the centrifugal or endothelial sprouting theory of Sabin (van der Putte, 1975).

The first evidence of the cervicofacial lymphatic system in the human is the appearance of paired jugular lymph sacs in the 6 week embryo (10 mm). These sacs sprout from the primitive venous plexus between the anterior cardinal (internal jugular) veins and the subclavian veins (Fig. 16–1A). Some of these channels lose their connections with the veins, become temporarily blind sacs, and later reopen into the internal jugular veins between the sixth and seventh week (embryos, 12–14 mm) (Patten, 1968). From the seventh week onward, the jugular sacs and channels spread to connect with the subclavian (axillary) lymph sacs. This juguloaxillary complex extends caudally to anastomose with the internal thoracic, paratracheal, and thoracic duct, forming the bilateral lymphatic drainage system of the dorsal body wall. By the ninth week, the thoracic duct is a continuous channel, opening at its cephalic end into the left jugular lymphatic sac and draining into the junction of the internal jugular and subclavian veins. Extensions of the jug-

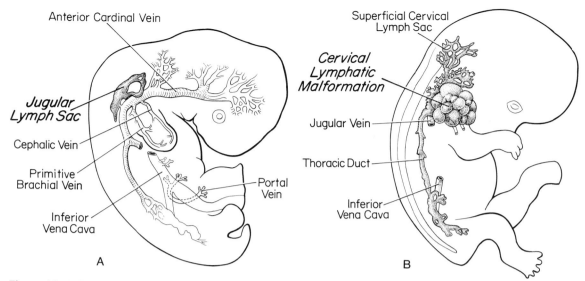

Figure 16–1. Embryology of cervical lymphatic malformation. A, Drawing to show relationship of the developing jugular lymph sac to the venous system in 10.5 mm human embryo (sixth week). (Redrawn after Sabin, F. R.: *In* Keibel, F., and Mall, F. P.: *Manual of Human Embryology*. Philadelphia, J. B. Lippincott, 1910, Vol. II.) *B*, Diagrammatic representation of cystic cervical lymphatic anomaly in 30 mm human embryo (beginning of ninth week). This may result from failure of reconnections between the jugular sac system and the internal jugular vein. (Redrawn after Sabin, F. R.: *In* Keibel, F., and Mall, F. P.: *Manual of Human Embryology*. Philadelphia, J. B. Lippincott, 1910, Vol. II.)

ular sac channels propagate into the head, neck, and upper limb and connect with lymphatic channels that have sprouted from peripheral veins.

Theories of Abnormal Development of Cervicofacial Lymphatics

By the preceding discussion, it can be envisioned that the cystic types of cervicofacial and axillary lymphatic anomalies ("cystic hygroma") are the result of maldevelopment of the primitive jugular, subclavian, and axillary sacs. This could be caused by a failure to reestablish venous connections (Fig. 16–1*B*). Later interruption of the peripheral lymphatics produces the diffuse, small channel anomalies, i.e., "lymphangiomas," lymphangiectasia, dermal-vesicular lesions, and congenital facial lymphedema. Bill and Sumner suggested that the anatomical location predetermines the various morphological types of lymphatic malformations (Bill and Sumner, 1965). Lesions occurring in areas with distinct tissue planes and loose areolar tissue are able to expand. Thus, in the neck, axilla, and mediastinum these malformations become cystic ("cystic hygroma") and insinuate along vessels and nerve trunks. In contrast, more compact lymphatic anomalies, arising in areas with restrictive tissue architecture, e.g., lips, cheeks, and tongue, cannot expand to cystic proportions; thus "lymphangiomatosis" might occur in these locations.

The Question of Postnatal Proliferation

Although the mechanism is unknown, these errors in the morphogenesis of the lymphatic system must occur sometime between the sixth and ninth week of gestation. Once established, the anomalous lymphatic spaces continue to grow and expand during late embryonic and fetal life. The debate continues over whether or not lymphatic anomalies have the capability for endothelial proliferation postnatally. Although Goetsch accepted that these are developmental lymphatic anomalies, he was convinced that the cyst walls retain their "embryonic power" for neoplastic growth (Goetsch, 1938). His microscopic sections of excised specimens were interpreted as showing proliferation of endothelial fibrillar sprouts with penetration and destruction of tissue surrounding the periphery of the lesion. Goetsch believed that this propagation and canalization to form new cysts were analogous to growth of the developing lymphatic system. Other investigators maintained that rapid growth of lymphatic anomalies is due to excessive secretion from the endothelial lining (Thompson and Keiller, 1923) and not to cellular infiltration (Singleton, 1937). Willis also disagreed with Goetsch and stated that lymphatic malformations do not grow by a proliferative invasive process, but rather expand secondary to fluid accumulation, cellulitis, or inadequate drainage of the anomalous lymphatic channels (Willis, 1960). Thymidine labelling studies of excised lymphatic anomalies do not show increased cellular turnover (Mulliken and Glowacki, 1982). Attempts to grow endothelium from tissue specimens of lymphatic anomalies using a medium and conditions favorable for capillary endothelium were unsuccessful (Mulliken et al., 1982). However, Bowman and colleagues report culture of an endothelial cell line from the lining of a congenital lymphatic cyst. These authors offer this as evidence of the possibility that a lymphatic anomaly can grow by endothelial proliferation (Bowman et al., 1984).

Histology

Microscopic studies show that the spaces of the unilocular, multilocular, and diffuse forms of lymphatic anomalies are lined with a single layer of flattened endothelium. The pale yellow fluid found in cystic lesions microscopically appears to be acidophilic and protein rich (Fig. 16–2A). Blood cells within the anomalous spaces may indicate recent hemorrhage into the specimen, or the lesion may, in fact, be a combined lymphatic-venous malformation. Mural thrombi are often noted in these combined lesions. Nodular collections of lymphocytes, including follicles with germinal centers, are frequently observed in the connective tissue surrounding a lymphatic malformation (Fig. 16–2B). The vessel walls are of variable thickness; some are quite thin, but more often the walls are fibromuscular with both striated and smooth muscle elements. The abnormal lymphatic tissue also can be seen within large nerves and the walls of local blood vessels. Sawyer and Woodruff's suggestion that the thickness and fibrosis of the cyst wall are proportionate to the patient's age has not been confirmed (Sawyer and Woodruff, 1951).

Clinical Findings

Lymphatic anomalies occur with equal frequency in both sexes and in all races (Gross, 1953). The cervicofacial location, including the axilla, is the most common, followed in frequency by the extremities and trunk (Bhattacharyya et al., 1981; Ninh and Ninh, 1974). Cystic lymphatic anomalies can be diagnosed *in utero* by ultrasonography as early as 12 weeks of gestation (Garden et al., 1986) (Fig. 16–3). The majority of lymphatic malformations are first seen in the newborn nursery. In Gross' series, 65% of lymphatic anomalies were noted at birth, 80% were manifested during the first year of life, and 90% were seen by the second year (Gross, 1953). The oldest patient in this group was age 14; however, lymphatic anomalies can also emerge in adulthood (Nussbaum and Buchwald, 1981).

Lymphatic vascular anomalies present in diverse forms, from tiny cutaneous or mucosal blebs (likened to salmon eggs or frog spawn) to large channel or multilocular lesions (Fig. 16–4). The various clinical manifestations can be explained by the diversity of abnormal channel morphology and the degree of fibrous tissue reaction, as well as the depth and extent of primary involvement. There may be generalized swelling or edema of the involved facial area, or a distinctly localized multilocular cystic lesion. The large cystic lesions are usually translucent. Occasionally these anomalies are manifested following intralesional hemorrhage as opaque, firm to tense swellings. A true neoplasm must be considered if a mass appears in the parotid region.

The cystic variety, commonly called "cystic hygroma" or "cavernous lymphangioma," most frequently occurs in the anterior cervical triangle (Ninh and Ninh, 1974). Cystic lymphatic malformations also present in the posterior cervical triangle, shoulder, axilla, and lower face, in decreasing order of frequency. Cystic anomalies can also involve the mediastinum, and radiographic examination may demonstrate displacement of the trachea, esophagus, or pharynx. This finding occurs in approximately 2% of cystic cervical anomalies (Ravitch and Rush, 1985). In addition to chest roentgenography, ultrasonography is helpful in documenting mediastinal involvement. Hemorrhage, fibrosis, and chronic inflammation can alter a cystic lym-

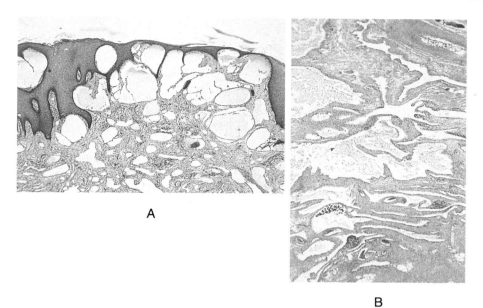

Figure 16–2. Histologic findings in lymphatic anomalies. *A,* Lymphatic malformation of cheek. Deep and superficial channels; contain pale acidophilic fluid. Epidermal involvement causes mucosal "bleb" (H&E × 10). *B,* Cervical lymphatic malformation. Both large and small channels with barely discernible endothelial lining. Fibrous walls of variable thickness; note lymphoid aggregates (H&E × 10).

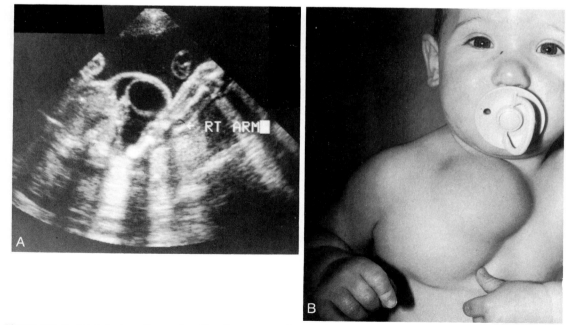

Figure 16–3. Intrauterine diagnosis with ultrasonography. *A,* Sonogram at 15 weeks gestation reveals multicystic anomaly of axillary and cervical region. *B,* Child in *A* with cystic lymphatic malformation.

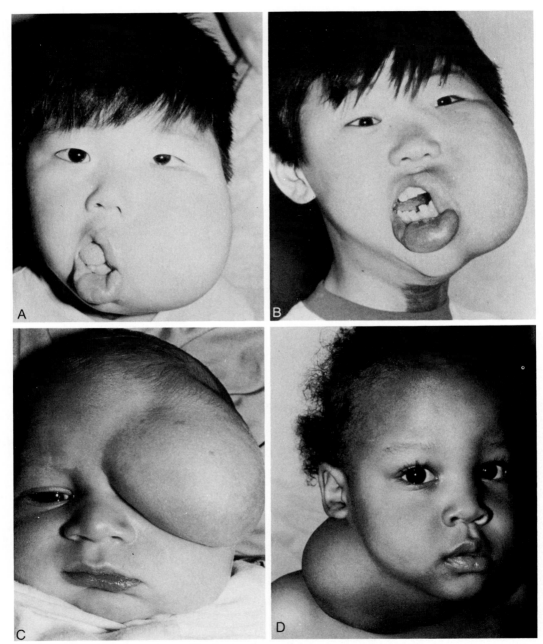

Figure 16–4. Different lymphatic malformations in head/neck region. *A,* Hemifacial anomaly in 3 year old child. Cervical pigmented nevus barely visible. *B,* Twelve years later, malformation has grown commensurately with patient shown in *A.* Note cervical nevus (congenital) and dental malocclusion. *C,* Forehead anomaly; involves adnexa oculi and intraorbital tissues and obstructs visual axis. *D,* Cervical anomaly; this common variant has a cystic quality to palpation and is easily transilluminated.

phatic anomaly of the neck and mediastinum and belie its true nature (Sumner et al., 1981).

The characteristic history of lymphatic malformations is enlargement commensurate with the child's growth (Fig. 16–4A and B). Therefore, determination of a lesion's growth pattern is the critical step to a proper diagnosis. This may require multiple office visits, retrospective study of early photographs, and other means of historical documentation. Periodic minor variations in size of a lymphatic anomaly are common, but proportionate growth is the rule. Not infrequently, however, a lymphatic malformation can suddenly expand; often this occurs coincident with an upper respiratory tract infection.

Bacterial infection (cellulitis) within a cervicocephalic lesion is a typical complication. Inflammation occurred in 16% of Ninh's series of 126 cases (Ninh and Ninh, 1974). Enlarged cervical lymph nodes are often found adjacent to and within inflamed lymphatic anomalies. It is likely that the anomalous lymphatic tissue is unable to control the periodic seeding with common oral microorganisms. The inflamed lymphatic lesion is typically tense, warm, and erythematous. Acute infection within a diffuse lymphatic abnormality of the tongue or floor of the mouth may lead to rapid enlargement and consequent upper airway obstruction and/or interference with swallowing. There are also reports of alarming respiratory distress secondary to extrinsic compression of the trachea and pulmonary parenchyma by infected lymphatic malformation (Sumner et al., 1981; Grosfeld et al., 1982). Superior vena caval obstruction, chylothorax, chylopericardium, and pulmonary hypoplasia have been reported as complications. Death may occur secondary to respiratory embarrassment and recurrent infections (Groves and Effler, 1954; Stratton and Grant, 1958; Csicsko and Grosfeld, 1974). In the pre-antibiotic era, Figi suggested that the high mortality rate in these situations accounts for the rarity of large lymphatic anomalies in adults (Figi, 1929). Repeated bouts of inflammation can cause fibrosis within the involved area, leading to further expansion of the lymphatic anomaly.

Lymphatic anomalies may also abruptly enlarge as a result of hemorrhage—this occurred in 8% of Broomhead's series of cystic cervicofacial lesions, including one fatality (Broomhead, 1964). Ninh and Ninh found evidence of hemorrhage in 12.6% of lymphatic lesions at time of excision (Ninh and Ninh, 1974).

Lymphatic anomalies of the orbit, lids, and conjunctiva present within the purview of ophthalmologists (Jakobiec and Jones, 1979). A characteristic feature of lesions in this location is exacerbation of exophthalmos concomitant with an upper respiratory tract infection. Cellulitis within a facial lymphatic anomaly can spread quickly to the orbit. Rupture and hemorrhage into lymphatic spaces can give rise to subconjunctival "chocolate cysts" or ocular proptosis. Muscle imbalance may also occur; exotropia is more frequent than esotropia.

Associated Abnormalities

Soft Tissue and Skeletal Hypertrophy

Lymphatic malformation is the most common pathological basis for a large lip (*macrochelia*), a large ear (*macrotia*), or a large tongue (*macroglossia*) (Fig. 16–5A to C). Lymphatic abnormality of the cheek tissue also causes skeletal and soft tissue hypertrophy of the malar eminence (*macromala*) and large teeth (*macrodontia*). Typically, the involved tongue is enlarged and covered with clear vesicles ("salmon eggs") or hemorrhagic vesicles ("caviar spots"). Multiple, brownish vesicopapules are seen on the buccal mucosa; these periodically exude clear or blood-stained fluid, especially when traumatized. In time, the tongue may protrude through the lips with resultant desiccation, ulceration, and necrosis (Fig. 16–5C).

Lymphatic anomalies of periorbital tissues can cause secondary expansion of the growing orbital cavity. This is probably a mass effect, similar in mechanism to that studied in rabbits (Wessely, 1920) and in transplanted newt eyes (Harrison, 1929).

Boyd and coworkers document skeletal hypertrophy and distortion in 80% of cervicofacial lymphatic lesions by age 10 (Boyd et al., 1984). This skeletal overgrowth may be noted soon after birth, and it is progressive. Typically there is maxillary and/or mandibular enlargement, resulting in prognathism, open bite, or other complex malocclusions (Fig. 16–5C and D). In one case, localized maxillary overgrowth was the presenting

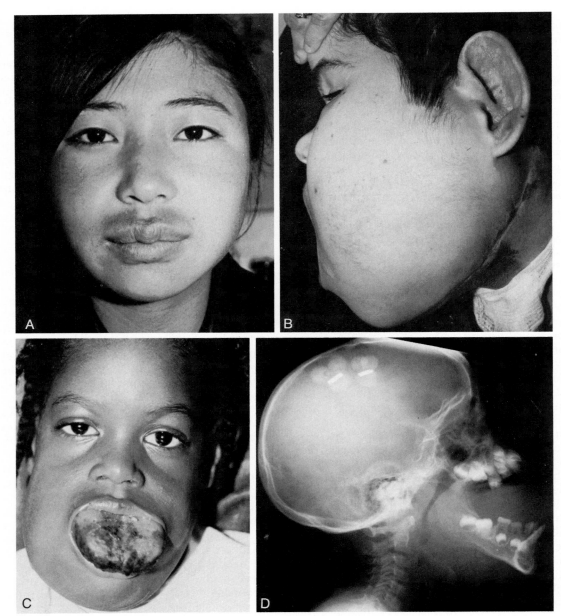

Figure 16–5. Soft tissue and skeletal changes with lymphatic malformations. *A, Macrochelia:* diffuse lymphatic anomaly of upper lip causes subtle enlargement and periodic swelling. *B, Macrotia:* diffuse lymphatic anomaly of lower face, necessitating tracheostomy. Note large auricle and enlargement of facial bones. This boy also has an epidermal nevus of the neck. *C, Macroglossia:* hemorrhagic vesicles on protruding tongue. Note mandibular prognathism with open bite. The malocclusion is, in part, secondary to the large tongue; however, skeletal enlargement also can be noted in infancy. (Courtesy of George H. Gifford, Jr., M.D.) *D,* Lateral radiograph of patient in C demonstrates mandibular overgrowth, particularly in body region.

complaint in a child; only with time, with swelling of the cheek and lip, did the lymphatic anomaly of the face become obvious. Scintigraphic studies show that these osseous changes are probably not the result of increased blood flow (Boyd et al., 1984).

There are several clues to suggest that cervicofacial lymphatic anomalies are somehow linked with abnormal development of neuroectoderm. For example, a congenital pigmented nevus is sometimes seen with lymphatic malformations and associated bone overgrowth (see Fig. 16–4B). The child shown in Figure 16–5B has a lymphatic anomaly in association with an epidermal nevus. Another clue to the puzzle is the "epidermal nevus syndrome," i.e., verrucous nevi, skeletal hypertrophy, and cutaneous and central nervous system vascular anomalies (Solomon et al., 1968). For further discussion of combined skeletal and vascular malformations, the reader is referred to Chapter Fourteen.

Midline Posterior Cervical Lymphatic Cysts and Genetic Abnormalities

There is a well-established association between cystic lymphatic lesions of the midline posterior cervical region and chromosomal abnormalities, particularly Turner's syndrome (Chervenak et al., 1983; Garden et al., 1986). This is a highly lethal anomaly that can be diagnosed by ultrasonography as early as 12–14 weeks of gestation. The sonographic hallmarks are a thin-walled, multiseptated, fluid-filled mass in the fetal head or nuchal region, located asymmetrically with respect to the long axis of the spine (Phillips and McGahan, 1981). There may be a midline septum that corresponds to the nuchal ligament (Fig. 16–6A). Fetal hydrops is seen on sonography as ascites and edematous skin (Fig. 16–6B). In this setting, amniocentesis for karyotyping is essential for parental counseling. Garden and coworkers reviewed the cytogenetic findings in published series and found that approximately one half of such fetuses had Turner's syndrome (Garden et al., 1986). There are also reports linking posterior cervical lymphatic anomalies with trisomy 18 and 21, trisomy 13, and Roberts' syndrome (Garden et al., 1986; Graham et al., 1983; Greenberg et al., 1983). The prognosis for a fetus with this complex is poor, particularly in the presence of hydrops.

Chervenak and coworkers found that 9 of 15 fetuses died either *in utero* or in the early neonatal period (Chervenak et al., 1983) (Fig. 16–6B). Of interest, Bohl reported a case of a 28 year old woman with Turner's syndrome who also had a combined extra- and intracranial lymphatic malformation involving the orbit (Bohl et al., 1981). There is no evidence that anterior cervical-axillary lymphatic anomaly is linked to aneuploidy.

The association of cystic nuchal lymphatic anomalies in hydropic fetuses was first studied by Singh and Carr (Singh and Carr, 1966) and later by van der Putte (1977). Stimulated by these papers, Graham and Smith hypothesized a "jugular lymphatic obstruction sequence" to explain the findings (Smith, 1982). They reasoned that if the jugular lymph sacs fail to communicate with the internal jugular veins, the posterior skin of the fetus would become distended. Later, with re-establishment of lymphatic-venous drainage, the jugular lymph sac would collapse, leaving a webbed neck and puffiness of the distal extremities, typical of adult Turner's syndrome patients.

Another curious correlation is that patients with Turner's syndrome may have capillary-venular ectasia of the small and large bowel (Burge et al., 1981; Rutlin et al., 1981). These vascular abnormalities can cause life-threatening gastrointestinal hemorrhage that is usually confined to childhood.

Diminution in Size

Growth, in proportion to the child, is the characteristic natural history of lymphatic anomalies of the head and neck region. No instances of spontaneous improvement were documented in a long term follow-up analysis of 122 patients with cervicofacial lymphatic anomalies (Saijo et al., 1975). Nevertheless, there are isolated reports of remarkable "regression" (Williams, 1979). Broomhead noted spontaneous resolution in 7 of 44 cases of cervical lymphatic anomalies without an intervening history of infective episodes. The improvement usually began early in life, continued steadily, and was complete by age 2 years (Broomhead, 1964). Grabb and colleagues followed 70 cases and noted improvement in 15–90% (Grabb et al., 1980). Ninh found 2 cases of shrinkage in 126 patients (Ninh and Ninh, 1974). Figure 16–7A and B

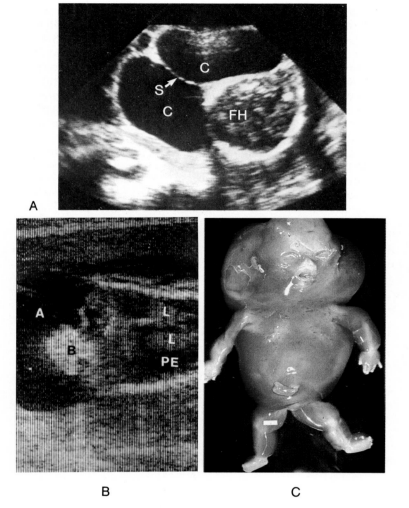

A

B   C

Figure 16–6. Lethal posterior cervical lymphatic anomaly. A, Sonogram of 22 week fetus: fetal head (FH) on the right seen as a bright, echogenic skull. Adjacent is a bilobed cystic anomaly (C) with characteristic midlne septum (S). Fetus has Turner's syndrome, lymphangiectasia, and skin edema. (Courtesy of Beryl Benacerraf, M.D.) B, Longitudinal sonogram of 18 week fetus with posterior cystic lymphatic anomaly demonstrates generalized hydrops (L = lung, PE = pleural effusion, B = bowel, A = ascites). (Courtesy of Frank A. Chervenak, M.D.) C, Postmortem 20 week fetus with posterior lymphatic anomaly of cervico-cranium; note generalized hydrops. Karyotype 45 × 0. (Courtesy of Frank A. Chervenak, M.D.)

illustrates a case of posterior cervical cystic lymphatic anomaly that literally vanished overnight and has yet to reappear! Another example is a diffuse facial lesion, seen in Figure 16–7C and D, that gradually diminished with time.

Rather than label these cases as examples of "involution" or "regression," until the mechanism is elucidated, the vague terms resolution or deflation seem more appropriate. Perhaps venous-lymphatic shunts are responsible; they have been documented in both animals and humans (Sabin, 1909; McClure and Silvester, 1909). It is also possible for drainage to occur through unobstructed lymphatic channels. Other explanations for deflation that have been proposed include rupture of cystic lesions or sclerosis

secondary to infection (Figi, 1929; Gross and Goeringer, 1939).

Treatment of Lymphatic Malformations

The litany of ministrations for lymphatic anomalies includes (1) *sclerosing injections*, e.g., boiling water (Reder, 1920), sodium morrhuate (Harrower, 1933), hypertonic salt and sugar solutions (Gross and Goeringer, 1939), iodized oil (Vaughan, 1934; MacGuire, 1935), and bleomycin (Ikeda et al., 1977); (2) *cautery* (Noyes, 1893; Crawford and Vivakananthan, 1973); and (3) *irradiation* (New, 1924; Figi, 1929; Goetsch, 1938). None of these treatments can be recommended today.

The wide variety of clinical presentations for these anomalies makes it difficult to outline specific management programs. Often, the best therapy is to do nothing for fear of causing harm. As a general therapeutic statement, infections should be treated aggressively with antibiotics, and the mainstay of management is a well-planned, well-timed, and well-executed surgical excision.

Obstruction and Sepsis

In the newborn period, a cervicofacial lesion may present with rapid enlargement of the tongue or floor of the mouth, leading to respiratory obstruction. This situation demands immediate attention to the airway. In these cases, aspiration or incision and drain-

age of a cystic sublingual lesion can be useful as an emergency maneuver (Fonkalsrud, 1974). Drainage rarely will be more than a temporizing measure because these anomalies are multilocular with poor intercommunication (Chait et al., 1974). Concurrent cellulitis should be treated with systemic antibiotics directed at gram-positive microorganisms, specifically mouth organisms (Chait et al., 1974). Not infrequently, a large cervicofacial anomaly may necessitate tracheostomy because of swelling secondary to intralesional hemorrhage or sepsis. Large anomalies may also compromise function of the tongue and upper alimentary tract, compelling the placement of a feeding tube or gastrostomy.

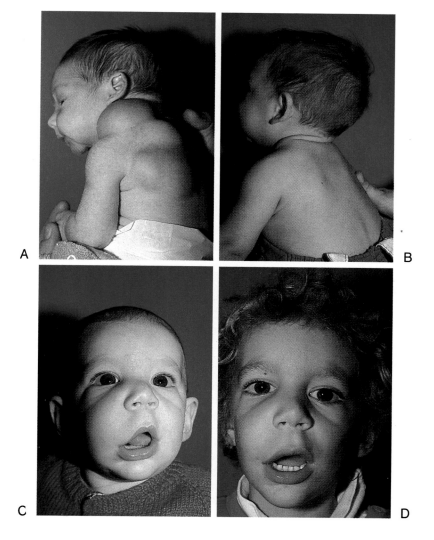

Figure 16–7. Natural shrinkage of lymphatic malformation. *A,* One month old child with multicystic lymphatic anomaly of posterior shoulder and thorax. *B,* Child in *A* at 3 months. The lymphatic anomaly "miraculously" disappeared (over a 48 hour period); now only tiny nodules can be palpated. The lesion has not re-expanded. *C,* Six month old boy with diffuse lymphatic anomaly of right face. *D,* Photograph of boy in *C* documents improvement in contour by age 4 years. The right maxilla is enlarged.

Every episode of cervicofacial swelling should be promptly treated with warm, moist soaks and penicillin—on the presumption that there is cellulitis and that intraoral organisms are responsible. In a patient who is unable to tolerate pencillin, either clindamycin or erythromycin should be used. For the older child with repeated bouts of infection, a supply of penicillin in the family medicine chest or an available prescription in the home can ensure prompt initiation of antibiotics by the parents. After the inflammation subsides, the involved area usually remains firm and edematous for a long period of time.

Carious primary teeth can be the source for bacterial contamination of a lymphatic anomaly. Dental care is an especially important prophylactic measure in these children. If the tonsils are suspected as the origin of repeated sepsis, tonsillectomy may be indicated.

Excision

The surgical management of cervicofacial lymphatic anomalies can be summarized in two words: *technique* and *timing*. Given the evidence that there is, indeed, improvement in some lesions, a plan of watchful waiting may be justified. This is particularly true for a small channel lesion with diffuse involvement throughout the face and neck, for which surgical excision is hazardous (Fig. 16–7C and D). At the other end of the spectrum, a well-localized cystic lesion is more amenable to excision and is less likely to deflate no matter how long it is observed.

The surgeon should keep in mind that a lymphatic anomaly is not neoplastic. It does not progressively invade normal tissues; rather, it typically involves adjacent tissues that are apparently normal. There are rare instances in which excision is necessary during the neonatal period. Tracheostomy can be life-saving and allows elective excision of a cervical lesion that is narrowing the upper airway. Figure 16–8C illustrates a case in which excision of a fronto-orbital lymphatic anomaly was performed during infancy in order to preserve vision. Excision should be undertaken only when the surgeon feels confident about executing the tedious dissection that is usually required. This injunction should be uppermost in mind when one is dealing with lymphatic anomalies that involve the parotid gland; seventh, tenth, and twelfth

cranial nerves; lingual nerves; and brachial plexus. A lymphatic malformation in the preauricular region requires complete exposure of the facial nerve and resection of the superficial portion of the parotid gland (Fig. 16–8A and B). The typical cervical lesion usually requires a radical neck type of dissection. Just as in cervical lymphadenectomy, the marginal mandibular branch of the facial nerve must be isolated early in the dissection. The internal jugular vein usually must be taken; sometimes the sternocleidomastoid muscle can be spared if it is not riddled with lymphatic cysts (Fig. 16–8D). All the important nerves in the neck must be identified during the course of dissection, including the vagus nerve and cervical sympathetic chain. The spinal accessory nerve and the great auricular nerve, in particular, are usually intimately adherent to the cyst walls and septa. The specimen can be divided during the course of excision in order to preserve these important nerves. Azzolini and coworkers recommend temporary occlusion of the external carotid artery during radical removal of a large cervicofacial lymphatic anomaly (Azzolini et al., 1984) (Fig. 16–9).

In fortunate cases, a well-localized cystic lesion that follows natural planes of cleavage can be removed easily with favorable long-term results (Grosfeld et al., 1982). For a large cervicofacial lesion, the resection is often incomplete, and persistent swelling is predictable. Staged excision, limiting each procedure to a defined anatomical area, is recommended for the diffuse anomaly that involves skin, subcutaneous tissue, muscle, and nerves. In the planning of such a subtotal resection, restrictions should be set, not only for the extent of dissection but also for the duration of the operation and acceptable blood loss. It is well known that repeated entry into areas previously resected becomes increasingly more difficult. Nerve damage is more likely with each procedure because dense scar tissue distorts the usual anatomical location of nerves, especially the facial, hypoglossal, lingual, phrenic, and spinal accessory.

The superficial subcutaneous-dermal lesion known as "lymphangioma circumscriptum" is usually seen in the posterior cervical area, shoulder, or axilla. It presents as multiple warty cutaneous excrescences, with repeated bleeding and often with purulent drainage and irritation. These same verru-

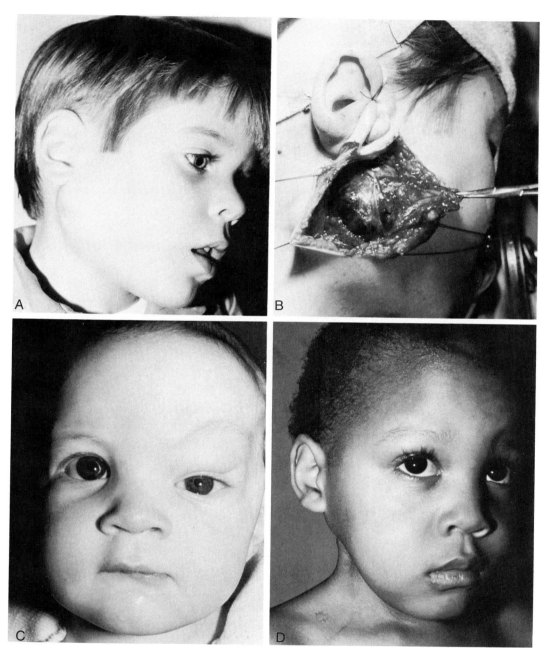

Figure 16–8. Operative treatment. *A,* Five year old boy was presented with 2 month history of rapid enlargement of right parotid mass. *B,* On exploration, hemorrhage is seen in a lymphatic anomaly within the deep portion of the parotid gland, lying beneath the seventh cranial nerve branches. Superficial portion of parotid gland is held by instrument. *C,* Following subtotal excision of forehead lymphatic malformation shown in Figure 16–4C to prevent amblyopia ex anopsia. There is a residual peri- and intraorbital anomaly. *D,* Postoperative appearance following resection of cervical lymphatic malformation seen in Figure 16–4D. The sternocleidomastoid muscle could not be preserved. (*A* and *B* reproduced by permission from Mulliken, J. B., and Murray, J. E.: Natural history of vascular birthmarks. *In* Williams, H. B. (editor): *Symposium on Vascular Malformations and Melanotic Lesions,* St. Louis, 1983, The C. V. Mosby Co., pp. 58–73.)

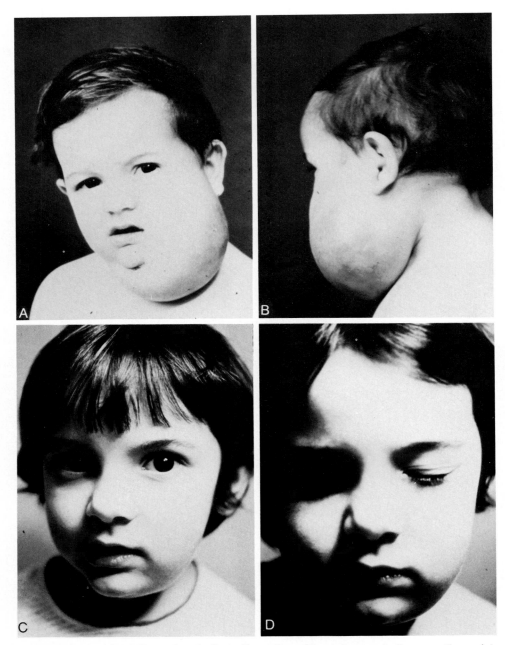

Figure 16–9. Radical excision of large lymphatic malformation without damage to the seventh cranial nerve. *A,* Cervicofacial lymphatic anomaly in 18 month old child. *B,* Oblique view showing posterior extent of lesion. *C,* Postoperative result, age 4 years. *D,* Photograph, taken during animation, demonstrating facial nerve function. (Courtesy of Prof. Alberto Azzolini.)

cous nodules also frequently occur in the surgical scar several months after subtotal excision of a lymphatic malformation. Whimster found that the abnormal superficial dermal vesicles communicate with muscle-coated lymphatic cisterns lying deep in the subcutaneous plane near the deep fascia (Whimster, 1976) (see Fig. 12–21). These cisterns fail to communicate with the deep lymphatic system. Removing only the involved skin leaves these anomalous channels behind, and recurrence of the vesicular lesions results. Whimster recommended excision of the deep tissue, preserving the superficial dermis/epidermis. More definitive treatment necessitates excision of both skin and subcutaneous tissue down to fascia. The wound usually requires primary closure with a split-thickness skin graft or a flap. Bauer suggests frozen section monitoring of the excision margin to ensure removal of abnormal tissue extending beyond the territory of skin vesicles (Bauer et al., 1981). If the abnormal lymphatic tissue is not completely removed, vesicles will appear in the linear closure scar or at the juncture of graft and skin. For this reason, Kinmonth preferred the term "lymphangioma diffusum" rather than "lymphangioma circumscriptum" for these lesions.

Operative reduction for macroglossia may be necessary to restore the tongue into the oral cavity. A vertical or transverse wedge resection of the tongue may also mitigate the development of open-bite deformity and prognathism (Dingman and Grabb, 1961). However, there is no evidence that surgical resection of a lymphatic anomaly of the tongue or cervicofacial tissues will prevent mandibular overgrowth. Recurrent vesicular excrescences in the scars of the tongue and oral mucosa are common. Argon laser can be used to coagulate oozing mucosal blebs (Apfelberg et al., 1985).

Skeletal hypertrophy and distortion may interfere with dental occlusion and cause facial asymmetry. Bone contour reduction and/or osteotomies of the craniofacial skeleton can be helpful. An orthognathic procedure may be necessary in the young adult with a malocclusion secondary to orofacial lymphatic malformation.

Complications of Lymphatic Anomalies

Common postoperative wound complications after excision of a lymphatic anomaly include serosanguineous fluid collection, prolonged serous drainage, and delayed healing. Early postoperative wound infection or delayed cellulitis within retained lymphatic tissue not infrequently occurs. In the pre-antibiotic era, postoperative infection was responsible for a high mortality rate. The postoperative mortality rate in the Gross series of 112 patients was 6% (Gross, 1953). In 126 operated cases from Children's Hospital in Saigon, there was an overall mortality rate of 3.1% (Ninh and Ninh, 1974).

An annoying late complication is the appearance of vesicular blebs bubbling into the excision scar. This is a typical healing pattern following transection of anomalous lymphatic channels. Persistent edema of the face or neck can also adversely affect the postoperative result.

The possibility of nerve damage cannot be overemphasized; facial nerve paralysis or weakness is an obvious concern. Devastating bilateral hypoglossal nerve loss may result from repeated excisions of an anterior cervical lymphatic anomaly.

Re-expansion of lymphatic cysts in the resected area may occur months to years following surgical removal of a lymphatic anomaly. Two possible mechanisms could account for this so-called "recurrence." Firstly, there may be dilatation of persistent or pre-existing channels resulting from scarring and obstruction of lymphatic drainage. Secondly, lymphatics have a remarkable ability to regenerate into healing wounds. Thus, incomplete excision may well stimulate the proliferation of lymphatic channels within the injured tissues. It remains to be proved whether or not regeneration of anomalous lymphatics can penetrate previously normal tissue. Histologic examination of a specimen removed after multiple extirpative attempts shows considerable fibrous tissue, often very thin lymphatic spaces, and no evidence of ongoing endothelial proliferation.

Enlargement of a lymphatic malformation may also be the result of hemorrhage into anomalous channels and spaces. This may occur during the natural course of a lymphatic anomaly or may happen as a late postoperative complication. Patients with dermal involvement frequently present with microscopic bleeding into lymphatic blebs. The case illustrated in Figure 16–10 raises the question of a rigid distinction between venous and lymphatic type low flow anomalies. Anytime after incomplete surgical excision, persistent lymphatic cysts can expand with venous blood, giving a grotesque appearance (Fig. 16–10C). This phenomenon may be the result of rupture of vessels in the lymphatic walls or the consequence of lymphatic-venous connections (combined low flow vascular anomaly).

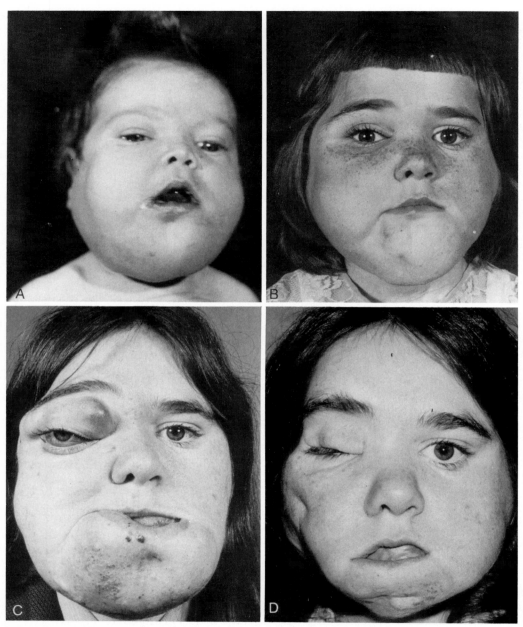

Figure 16–10. Expansion of a combined venous-lymphatic craniofacial anomaly. (Reproduced by permission from Mulliken, J. B., and Murray, J. E.: Natural history of vascular birthmarks. *In* Williams, H. B. (editor): *Symposium on Vascular Malformations and Melanotic Lesions*, St. Louis, 1983, The C. V. Mosby Co., pp. 58–73.) *A*, Infant with diffuse lymphatic malformation of lower face, floor of mouth, tongue, and neck. Treated with radiation (1800 R) and bilateral neck excision. *B*, Age 5: after multiple cervical resections. Histologic diagnosis: "cystic hygroma." *C*, Age 20: expansion of vascular malformation with overgrowth of mandible and proptosis O.D. Note hemorrhagic vesicles on chin, lip, and tongue. Multiple phleboliths are seen on plain radiographs. Angiographic studies demonstrated venous malformation of orbit, ethmoid and maxillary sinuses and lower jaw, and another low-flow vascular anomaly in right parieto-occipital cerebrum. *D*, Age 21: following two subtotal resections of combined venous-lymphatic malformation of orbit and face.

VENOUS AND COMBINED (LOW FLOW) MALFORMATIONS

Terminology

Unfortunately and erroneously, the venous anomalies have often been included under the generic mantle of "hemangioma" and labelled "cavernous hemangioma," "varicose hemangioma," or "lymphangiohemangioma." They are not true hemangiomas, because they do not demonstrate endothelial proliferation. Instead, they are developmental abnormalities of veins, dysmorphic in configuration and structure. They usually occur in pure form, or they may be combined as capillary-venous or lymphatic-venous anomalies. They are best subclassified in this manner and further described as localized or diffuse, deep or superficial.

Clinical Findings

Venous anomalies of the head and neck region present in a wide spectrum from isolated skin varicosities or ectasias, to localized spongy masses, to complex lesions permeated throughout tissue planes and involving the upper trunk and mediastinum (Fig. 16–11A to C). The skin overlying a venous malformation may appear quite normal, although more often there is a bluish hue. Combined capillary-venous malformations of the skin have a dark red to purple color. The combined lymphatic-venous lesions exhibit superficial lymphatic vesicles overlying deep venous channel anomalies.

Venous anomalies are soft, decompressible, and non-pulsatile. Venous lesions characteristically expand with a Valsalva maneuver, when the patient bends over with the head in a dependent position, or with jugular vein compression (Fig. 16–11D and E). They usually grow in proportion to the child, and they have little tendency to expand unless interfered with. Rapid enlargement may occur following injury or partial surgical resection, or may occur coincident with puberty, pregnancy, or antiovulant medication. Occasionally, following trauma, a quiescent venous abnormality may evidence arteriovenous shunting. In such a case, the anomaly must be reclassified as an arteriovenous malformation. Phlebothrombosis is common within venous anomalies, and recurrent localized pain and tenderness are frequent presenting complaints. In older lesions, phleboliths can be palpated or seen on plain film radiographic examination (Fig. 16–12A).

Microscopic examination of a resected venous anomaly often reveals fibrous organization and canalization of thrombi. Sections of a recent thrombus may demonstrate hypercellularity and mitoses as endothelium grows into the thrombosed lumen. This should not be interpreted as neoangiogenesis within the malformation, nor should it be confused with angiosarcoma. It is usually termed "pseudosarcomatous endothelial proliferation" (Jakobiec and Jones, 1979).

Venous and combined low flow anomalies may be found in skeletal muscle without involvement of the overlying skin. In a review of 393 intramuscular vascular anomalies, 13.5% presented in the head and neck region (Scott, 1957). Intramasseteric venous anomalies are the most common; Welsh and Hengerer collected 23 cases (Welsh and Hengerer, 1980). Venous malformations of the temporalis muscle are even more rare (Joehl et al., 1979). These intramuscular lesions, frequently mislabelled "hemangiomas," characteristically present before the third decade and are usually not diagnosed until operative exposure. Clinically, intramuscular venous anomalies enlarge with muscle contraction. If a presumed vascular lesion within the cheek becomes more prominent by tensing of the masseter, the anomaly may be either intramuscular or within the parotid gland (Faber et al., 1978). The diagnosis is confirmed if phleboliths are palpated or seen radiographically.

There are also rare instances of venous malformation within the cranial or facial bones. Vascular anomalies of the frontal and parietal skull are discussed in several papers (Wyke, 1949; Gupta, 1975; Kirchhoff, 1978). The principal vascular supply is from the middle meningeal artery and oftentimes the superficial temporal artery (Davis et al., 1966; Rosenbaum et al., 1969). Kanter and colleagues reviewed the literature and found 23 cases of vascular anomalies in the nasal bones (Kanter et al., 1985). There are only a few cases of tiny zygomatic vascular anomalies (Marshak, 1980; Schmidt, 1982). The most common intraosseous craniofacial location is the mandible, and less often the maxilla. These lesions are usually referred to in the oral surgery literature as "central heman-

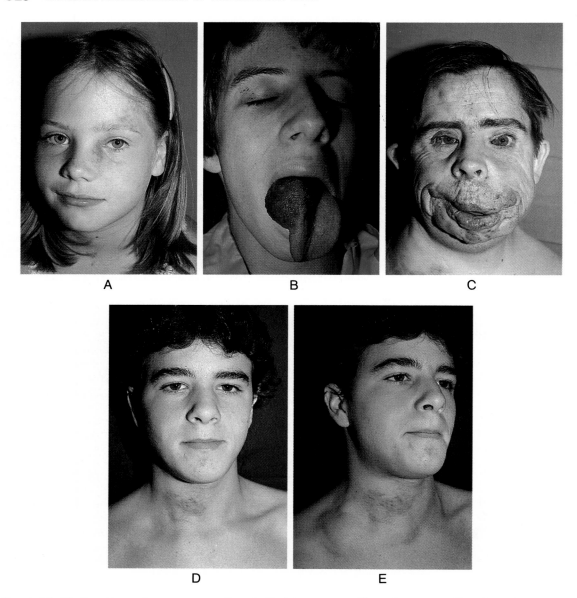

Figure 16–11. Spectrum of venous anomalies. *A,* Facial venous malformation, a manifestation of the blue-rubber bleb syndrome. Erosion of the outer cortex of the temporoparietal cranium can be palpated. See Figure 11–8*E* for the extremity lesions in this young girl. *B,* Localized venous malformations of the tongue. *C,* Diffuse venous anomaly involves face, including mandible, trunk, and extremities. *D,* Cervical venous malformation with telangiectatic vessels in overlying skin. *E,* Malformation more obvious with Valsalva maneuver.

gioma" (Sadowsky et al., 1981). The majority of reported cases are venous in type, although arteriovenous anomalies in the mandible have also been documented (Hoey et al., 1970; Kaban and Mulliken, 1986). The venous lesions usually appear in the second decade as painless, slowly growing jaw masses. There may also be increased mobility of teeth, expansion of the buccal cortex, or spontaneous bleeding around the gingival necks of the teeth; these lesions seldom cause paresthesia (Sadowsky et al., 1981). Unexpected hemorrhage can follow tooth extraction or intervention for biopsy. The bleeding may be either from the intraosseous vascular malformation or secondary to a localized coagulopathy, as a result of stasis within the venous anomaly (Kaban and Mulliken, 1986).

The radiographic appearance of the craniofacial intraosseous vascular anomalies is usually pathognomonic (Sherman and Wilner, 1961). Plain films demonstrate a local rarefied area with a "soap bubble" or "honeycomb" appearance, reflecting the venous sinuses, supported by connective tissue stroma and bony trabeculae (Fig. 16–12B). Profile or tangential films show spicules of bone radiating in a "sunburst" pattern. Computed tomography helps demonstrate intact periosteum, cortical expansion, and the bone trabeculae within the anomaly. Bone erosion is more typical of an arteriovenous anomaly.

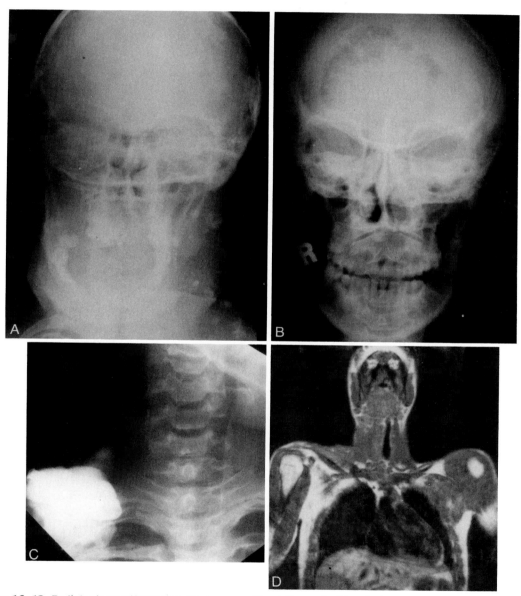

Figure 16–12. Radiologic manifestations of venous malformations. *A,* AP cephalogram of patient in Figure 16–11C demonstrates multiple bilateral phleboliths, characteristic of venous malformation. Also note extensive erosion of mandible. *B,* Venous malformation of frontal bone exhibits characteristic "honeycomb" or "sunburst" pattern. *C,* Direct intralesional dye injection of vascular anomaly in Figure 16–11D shows large multilocular venous malformation involving brachial plexus; however, it fails to fill more proximal channels in neck. *D,* Magnetic resonance image demonstrates that the venous anomaly in Figure 16–11D is more extensive, involving cervical and hypopharyngeal areas and deviating the trachea.

Skeletal alteration without actual intraosseous involvement frequently occurs in association with cutaneous venous anomalies, particularly in combined lymphatic-venous forms. Bone distortion and hypertrophy are the most commonly seen patterns (Boyd et al., 1984). Hypertrophy of the facial bones also occurs in various complex vascular anomalies, e.g., Sturge-Weber, Proteus, and epidermal nevus syndromes.

Treatment of Venous and Combined Low Flow Anomalies

Venous malformations have been assailed with *irradiation, electrocoagulation* (Figi, 1948), and *freezing techniques* (Goldwyn and Rosoff, 1969; Huang et al., 1972; Jarzab, 1975; Ohtsuka et al., 1980). *Intravascular magnesium needles* (Wilflingseder et al., 1981) have been tried, as well as a long list of *sclerosants*: boiling water (Wyeth, 1903; Cole and Hunt, 1949), alcohol, solutions of sodium salicylate, sodium morrhuate, quinine, urethan (solution of quinine and ethyl carbamate), silver nitrate, and iron or zinc chloride (Bowman, 1940).

Total excision is the definitive treatment for cervicofacial venous anomalies. Although this may be very successful in dealing with small to moderate-sized lesions, all too often only subtotal or contour resection is possible. Intralesional sclerotherapy by direct percutaneous injection is an old modality that presently appears to have an expanding role. Argon laser coagulation is useful only for the tiny lesions located in the upper 1.5 mm of the dermis.

The steps in planning therapy are (1) determine the lesion's rheologic character, (2) delineate the anatomical boundaries and channel size, and (3) evaluate the coagulation parameters. Does the vascular anomaly belong in the low flow category, i.e., capillary, venous, or lymphatic-venous? For the pure venous or capillary-venous anomaly, direct venography under fluoroscopic control is the best way to document the anatomy of the lesion (Boxt et al., 1983). It should be kept in mind that the actual extent of the lesion may be underestimated if there is incomplete filling of all of the abnormal veins or sinusoids that constitute the malformation (Fig. 16–12C). Arteriography, either a selective or a superselective study, may be necessary to rule out an arterial component manifested by microarteriovenous shunting. In a large venous anomaly, superselective angiography may demonstrate the entire lesion, but only if sufficient contrast material is injected over a relatively long period of time. In such a case, there should be no abnormal "feeding" arteries seen. Delayed films show saccular pooling of the contrast material, often just in a portion of the lesion. It is for this reason that direct percutaneous injection of contrast material may be necessary. Digital subtraction angiography, although not yet employed in a large clinical series, is a helpful technique for delineation of anomalous venous anatomy. Magnetic resonance imaging is just beginning to be applied to the study of vascular anomalies (Fig. 16–12D).

Localized Intravascular Coagulopathy

Large or extensive venous anomalies are frequently associated with a low grade localized intravascular coagulopathy. A thorough hematologic evaluation should be carried out. PT and PTT are often within normal limits; fibrin split products and fibrinopeptide-A may be elevated, with concomitant decreased fibrinogen and platelet levels. Unless the coagulopathy is corrected preoperatively, even dental extraction in the presence of gingival venous lesions can result in life-threatening hemorrhage. Severe systemic consumption coagulopathy may require heparin therapy before a surgical procedure can be safely performed. Another approach is to begin heparin first, and follow with antifibrinolytic therapy using episilon-aminocaproic acid. Warrell and Kempin report that aminocaproic acid combined with cryoprecipitate is effective therapy for localized coagulopathy and also resulted in thrombosis and shrinkage of an extensive venous anomaly of the chest wall (Warrell and Kempin, 1985).

Resection

Total excision of the venous anomaly is the therapeutic goal. Usually, venous anomalies are extensive, and surgical removal must be restrained by anatomical considerations, both aesthetic and functional. Subtotal resection always carries a risk of postoperative expansion of remaining malformed channels—often incorrectly called "recurrence." The patient seen in Figure 16–13 illustrates this problem. He presented with massive in-

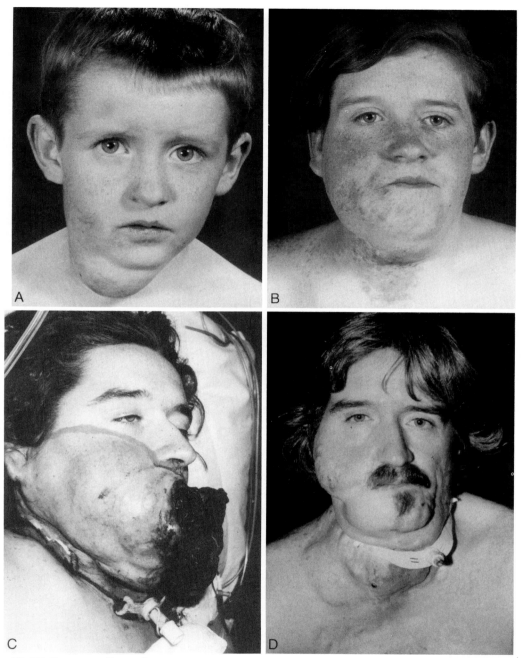

Figure 16–13. Venous malformation: a temporary solution to an insoluble problem. (From Mulliken, J. B., et al.: Surg. Gynec. Obstet. *146:*168, 1978. By permission of Surgery, Gynecology & Obstetrics.) *A,* Six year old boy with venous anomaly of cervicofacial area. *B,* Age 13, after several partial excisions; lesion continues to enlarge. *C,* Age 20; patient presented, following dental extraction, with uncontrolled hemorrhage from mouth. Note massive enlargement of tongue. He required emergency tracheostomy and semi-emergent resection of oral floor and cheek under cardiopulmonary bypass and deep hypothermic arrest. *D,* Reconstruction with tubed abdominal flap, migrated to cheek. Venous malformation continued to expand, in mediastinum, deviating trachea. This courageous man died at age 33.

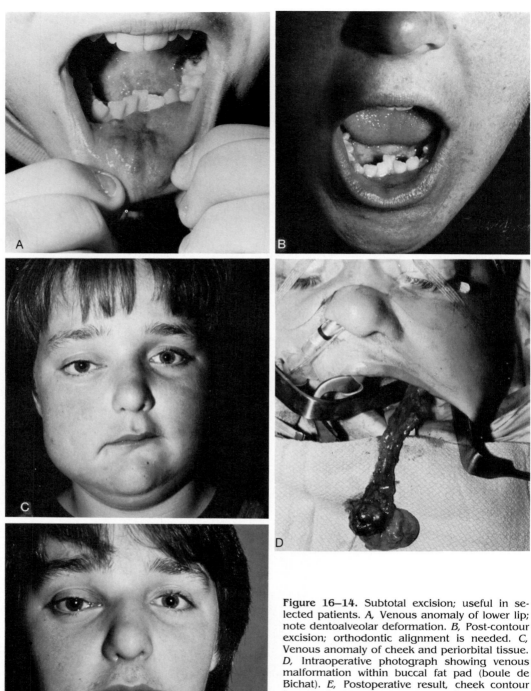

Figure 16–14. Subtotal excision; useful in selected patients. *A,* Venous anomaly of lower lip; note dentoalveolar deformation. *B,* Post-contour excision; orthodontic alignment is needed. *C,* Venous anomaly of cheek and periorbital tissue. *D,* Intraoperative photograph showing venous malformation within buccal fat pad (boule de Bichat). *E,* Postoperative result, cheek contour improved; venous anomaly remains in subconjunctival and periorbital tissues. There is secondary orbital enlargement.

traoral bleeding that could only be controlled by extensive resection with the patient under hypothermic cardiopulmonary bypass (Mulliken et al., 1978). In the years following flap reconstruction of the face and neck, the venous anomaly continued to expand inexorably and was eventually fatal. This extensive venous anomaly may have contained microscopic arteriovenous shunts that were not documented, even with selective angiography.

Subtotal removal can usually be safely accomplished in selected cases of venous, lymphatic-venous, and capillary-venous lesions. Resection is indicated to reduce bulk and improve contour and function—for example, a lesion that interferes with dental occlusion (Fig. 16–14A and B). In some instances, limited excision is necessary to treat painful areas. Removal of a venous anomaly within the buccal fat pad will improve cheek contour (Fig. 16–14C and E). Excision with CO_2 laser has been useful for small oral mucosal venous lesions (Apfelberg et al., 1985).

Resection is also the ideal treatment of venous anomalies of the craniofacial skeleton. Total excision is usually possible for low flow lesions of the skull, followed by primary or secondary cranioplasty (Kirchhoff, 1978). There is a reported case in which a girl's headaches and petit mal epilepsy were cured by removal of a venous anomaly of the scalp and outer table of calvaria (Wojtanowski and Mandel, 1979). Venous malformations of the zygoma, nasal bones, or jaws can usually be

managed by curettage and packing with hemostatic material.

Bone hypertrophy and distortion secondary to venous or lymphatic-venous anomalies are managed by craniomaxillofacial procedures. The soft tissue deformity may be treated prior to, or after, the skeletal correction.

Sclerosant Therapy

Selective angiography and embolization techniques have a deserved place in the management of arteriovenous anomalies. However, embolic occlusion of the arterial inflow to a venous anomaly often causes necrosis of adjacent tissue and overlying skin (Demuth et al., 1984). A far more appealing concept is direct injection of the sclerosing solution into the epicenter of a venous anomaly while the arterial inflow and venous outflow are occluded.

Endovascular obliteration of these anomalies has had a past history of checkered success. Older sclerosing agents, including sodium morrhuate and ethyl carbamate (urethan), have not been particularly successful, except for small local ectasias (Morgan and Schow, 1974). A newer material, Ethibloc (Ethicon Laboratories), has been used extensively in France and Germany and appears to be particularly effective for capillary-venous anomalies (Riché et al., 1983) (see Chapter Twenty-One) (Fig. 16–15A and B). Sodium tetradecyl sulfate (United States),

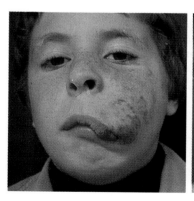
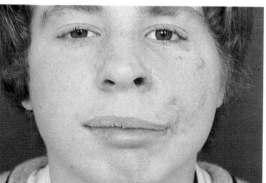

A   B

Figure 16–15. Sclerosant therapy of venous malformation. A, Ethibloc treatment. Sixteen year old male with capillary-venous malformation of upper lip and left cheek. B, Result after single Ethibloc injection and excision through melolabial fold, 2 years postoperative. (From Riché, M. C., et al.: Treatment of capillary-venous malformations using a new fibrosing agent. Plast. Reconstr. Surg. 71:607, 1983.)

ethanolamine oleate (Great Britain), and polidocanol (Germany) are successfully used for endovascular obliteration of esophageal varices (Brooks, 1984). The injection of sodium tetradecyl sulfate for congenital venous anomalies is reported in a small number of patients (Minkow et al., 1979; Woods, 1987). Ethanol sclerotherapy is also at the stage of clinical investigation (Lasjaunias, 1984).

A clinical trial using percutaneous electrodes to induce thrombosis within facial vascular anomalies is reported by Ogawa and Inoue (Ogawa and Inoue, 1982). Photocoagulation with argon or yttrium aluminum garnet (YAG) laser may be effective for small superficial venous or capillary-venous lesions.

ARTERIOVENOUS MALFORMATIONS

Terminology

The studies of acquired aneurysm by William and John Hunter undoubtedly influenced their fellow Scotsman John Bell. It was he who coined the term "aneurysm by anastomosis" (Bell, 1815), a term that later became synonymous with "pulsating angioma," "racemose aneurysm," "cirsoid aneurysm," and "fungus hematodes." Nineteenth century physicians were well aware of the "malignant" behavior of these pulsatile birthmarks, in contrast to the benign *naevi materni*. The congenital "aneurysm by anastomosis" was feared because of its propensity for hemorrhage, ulceration, and rapid enlargement, particularly following attempted extirpation. However, this old concept, that these lesions are neoplastic tumors capable of independent growth and even metastases, must be laid to rest. These anomalies enlarge, not by cellular hyperplasia but by hemodynamic mechanisms. An arteriovenous malformation, with its multiple, low resistance shunts, acts to siphon regional blood flow and thus promote collateral formation and dilatation of abnormal as well as normal adjacent vasculature.

Clinical Findings

Arteriovenous malformations of the head and neck region are quite rare in contrast to low flow vascular anomalies. The largest series of 15 cases was reported by Malan and

Azzolini in 1968 (Malan and Azzolini, 1968). The other well-known papers on this subject are based on an experience with 6 cases or less (Callander, 1920; Reid, 1925a; Pemberton and Saint, 1928; Coleman and Hoopes, 1971). Arteriovenous malformations are 20-fold more common in the intracerebral vasculature than in extracerebral sites (Olivecrona and Ladenheim, 1957).

Cervicofacial arteriovenous anomalies are sometimes noted soon after birth. Usually, years may go by before they pose a threat to the patient as the signs and symptoms of their high flow nature become ominous. Typically these anomalies grow proportionately during childhood, and many go unnoticed. Then there is rapid expansion following local trauma, attempted excision/ligation, or hormonal changes associated with puberty or pregnancy. Some lesions lie hidden within the masticatory muscles or beneath an innocent-appearing cutaneous stain. The fistulae, particularly those in the cheek and mastoid area, produce murmurs that because of their location are best heard by the patient. A distressing *buzzing sound* in the ears was present in 6 of 15 patients with craniofacial arteriovenous malformations reported by Malan and Azzolini (1968). A rhythmic throbbing sensation is also common in patients with vertebral artery arteriovenous malformations (Lawson and Newton, 1970; Storrs and King, 1973). This blowing sound often prevents concentration or deprives the patient of sleep (Coleman, 1973). *Pain,* frequently sudden and stabbing in nature, can also be very distressing to the patient (Malan and Azzolini, 1968). Malan and Azzolini speculate that this type of pain is due to congestion in the vascular malformation. Perhaps the pain is caused by encroachment on sensory nerves. Coleman also finds pain to be a common presenting complaint, especially when the vascular anomaly lies within the facial bones (Coleman, 1973). He also notes cases of toothache and earache associated with trismus, implicating intraosseous fistulae of the mandible. Coleman also reports on manifestations of internal carotid involvement, causing repeated epistaxis in one case; and in another, blurred vision, progressing to thrombosis of the retinal artery (Coleman, 1973).

The involved skin has an *elevated temperature*, and frequently dermal staining is obvious. Palpation reveals a *thrill*, often transmitted along the vessels of the ipsilateral side of the neck and head. In older lesions, pulsating veins, congestion, and tortuosity of the abnormal vessels may be seen. The presence of a *bruit* on auscultation, a constant machinery-like murmur that is accentuated during systole, confirms arteriovenous shunting in the vascular anomaly.

There are rare cases in which a patient with congenital arteriovenous fistulae may present with *congestive heart failure* in infancy (Norman et al., 1950). Usually it requires years for the patient to manifest the physiological effects of an increased load on the heart. Arteriovenous shunting can diminish nutritive flow to the skin, so that *ischemic necrosis* occurs. Repeated episodes of *hemorrhage*, often precipitous, following minor trauma may lead to a life-threatening emergency.

Destruction of adjacent osseous structures and/or actual bone involvement also occurs with facial arteriovenous anomalies. When located in the mandible or maxilla, these anomalies have been referred to as "central" or "pulsating" "hemangioma." These may be asymptomatic or may present with pulsatile swelling in the jaw, localized throbbing pain, or unexpected hemorrhage. The radiographic finding may be an ill-defined radiolucency or a well-defined multilocular lesion, quite similar to a low flow venous jaw anomaly. There is an entity called "unilateral retinocephalic" facial vascular anomaly with involvement of the nose, maxilla, or mandible, along with the retina and anterior cranial fossa (Théron et al., 1974). This is called the Wyburn-Mason syndrome or Bonnet-Dechaume-Blanc syndrome and is discussed further in Chapter Fifteen.

Disseminated intravascular coagulation, secondary to thrombotic consumption or destruction of clotting factors, may be a chronic problem with large arteriovenous anomalies.

Pathogenesis

Arteriovenous malformations were not overlooked during those remarkable early years at the Johns Hopkins Hospital and the School of Medicine. Florence Sabin was fascinated by the subject of growth and morphogenesis of the cervicofacial vasculature (Fig. 16–16). Sabin wrote to Halsted, upon his request, to tell him about her observations

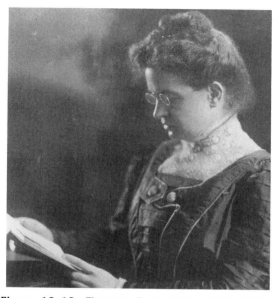

Figure 16–16. Florence Rena Sabin (1871–1953) made original contributions to our knowledge of blood vessel development, particularly that lymphatics arise from veins by endothelial sprouting. She was the first woman professor at the Johns Hopkins Medical School (1917) and the first woman elected to the National Academy of Sciences (1925). (Courtesy of the Alan Mason Chesney Medical Archives of The Johns Hopkins Medical Institutions.)

on the development of head and neck vasculature in pig embryos (Halsted, 1919). Sabin pointed out that during the embryonic period, vessels that once served as primitive arteries may become veins, and *vice versa*. She also noted that there are evanescent communications between the middle segment of the internal jugular vein and the internal carotid artery. Sabin concluded her letter to Halsted: ". . . the underlying principle that arteries and veins develop out of a common capillary plexus forms the basis for the persistence of direct connections between them" (Halsted, 1919). Later, Woollard also observed these multiple connections between the subclavian artery and vein during embryonic development (Woollard, 1922).

Halsted's last resident, William Reinhoff, examined pig embryos after injection of India ink, noting multiple communications between the internal carotid arteries and the anterior cardinal veins (Fig. 16–17). He also cultured chick embryonic tissue and watched the *in vitro* development of the primitive capillary network of the *area vasculosa*. In a letter to Reinhoff, Sabin had described ex-

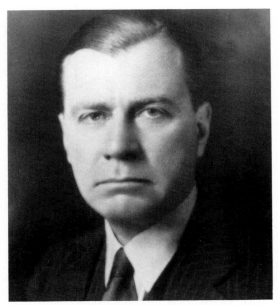

Figure 16–17. William Francis Reinhoff, Jr. (1894–1981), inquisitive Johns Hopkins surgeon best known for clinicopathologic research in hyperthyroidism. He should also be remembered for his embryologic studies of vascular anomalies and his clear perception that these lesions are errors of vascular morphogenesis. (Courtesy of the Alan Mason Chesney Medical Archives of The Johns Hopkins Medical Institutions.)

changes in the vessel walls, specifically dilatation of the proximal artery and progressive fibrosis, thinning of the media, and diminished elastic tissue. Even more remarkable was hyperplasia, thinning, and dilatation of the involved veins that are subjected to increased pressure (Reid, 1925b). Microscopic sections of the veins revealed increased smooth muscle within the media, intimal thickening, and dilatation of the vasa vasorum. Reid believed that these thin-walled arteries and veins could rupture into one another, forming new fistulous channels. This was his explanation for the rapid enlargement of arteriovenous anomalies that occurs following trauma or during pregnancy (Reid, 1925c). He also speculated that arteriovenous anomalies of the scalp may originate from pressure exerted on the skull during childbirth (Reid, 1925b).

Physiology

Our understanding of the natural history of congenital arteriovenous malformations is

periments she had performed with Cunningham, in which they produced an arteriovenous fistula in the *area vasculosa* between the chick omphalomesenteric artery and vein, using broth culture of *Bacillus typhosus* (Reinhoff, 1924). Reinhoff tried various "methods of irritation," but he was unable to induce a vascular malformation *in vivo*. Based on his observations, Reinhoff espoused the theory that arteriovenous malformations were abnormalities of normal embryonic vascular connections that could be arterial, venous, or combined arteriovenous in type (Reinhoff, 1924). Reinhoff's microscopic studies of surgical specimens showed "not the slightest suggestion of a new growth of blood vessels in the sense of a neoplasm." He pleaded that investigators discard the confusing and inaccurate terms such as "aneurysm by anastomosis," "cirsoid aneurysm," "venous tumor," and "pulsating nevus."

Mont Reid, another Halsted resident, is the third Hopkins contributor to our understanding of cervicofacial arteriovenous malformations (Fig. 16–18). He observed that with time these anomalies demonstrate

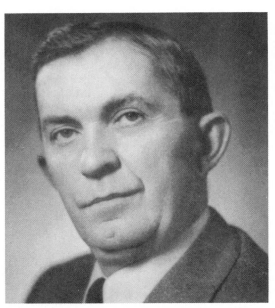

Figure 16–18. Mont Rogers Reid (1889–1943) was stimulated to study vascular malformations while a resident under W. S. Halsted at the Johns Hopkins Hospital (1912–1922). His classic papers, published in 1925, describe the clinical findings and pathophysiology of congenital arteriovenous communications. He maintained his interest in the surgery of large vessels during a distinguished career at the University of Cincinnati.

aided by examination of post-traumatic and artificially constructed arteriovenous fistulae. These studies are found in the classic monograph by Emile Holman (Holman, 1968) and in papers by Pemberton and Saint (1928) and by Reid (1925b). To some degree, congenital fistulae physiologically resemble the acquired lesions. There are differences, as Holman points out; for example, congenital fistulae are more numerous and often microscopic in size, in comparison with acquired connections (Holman, 1968). Nevertheless, just as in acquired fistulae, congenital fistulae, over a long period of time, can cause cardiac enlargement as a result of the direct communication between the high resistance, high pressure, arterial system and the low pressure, low resistance venous system. The fistulae enlarge slowly and the distal vascular bed dilates as more blood is sequestered into the fistulous circuits, causing distension of the fistulae and communicating veins. The involved arteries gradually dilate further (perhaps their walls are structurally faulty), and they become more tortuous. The veins dilate as well. In fact, most authors agree that the dilated and tortuous vessels ("cirsoid aneurysm") are veins rather than arteries (Reid, 1925b). Malan used the term "angiectatic action" for this process (Malan and Azzolini, 1968). With time, cardiac output increases to keep up with the demand; blood volume also increases, and heart failure may ensue. Just as William Hunter demonstrated, arteriovenous fistulae stimulate the development of collateral circulation in the area. If the fistulae between the arterial and venous circuit are quickly occluded, the heart slows—the bradycardiac phenomenon was first observed by Nicoladoni in 1875 (Nicoladoni, 1875). This reflex is difficult to elicit in a head/neck vascular anomaly, particularly one in which numerous small fistulae exist.

Treatment

The management of craniocervicofacial arteriovenous anomalies is hazardous, and the results are frequently disappointing. Therefore, it is usually not wise to tackle a high flow anomaly that is quiescent. The patient should be seen periodically and warned about danger signs and how to avoid trauma to the region. Therapy for a purely cosmetic deformity may have to be postponed until more serious complications arise. Intervention is indicated for life-threatening problems such as repeated hemorrhage, pain, pressure, ischemic ulceration, and heart failure. The therapeutic strategy for these lesions is (1) selective embolization, (2) surgical removal, or (3) a combination of both.

Angiography

Angiography is absolutely necessary before one embarks on a management plan. Malan and Azzolini emphasize that the complicated anatomy and rapid flow in these anomalies make radiographic visualization of microarteriovenous fistulae difficult (Malan and Azzolini, 1968). There is a rheologic tendency for contrast medium to shunt preferentially through the most proximal arteriovenous fistulae and fail to demonstrate the more peripheral fistulae. Failure to recognize minor arterial feeders may also relate to a "washout" phenomenon, owing to dye dilution within large pools of non-opacified blood in the malformation (Storrs and King, 1973). In addition, many of the shunts may be nonfunctional at the time of arteriography. Malan and Azzolini list five indirect radiographic signs of arteriovenous fistulae in head/neck vascular anomalies (Malan and Azzolini, 1968):

1. Dilatation and lengthening of afferent arteries
2. Early and preferential flow of contrast medium toward the shunts
3. Delayed and diminished filling of the other arteries originating from the external carotid artery
4. Early opacification of the efferent veins, the visualization beginning at the level of the proximal fistulae
5. Abnormal and rapid opacification of the collateral circulation

Because the complex facial skeleton obscures the vascular anatomy, subtraction techniques and selective angiography are helpful to the radiographic assessment. In case a major vessel may need to be sacrificed, the study must include the intracerebral circulation in order to assess the possibility of shunting between the external and internal carotid systems, flow within the circle of Willis, and relative contributions of the vertebral and internal carotid vessels.

Operative Management

The Fallacy of Proximal Ligation. Operative management of a cervicofacial arteriovenous malformation is, and always has been, a daunting challenge. The oldest surgical approach to these lesions can be traced to John Hunter's successful ligation for degenerative popliteal aneurysm (Home, 1793). John Bell halfheartedly tried local ligatures for "aneurysm by anastomosis" (Bell, 1815), and there are reported cases in which figure-of-eight sutures were used by Brodie (1829), Scarpa (1830), and Warren (1867). Proximal ligation was more successfully applied in cases of mycotic, atherosclerotic, syphilitic, or post-traumatic aneurysm throughout the nineteenth and early twentieth centuries. There is a direct tutorial lineage of proximal ligators from Hunter to his pupil Astley Cooper, who, in turn, trained the Americans John Collins Warren and Valentine Mott. In 1845, Warren's son, Jonathan Mason Warren, employed proximal carotid ligation for a "remarkable erectile tumor" (a term he learned from Dupuytren) (Warren, 1846). The color lithographs accompanying this article show an extraordinary result in the short term evaluation (Fig. 16–19).

Halsted reported a case of ligation of anomalous communications between the external carotid and venous cervical plexus (Halsted, 1919). The first procedure was in 1911; the patient was operated upon again in 1918 for persistent fistulae by Mont Reid (in Halsted's presence); and 48 years later, *en bloc* resection was performed by Ravitch (Ravitch and Gaertner, 1960). Reinhoff apparently cured a unique patient by ligating eight anomalous communicating channels between the external carotid artery and external jugular vein (Reinhoff, 1924). Gerbode and Holman tried ligation and a transarterial embolus of sternocleidomastoid muscle to occlude a congenital fistula between the internal maxillary artery and pterygoid venous plexus in a 6 year old girl (Gerbode and Holman, 1947). A faint bruit was still heard 2 months postoperatively. Clay and Blalock were reluctant to resect an arteriovenous malformation within the mandible; instead, they simply excised an anomalous feeding vessel originating from the external carotid artery (Clay and Blalock, 1950).

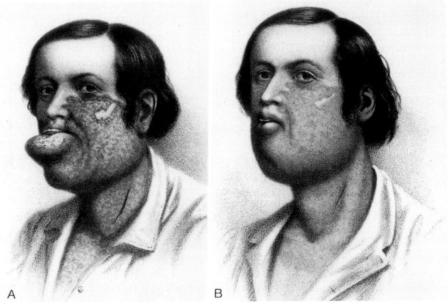

Figure 16–19. *A,* Jonathan Mason Warren's case of "A Remarkable Erectile Tumor." A 23 year old Maine man with vascular anomaly of the face, present since birth, presented with enlargement and ulceration. After consultation with his father, Dr. John C. Warren, Mason Warren tied the left carotid on October 5, the right carotid on November 7, then performed V-excision of the lip on November 26, 1845. *B,* Post-operative lithograph, December 1845. A later follow-up evaluation would probably not be so remarkable. (From Warren, J. M.: *Surgical Observations, etc.,* 1867.)

Such cases of isolated arteriovenous fistulae, potentially curable by ligation, are exceedingly rare. In fact, the hunterian concept of proximal ligation for treatment of arteriovenous malformations proved to be disastrous. John Hunter surely could have predicted this, for he was well aware of the potential for collateral circulation (Fig. 16–20). In 1785, Hunter, who had just suffered another heart attack, undertook an investigation of how antlers are shed and regrown each year. His first experiment was to ligate the carotid artery in a young stag snared in Richmond Park, a privilege accorded to Hunter by George III. He expected that the cold antler, corresponding to the ligated artery, would soon wither. Instead, one week later, he was astonished to find that the antler was warm again and growing. He ordered the stag killed. His dissection revealed that the ligature was intact and that collateral vessels had enlarged above and below the ligature. From this simple observation, Hunter deduced the principle of collateral circulation: that small tributary arteries, under the "stimulus of necessity," will assume the function of a larger vessel (Kobler, 1960).

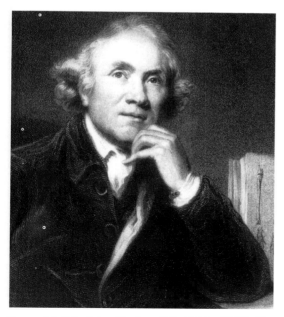

Figure 16–20. John Hunter, FRS (1728–1793). The father of scientific surgery would not want to be remembered for the technique of proximal ligation, but rather for his experimental demonstration of the principle of collateral circulation. (Engraving by W. Hall, from the 1786 portrait by Sir Joshua Reynolds.)

Interruption of the external carotid artery results in a pressure drop in the distal branches and causes collateral formation and diversion of flow from the internal carotid artery system in a retrograde direction. This occurs particularly in the ophthalmic artery, because it is the most direct channel and has the greatest number of communications with the external carotid system. This "steal phenomenon" also occurs, to a lesser degree, from other anastomotic branches, particularly the meningeal arteries. With time, the arteriovenous malformation becomes larger and more expansive than ever, as collateral channels open from ipsilateral as well as contralateral vessels. Azzolini and Lechi recount two cases of severe atherosclerotic lesions in the supratentorial internal carotid system, in both the main trunk and intracranial branches, following such ill-advised ligation of the external carotid system (Azzolini and Lechi, 1968). They also report two cases in which carotid interruption caused chronic hemispherical ischemia and frank cerebral atrophy (Azzolini and Lechi, 1968). Horrendous examples of expansion and tissue destruction following proximal ligation for arteriovenous malformation are well documented in the literature (Coleman and Hoopes, 1971; Habal and Murray, 1972).

Embolization. Embolic therapy for arteriovenous malformations can be curative, palliative, or preoperative (Leikensohn et al., 1981). On first reflection, embolization would seem to carry the same hemodynamic hazards as proximal ligation. However, the therapeutic principle in embolization is to deliver the embolic material into the center of the vascular anomaly (the nidus) in an attempt to block the smallest vessels first, from the inside out (Leikensohn et al., 1981). Selective angiography has shown that embolic occlusion of one feeding vessel causes an immediate increased flow from another facial vessel. Therefore, in theory, *all* micro- and macrofistulae must be obliterated in order to collapse the arteriovenous malformation permanently.

For extensive lesions, in which surgical resection would be too destructive, or for inaccessible lesions, embolization can be used as a primary treatment modality. By blocking a large proportion of shunts, diminution in size of the lesion may happen, and collateral vessels can develop very slowly. However, primary embolization should be regarded as only potentially curative, for in time, all too often, recanalization and re-expansion will occur.

Preoperative embolization should be considered by any surgical candidate in order to diminish blood loss and facilitate extirpation. Presurgical embolization should not be used in hopes of reducing the extent of resection. The surgeon must be involved in the selection of the embolic material and must fully understand the specific indications and risks. In most instances, temporary occlusive embolic material is favored, and the excision is planned for 48–72 hours following embolization (Azzolini et al., 1982). Figure 16–21 illustrates a well-localized arteriovenous malformation of the upper lip treated with embolization and excision. Two years following this combined therapy, there has been no re-expansion of the lesion. More remarkable short term results are possible, even with extensive high flow anomalies, using combined embolization and resection; three such cases are reported by Schrudde and Petrovici (Schrudde and Petrovici, 1981).

Palliative embolization may be indicated for relief of symptoms when the lesion cannot be surgically removed, e.g., for hemorrhage, pain, or ischemic ulceration. The reader is referred to Chapter Twenty-One for a more thorough presentation of this subject.

Resection. John Bell, in his 1815 textbook, emphasized that an arteriovenous malformation ("aneurysm from anastomosis") is quite a different problem from an acquired fistula. He noted:

This aneurism is a mere congeries of active vessels, which will not be cured by opening it; all attempts at obliterating them with caustics, after a simple incision, have proved unsuccessful, nor does the interrupting of particular vessels which led to it affect the tumor; the whole group of vessels must be extirpated.

Thus, the only therapeutic approach that carries any hope for long-term success is total resection of tissue that is clinically involved with the arteriovenous anomaly (Pemberton and Saint, 1928; Malan and Azzolini, 1968; Coleman, 1973). Leaving behind residual and dormant anomalous channels beyond the resection margin only invites further collateral formation, shunting, and expansion.

Obvious aesthetic and functional considerations in the facial region make it imperative for the surgeon to limit unnecessary sacrifice of tissue. Nevertheless, the goal remains total removal of the malformation. Experienced authors agree that the resection must be radical, just as if dealing with cancer (Malan and Azzolini, 1968; Coleman, 1973). Feeding vessels can be temporarily occluded in order to diminish blood loss during the resection; however, these feeding vessels should *never* be permanently ligated. These very same vessels may be needed later for embolic therapy. What are the boundaries for resection? Uppermost in the surgeon's mind should be the questions: Which vessels are truly part of the primary vascular anomaly, and which tissues and tortuous vessels are secondarily involved? To this end, the Doppler ultrasonic flow detector can be quite useful, both preoperatively to discover and intraoperatively to determine the limits of resection and unsuspected fistulous areas (Withers et al., 1979). The classic to and fro sound of shunting flow is not heard over collateral vessels.

There are several maneuvers that can be employed to minimize intraoperative hemorrhage. Placement of temporary mattress sutures around the periphery of the excision margin is a frequently rediscovered old technique. Percutaneous transcatheter balloon occlusion of feeding vessels has been used to facilitate excision of two large scalp arteriovenous lesions (Haller et al., 1980). The maximum diameter of vessels that can be occluded with currently available balloons is 4 mm. Profound hypotensive anesthesia (Munro and Martin, 1980) and cardiopulmonary bypass with deep hypothermic circulatory arrest (Mulliken et al., 1978) should be considered for an extensive resection.

Arteriovenous malformations of the scalp can be widely excised (usually down to pericranium) and the defect closed primarily with a split-thickness skin graft or local flap. A simple stain of the auricle, more often than not, belies an underlying arteriovenous malformation. The natural history of these anomalies is well described by Dingman and Grabb (Dingman and Grabb, 1965). In a typical case, there is an innocent pinkish stain seen in infancy; over the first two decades, the ear enlarges, and the telltale signs of an arteriovenous anomaly become all too obvious. Treatment usually necessitates total amputation of the external ear and if necessary, dissection of the seventh cranial nerve (Fig. 16–22).

The more extensive and complicated cases of head/neck vascular anomalies often pre-

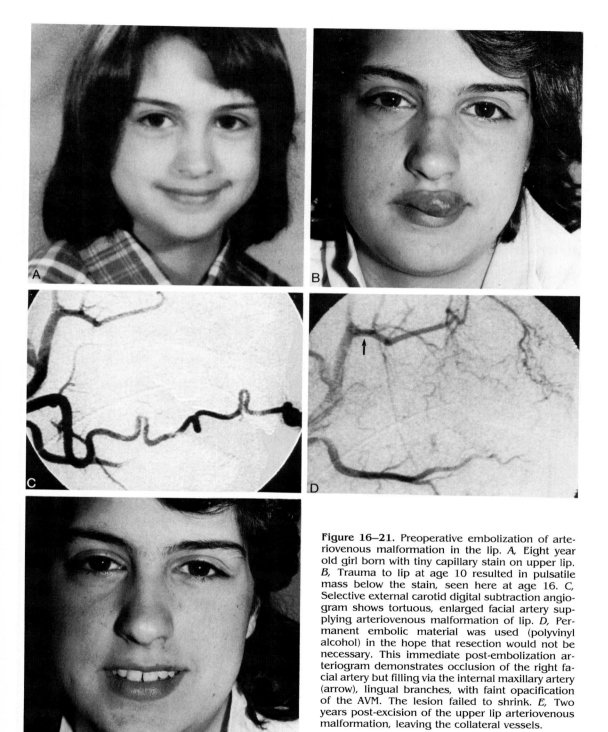

Figure 16–21. Preoperative embolization of arteriovenous malformation in the lip. *A,* Eight year old girl born with tiny capillary stain on upper lip. *B,* Trauma to lip at age 10 resulted in pulsatile mass below the stain, seen here at age 16. *C,* Selective external carotid digital subtraction angiogram shows tortuous, enlarged facial artery supplying arteriovenous malformation of lip. *D,* Permanent embolic material was used (polyvinyl alcohol) in the hope that resection would not be necessary. This immediate post-embolization arteriogram demonstrates occlusion of the right facial artery but filling via the internal maxillary artery (arrow), lingual branches, with faint opacification of the AVM. The lesion failed to shrink. *E,* Two years post-excision of the upper lip arteriovenous malformation, leaving the collateral vessels.

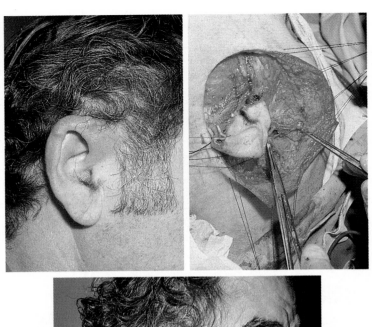

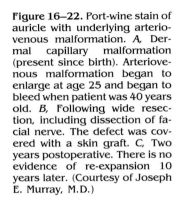

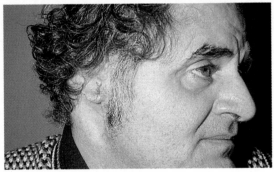

Figure 16–22. Port-wine stain of auricle with underlying arteriovenous malformation. A, Dermal capillary malformation (present since birth). Arteriovenous malformation began to enlarge at age 25 and began to bleed when patient was 40 years old. B, Following wide resection, including dissection of facial nerve. The defect was covered with a skin graft. C, Two years postoperative. There is no evidence of re-expansion 10 years later. (Courtesy of Joseph E. Murray, M.D.)

sent with a history of ill-advised attempts at piecemeal resection and proximal ligation. A lesion's extent or inaccessibility may preclude total extirpation. The widest possible removal of the central area of the arteriovenous malformation may have to suffice. Such a case is illustrated in Figure 16–23—a 22 year old woman with a history of multiple attempts to treat a complex arteriovenous anomaly of the face. The lower cheek, lip, and hemimaxilla were resected, leaving behind collateral vessels in the face and a residual capillary anomaly of the nasal skin. The upper lip was reconstructed with a tubed arm flap and tubed mucosal flaps.

Excellent exposure to anomalies of the temporalis, masseter, and pterygoid muscles is provided by a transtemporal subfascial approach first described by Azzolini (Malan and Azzolini, 1968; Azzolini et al., 1982).

Arteriovenous anomalies of the jaws can present with frightening hemorrhage, often following tooth extraction. Bleeding can be

fatal in these cases (Lamberg et al., 1979). The most effective measure is immediate packing and pressure. There is no place for proximal ligation, except perhaps as a life-saving maneuver. Azzolini recommends elective temporary occlusion of both external carotid vessels, dental extraction, and extensive curettage and packing with absorbable hemostatic material (Azzolini et al., 1982). Preoperative embolization is also useful for mandibular arteriovenous malformations (Hoey et al., 1970; Bryant and Maull, 1975) (Figs. 16–24 and 16–25). If these approaches fail, hemimandibulectomy is clearly indicated.

Closure. After all tissue that contains the primary vascular anomaly is removed, there may be insufficient skin remaining for linear closure. Thus, primary closure with a skin graft or flap is often necessary. Delayed primary closure with a skin graft is particularly useful if bleeding is excessive, provided that vital structures are not exposed. Primary or delayed coverage with a local cutaneous or musculocutaneous flap may involve abnormal collateral vessels. Microvascular transfer of cutaneous, musculocutaneous, or fasciocutaneous flaps should be considered for coverage of these large wounds. Potential donor vessels for microanastomoses must be recognized in the planning for preoperative embo-lization and must be preserved, if possible, during the resection. If the resection of an arteriovenous anomaly is incomplete, in time the malformation will surely re-expand and may entangle the skin graft or flap tissue used for coverage (Puglionisi and Azzolini, 1963). Hurvitz and Kerber suggest that arterialized flaps can minimize the late dilata-

Text continued on page 338

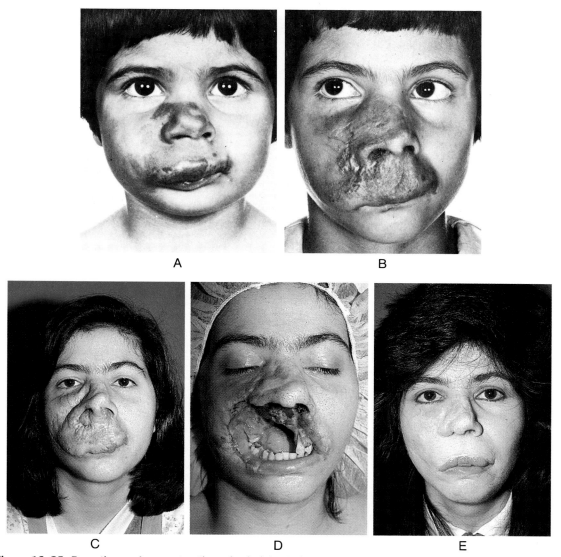

A B

C D E

Figure 16–23. Resection and reconstruction of a facial arteriovenous anomaly. *A,* Three year old girl with port-wine stain of nose and lip with underlying arteriovenous malformation. *B,* Age 7, following irradiation, hypertonic saline injections, and two resections. (Courtesy of Mr. David N. Matthews, M.Ch., FRCS, and the Hospital for Sick Children, London.) *C,* Age 22, following eight subtotal resections. The patient has frequent nose bleeds, and the right maxillary teeth are loose. *D,* Hemi-maxillectomy and resection of upper lip and lower cheek performed 48 hours post-embolization of right internal maxillary artery (with Gelfoam). *E,* Five years post-staged reconstruction with tubed upper-inner arm flap and tubed buccal mucosal flaps. Capillary-venous component in nasal skin remains quiescent.

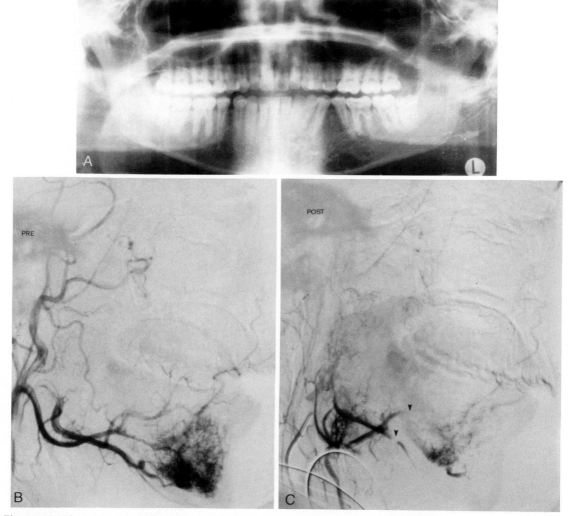

Figure 16–24. Intraosseous arteriovenous malformation of mandible. *A,* Panographic study shows roots of bicuspids symmetrically splayed by radiolucent, multilocular mass in left mandibular body. *B,* Selective external carotid angiogram (at 3 seconds) shows dense opacification of arteriovenous malformation within mandible. *C,* Angiogram following partial occlusion of main feeding branches (mandibular and lingual, arrows) with Gelfoam. (Courtesy of Kenneth E. Fellows, M.D.)

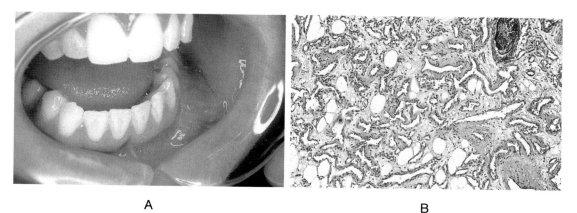

A   B

Figure 16–25. *A*, Intraoral photograph of 17 year old female with arteriovenous malformation of mandible seen in Figure 16–23 shows expansion of buccal cortex. *B*, Histologic examination of curetted specimen shows anomalous channels with fibromuscular walls of variable thickness. Note Gelfoam embolus in upper right hand corner (H&E × 100).

Figure 16–26. Arteriovenous malformation of the left face. *A*, Wedding photograph of the patient at age 21. His left ear, pink and warm since birth, is a little larger than the right ear. He began to bleed from the ear within 5 years, setting into motion a cascade of operations. *B*, Age 50, following staged ligations of both vertebral arteries and both external carotid vessels. Patient is bleeding constantly; the ulceration that appeared after resection of the ear failed to heal.

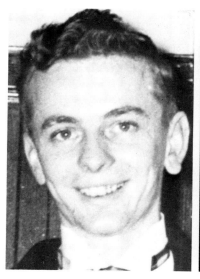

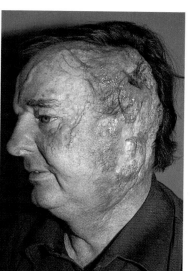

A   B

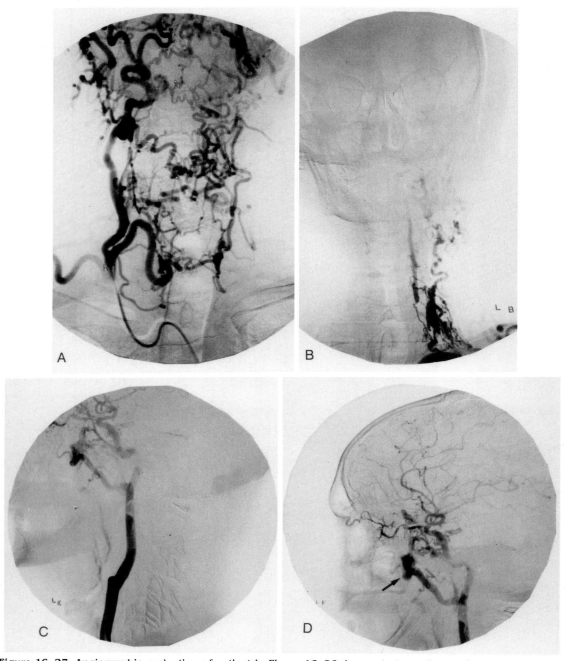

Figure 16–27. Angiographic evaluation of patient in Figure 16–26 demonstrates collateral flow around ligated vessels. *A,* Right thyrocervical trunk is greatly enlarged, as are ascending cervical arteries feeding the ipsilateral and contralateral external carotid branches. *B,* Frontal view of ligated left vertebral artery with flow reconstituted via large thyrocervical branches. *C,* Ligated left external carotid artery with collateral flow into external carotid branches. *D,* View of collaterals via dural branches of internal carotid artery exiting from foramen ovale and foramen rotundum. Huge internal maxillary artery (arrow) with retrograde flow through middle meningeal artery.

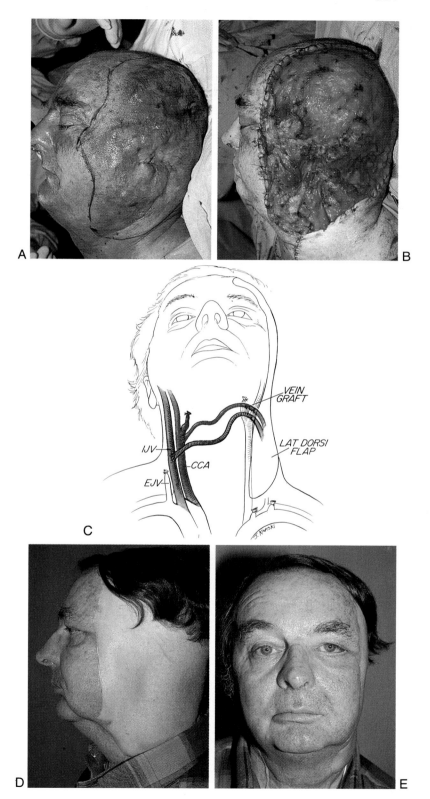

Figure 16–28. Resection and reconstruction with microvascular flap transfer. *A,* Margins of resection, drawn in the operating room. *B,* Intraoperative photograph following excision of arteriovenous malformation, including facial nerve. *C,* Drawing to illustrate plan for microvascular anastomoses. The resected (ligated) facial vessels made it necessary to span the neck with vein grafts to the contralateral proximal common carotid and jugular vessels. *D,* Latissimus dorsi musculocutaneous free flap used to cover defect. (Courtesy of Joseph Upton, M.D.) *E,* Appearance following fascial sling suspension of mouth, lower eyelid, and brow to ameliorate facial palsy (3 years postoperative).

tion and collateral formation at the site of an incompletely resected arteriovenous anomaly (Hurvitz and Kerber, 1981). This concept has yet to be validated. However, there is no doubt that axial flaps, if necessary as a microsurgical free tissue transfer, facilitate wide resection and closure in a case of a large craniofacial arteriovenous malformation (Figs. 16–26 to 16–28).

Results of Treatment

Subtotal resection of cervicofacial arteriovenous anomalies gives a suboptimal result. The vascular malformation will "recur," often larger than ever. These frightful cases have led to the pessimistic belief that these lesions can never be completely eradicated. Acceptance of these patients for treatment is a major commitment. Under proper indications and with very careful planning, extensive resection is justified and potentially curative.

EPILOGUE

All too often, patients with complex vascular anomalies become, in a sense, medical orphans, wandering from place to place seeking help. Very few of the large, sometimes grotesque vascular malformations will be seen in any one practitioner's lifetime. These patients, with lesions both large and small, deserve care by a multidisciplinary group in a hospital or referral center. The front line of this team should include the vascular radiologist, hematologist, and surgeon; other important members are a psychologist, dental prosthetist, social worker, and nurse specialist. Unfortunately, as this chapter attests, a total cure for many patients with vascular malformations is not possible. In the minds of some observers, these anomalies are dismissed as insoluble problems.

An interdisciplinary group devoted to vascular anomalies should serve to minimize the complications resulting from injudicious therapy in these patients. A *vascular anomalies team* serves as a focus for studies of new therapeutic strategems and research into pathogenesis and pathophysiology. There is so much to be learned. This is *terra incognita*. At the clinical level, studies are needed to document rheologic patterns and physiological responses in the various types of chan-

nel anomalies. Hematological disturbances should be categorized and specific pharmacologic therapies devised. At the tissue level, investigations could focus on the dysmorphic vessel wall, with particular attention paid to the neural and smooth muscular elements. The mechanisms of soft tissue and skeletal overgrowth, progressive vascular ectasia, and collateral formation are other subjects worthy of study. Only through such clinical-laboratory inquiries into vascular anomalies will improved therapy be possible for these medical orphans. In the meantime, as O. W. Holmes once said, "It is the duty of the physician to heal sometimes, but encourage always."

References

Lymphatic Malformations

Apfelberg, D. B., Maser, M. R., Lash, H., and White, D. N.: Benefits of CO_2 laser in oral hemangioma excision. Plast. Reconstr. Surg. 75:46, 1985.

Arnold, J.: Zwei Fälle von Hygroma colli cysticum congenitum und deren fragliche Beziehung zu dem Ganglion intercaroticum. Virch. Arch. f. Path. Anat. 33:209, 1865.

Azzolini, A., Salimbeni Ughi, G., and Riberti, C.: Present approach to large lymphangiomatous malformations of parotid and submandibular regions in infancy and childhood. Chir. Plast. 7:233, 1984.

Batsakis, J. G.: *Tumors of the Head and Neck: Clinical and Pathological Considerations*, 2nd ed. Baltimore: Williams and Wilkins, 1979, p. 301.

Bauer, B. S., Kernahan, D. A., and Hugo, N. E.: Lymphangioma circumscriptum—a clinicopathological review. Ann. Plast. Surg. 7:318, 1981.

Bhattacharyya, N. C., Yadav, K., Mitra, S. K., and Pathak, I. C.: Lymphangiomas in children. Aust. N. Zeal. J. Surg. 51:296, 1981.

Bill, A. H., and Sumner, D. S.: A unified concept of lymphangioma and cystic hygroma. Surg. Gynec. Obstet. 120:79, 1965.

Bohl, J., Wallenfang, T., and Schroder, J. M.: Faziozerebrales Lymphangiom bei Ullrich-Turner Syndrom. Neurochirurgia 24:176, 1981.

Bowman, C. A., Witte, M. J., Witte, C. L., et al.: Cystic hygroma reconsidered: hamartoma or neoplasm? Primary culture of an endothelial cell line from a massive cervicomediastinal hygroma with bony lymphangiomatosis. Lymphology 17:15, 1984.

Boyd, J. B., Mulliken, J. B., Kaban, L. B., et al.: Skeletal changes associated with vascular malformations. Plast. Reconstr. Surg. 74:789, 1984.

Broomhead, I. W.: Cystic hygroma of the neck. Brit. J. Plast. Surg. 17:225, 1964.

Burge, D. M., Middleton, A. W., Kamath, R., and Fasher, B. J.: Intestinal haemorrhage in Turner's syndrome. Arch. Dis. Child. 56:557, 1981.

Chait, D., Yonkers, A. J., Beddoe, G. M., and Yarington, C. T.: Management of cystic hygromas. Surg. Gynec. Obstet. 139:55, 1974.

Chervenak, F. A., Isaacson, G., Blakemore, K. J., et al.: Fetal cystic hygroma. Cause and natural history. New Engl. J. Med. *309*:822, 1983.

Crawford, B. S., and Vivakananthan, C.: The treatment of giant cystic hygroma of the neck. Brit. J. Plast. Surg. *26*:69, 1973.

Csicsko, J. F., and Grosfeld, J. L.: Cervicomediastinal hygroma with pulmonary hypoplasia in the newly born. Am. J. Dis. Child. *128*:557, 1974.

Dingman, R. O., and Grabb, W. C.: Lymphangioma of the tongue. Plast. Reconstr. Surg. *27*:214, 1961.

Dowd, C. N.: Hygroma cysticum colli: Its structure and etiology. Ann. Surg. *58*:112, 1913.

Figi, A. F.: Radium in the treatment of multilocular lymph cysts of the neck in children. Amer. J. Roentgenol. *21*:473, 1929.

Fonkalsrud, E. W.: Surgical management of congenital malformations of the lymphatic system. Amer. J. Surg. *128*:152, 1974.

Garden, A. S., Benzie, R. J., Miskin, M., and Gardner, H. A.: Fetal cystic hygroma colli: Antenatal diagnosis, significance and management. Amer. J. Obstet. Gynec. *154*:221, 1986.

Goetsch, E.: Hygroma colli cysticum and hygroma axillare. Pathologic and clinical study and report of twelve cases. Arch. Surg. *36*:394, 1938.

Grabb, W. C., Dingman, R. O., Oneal, R. M., and Dempsey, P. D.: Facial hamartomas in children: Neurofibroma, lymphangioma, and hemangioma. Plast. Reconstr. Surg. *66*:509, 1980.

Graham, J. M., Jr., Stephens, T. D., and Shepard, T. H.: Nuchal cystic hygroma in a fetus with presumed Roberts syndrome. Am. J. Med. Genet. *15*:163, 1983.

Greenberg, F., Carpenter, R. J., and Ledbetter, D. H.: Cystic hygroma and hydrops fetalis in a fetus with trisomy 13. Clin. Genet. *24*:389, 1983.

Grosfeld, J. L., Weber, T. R., and Vane, D. W.: One-stage resection for massive cervicomediastinal hygroma. Surgery *92*:693, 1982.

Gross, R. E.: Cystic hygroma. In *The Surgery of Infancy and Childhood.* Philadelphia: W. B. Saunders Co., 1953, pp. 960–970.

Gross, R. E., and Goeringer, C. F.: Cystic hygroma of the neck. Report of twenty-seven cases. Surg. Gynec. Obstet. *69*:48, 1939.

Groves, L. K., and Effler, D. B.: Primary chylopericardium. N. Engl. J. Med. *250*:520, 1954.

Harkins, G. A., and Sabiston, D. C., Jr.: Lymphangioma in infancy and childhood. Surgery *47*:811, 1960.

Harrison, R. G.: Correlation in the development and growth of the eye studied by means of heteroplastic transplantation. Arch. Entw. Mech. Org. *129*:1, 1929.

Harrower, G.: Treatment of cystic hygroma of the neck by sodium morrhuate. Brit. Med. J. *2*:148, 1933.

Huntington, G. S., and McClure, C. F. W.: The development of the main lymph channels of the cat in their relation to the venous system. Anat. Rec. *1*:36, 1906–1908.

Huntington, G. S., and McClure, C. F. W.: The anatomy and development of the jugular lymph sacs in the domestic cat (Felis domestica). Am. J. Anat. *10*:177, 1910.

Ikeda, K., Suita, S., Hayashida, Y., and Yakabe, S.: Massive infiltrating cystic hygroma of the neck in infancy with special reference to bleomycin therapy. Zeit. Kinderchir. *20*:227, 1977.

Jakobiec, F. A., and Jones, I. S.: Vascular tumors, malformations, and degenerations. In Jones, I. S., and

Jakobiec, F. A. (eds.): *Diseases of the Orbit.* Hagerstown, MD: Harper and Row, 1979, pp. 276–283.

Kampmeier, O. F.: The development of the jugular lymph sacs in the light of vestigial, provisional and definitive phases of morphogenesis. Am. J. Anat. *107*:153, 1960.

Koester, K.: Ueber hygroma cysticum colli congenitum. Verh. Phys. Med. Ges. Wurzburg *3*:44, 1872.

Lewis, F. J.: The development of the lymphatic system in rabbits. Am. J. Anat. *5*:95, 1905.

MacGuire, D. P.: Cystic hygroma of the neck. Arch. Surg. *31*:301, 1935.

McClure, C. F. W.: The development of the lymphatic system in the light of the more recent investigations in the field of vasculogenesis. Anat. Rec. *9*:563, 1915.

McClure, C. F. W., and Silvester, C. F.: A comparative study of the lymphaticovenous communications in adult mammals. Anat. Rec. *3*:534, 1909.

Morris, M.: Lymphangioma circumscriptum. In Unna, P. G., Morris, M., Duhring, L. A., et al. (eds.): *International Atlas of Rare Skin Diseases.* London: H. K. Lewis, 1889, p. 2.

Mulliken, J. B., and Glowacki, J.: Hemangiomas and vascular malformations in infants and children: A classification based on endothelial characteristics. Plast. Reconstr. Surg. *69*:412, 1982.

Mulliken, J. B., Zetter, B. R., and Folkman, J.: *In vitro* characteristics of endothelium from hemangiomas and vascular malformations. Surgery *92*:348, 1982.

New, G. B.: Hygroma cystica treated with radium. Surg. Clin. North Am. *4*:527, 1924.

Ninh, T. N., and Ninh, T. X.: Cystic hygroma in children: Report of 126 cases. J. Pediatr. Surg. *9*:191, 1974.

Noyes, A. W. F.: A case of lymphangioma circumscriptum. Brit. Med. J. *1*:1189, 1893.

Nussbaum, M., and Buchwald, R. P.: Adult cystic hygroma. Amer. J. Otolaryng. *2*:159, 1981.

Patten, B. M.: *Human Embryology,* 3rd ed. New York: McGraw-Hill Book Co., 1968, pp. 532–537.

Phillips, H. E., and McGahan, J. P.: Intrauterine fetal cystic hygromas: Sonographic detection. AJR *136*:799, 1981.

Ravitch, M. M., and Rush, B. F., Jr.: Cystic hygroma. In Welch, K. J., Randolph, J. G., Ravitch, M. M., et al. (eds.): *Pediatric Surgery,* 4th ed. Chicago, Year Book Medical Publishers, 1986, pp. 533–539.

Redenbacker, E. A. H.: De ranula sub lingua, speciali, cum casu congenito. Monachii: Lindhauer, 1828.

Reder, F.: Hemangioma and lymphangioma, their response to the injection of boiling water. Med. Rec. N.Y. *98*:519, 1920.

Reid, M. R.: Abnormal arteriovenous communications, acquired and congenital. II. The origin and nature of arteriovenous aneurysms, cirsoid aneurysms, and simple angiomas. Arch. Surg. *10*:996, 1925.

Rutlin, E., Wisloff, R., Myren, J., and Serck-Hannssen, A.: Intestinal telangiectasia in Turner's syndrome. Endoscopy *56*:557, 1981.

Sabin, F. R.: On the origin of the lymphatic system from the veins and the development of the lymph hearts and thoracic duct in the pig. Am. J. Anat. *1*:367, 1902.

Sabin, F. R.: On the development of the superficial lymphatics in the skin of the pig. Am. J. Anat. *3*:183, 1904.

Sabin, F. R.: The development of the lymphatic nodes in the pig and their relation to the lymph hearts. Am. J. Anat. *4*:355, 1905.

Sabin, F. R.: The lymphatic system in human embryos, with a consideration of the morphology of the system as a whole. Am. J. Anat. *9*:43, 1909.

Saijo, M., Munro, I. R., and Mancer, K.: Lymphangioma. A long-term follow-up study. Plast. Reconstr. Surg. *56*:642, 1975.

Sawyer, K. C., and Woodruff, R.: Cystic hygromas of the neck. Arch. Surg. *63*:83, 1951.

Singh, R. P., and Carr, D. H.: The anatomy and histology of XO human embryos and fetuses. Anat. Rec. *155*:369, 1966.

Singleton, A. O.: Congenital lymphatic diseases—lymphangiomata. Ann. Surg. *105*:952, 1937.

Smith, D. W.: *Recognizable Patterns of Human Malformation: Genetic, Embryologic and Clinical Aspects*, 3rd ed. Philadelphia: W. B. Saunders Co., 1982, p. 472.

Solomon, L. M., Fretzin, D. F., and Dewald, R. L.: The epidermal nevus syndrome. Arch. Derm. *97*:273, 1968.

Stratton, V. C., and Grant, R. N.: Cervicomediastinal cystic hygroma associated with chylopericardium. Arch. Surg. *77*:887, 1958.

Sumner, T. E., Volberg, F. M., Kiser, P. E., and Schaffner, L. de. S.: Mediastinal cystic hygroma in children. Ped. Radiol. *11*:160, 1981.

Thompson, J. E., and Keiller, V. H.: Lymphangioma of the neck. Ann. Surg. *77*:385, 1923.

van der Putte, S. C. J.: The development of the lymphatic system in man. Adv. Anat. Embryol. Cell Biol. *51*:1, 1975.

van der Putte, S. C. J.: Lymphatic malformation in human fetuses. A study of fetuses with Turner's syndrome or status Bonnevie-Ullrich. Virch. Arch. Path. Anat. *376*:233, 1977.

Vaughan, A. M.: Cystic hygroma of the neck. Amer. J. Dis. Child *48*:149, 1934.

Virchow, R.: *Die Krankhaften Geschwülste*. Berlin: A. Hirschwald, 1863, Vol. III, p. 170.

Wegner, G.: Ueber Lymphangiome. Arch. Klin. Chir. *20*:641, 1877.

Wernher, A.: *Die angebornen Kysten-hygrome und die ihnen verwandten Geschwülste in anatomischer, diagnosticher und therapeuticscher Beziehung*. Giessen, G. F. Heyer, Vater, 1843.

Wessely, L.: Über Korrelationen des Wachstums (nach Versuchen am Auge). Z. Augenheilkd *43*:654, 1920.

Whimster, I. W.: The pathology of lymphangioma circumscriptum. Brit. J. Surg. *94*:473, 1976.

Williams, H. B.: Facial bone changes with vascular tumors in children. Plast. Reconstr. Surg. *63*:309, 1979.

Willis, R. A.: *Pathology of Tumors*, 3rd ed. London: Butterworth and Co., Ltd., 1960, p. 716.

Venous and Combined (Low Flow) Malformations

Apfelberg, D. B., Maser, M. F., Lash, H., and White, D. N.: Benefits of CO_2 laser in oral hemangioma excision. Plast. Reconstr. Surg. *75*:46, 1985.

Bowman, G.: A clinico-histologic investigation on hemangioma. Acta Chir. Scand. *83*:185, 1940.

Boxt, L. M., Levin, D. C., and Fellows, K. E.: Direct puncture angiography in congenital venous malformations. AJR *140*:135, 1983.

Boyd, J. B., Mulliken, J. B., Kaban, L. B., et al.: Skeletal changes associated with vascular malformations. Plast. Reconstr. Surg. *74*:789, 1984.

Brooks, W. S.: Variceal sclerosing agents. Amer. J. Gastroent. *79*:424, 1984.

Cole, P. P., and Hunt, A. H.: The treatment of cavernous haemangiomas and cirsoid aneurysms by the injection of boiling water. Brit. J. Surg. *36*:346, 1949.

Davis, D. O., Rumbaugh, C. L., and Petty, J.: Calvarial hemangioma: Tumor stain and meningeal artery blood supply. J. Neuro. *25*:561, 1966.

Demuth, R. J., Miller, S. H., and Keller, F.: Complications of embolization treatment for problem cavernous hemangiomas. Ann. Plast. Surg. *13*:135, 1984.

Faber, R. G., Ibrahim, S. Z., Drew, D. S., and Hobsley, M.: Vascular malformations of the parotid region. Brit. J. Surg. *65*:171, 1978.

Figi, F. A.: Treatment of hemangiomas of the head and neck. Plast. Reconstr. Surg. *3*:1, 1948.

Goldwyn, R. M., and Rosoff, C. B.: Cryosurgery for large hemangiomas in adults. Plast. Reconstr. Surg. *43*:605, 1969.

Gupta, S. D., Tiwari, I. N., and Pasurathy, N. K.: Cavernous haemangioma of the frontal bone: Case report. Brit. J. Surg. *62*:330, 1975.

Hoey, M. F., Courage, G. R., Newton, T. H., and Hoyt, W. F.: Management of vascular malformations of the mandible and maxilla. Review and report of two cases treated by embolization and surgical obliteration. J. Oral Surg. *28*:696, 1970.

Huang, T., Kim, K. A., Lynch, J. B., et al.: The use of cryotherapy in the management of intra-oral hemangiomas. South. M. J. *65*:1123, 1972.

Jakobiec, F. A., and Jones, I. S.: Vascular tumors, malformations, and degenerations. In Jones, I. S., and Jakobiec, F. A. (eds.): *Diseases of the Orbit*. Hagerstown, MD, Harper and Row, 1979, p. 286.

Jarzab, G.: Clinical experience in the cryosurgery of haemangioma. J. Max-Fac. Surg. *3*:146, 1975.

Joehl, R. J., Miller, S. H., Davis, T. S., and Graham, W. P., III: Hemangioma of the temporalis muscle: A case report and review of the literature. Ann. Plast. Surg. *3*:273, 1979.

Kaban, L. B., and Mulliken, J. B.: Vascular anomalies of the maxillofacial region. J. Oral Maxillofac. Surg. *44*:203, 1986.

Kanter, W. R., Brown, W. C., and Noe, J. M.: Nasal bone hemangiomas: A review of clinical, radiologic and operative experience. Plast. Reconstr. Surg. *76*:774, 1985.

Kirchhoff, D., Eggert, H. R., and Agnoli, A. L.: Cavernous angiomas of the skull. Neurochirurgia *21*:53, 1978.

Lasjaunias, P., and Berenstein, A.: *Surgical Neuroangiography*. Heidelberg: Springer-Verlag, Volume II, 1987, Chap. 9, p. 394.

Marshak, J. A.: Hemangioma of the zygomatic bone. Arch. Otolaryng. *106*:581, 1980.

Minkow, B., Laufer, D., and Gutman, D.: Treatment of oral hemangiomas with local sclerosing agents. Int. J. Oral Surg. *8*:18, 1979.

Morgan, J. F., and Schow, C. E.: Use of sodium morrhuate in the management of hemangiomas. J. Oral Surg. *32*:363, 1974.

Mulliken, J. B., Murray, J. E., Castaneda, A. R., and Kaban, L. B.: Management of a vascular malformation of the face using total circulatory arrest. Surg. Gynec. Obstet. *146*:168, 1978.

Ogawa, Y., and Inoue, K.: Electrothrombosis as a treatment of cirsoid angioma in the face and scalp and varicosities of the leg. Plast. Reconstr. Surg. *70*:310, 1982.

Ohtsuka, H., Shioya, N., and Tanaka, S.: Cryosurgery for hemangiomas of the body surface and oral cavity. Ann. Plast. Surg. *4*:462, 1980.

Riché, M. C., Hadjean, E., Tran-Bay-Huy, P., and Merland, J. J.: The treatment of capillary-venous malformations using a new fibrosing agent. Plast. Reconstr. Surg. 71:607, 1983.

Rosenbaum, A. E., Rossi, P., Schechter, M. M., and Sheehan, J. P.: Angiography of haemangiomata of the calvarium. Brit. J. Radiol. 42:682, 1969.

Sadowsky, D., Rosenberg, R. D., Kaufman, J., et al.: Central hemangioma of the mandible. Oral Surg. 52:471, 1981.

Schmidt, G. H.: Hemangioma in the zygoma. Ann. Plast. Surg. 3:330, 1982.

Scott, J. E. S.: Hemangiomata in skeletal muscle. Brit. J. Surg. 44:496, 1957.

Sherman, R. S., and Wilner, D.: The roentgen diagnosis of hemangioma of bone. Amer. J. Roentgenol. 86:1146, 1961.

Warrell, R. P., Jr., and Kempin, S. J.: Treatment of severe coagulopathy in the Kasabach-Merritt syndrome with aminocaproic acid and cryoprecipitate. N. Engl. J. Med. 313:309, 1985.

Welsh, D., and Hengerer, A. S.: The diagnosis and treatment of intramuscular hemangiomas of the masseter muscle. Am. J. Otol. 1:186, 1980.

Wilflingseder, R., Martin, R., and Papp, Ch.: Magnesium seeds in the treatment of lymph- and haemangiomata. Chir. Plast. 6:105, 1981.

Wojtanowski, M. H., and Mandel, M. A.: Seizures abolished by excision of a cavernous hemangioma of the scalp and skull. Case report. Plast. Reconstr. Surg. 64:831, 1979.

Woods, J. E.: Extended use of sodium tetradecyl sulfate in treatment of hemangiomas and other related conditions. Plast. Reconstr. Surg. 79:542, 1987.

Wyeth, J. A.: The treatment of vascular tumours by the injection of water at a high temperature. JAMA 40:1778, 1903.

Wyke, B. D.: Primary hemangioma of the skull: A rare cranial tumor. Am. J. Roent. 61:302, 1949.

Arteriovenous Malformations

Azzolini, A., and Lechi, A.: Circoli anastomotici dall'arteria carotide interna all'esterna nelle malformazioni artero-venose della faccia. Min. Cardioang. 16:182, 1968.

Azzolini, A., Bertani, A., and Riberti, C.: Superselective embolization and immediate surgical treatment: Our present approach to treatment of large vascular hemangiomas of the face. Ann. Plast. Surg. 9:42, 1982.

Bell, J.: The Principles of Surgery. London: Longman, Hurst, Rees, etc., 1815, p. 459.

Brodie, B. C.: An account of a case of aneurism by anastomosis of the forehead treated by the application of ligatures. Medico-Chir. Trans. 15:177, 1829.

Bryant, W. M., and Maull, K. I.: Arteriovenous malformations of the mandible. Plast. Reconstr. Surg. 55:690, 1975.

Callander, C. L.: Study of arteriovenous fistula with an analysis of 447 cases. Ann. Surg. 71:428, 1920.

Clay, R. C., and Blalock, A.: Congenital arteriovenous fistulas in the mandible. Surg. Gynec. Obstet. 90:543, 1950.

Coleman, C. C., Jr.: Diagnosis and treatment of congenital arteriovenous fistulas of the head and neck. Amer. J. Surg. 126:557, 1973.

Coleman, C. C., Jr., and Hoopes, J. E.: Congenital arteriovenous anomalies of the head and neck. Plast. Reconstr. Surg. 47:354, 1971.

Dingman, R. O., and Grabb, W. C.: Congenital arteriovenous fistulae of the external ear. Plast. Reconstr. Surg. 35:620, 1965.

Gerbode, F., and Holman, E.: Congenital arteriovenous fistula between the internal maxillary artery and pterygoid plexus. Surgery 22:209, 1947.

Habal, M. B., and Murray, J. E.: The natural history of a benign locally invasive hemangioma of the orbital region. Plast. Reconstr. Surg. 49:209, 1972.

Haller, J. A., Jr., Pickard, L. R., Kumar, A. J., and White, R. I., Jr.: A new percutaneous technique for occluding arterial flow to massive congenital A-V malformations to prevent major hemorrhage during resection. J. Ped. Surg. 15:523, 1980.

Halsted, W. S.: Congenital arteriovenous and lymphaticovenous fistulae: Unique clinical and experimental observations. Trans. Am. Surg. Assoc. 37:262, 1919.

Hoey, M. F., Courage, G. R., Newton, T. H., and Hoyt, W. F.: Management of vascular malformations of the mandible and maxilla: Review and report of two cases treated by embolization and surgical obliteration. J. Oral Surg. 28:696, 1970.

Holman, E.: Abnormal Arteriovenous Communications. Springfield, IL: Charles C Thomas, 1968, p. 169.

Home, E.: An account of Mr. Hunter's method of performing the operation for the cure of the popliteal aneurism. Trans. Soc. Impr. Med. Chir. Know. Vol. I, p. 138, 1793.

Hurwitz, D. J., and Kerber, C. W.: Hemodynamic considerations in the treatment of arteriovenous malformations of the face and scalp. Plast. Reconstr. Surg. 67:421, 1981.

Kobler, J.: The Reluctant Surgeon: A Biography of John Hunter. Garden City, N.Y.: Doubleday and Co., 1960, p. 267.

Lamberg, M. A., Tasanen, A., and Jääskeläinen, J.: Fatality from central hemangiomas of the mandible. J. Oral Surg. 37:578, 1979.

Lawson, T. L., and Newton, T. H.: Congenital cervical arteriovenous malformations. Radiology 97:565, 1970.

Leikensohn, J. R., Epstein, L. I., and Vasconez, L. O.: Superselective embolization and surgery of noninvoluting hemangiomas and A-V malformations. Plast. Reconstr. Surg. 68:143, 1981.

Malan, E., and Azzolini, A.: Congenital arteriovenous malformations of the face and scalp. J. Cardiovasc. Surg. 9:109, 1968.

Mulliken, J. B., Murray, J. E., Castaneda, A. R., and Kaban, L. B.: Management of a vascular malformation of the face using total circulatory arrest. Surg. Gynec. Obstet. 146:168, 1978.

Munro, I. R., and Martin, R. D.: The management of gigantic benign craniofacial tumors: The reverse facial osteotomy. Plast. Reconstr. Surg. 65:777, 1980.

Nicoladoni, C.: Phlebariectasie der rechten oberen Extremität. Arch. f. Klin. Chir. 18:252, 1875.

Norman, J. A., Schmidt, K. W., and Grow, J. B.: Congenital arteriovenous fistula of cervical vertebral vessels with heart failure in infant. J. Pediatr. 36:598, 1950.

Olivecrona, H., and Ladenheim, J.: Congenital Arterio-Venous Aneurysms of the Carotid and Vertebral Arterial Systems. Berlin: Springer-Verlag, 1957, p. 14.

Pemberton, J. D., Jr., and Saint, J. H.: Congenital arteriovenous communications. Surg. Gynec. Obstet. 46:470, 1928.

Puglionisi, A., and Azzolini, A.: Caratteri dei nevi vascolari e transformazione angiomatosa di innesti e trapianti cutanei in soggetti portatori de fistole arterovenose congenite. Min. Cardioang. 11:493, 1963.

Ravitch, M. M., and Gaertner, R. A.: Congenital arteriovenous fistula in the neck—48 year follow-up of a patient operated upon by Dr. Halsted in 1911. Johns Hopkins Hosp. Bull. *107*:31, 1960.

Reid, M. R.: Studies on abnormal arteriovenous communications, acquired and congenital. I. Report of a series of cases. Arch. Surg. *10*:601, 1925a.

Reid, M. R.: Abnormal arteriovenous communications, acquired and congenital. II. The origin and nature of arteriovenous aneurysms, cirsoid aneurysms, and simple angiomas. Arch. Surg. *10*:996, 1925b.

Reid, M. R.: Abnormal arteriovenous communications, acquired and congenital. III. The effects of abnormal arteriovenous communications on the heart, blood vessels and other structures. Arch. Surg. *11*:25, 1925c.

Reinhoff, W. F.: Congenital arteriovenous fistula. An embryologic study, with report of a case. Johns Hopkins Hosp. Bull. *35*:271, 1924.

Scarpa, A.: Memoria del Cav. Prof. Scarpa sull'aneurisma detto per anastomosi. In *Annali Universali di Medicina*, Milano, 1830, Vol. 54, p. 501.

Schrudde, J., and Petrovici, V.: Surgical treatment of giant hemangioma of the facial region after arterial embolization. Plast. Reconstr. Surg. *68*:878, 1981.

Storrs, D. G., and King, R. B.: Management of extracranial congenital arteriovenous malformations of the head and neck. J. Neurosurg. *38*:584, 1973.

Théron, J., Newton, T. H., and Hoyt, W. F.: Unilateral retinocephalic vascular malformations. Neuroradiology 7:185, 1974.

Warren, J. M.: Ligature of both carotid arteries for a remarkable erectile tumour of the mouth, face and neck. Amer. J. Med. Sci. *11*:281, 1846.

Warren, J. M.: *Surgical Observations with Cases and Operations*. Boston: Ticknor and Fields, 1867, pp. 441–464.

Withers, E. H., Franklin, J. D., and Lynch, J. B.: Resection of a massive arteriovenous malformation of the head and neck. Plast. Reconstr. Surg. *63*:566, 1979.

Woollard, H. H.: The development of the principal arterial stems in the forelimb of the pig. Contrib. Embryol., Carnegie Inst. *14*:139, 1922.

CHAPTER SEVENTEEN

Vascular Malformations of the Upper Limb

Joseph Upton

INTRODUCTION

Hemangiomas

In our series of 291 vascular lesions of the upper limb, 174 were classified as true *hemangiomas* (Upton et al., 1985). In a surgical context, these lesions are not major problems. Although a hemangioma grows remarkably during the first year of life, it begins to involute slowly before age 1 and is quiescent by age 5 years. This characteristic growth and regression and a physical examination differentiate hemangiomas from vascular malformations (Mulliken and Glowacki, 1982a, b; Finn et al., 1983) (Table 17–1).

Approximately 30% of upper limb hemangiomas ulcerate. Infection and maceration of lesions in the upper arm and forearm are not as problematic as those within the hand. A fingertip hemangioma may present with an acute or chronic paronychial infection, especially in a finger-sucker (Fig. 17–1A). Local wound care is all that is needed for an ulcerated hemangioma: cleaning; application of topical antibiotic ointment; and sometimes "wet-to-dry" dressings, changed three or four times a day. Ulcerations within the interdigital webspaces are frequently macerated and are difficult to dress in the child who is between the ages of 18 months and 3 years. Splints may be needed until the ulcer epithelializes. Active youngsters should have their limb immobilized with splints that extend above the flexed elbow, or with the special sleeves used in the postoperative period with cleft palate patients. Rigid supports within these garments keep the elbows extended and the fingers away from the child's mouth.

Extensive upper extremity hemangiomas do not cause compression syndromes, nerve palsies, or significant compromise of major muscle tendon units.

The parents must be convinced that watchful waiting is almost always the best course of treatment for hemangiomas (Fig. 17–1B and Fig. 17–2).

In our series, only 6% of children with hemangiomas required excision of redundant fibrofatty tissue after involution was complete to improve contour and/or digital function.

During the first decade of our study, 39 of 174 hemangiomas were treated with low dose irradiation, administered in one or two 300–400 rad doses. In retrospect, all these lesions

Table 17–1. UPPER EXTREMITY VASCULAR ANOMALIES*

Hemangiomas	174	
Malformations	117	
	291	

Malformations	*Low Flow*	*High Flow*
Capillary	10	2
Venous	41	0
Lymphatic	27	0
Lymphatic-venous	21	0
Arteriovenous	0	16
	99	18

*Data from Children's Hospital, Boston, MA.

343

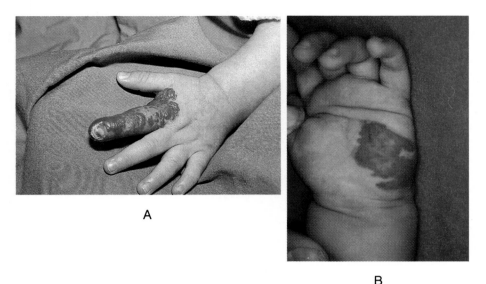

Figure 17–1. Hemangioma: proliferative phase. *A,* This hemangioma was the source of a chronic paronychial infection aggravated by finger sucking in this infant. *B,* Hypothenar lesion in a 2 year old child is beginning to involute, as evidenced by graying of surface.

would have involuted; irradiation is no longer recommended for this benign condition. Although compression therapy is occasionally mentioned (Moore, 1964; Miller and Smith, 1976), there is no convincing evidence that this accelerates regression of hemangiomas.

Vascular Malformations

The primary topic of this chapter is the diagnosis and treatment of errors of vascular morphogenesis, a subject that has confounded hand surgeons for decades. This chapter outlines the management of all grades of vascular malformation, from asymptomatic low flow lesions to highly symptomatic high flow arteriovenous catastrophes; yet, one must realize that combinations of these different types can exist in the same patient within the same extremity. In our series, the most common type of vascular abnormality of the upper limb was venous, followed in frequency by lymphatic and combined lymphatic-venous lesions (Table 17–1).

Although only 10–15% of all vascular anomalies (hemangiomas and malformations) involve the upper limb (Watson and McCarthy, 1940; Johnson et al., 1956; Stout, 1953), those that do occur may have major functional and/or aesthetic consequences.

The importance of function cannot be overemphasized when one is dealing with upper limb anomalies. For example, the deficit caused by a painful, thrombosed lesion located within the palm of the hand may be much greater than that associated with a massive malformation with limb hypertrophy. Careful assessment of function must precede setting priorities for the management of multiple vascular anomalies in the same patient.

EVALUATION OF A VASCULAR MALFORMATION

Clinical History and Observation

Evaluation begins with a careful history and physical examination. The rapid growth and involution that characterize a hemangioma are seen in one half of all upper extremity vascular anomalies. Vascular malformations, in contrast, grow commensurately with the child. Although by definition malformations are present at birth, many are inconspicuous and some do not appear until late childhood. Dermal ectasias, such as the port-wine stain, are usually noted at birth; only later in life does it become obvious that there is an associated low flow venous or lymphatic anomaly; or much less frequently, a high flow arteriovenous malformation. The

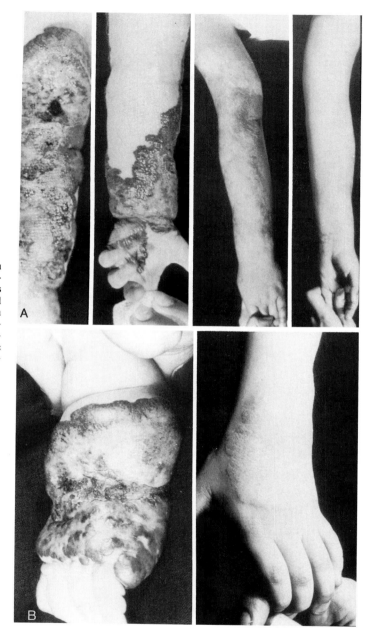

Figure 17–2. Hemangioma: ulceration and predictable involution. *A,* The secondary infection and maceration in this extensive forearm lesion were treated with local wound care. Only pigmentation abnormalities remain 10 years later. Excision was unnecessary; there is no functional loss. *B,* Same result in an extensive hand and wrist lesion. (Courtesy of Joseph E. Murray, M.D.)

extent of the "stain" does not change with growth, and there is no tendency for involvement of specific trigeminal dermatome patterns, as seen in the face. Venous and lymphatic malformations often coexist and may be quite insidious in their initial presentation. Venous malformations may barely be seen until late childhood or adolescence, but large lesions are usually obvious within the first 4–8 years of life.

Venous malformations are easy to differentiate from lymphatic lesions, because they enlarge dramatically when the limb is held in a dependent position and decompress completely when the limb is elevated. In large malformations, the redundant skin may have a prune-like appearance (Fig. 17–3). Palpation of a phlebolith confirms that a lesion is a venous malformation.

Lymphatic anomalies present as diffuse lymphedema or as localized swellings, particularly in the digits and dorsum of the hand. Although large communicating cystic cavities may be associated with fluid shifts and altered

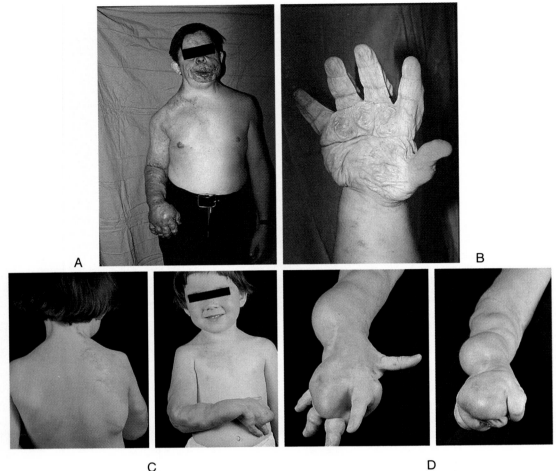

Figure 17–3. *A,* The size of the hand and limb in this man with a predominantly venous malformation, with extremity held in a dependent position. *B,* The appearance with the limb elevated and all blood drained from its large, saccular spaces. *C* and *D,* Similar extensive venous malformation in a younger child.

appearance in the neck and axilla, this does not occur in the lower arm, forearm, or hand, where the lymphatic spaces are much smaller and have less effective intercommunication. Local trauma or bleeding within a lymphatic malformation sometimes results in a painful, rubbery mass that will resolve with time. These masses are hard to differentiate from the equally painful localized thrombosis or hemorrhage that may occur within a predominantly venous lesion. Epidermal vesicle formation or "bubbling" of clear serous fluid is pathognomonic of a lymphatic lesion, particularly when it appears in an incisional scar. Deep lymphatic malformations do not necessarily involve the overlying dermis (Blair et al., 1983).

Low flow lesions are usually not sympto-

matic but instead present problems in terms of bulk and contour. Capillary, venous, lymphatic, and combined lymphatic-venous malformations belong in this category. Severe pain may result from intralesional bleeding or from thrombosis and/or calcification involving peripheral nerves. Nerve palsies, compression neuropathies, or systemic cardiovascular alterations generally do not occur.

In contrast, *a high flow* arteriovenous malformation presents with dramatic rheologic findings, occasionally with severe pain. Increased warmth, subcutaneous pulsations or throbbing, a thrill, and a bruit typify the arteriovenous malformation. A large lesion proximal to the wrist may demonstrate a positive Nicoladoni-Branham sign—a paradoxical reduction in heart rate when a tourniquet excludes the involved extremity from the general circulation (Nicoladoni, 1875; Branham, 1890). In time, neurologic symptoms or distal gangrene may occur, secondary to short-circuiting of blood flow through the malformation (Lewis, 1930; Holman, 1965, 1968).

Diagnostic Investigation

Expensive diagnostic studies are unnecessary in the case of a diffuse, asymptomatic malformation or a small, low flow lesion amenable to simple excision and closure. When a patient is symptomatic or if an operation is being considered for a large vascular anomaly, one should learn as much as possible about the size, extent, and depth of involvement and gain specific information about the location, caliber, and flow characteristics of abnormal channels (Table 17–2). *Angiography* is still the single most important diagnostic test (Malan and Puglionisi, 1964, 1965; Erikson and Hemmingsson, 1973; Bliznak and Staple, 1974; McNeill et al., 1974). Important technical modifications include biplanar (anteroposterior and lateral) magnification views of the hand and digits, rapid change cassettes, selective catheterization, and proximal compression to accentuate the venous phase (Horton and Ghormley, 1935; Greenspan et al., 1967; Geiser and Eversmann 1978; May et al., 1979). The femoral approach is preferred, but occasionally axillary insertion of the catheter is necessary. Brachial catheterization should not be performed, for fear of spasm, thrombosis, and distal ischemia. By using a femoral catheter and a pharmacologic sympathectomy prior to dye injection, our radiologists have avoided problems with spasm, which were frequently seen in the past with brachial punctures, particularly in young females. Digital subtraction angiography (DSA) gives rapid visualization with less contrast dye; it is particularly indicated if embolization is being considered. We have not routinely used regional anesthesia or direct intralesional injections.

Xerograms and *computerized axial tomography* with dye enhancement help define osseous involvement and delineate soft tissue planes.

Thermography, skin temperature recordings, pulse volume recordings, oxygen saturation studies, and bone scans may yield some objective information about blood flow, but these studies are often more confirmatory than diagnostic.

Subtraction views of particularly diagnostic films are useful in planning the surgical approach. Although angiography may not yield firm information about the potential expansion of collateral vessels following excision, careful scrutiny of the films may resolve diagnostic uncertainties. Separate maps of normal and abnormal vessels within the area to be dissected are prepared and are used for intraoperative reference. These permit careful planning of the surgical procedure so that as thorough an excision as possible is performed without unnecessary sacrifice of nerves, arteries, tendons, ligaments, and joints. Such maps help keep the surgeon from straying outside the planned area of dissection and allow improved hemostasis.

PRINCIPLES OF MANAGEMENT

The initial therapy of a vascular malformation of the upper limb should not be an operation. Indeed, excision normally is contemplated only after conservative measures have failed to control either bulk or symptoms. The plan of management can only be devised after a thorough history and physical examination, which should correlate the patient's age, first appearance of the vascular anomaly, function of the limb, size, activities of daily living, response to previous treatment, and assessment of the patient's needs and expectations (Curtis, 1953; Newmeyer, 1984). Angiograms and other invasive diagnostic tests are not considered unless there are real symptoms or loss of function. For example, a patient with a large, soft, diffuse, asymptomatic venous lesion may never require these studies. Parents of young children often request operative procedures for aesthetic reasons. The surgeon should avoid

Table 17–2. DIAGNOSTIC AIDS FOR VASCULAR MALFORMATIONS

Doppler flow studies
Plethysmography
Thermography
Roentgenography
  Computed tomography
  Arteriography
  Venography
  Xeroradiography

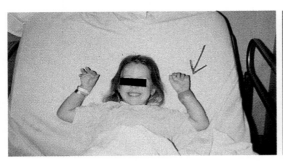
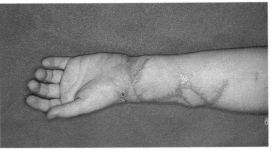

A   B

Figure 17–4. Complication: venous malformation. *A* and *B,* Appearance of a multi-scarred and surgically violated arm and hand in a child born with a low-flow venous anomaly. After repeated procedures, histologic findings were misinterpreted as "angiosarcoma" in several institutions. Poor planning of incisions resulted in unfortunate scarring. The gross appearance of the lesion prior to the operative intervention was consistent with that of predominantly venous vascular malformation.

such temptation, as he or she cannot improve upon an asymptomatic lesion and, in trying to do so, may cause a conspicuous scar as objectionable to the parent as the original contour deformity (Fig. 17–4).

Surgical Management

Although an operation in the upper limb is usually controlled and predictable, excision of a vascular malformation is beset with potential pitfalls. Experience with approximately 100 operations on both high and low flow anomalies of the upper limb, and the management of many postoperative complications, have taught certain principles common to all vascular malformations. *Adherence to these principles in the preoperative planning phases as well as in intraoperative execution cannot be overemphasized.*

Careful preoperative planning should include correlation of the size, extent, and involvement of structures with the physical examination and angiograms. All studies should be reviewed preoperatively; serial studies of growing children are often invaluable in demonstrating the true extent of involvement of the extremity. A thorough explanation of all potential complications

must be given to the patient and/or parents.

Preoperatively, the surgeon should outline a border for the excision and abide by it. The use of the pneumatic tourniquet and complete exsanguination enable the surgeon to visualize normal and abnormal structures clearly, despite the size of the malformation.

The placement of incisions is important, particularly in children. A high midaxial incision in the digit is preferred. With growth, palmar scar in or near the palm can lead to contracture. If a palmar approach is chosen, a zigzag incision is preferred. If multiple debulking procedures are contemplated in the upper arm or forearm, each incision should be planned carefully to avoid unnecessary scarring.

The use of magnification, either loupe or microscope, makes a tremendous difference in the identification and preservation of normal neurovascular structures.

A thorough dissection of a specified area should be performed so that subsequent surgical re-entry into a densely scarred bed will be unnecessary. Often the malformation extends well beyond its anticipated limits. In specific regions, staged excisions are better than one extensive and protracted dissection that leaves behind tissue containing abnormal vasculature (Fig. 17–5).

Figure 17–5. Venous malformation. *A* and *B,* Extensive low-flow malformation in a 2 year old child in whom ray resection of the ulnar two digits had been recommended. The purple discoloration of the skin is not a port-wine stain and represents almost complete skin and soft tissue replacement by a combined capillary-venous anomaly. *C* and *D,* Staged excisions started with thorough dissections of the palm over the first three metacarpals and the long finger, followed by dissection of the dorsum of the long and ring finger 1 year later. *E,* One year later, the ulnar half of the palm and palmar surface of the fifth finger were excised as the ulnar artery and nerve with its major branches were preserved with the the help of the operating microscope. *F* and *G,* Resurfacing was accomplished with a free vascularized parietotemporal fascial flap joined end-to-end into the ulnar artery and a local wrist vein. *H,* Three years later, the skin grafted surface remains durable; protective sensation is present from the digital nerves, which were splayed out directly beneath the fascia. (From *Journal of Hand Surgery 10A:*970, 1985.)

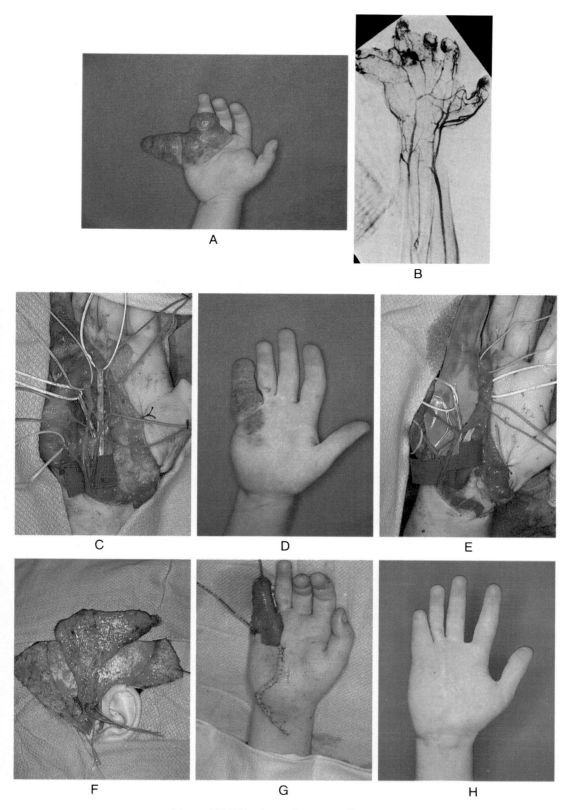

Figure 17–5 *See legend on opposite page*

To avoid vascular compromise, only one half of a digit should be dissected at a time. If possible, at least one or two large dorsal veins per finger should be preserved to enhance venous drainage, especially when one is dealing with diffuse lymphatic lesions (see Fig. 17–18). When a critical arterial segment is resected, this digit should be reconstructed with a vein graft so that at least one digital artery is preserved per digit and one major artery supplies the hand with a functional palmar arch.

Intraneural dissection should be avoided, whenever possible, despite gross involvement. Although many malformations, particularly the venous type, are entangled in nerves, dissection often leaves incontinuity neuromas with partial or complete loss of distal sensory or motor function and often creates symptoms that are much worse than the initial ones.

Skin flaps should not be coapted under tension, and non-viable skin should be replaced with skin grafts or a flap (Fig. 17–6).

Drains should be used liberally, and delayed primary closure of the surgical wound should be considered. Persistent postoperative bleeding is usually best treated with direct pressure, elevation, and immobilization, rather than with re-exploration.

The surgeon who has the courage to treat difficult high flow lesions should also be prepared to amputate a symptomatic, non-functional, or painful digit, hand, or limb following unsuccessful attempts for palliation. The reconstructive surgeon should not necessarily view amputation as a failure, or consider this option as a last resort for a difficult problem.

Regardless of the particular type of malformation, size, and hemodynamic activity, follow-up evaluation should be performed compulsively at yearly intervals. Early childhood, adolescence, and pregnancy are times when change may occur in vascular malformations, and patients and parents often have questions that are not easily answered by their family physician (owing to the paucity of information available in the medical literature).

CAPILLARY MALFORMATION

Clinical Presentation

In 39 patients with cutaneous port-wine stains, the area of involvement varied from multiple digits to the entire extremity and sometimes the entire hemithorax (Upton et al., 1985). Upper extremity stains are frequently associated with deeper anomalous vascular elements: arterial, venous, and/or lymphatic (Mulliken and Glowacki, 1982a) (Fig. 17–7). In our study group, 12 of the 20 patients with extensive "port-wine stains" had underlying high flow arterial lesions (Upton et al., 1985) (Figs. 17–8 and 17–9). In contrast to a venous lesion, a capillary malfor-

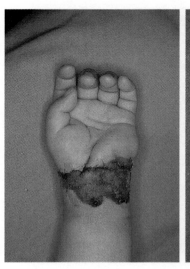 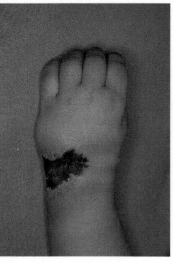

A   B

Figure 17–6. Complication: lymphatic malformation. A and B, Skin necrosis following subtotal excision of a lymphatic malformation with excessively thinned flaps and a postoperative hematoma. No drains had been used, and the incision involved almost 300 degrees of the wrist circumference.

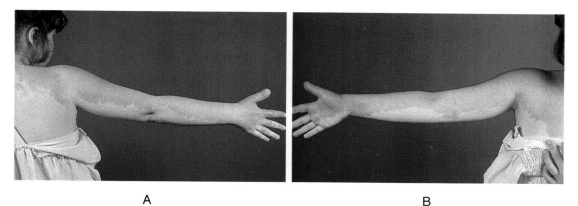

A   B

Figure 17–7. Capillary malformation. *A* and *B,* Extensive involvement of the entire limb and the ipsilateral side of the body is not unusual with this dermal capillary malformation, or port-wine stain. To date, associated deep vascular anomalies are not apparent and there are no functional problems.

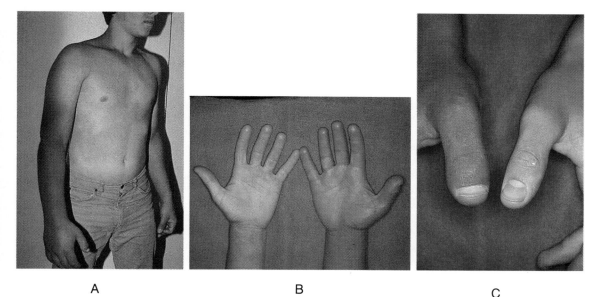

A   B   C

Figure 17–8. Capillary malformation. *A* and *B,* This teenager's extremity malformation has a brighter hue and is very warm compared with that on his chest and abdomen. The arm is enlarged, and there is underlying microarteriovenous shunting. Despite the soft tissue and skeletal enlargement, there have been no functional problems. *C,* His fingernails on the involved hand are broad, short, and thick. He has had no infections. Sensation is normal.

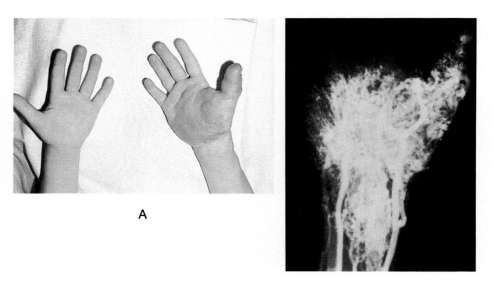

Figure 17–9. Arteriovenous malformation. *A,* Appearance of a high-flow malformation in a 7 year old child. The associated port-wine stain has not changed since birth, and the malformation has not been symptomatic and is controlled with a compression garment. *B,* Very early filling of dynamic shunts is seen involving all tissues within the palm in three dimensions. This lesion is not surgically resectable.

mation changes little with growth. Early in life the skin has a characteristic pink color, accounting for the name "nevus flammeus." With aging, the stain becomes a purple hue and the abnormal skin develops a cobblestone appearance.

Management

Treatment of upper extremity stains has been and should continue to be conservative. Many modalities have been tried for port-wine marks of the face: cryosurgery (Morel-Fatio, 1964), tattooing (Grabb et al., 1977), and argon laser therapy (Apfelberg et al., 1976; Cosman, 1980). Camouflage with special cosmetic preparations still has a role in covering facial vascular stains; it certainly has not been used extensively for capillary lesions in the upper extremity. Argon laser and a tunable dye laser are the most currently publicized treatments for port-wine stains. The principle is that high energy light is converted into heat, causing either thrombosis or perivascular narrowing, thus diminishing the size of the capillary malformation with, it is hoped, minimal attendant dermal scar formation.

Hypertrophic scarring with argon laser has been a problem in the face, especially in children (Noe et al., 1980). It will also predictably occur in the upper extremity because there are fewer adnexal appendages as a source for epithelial cell regeneration. Port-wine stains, even those in the most aesthetically obvious dorsal surface of the hand, have not been treated with laser in our patients.

Excision and resurfacing with split-thickness skin grafts may be considered for hypertrophic port-wine stains in older patients. This approach has been primarily used in the face (Clodius, 1977). Occasionally, there may be oozing from hyperkeratosis or vesicles within a port-wine stain. In this situation, local cauterization or excision with or without split-thickness skin grafting can be beneficial. One should remember that the local symptoms may indicate a deep arterial, venous, or lymphatic anomaly.

VENOUS MALFORMATION

Clinical Presentation

The venous type of low flow anomaly is the most common vascular malformation seen in the upper limb. Forty-one of our 118 patients with extensive lesions were categorized in this group (Upton et al., 1985). Small, localized lesions within a web space, the volar forearm, or axilla may remain unnoticed for many years. Large, saccular lesions become more obvious when they are engorged with blood when the limb is held in a dependent position (see Fig. 17–3). Typically, venous anomalies enlarge proportionately as the child grows. Expansion can occur with the pubertal growth spurt, during pregnancy, following trauma, while the patient is on birth control medication, or after subtotal excision (Mulliken, 1983).

Venous malformations may involve any tissues within the extremity, including skin, bone, nerve, arterial wall, muscle, tendon, fat, or fascia. The true extent of the vascular anomaly is often not obvious. Painful subcutaneous thrombi and occasionally calcifications are typically found. Subcutaneous thrombi are less symptomatic in non-percussive surfaces (David, 1936). Although skin ulceration rarely occurs, patients with massively involved soft tissues may present with intertriginous infections and skin maceration (Fig. 17–10). Children with extensive skin involvement often complain of itching in the summer months and need skin lubrication. Functional problems are related to the size, weight, and location of the malformation. For example, an egg-sized mass is usually asymptomatic within the arm or forearm but not within the thumb–index finger web space. A large vascular anomaly is better tolerated in the proximal extremity than in the more mobile wrist or hand. Increased

weight and bulk are bothersome to all patients to some degree, regardless of attendant pain (Figs. 17–10 and 17–11). Demineralization and hypoplasia of the underlying skeleton are frequently seen in association with extremity venous malformations (Boyd et al., 1984).

Treatment

Treatment should be conservative for the upper extremity venous lesions; this is especially true for the hand because of its complex anatomical and functional characteristics. The management of venous anomalies depends on size and symptoms. Localized pain frequently occurs; it is unclear whether this is the result of intravascular coagulation, localized phlebothrombosis, or some other process. Aspirin or acetaminophen, elevation, and elastic support should be the initial treatment for pain. Chronic pain in small, localized malformations on the dorsum of the hand or a digit can be helped by excision and linear closure (Fig. 17–12).

More extensive, albeit subtotal, resection may be necessary for functional and aesthetic reasons (Figs. 17–13 and 17–14). The size and three-dimensional extent of a lesion determine the difficulty of dissection and potential postoperative problems. Diffuse venous anomalies cannot be completely excised, but they can usually be safely debulked (Glanz, 1969; Upton et al., 1985). The decision to operate on an extensive lesion is

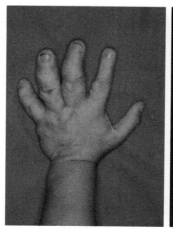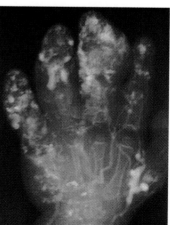

Figure 17–10. Venous malformation. *A* and *B,* Typical appearance of an extensive venous malformation, present since birth. This boy's symptoms of heaviness, aching, and pain are related to engorgement when the limb is held in a dependent position or to local intralesional thromboses, both of which are alleviated with a compression glove. Only the hand has been symptomatic despite extensive ipsilateral involvement of the extremity and chest wall.

A   B

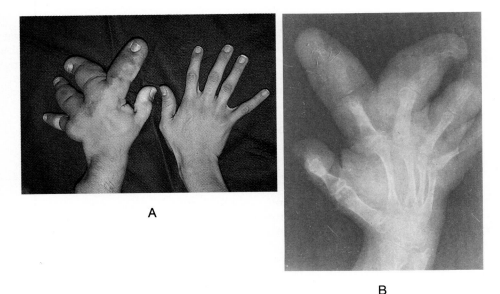

Figure 17–11. Venous malformation. *A* and *B,* The palmar appearance of the hand and corresponding radiograph of this boy demonstrate gross overgrowth associated with a diffuse low-flow venous malformation. Note the associated intradermal capillary malformation. Bone hypertrophy is diffuse, with increased length, breadth, and circumference. Joint distortion is asymmetrical, and large venous channels course through the skeleton. The capillary (port-wine staining) and venous malformation, skeletal hypertrophy, and associated lymphatic malformations place him in the category of the Klippel-Trenaunay syndrome. Comparison with the opposite and more functional hand is shown. This boy also has associated hepatic, gastrointestinal, lower extremity, and buttock capillary-lymphatic-venous malformations.

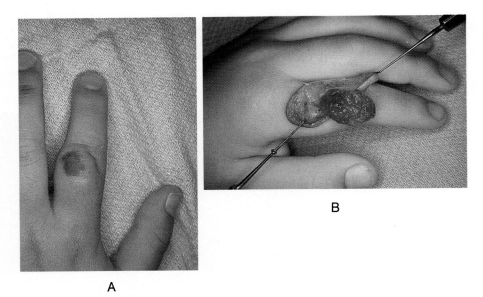

Figure 17–12. Venous malformation. *A* and *B,* A well-localized capillary malformation with underlying venous malformation of the digit is effectively treated with simple excision and closure. Preoperative angiograms or expensive non-invasive flow studies are not necessary in this situation.

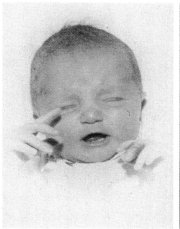 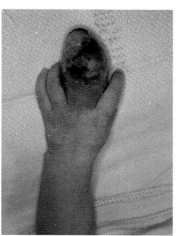

Figure 17–13. Venous malformation. *A* and *B,* An unusual ulcerating malformation in the left long finger of this newborn hemorrhaged, thrombosed within the first few months of life, and resulted in skin loss and required amputation. Histology revealed dilated vascular channels throughout the skin (venous malformation).

A   B

difficult and should not be made without arterial and venous angiography, as anomalous vascular anatomy within these extremities is the rule rather than the exception. These abnormalities correlate with incomplete differentiation of the classic descriptions of vascular development (Sabin, 1917; Woollard, 1922). There are several findings commonly noted in the angiographic evaluation of venous anomalies. Arterial anatomy at the brachial, palmar, and digital level is usually normal, and afferent feeding vessels to a malformation are small and branch at multiple levels. There are no pulsating arteriovenous shunts. Slow venous pooling occurs in large saccular dilatations or varices, which are usually located on the dorsum and within the intermetacarpal spaces of the hand and are difficult areas to approach surgically (see Fig. 17–10). Smaller veins are normally found on the palmar side of the hand. During angiography, proximal venous compression of the limb can be used to accentuate the venous phase, but this maneuver also obliterates the fine detail of the lesion because the varicosities fill faster and more completely (Geiser and Eversmann, 1978). The angiographic extent of the venous anomaly is usually greater than that deduced by clinical examination. Patients with venous malformations are usually asymptomatic when their extremity is elevated or compressed within a garment.

Subcutaneous thrombi may be difficult to locate clinically. Calcifications are easily seen on plain radiograms and tend to occur in lesions that are diffuse and contain smaller caliber vascular channels. Calcifications do not have a predilection for either the palmar or dorsal surfaces, and they may be seen wherever there is a vascular malformation (Fig. 17–15).

A strategy of staged operations is appropriate for the upper extremity so that only one dissection will ever be needed in a particular anatomical region. With extensive malformations, staged procedures should begin distally and progress proximally. The major principles of surgical management, previously noted for all vascular anomalies, are important. For a large venous or combined lymphatic-venous lesion, a preoperative clotting assessment should include CBC, platelets, PT, PTT, fibrinogen, and fibrin split products. Particular attention should be focused on planning the incisions, particularly when large segments of skin and soft tissue will be excised. Intraoperatively, there should be meticulous attention to hemostasis, especially in the intermetacarpal region, and avoidance of unnecessary sacrifice of collateral ligaments. Median and ulnar nerves are routinely decompressed at the wrist level coincident with extensive dissection of the distal forearm and palm. Intraneural dissection of saccular veins within fascicular groups is unrewarding and may result in neurologic damage. In spite of attention to these intraoperative details, staged debulking of large venous anomalies carries a considerable risk

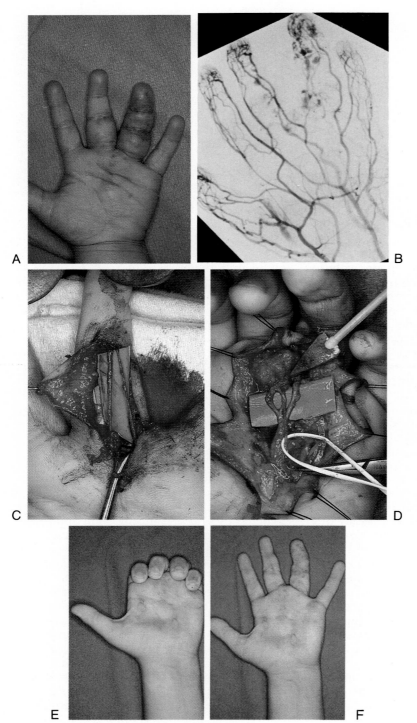

Figure 17–14. Venous malformation. *A,* Appearance of a typical diffuse low-flow malformation in a 4 year old child's palm and central digits. *B,* Angiograms show normal arterial anatomy with very little extrinsic distortion, but lateral films demonstrate diffuse varicosities and saccular lakes. Application of a venous tourniquet is often helpful in demonstrating the full extent of these lesions, which are often not completely visualized on selective angiograms. *C* and *D,* Three staged excisions were performed on the ulnar side of the ring finger, the long-ring webspace, and the palm, in that order. The operating microscope was an invaluable aid during these dissections. *E* and *F,* Flexion and extension 9 years later. The patient remains asymptomatic with good function, although small areas of anomalous vessels are still present. She has not experienced any enlargement during adolescence.

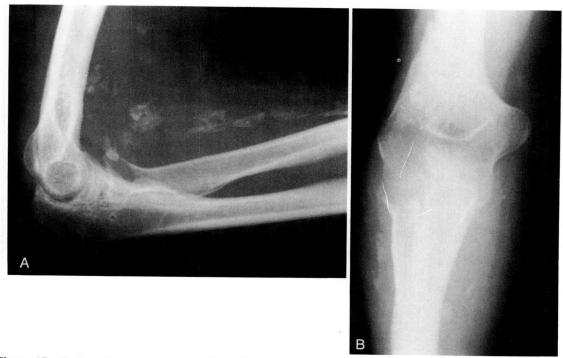

Figure 17–15. Complication: venous malformation. *A* and *B,* Painful intralesional calcifications in this young woman prompted multiple excisions during adolescence to alleviate pain. Dissections around (but not within) nerves resulted in a temporary radial nerve palsy and a protracted sympathetic dystrophy syndrome. The patient has never regained any elbow motion, and 10 years later still has pain, which requires daily analgesics.

and requires assiduous preoperative planning and surgical execution if optimal functional benefits are to be achieved (deTakats, 1932; Ward and Horton, 1940; Malan and Puglionisi, 1964; Szilagyi et al., 1965; Nevaiser and Adams, 1974; Szilagyi et al., 1976).

Complications of Treatment

Complications usually are attributable to operative damage to nerves, scar formation around gliding tendons, sacrifice of supporting ligaments, or ischemic necrosis of the skin (Figs. 17–15 and 17–16; see also Fig. 17–4). The early postoperative problem of hematoma and wound dehiscence can be minimized by drainage of the wound and delayed primary closure. Debulking of large regions within the palm and especially in the forearm and arm carries considerable risk. Excessive trauma to arteries may result in thrombosis and ischemic necrosis.

A low grade disseminated intravascular coagulopathy may occur intra- or postoperatively. In our series, this complication always happened in patients with extensive lesions and in whom there was a high index of suspicion preoperatively. We have also seen intralesional or intramuscular bleeding secondary to inflation of a tourniquet above an incompletely exsanguinated extremity. One such patient with a lower limb malformation developed a complete sciatic nerve loss secondary to an intraneural hematoma. Nerve palsy and muscle necrosis may also occur with excessively long and repeated tourniquet times, which are inevitable whenever bleeding is out of control.

LYMPHATIC MALFORMATION

Clinical Presentation

Lymphatic malformations may present as lymphedema or as circumscribed lesions known, in the past, as "lymphangiomas." These malformations may involve a single digit, the dorsum of the hand, the forearm, the upper arm, or the entire extremity. An extensive lymphatic anomaly of the upper

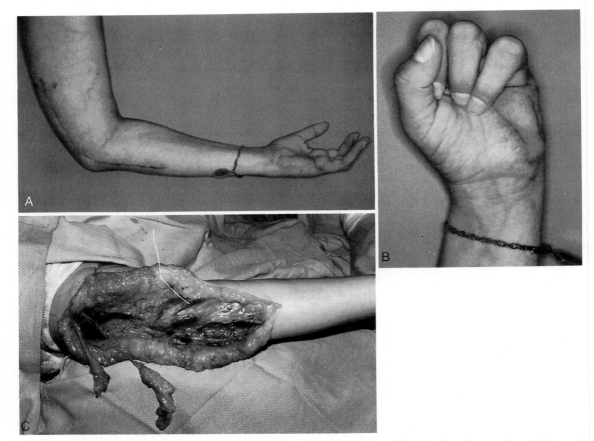

Figure 17–16. Complication: venous malformation. *A* and *B,* Appearance of the hand and arm of a middle aged female following 12 previous operations, including a multistage abdominal flap for an extensive venous lesion that involved her hand and forearm. *C,* Following amputation of the ulnar two digits, her chronic pain and sympathetic dystrophy syndrome were alleviated by excision and rerouting of the heavily scarred ulnar nerve at the elbow and the medial antebrachial cutaneous nerves of the forearm.

limb commonly is also within the ipsilateral chest wall, neck, and mediastinum (Fig. 17–17*A* to *C*) (Young, 1978). Skeletal hypertrophy may be present at an early age (Boyd et al., 1984). The abnormal lymphatic channels vary tremendously in size from large cysts, freely communicating catacombs in the upper arm, axilla, and chest wall, to small, spongy spaces in the forearm and hand. The fact that large cystic channels do not occur in the hand and digits may account for the diminished effectiveness of compression garments in the more distal extremity. The skin overlying a lymphatic malformation may be studded with epidermal blebs filled with serous or bloody fluid. A capillary or venous malformation may be seen in association with a lymphatic anomaly (Fig. 17–19).

Symptoms are related to the size and location of the malformation and the extent of skin involvement. Pain is rarely a problem.

When the skin is implicated, there may be recurrent infection or persistent leakage of serous fluid. Skin incisions made in such areas will frequently break down postoperatively and discharge fluid from deeper cystic pockets (Fig. 17–20). *Beta-hemolytic streptococcus* is responsible for most cellulitic episodes. The weight and bulk of large lymphatic lesions may overwhelm the proximal supporting musculature of the extremity and render a limb functionless. Wrist and small joint motion within the hand can be severely restricted by the bulk of the lesion. Sensation is not altered, and compression neuropathies have not been noted. Children with extensive lymphatic anomaly of more than one extremity sometimes have "diffuse lymphangiectasia" involving the pulmonary system, liver, and gastrointestinal tract. In these cases, malabsorption and protein-losing enteropathy may become a life-threatening problem.

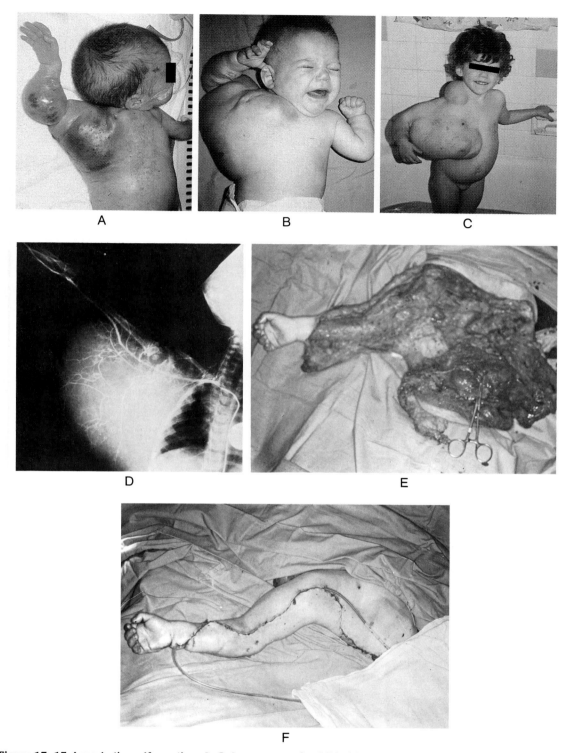

A

B

C

D

E

F

Figure 17–17. Lymphatic malformation. *A–C,* Appearance of a child with a large lymphatic malformation at birth *(A),* age 6 months *(B),* and at 4 years of age *(C),* when the weight and bulk of the mass affected her ambulation and extremity function. There was no intrathoracic extension or respiratory airway difficulty. *D,* Angiogram revealed normal arterial patterns greatly distorted by the mass of anomalous tissue and large dilated collecting veins. *E* and *F,* An aggressive surgical approach was used initially, with excision of the chest wall mass with a portion of the latissimus dorsi muscle and debulking of the axilla with preservation of the brachial plexus and axillary and brachial arteries. Large cystic communications were present between the neck and axilla.

Illustration continued on following page

359

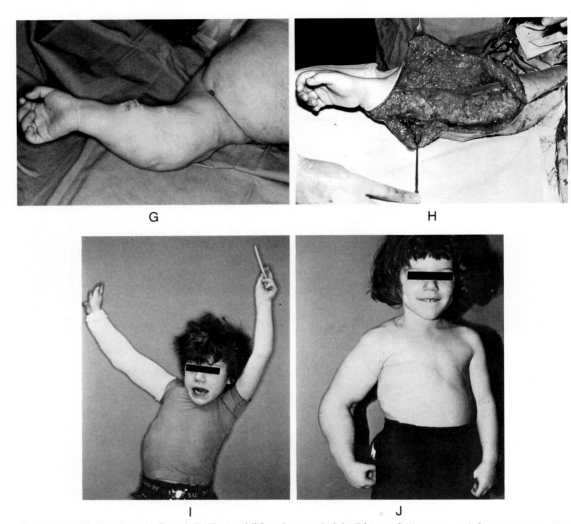

G

H

I

J

Figure 17–17 *Continued. G* and *H,* Two additional staged debulkings of the arm and forearm were then performed at yearly intervals, with preservation of all flexor and extensor muscle groups, as well as the median, ulnar, and radial nerves. *I,* The surgical result is maintained with a compression garment. Hand and forearm function is normal. *J,* Appearance of patient at age 7. She has occasional bubbling of her thoracic suture line and develops episodic infections during the winter months, when she has tonsillitis or pharyngitis; all are treated with penicillin.

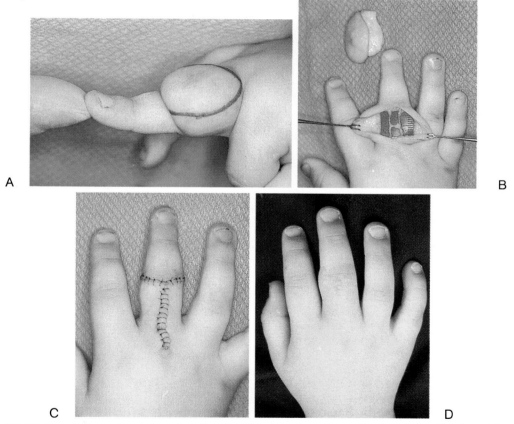

Figure 17–18. Lymphatic malformation. *A*, A "localized" lymphatic malformation isolated to the dorsal finger is treated by *B* and *C*, total excision of the lesion with preservation of dorsal veins under magnification. *D*, Postoperative appearance 2 years later. Such a localized lesion is an unfortunately rare opportunity with lymphatic anomalies.

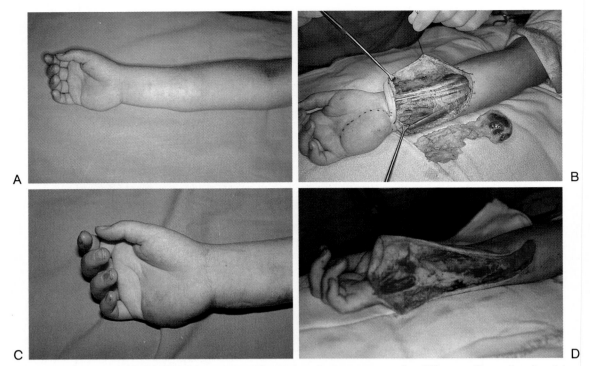

Figure 17–19. Combined lymphatic-venous malformation. *A,* Appearance of a diffuse malformation involving the ulnar half of the forearm and hand. *B,* The forearm component was excised, along with a thorough tenosynovectomy, as the first stage. Several large cystic areas are seen in the proximal portion of the specimen. *C* and *D,* The hand portion with its smaller lymphatic channels and large venous component was removed 1 year later, and preservation of the ulnar nerve, including the deep motor branch, and ulnar artery was accomplished.

Management

Treatment is commonly necessary for episodic infections, and consists of elevation, immobilization, warmth, and systemic antibiotics. Localized abscess is infrequent; therefore, incision and drainage are usually not necessary. In fact, most infections present with no obvious portal of entry, and those that do, usually implicate a paronychia, intertriginous maceration, infected cut, insect bite, or abrasion. When repeated cellulitis is a problem, long-term prophylactic antibiotics may be needed. As with all patients with lymphedema of a limb, these individuals must take scrupulous care of the skin and nails.

Compressive garments definitely control swelling, but they are not as effective in diminishing bulk as for venous malformations. Home compression pumps can be recommended for patients with extensive involvement of the forearm and arm. Self-adherent tape (Coban) for wrapping the digits and palm at night is very effective in controlling digital swelling. Unfortunately, it is quite difficult to keep Coban on children under 5 years of age.

Figure 17–20. Lymphatic malformation with limb hypertrophy. *A* and *B,* Appearance of a massive malformation involving the neck, chest wall, axilla, and upper extremity, with radiographic demonstration of hypertrophy of the clavicle, scapula, and long bones of the arm and extrinsic pressure upon the thoracic cage. *C–F,* Following neck debulking to manage a compromised airway, the extremity was approached aggressively with distal to proximal radical debulkings of the dorsum of the hand, palm, and volar forearm in three stages. *G* and *H,* A direct approach to the volar forearm included excision of all tissue down to muscle and fascia, and 180 degree dissection circumferentially. Edema was impossible to control, as bulk and weight made the limb non-functional. Shoulder disarticulation with preservation of the scapula for cosmetic purposes was the final result. Now 7 years of age, this youngster wears a prosthesis.

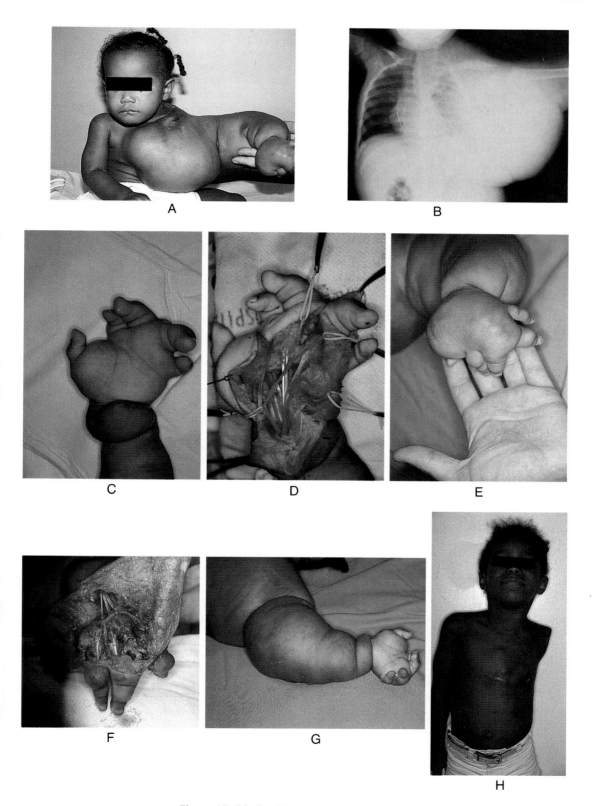

Figure 17–20. *See legend on opposite page*

Conservative treatment is the rule unless size or volume interferes with function. Staged surgical debulking can be performed (deTakats, 1932; Malan and Puglionisi, 1965; Upton et al., 1985). The most satisfactory results are obtained with the excisions of the dorsum of the hand and digits. Every effort should be made to preserve the cutaneous nerves, dorsal veins, and overlying skin. Although removal of all anomalous tissue is usually impossible, excision of as much involved tissue as feasible is recommended so that re-entry into a scarred region will not be necessary. The dorsal and palmar surfaces of the hand should be approached in separate stages. Strip excisions (Homans procedure) with or without excision of underlying muscle or fascia have had variable success in the forearm and arm (Fonkalsrud and Coulson, 1973; Miller, 1975). The dissection should not extend more than 180 degrees circumferentially around the limb, as the extent and depth of undermining skin are critical to the survival of these flaps. Intraoperative evaluation of flap viability with intravenous fluorescein may be helpful. Complete excision of the affected skin and subcutaneous tissue with skin graft replacement (Charles, 1912), useful as a salvage procedure in the lower limb, leaves an aesthetically unacceptable result with recurrent skin breakdown and contractures. This technique is not appropriate for use in the upper limb.

A lymphatic malformation in the upper arm is often continuous with anomalous tissue in the chest wall. A single staged chest wall and axillary dissection is often easier than multiple staged resections (see Figs. 17–17 and 17–19). Large cystic communications are located in and around the brachial plexus and subclavian, axillary, and/or brachial arteries and veins. Dissection within the plexus may cause scarring, nerve damage, and subsequent pain, and this pursuit is not recommended for an asymptomatic patient or an inexperienced surgeon.

Massive, diffuse lesions in functionless limbs may be best treated with amputation instead of multiple unsuccessful attempts at debulking.

Lymphatic-venous and lymph node–venous microvascular anastomoses have been, and still are, attempted but have *never* been shown to be effective for relief of lymphatic obstruction in congenital conditions.

Complications of Treatment

Postoperative complications include persistent fluid leakage from the incision, hematoma, seroma, and necrosis of excessively thinned flaps (Fig. 17–21; see also Fig. 17–6). Cellulitis within the limb, usually in the resected area, is another frequent postoperative occurrence. Skin excision and skin graft replacement are often complicated by late scarring, persistent ulceration, cutaneous vesicles, dermatitis, and contractures, which in the axilla, elbow, and wrist regions may be far worse than the original condition.

Compression garments are recommended in all patients postoperatively to maintain the surgical result. The most difficult areas within which to control persistent swelling are the thumb–index finger web space, palm of the hand, and base of the interdigital commissures.

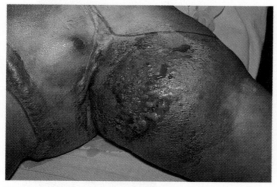

Figure 17–21. Complication: lymphatic malformation. Persistent "bubbling" of epidermal surface; a site of previous surgical incisions is commonly seen with residual lymphatic malformation. Same patient as in Figure 17–20.

COMBINED LYMPHATIC-VENOUS MALFORMATION

Clinical Presentation

A combination of venous and lymphatic anomalous channels is another low flow, hemodynamically stable malformation that affects the forearm, hand, and particularly the dorsum of the hand. These combined lesions are often associated with skeletal elongation and hypertrophy. When there is also a port-wine stain, the eponym Klippel-Trenaunay syndrome is applicable (Klippel and Trenaunay, 1900; Björkholm and Aschberg, 1900; Boyd et al., 1984). Size, weight, and abnormal contour dominate the clinical presentation in these patients, so that they (or the parents) often press for more than conservative therapy. The angioarchitecture of these malformations varies tremendously, and few generalizations can be made. When a hand is diffusely involved, venous channels are usually more prominent in the digits and the dorsal metacarpal region. Cystic lymphatic communications tend to be located in the palm (see Fig. 17–19). In a diffusely involved limb, large venous varicosities may be encountered within the forearm and arm with huge draining veins in the axilla. Arterial architecture is normal, but it is often distorted by the mass effect of the malformation. Angiograms and venograms usually demonstrate large, tortuous veins with interconnecting saccular regions and a conspicuous absence of smaller channels.

Symptoms are the same as in patients with purely venous or lymphatic malformations. Spontaneous infections, without an obvious portal of entry, are not as frequent in this group as in those with the lymphatic anomalies. Pain is usually not a presenting complaint. Weight, bulk, and contour deformities cause functional problems.

A rare and interesting type of gigantism of the upper limb is seen in the presence of lymphatic malformation (Pearse and Morton, 1930; Harris and Wright, 1930; Goldanich and Campanacci, 1962). We have documented seven patients who exhibited characteristic hemihypertrophy of their upper limbs as well as their lower limbs. Lymphatic malformation localized to the axilla or arm was present, but the enlargement was due to generalized hypertrophy of normal anatomical structures, particularly bone and muscle. Hand and forearm enlargement was the result of enlarged normal muscles, duplicated muscles, or atavistic intrinsic and extrinsic muscle groups (Fig. 17–22). No specific relationship between the enlargement and the lymphatic malformation has been established. Both may result from a failure of morphogenesis at a very early embryologic stage without any specific cause and effect relationship to each other.

Treatment

Surgical debulking of these combined low flow lesions can usually be safely accomplished. The principles of treatment are the same as with the more pure venous or lymphatic categories. Preoperative coagulation studies are important in patients with large, diffuse venous lesions. The resections should be as thorough as possible, with preservation of uninvolved neurovascular elements. Large venous lakes and varicosities must be completely excised or obliterated, to avoid postoperative bleeding problems, particularly in the metacarpal region. Early and late complications are the same as for more predominantly lymphatic and venous categories. Recurrent enlargement of a finger, hand, or limb, following what was thought to be a "thorough" resection, may occur and is probably due to redirection of flow or accumulation of lymphatic fluid within remaining abnormal vascular channels. With extensive lesions, it is often impossible to identify and remove all abnormal channels without resorting to amputation.

Overgrowth of the upper limb is usually not a functional problem, in contrast to the lower limb. Epiphysiodesis of the humerus, radius, metacarpals, and phalanges is rarely indicated in upper limb hypertrophy. In our series of patients, only one radial shortening was performed for progressive ulnar deviation of the carpus and hand. Growth arrest of metacarpals and proximal phalanges was done in only three instances to control excessive length before adolescence. When necessary, extraarticular ablation of the digital growth plate is performed through midlateral incisions.

ARTERIOVENOUS MALFORMATION

Clinical Presentation

Fortunately, high flow arteriovenous malformations of the upper limb are infrequent. Of 117 vascular malformations of the upper limb in our series, only 21 cases were in this diagnostic category. Patients with these anomalies are usually symptomatic at time of first presentation, and the symptoms correlate with the hemodynamic state of the fistulae (Reid, 1925a, b; Harris and Wright, 1930; Bertelsen and Dohn, 1953; Cross et al., 1958; Weinberg et al., 1960; Fry, 1974; Bogumill, 1977; Niechajev and Karlsson, 1982a; Newmeyer, 1984). There may be involvement of the entire arm, forearm, or hand; rarely is the malformation localized

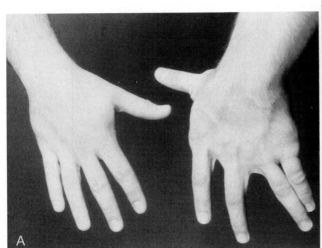

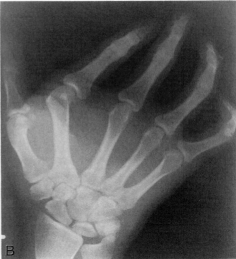

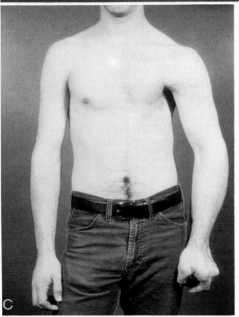

Figure 17–22. Hemi-hypertrophy with lymphatic malformation. *A* and *B,* Appearance and radiograph of an enlarged but functional hand in a teenager. The entire arm had been enlarged since birth. A large cystic lymphatic malformation had been removed from the ipsilateral axilla. *C,* Forearm is twice normal circumference and like the hand consists of enlarged or duplicated normal and atavistic muscles. Multiple procedures on the hand have been performed to release flexion contractures, lengthen flexor tendons, release tight intrinsic muscles, and realign splayed out metacarpals.

Figure 17–23. Arteriovenous malformation. *A–C,* Appearance of the hand of a young mother who first noticed a small bluish discoloration within her palm as a teenager. This gradually enlarged and became markedly worse during late adolescence and two subsequent pregnancies and is seen here with painful trophic ulcerations associated with a proximal "steal" phenomenon. *D,* Early angiographic films show rapid high-flow shunting through a diffuse arteriovenous malformation. *E,* Review of her first (left) and second (right) contrast studies, which were obtained before and after her pregnancies, shows a remarkable increase in the tortuosity and saccular dilatations of the feeding ulnar artery and its branches. Note the persistent median artery, which is common in these lesions. *F,* A massive and somewhat tortuous brachial artery was present.

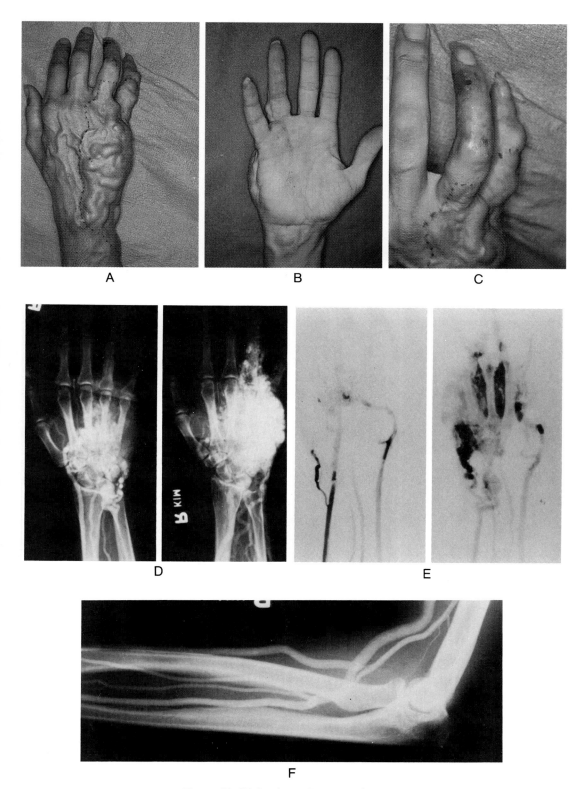

Figure 17–23 *See legend on opposite page*

Illustration continued on following page

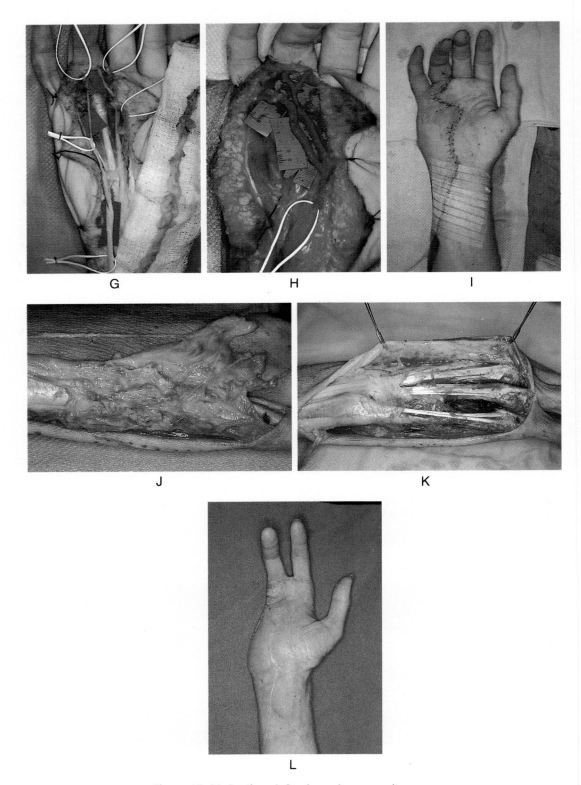

Figure 17–23 *Continued. See legend on opposite page*

within a single digit. Associated dermal capillary malformations are present in almost half of our patients with arteriovenous anomalies (see Fig. 17–9). One third of these lesions are noticed at birth, many are detected by the age of 2 years, and almost all are obvious by adolescence (Malan and Puglionisi, 1964).

All patients experienced increased warmth in the limb (Harris and Wright, 1930; Szilagyi et al., 1976); pain, paresthesias, hyperhidrosis, and compression neuropathies are also common (Coursley et al., 1956). Bruits and thrills are not always marked, but careful scrutiny of the lesion with a Doppler unit invariably demonstrates multiple micro- and macrofistulous tracts (Stephenson and Lichti, 1971; Pisko-Dubienski et al., 1975). For some patients, pulsating masses and accompanying thrills may be psychologically disturbing. Mottling of the skin, distal trophic ulcerations, and joint stiffness are other problems that occur secondary to peripheral ischemia. A paradoxical "steal phenomenon" shunts flow away from the distal portion of the limb (Malan and Puglionisi, 1965; Wakim and Janes, 1958) (Fig. 17–23). There may be associated vascular malformations in other anatomical regions, particularly the central nervous system, gastrointestinal tract, lower extremities, and head and neck, that may demand more urgent treatment (Callander, 1920; Gomes and Bernatz, 1970; Newmeyer, 1984). Patients with extensive lesions involving the entire extremity and ipsilateral chest wall often demonstrate a positive Nicoladoni-Branham sign (Nicoladoni, 1875; Branham, 1890). Patients with large hyperdynamic malformations are also at risk for cardiopulmonary overload and consumption coagulopathy (Rodriguez-Erdman et al., 1971). Intralesional bleeding can cause a compartment compression syndrome. Skeletal hypertrophy and elongation are present in half of these patients. In the lower limb, the Parkes Weber syndrome (Parkes Weber, 1918; Horton, 1932; Leonard and Vassos, 1951) consists of a high flow arteriovenous malformation, a dermal capillary malformation, and skeletal hypertrophy. Symptoms of arteriovenous malformations may be exacerbated by trauma (Curtis, 1953) and may change with alterations of flow during adolescence, during pregnancy, or while the patient is on oral contraceptive agents (Mulliken, 1983). Bone involvement carries an unfavorable prognosis but is not an absolute contraindication to operative therapy.

Diagnosis

Diagnostic studies, e.g., roentgenograms, xerograms, thermograms, plethysmograms, Doppler flow studies, bone scans, pulse volume recordings (Yao et al., 1973), blood gas determinations (Brown, 1929; Veal and McCord, 1936), computerized axial tomograms (CT scans), and other tests yield important information and tend to confirm the clinical diagnosis (Upton et al., 1985). The selective angiogram, with magnified views taken in two planes, provides the most important diagnostic information. In some cases, the anatomical extent of the malformation and the size, caliber, and flow dynamics of major shunts are clearly seen. Rapid change cassettes are necessary because fine detail is quickly obliterated in the presence of a large, active shunt (Fig. 17–23D). Often, however, the true potential extent of the malformation cannot be delineated by any of these methods because of small fistulae and secondary enlargement of inflow and outflow vessels. Angiograms have been obtained on all of our patients, although patterns are quite variable; usually, active shunting is noted through micro- and macrofistulous channels or both (Bliznak and Staple, 1974). Visualization of both normal and abnormal vascular anatomy may be inadequate or completely lost on angiograms in the presence of

---

Figure 17–23 *Continued. G–I,* In the first of two procedures, thorough excision within the palm with preservation of nerves and tendons was performed. Intercalated vein grafts were used to revascularize the ring and small fingers, which clearly would not have survived following this excision. *J and K,* The dorsum of the hand was approached at the second stage where the excision extended within the intermetacarpal space. Removal of all involved tissue was impossible. The fourth through sixth dorsal compartments with tendons are shown. Despite previous excision and ligation of the ulnar artery, banding of the median and radial arteries was necessary to control bleeding. *L,* Trophic ulcerations and pain persisted post-operatively, and a hemi-hand amputation was necessary.

significant proximal shunting of flow through the malformation, or by early filling of large arterialized veins on the dorsum of the hand. The true extent of these active lesions is never fully appreciated on a simple angiogram. They are always more extensive than they initially appear, and it is not unusual to see rapid local extension postoperatively as flow is redirected into other abnormal channels.

Abnormalities of major arteries are often seen in these limbs, e.g., giant feeding vessels, duplicated brachial arteries, or persistent interosseous or median arteries continuing to form the superficial arch within the palm. A large, pulsating, tortuous axillary and brachial artery is usually present with distal extensive lesions. Aneurysmal dilatations and tortuosity of arterial segments are frequently noted in adolescence and become progressively worse with age (Figs. 17–23 and 24). Communications between the radial and ulnar sides of the hand are often quite diffuse, obscuring the superficial and deep palmar arches. It is not unusual for a muscle group to be completely replaced by a mass of microfistulous shunts (Fig. 17–25). Vincular vessels within the digits will be present if there is a digital artery, but often they are completely obliterated by the malformation.

Management

The treatment of these difficult lesions must be carefully individualized. Young children should be trained to wear elastic compression garments with a pressure between 20 and 40 mmHg. Diffuse lesions with microfistulous connections seen by angiography are probably not amenable to excisional biopsy (see Fig. 17–9).

Symptoms that may prompt surgical intervention are severe pain, trophic ulcerations secondary to distal ischemia, intralesional bleeding causing a compartment compression syndrome, and mechanical factors such as size and weight affecting function. The decision to operate depends upon careful assessment of symptoms and functional loss. Preoperative information from all of the diagnostic studies, particularly the subtraction views of selected angiograms, should be carefully analyzed and a specific operation outlined. If the surgeon is trying to be flexible and non-committal, little is accomplished by

dissecting these malformations. Instead, specific preoperative objectives should be achieved during a safe tourniquet time. The problems that transpire when these procedures get out of control are well known to all surgeons who have operated on these malformations (Bernheim, 1925; Szilagyi, 1965; Szilagyi et al., 1976).

Each operation should be tailored to the patient's individual needs. In all but the most localized lesions, operations for arteriovenous malformations of the limb are palliative. Historically, four types of procedures have been performed: (1) proximal ligation, (2) deafferentation (or "skeletonization") (Malan and Puglionisi, 1965), (3) subtotal excision, and (4) amputation. In our series, proximal ligation has been totally unsuccessful for high flow lesions with both micro- and macrofistulous shunting (Figs. 17–27 and 17–29). Blood is rapidly redirected into new and sometimes unrecognized anomalous fistulous tracts along channels of least peripheral resistance (Norris, 1843; Pemberton and Saint, 1928). This flow alteration has been misinterpreted as metastasis in the past (Matas, 1940). Distal perfusion to the limb may be compromised, and the steal phenomenon may aggravate symptoms (Malan and Puglionisi, 1965; Matolo et al., 1971; Ozeran et al., 1972). Partial, staged, or subtotal excisions have been more successful, particularly when lesions have been well localized in the arm or forearm (deTakats, 1932; Seeger, 1938; Freeman, 1946; Curtis, 1953; Szilagyi et al., 1965; Malan and Puglionisi, 1965; Storey et al., 1969; Gelberman and Goldner, 1978; Upton et al., 1985).

The general principles of treatment (outlined earlier in the introductory section) apply to high flow anomalies. There is no predictable procedure that when performed in childhood will keep the malformation from growing with the child. Usually, neurologic symptoms, distal gangrene, increasing steal phenomenon, and complications secondary to bleeding are the precipitating events prior to an operation. Most patients undergo excision as a last resort prior to amputation. A preoperative coagulation work-up is essential when one is dealing with any symptomatic lesion of significant size; these tests include CBC, platelet count, PT, PTT, bleeding time, fibrinogen, and fibrin split products. In few other areas of hand surgery is careful explanation of potential complications so impor-

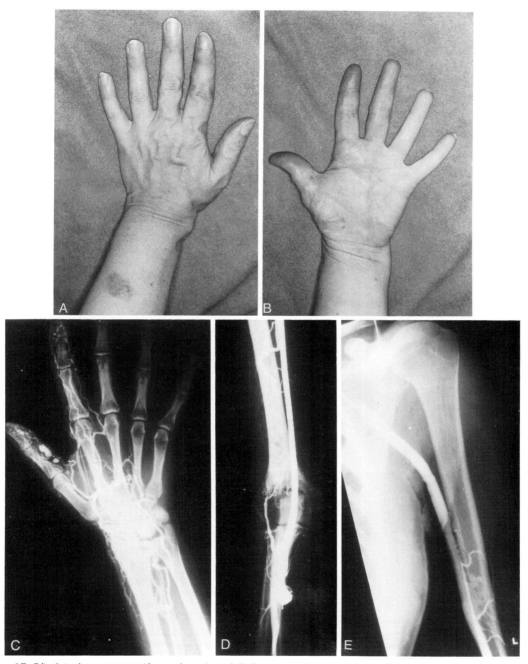

Figure 17–24. Arteriovenous malformation. *A* and *B,* Dorsal and palmar views of the hand of a young woman who since early childhood had multiple pulsatile regions in the palm, forearm, and upper arm. The skin lesion on the dorsal forearm was excised and found to be a "malignant acrospiroma," a locally aggressive tumor of sweat duct origin. *C* and *D,* Angiograms show distorted arterial anatomy with multiple prominent saccular aneurysms. Only the lesion in the forearm has been excised and replaced with an autogenous vein graft. *E,* The intermittent pain she experiences as an adult is probably related to the interosseous malformation, which has not changed in the 12 years between angiograms.

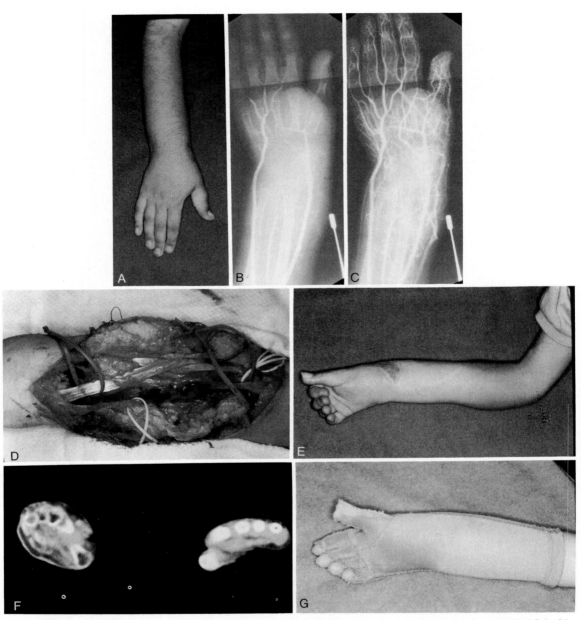

Figure 17–25. Complication: arteriovenous malformation. *A–C,* The hand and forearm of a 4 year old child with a slowly progressive arteriovenous malformation causing enlargement and radial deviation of the distal forearm and limited function of the flexor muscle mass. Angiograms show a diffuse malformation with very small but dynamic microfistulous shunts. *D* and *E,* Despite resection, which included the flexor pollicis longus, the malformation persists. Dark loop on left is around extensor pollicis longus. White loop in middle encircles sensory branches of the radial nerve. Distal flap necrosis occurred following this aggressive resection. *F,* Subsequent CT scan at the proximal metacarpal level shows diffuse soft tissue enlargement, which corresponded to progressive diminution of function. Ulnar deviation of the hand and carpus is secondary to overgrowth of the distal radius. *G,* Despite constant use of an elastic garment, her symptoms and enlargement persist.

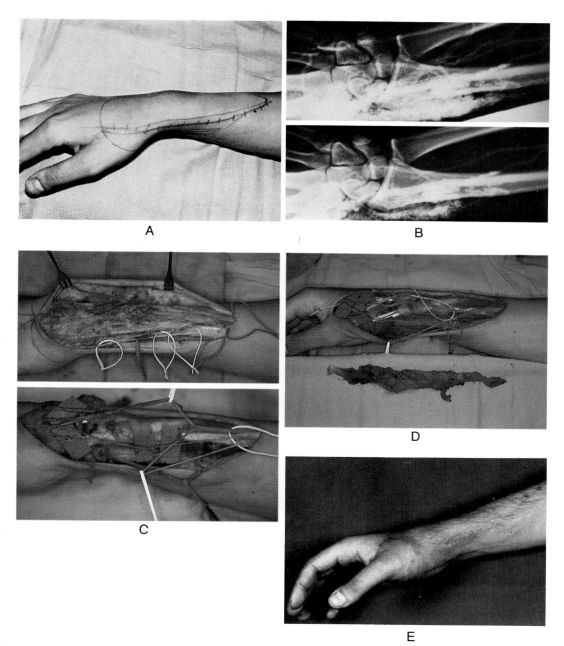

Figure 17–26. Arterial malformation: high-flow. *A,* Distribution of a well localized, warm, pulsating mass that had been present for 10 years in a teenage boy. Symptoms included paresthesias in the cutaneous branches of the radial nerve, which were precipitated by local repetitive trauma. *B,* Angiograms demonstrate rapid filling of large arterial saccular dilatations at less than 3 seconds. The malformation is fed by the radial artery. *C* and *D,* Surgical exposure (above) shows the malformation originating from and involving the radial artery, which was excised in continuity with the mass. All sensory branches of the radial nerve (below) were preserved. *E,* Five years later, patient is asymptomatic and has not developed recurrent enlargement. Tendon and nerve function is normal.

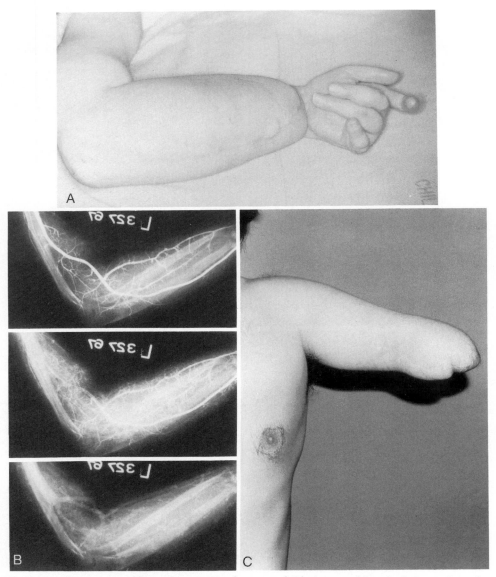

Figure 17–27. Arteriovenous malformation. *A,* The forearm of this teenaged boy had always been large, with pulsations and bruit. A massive intravascular bleed within the flexor compartment resulted in severe pain, anesthesia in the median and ulnar nerve distributions, and flexion contractures. *B,* Serial angiograms show early, active fistulization throughout the entire forearm. Previous surgical attempts to control pain with proximal vessel ligation or debulking were unsuccessful. *C,* Above elbow amputation alleviated most of the patient's symptoms. Phantom limb pain resolved in 2–3 years. He now wears a prosthesis. (Courtesy of Joseph E. Murray, M.D.)

tant. The patient with a diffuse arteriovenous malformation causing cardiopulmonary overload will probably not respond to any type of staged excision; the patient with more quiescent lesions that have been present for a long period of time may respond quite well.

Attempts at partial excisions and deafferentation should not be made in these patients. Instead, a thorough dissection of one particular region should be planned from the outset. Although revascularization is not usually necessary, one must be prepared to use microvascular techniques to establish at least one major artery per digit and at least one artery feeding a patent palmar arch (if one exists). Knowledge of normal and abnormal anatomy is crucial. Major intraosseous and median arteries are frequently seen, along with duplication and bizarre tortuosities at the brachial level. The surgeon must work efficiently because bleeding after deflation of the tourniquet precludes another chance for precise dissection and identification of structures. During the tissue dissection, it is best to ligate or cauterize as many potential bleeding points as possible. Desperate clamping within the avalanche of blood that follows tourniquet deflation invariably causes nerve damage. The dissection should not be beyond planned limits, opening up areas that cannot be adequately handled within reasonable tourniquet times of 90 minutes. With repeated tourniquet inflation, additional complications may arise for both surgeon and anesthesiologist. Preoperative cooling of the extremity will safely allow ischemia times in the range of 120 minutes. Torrential bleeding following tourniquet release can be controlled with direct pressure and elevation, followed by control of individual vessels in a systematic fashion. Clotting parameters should be monitored intraoperatively with the assistance of a hematologist, particularly if there is preoperative intravascular coagulopathy.

The major intraoperative dilemma is the question, "What to do in the face of diffuse involvement of all tissue planes?" The most satisfactory results in our patients have followed complete excision of the anomalous soft tissue within a given region with preservation of nerves, skeletal structures, and joints. Involved muscle tendon units, skin, and subcutaneous tissue may be reconstructed and/or replaced. Curettage of interosseous vascular malformations and packing

with autogenous bone have been suggested by other investigators (Nisbet, 1954) and may be of value for the large bones of the extremity. Because radical excision invariably includes major arterial structures, revascularization (utilizing microvascular techniques) may be necessary; this has been accomplished in three of our patients. Veins from the dorsum of the foot or arterialized veins from the dorsal forearm are satisfactory arterial grafts. When the flow to the forearm or hand is still excessive in a patient with only one major vessel remaining, circumferential banding can be useful. In patients with localized pulsating lesions, the malformation may be excised after ligation of multiple feeding vessels. Removal of the involved segment of an axial vessel is recommended, especially if it shows any sign of tortuosity or aneurysmal dilatation. In two of our cases in which this segment was saved, progressive deterioration occurred, and the segment was ultimately removed because of large pulsating saccular aneurysms (see Fig. 17–24).

The liberal use of drains and delayed primary closure will help minimize complications and tissue loss. When digit or flap compromise occurs in the early postoperative period, the surgeon must have an alternative plan for excision, revascularization, or closure. The simplest methods are usually the best.

Soft tissue replacement may be required following radical excision. Split-thickness skin grafts are often the most expeditious coverage (primary or delayed primary closure). Local or distant flaps are reserved for secondary coverage.

Selective embolization has been useful in the head and neck region, but not in the hand and upper extremity owing to the danger of distal thrombotic ischemia (Dotter et al., 1975; Olcott et al., 1976; Griffin et al., 1978; Moore and Weiland, 1985). There are unpublished examples of embolization causing distal gangrene.

Amputation may be the only way to cure a patient with a non-functional limb, but even this procedure may not be the solution. Amputation has been life saving in three of our patients with extensive malformations who had developed consumptive coagulopathy (see Figs. 17–23, 17–24, and 17–29). Intractable pain, functional loss of the affected part of the extremity, failed previous operations, and chronically infected trophic ulcerations

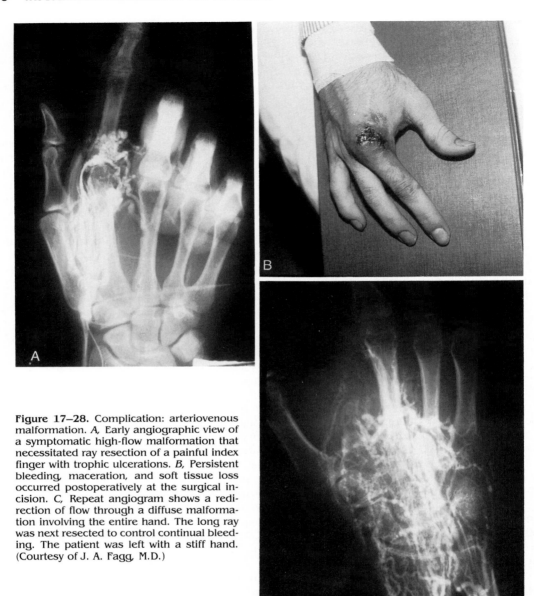

Figure 17–28. Complication: arteriovenous malformation. *A,* Early angiographic view of a symptomatic high-flow malformation that necessitated ray resection of a painful index finger with trophic ulcerations. *B,* Persistent bleeding, maceration, and soft tissue loss occurred postoperatively at the surgical incision. *C,* Repeat angiogram shows a redirection of flow through a diffuse malformation involving the entire hand. The long ray was next resected to control continual bleeding. The patient was left with a stiff hand. (Courtesy of J. A. Fagg, M.D.)

Figure 17–29. Arteriovenous malformation. *A,* Appearance of a young boy with a diffuse malformation involving the left side of his body present almost since the time of birth. His hand and forearm had always been warm and painful. Thirty years ago, this was called a "varicose hemangioma." *B* and *C,* At age 18 years, pain persisted despite several attempts to control flow by proximal ligation. Below elbow amputation was performed as a life-saving maneuver in the face of severe pain and intralesional bleeding precipitated by a disseminated intravascular coagulopathy. *D,* The operative exposure shows anomalous vascular channels and intravascular calcifications within the antecubital fossa. *E* and *F,* Appearance of thorax at age 18 and 31, where no procedures have been performed. The patient has had repeated hospitalizations for problems involving the central nervous system and gastrointestinal tract and for persistent ulcerations in the left leg. (Courtesy of J. A. Fagg, M.D.)

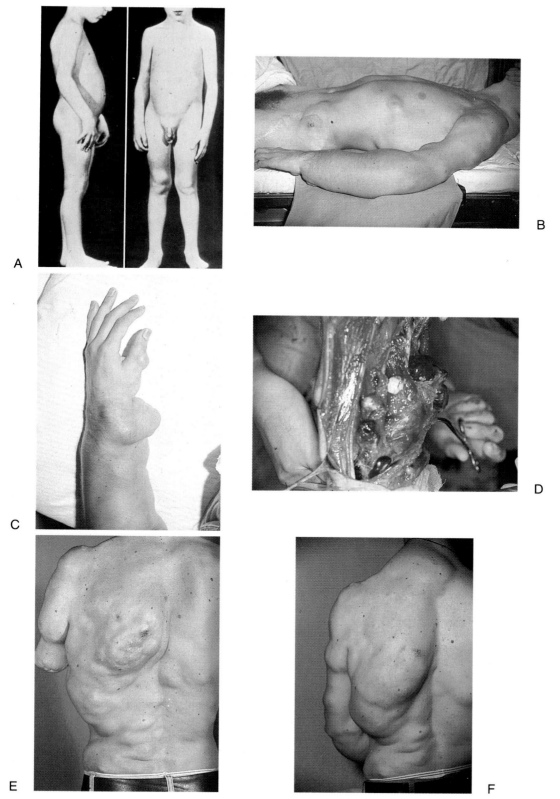

Figure 17–29 *See legend on opposite page*

may all warrant ablation (Fig. 17–28). Each case must be assessed individually, but the surgeon should not persist in trying to save a functionless extremity. Fortunately, all of our amputations have been unilateral. One patient wears a prosthesis, and all have a normal contralateral upper limb.

Complications of Treatment

In few other areas of hand and upper extremity surgery are the incidence of early and late complications as high—there is at least a 50% complication rate. Persistent oozing from the incision sites, wound breakdown, hematoma, infection, marginally vascularized tissues, or skin necrosis following the devascularization of a radical excision may all occur early. Incomplete excision invariably results in proximal expansion of the lesion. Occasionally, a clinician, impressed by the aggressive expansion of a malformation, and a pathologist, impressed by the invasive appearance of the vascular channels, despite a low mitotic index, may reach a diagnosis of "angiosarcoma," an ominous diagnosis that requires radical amputation. In fact, sarcomatous degeneration within a congenital vascular anomaly is almost unknown (see Fig. 17–4).

Late problems relate to incomplete excision, distal ischemia, or injury to anatomical structures during the surgical dissection. Trophic ulceration of the fingertips, skin mottling, and ischemic pain may occur following aggressive excision without revascularization, or incomplete excision with aggravation of the steal phenomenon. Many of these hemodynamic problems can be avoided by careful preoperative planning.

Severe pain following dissection of major neurovascular structures has been a particularly annoying complication in the high flow group. Three instances of post-traumatic sympathetic dystrophy occurred in 15 patients, who had operations for very unstable malformations; for this reason, intraneural dissections are now avoided. Scar contracture and adherence of tendons within the hand and forearm may occur in the patient who has had an extensive dissection and prolonged postoperative immobilization.

References

Apfelberg, D. B., Maser, M. R., and Lash, H.: Argon laser management of cutaneous vascular deformities: A preliminary report. West J. Med. *124*:99, 1976.

Bernheim, B. M.: Congenital arteriovenous fistula in left brachial artery and vein with secondary arterial blood supply to arm. Ann. Surg. *81*:465, 1925.

Bertelsen, A., and Dohn, K.: Congenital arteriovenous communications of the extremities. Clinical and pathophysiological investigations. Acta Chir. Scand. *105*:448, 1953.

Björkholm, M., and Aschberg, S.: Functional aspects of the Klippel-Trenaunay and related syndromes. Acta Derm. Venereol. (Stockh.) *60*:409, 1980.

Blair, W. F., Buckwalter, J. A., Michelson, M. R., and Omer, G. E.: Lymphangioma of the forearm and hand. J. Hand Surg. *8*:399, 1983.

Bliznak, J., and Staple, T. W.: Radiology of angiodysplasias of the limb. Radiology *110*:35, 1974.

Bogumill, G. P.: Clinico-pathological correlation in a case of congenital arteriovenous fistula. Hand *9*:60, 1977.

Boyd, J. B., Mulliken, J. B., Kaban, L. B., Upton, J., and Murray, J. E.: Skeletal changes associated with vascular malformations. Plast. Reconstr. Surg. *74*:789, 1984.

Branham, H. H.: Aneurismal varix of the femoral artery and vein following a gunshot wound. Int. J. Surg. *3*:250, 1890.

Brown, G. E.: Abnormal arteriovenous communications diagnosed from the oxygen content of the blood of the regional veins. Arch. Surg. *18*:807, 1929.

Callander, C. L.: Study of arteriovenous fistula with an analysis of 447 cases. Johns Hopkins Hosp. Rep. *19*:259, 1920.

Charles, R. H.: *A System of Treatment.* London: Churchill, Vol. 3, 1912.

Clodius, L.: Excision and grafting of extensive facial hemangiomas. Brit. J. Plast. Surg. *30*:185, 1977.

Cosman, B.: Experience in the argon laser therapy of port wine stains. Plast. Reconstr. Surg. *65*:119, 1980.

Coursley, G., Ivins, J. C., and Barker, N. W.: Congenital arteriovenous fistulas in extremities: An analysis of 69 cases. Angiology *7*:201, 1956.

Cross, F. S., Glover, D. M., Simeone, F. A., and Oldenburg, F. A.: Congenital arteriovenous aneurysms. Ann. Surg. *148*:649, 1958.

Curtis, R. M.: Congenital arteriovenous fistulae of the hand. J. Bone Joint Surg. *35A*:917, 1953.

David, V. C.: Aneurysm of the hand. Arch. Surg. *33*:267, 1936.

deTakats, G.: Vascular anomalies of the extremities. Report of five cases. Surg. Gynecol. Obstet. *55*:227, 1932.

Dotter, C. T., Goldman, M. L., and Rösch, J.: Instant selective arterial occlusion with isobutyl 2-cyanoacrylate. Radiology *114*:227, 1975.

Erikson, U., and Hemmingsson, A.: Congenital vascular malformations of the hand. Acta Radiol. Diag. *14*:753, 1973.

Finn, M. C., Mulliken, J. B., and Glowacki, J.: Congenital vascular lesions: Clinical application of a new classification. J. Pediat. Surg. *18*:894, 1983.

Fonkalsrud, E. W., and Coulson, W. F.: Management of congenital lymphedema in infants and children. Ann. Surg. *177*:280, 1973.

Freeman, N. E.: Arterial repair in the treatment of aneurysms and arteriovenous fistulae. A report of eighteen successful restorations. Ann. Surg. *124*:888, 1946.

Fry, W. J.: Surgical considerations in congenital arteriovenous fistula. Surg. Clin. North Am. *54*:165, 1974.

Geiser, J. H., and Eversmann, W. W., Jr.: Closed system venography in the evaluation of upper extremity hemangiomas. J. Hand Surg. *3*:173, 1978.

Gelberman, R. H., and Goldner, J. L.: Congenital arteriovenous fistulas of the hand. J. Hand Surg. *3*:451, 1978.

Glanz, S.: The surgical treatment of cavernous hemangiomas of the hand. Brit. J. Plast. Surg. *22*:293, 1969.

Goldanich, I. F., and Campanacci, M.: Vascular hamartomata and infantile angioectatic osteohyperplasia of the extremities: A study of ninety-four cases. J. Bone Joint Surg. *44A*:815, 1962.

Gomes, M. R., and Bernatz, P. E.: Arteriovenous fistulas: A review and ten year experience at the Mayo Clinic. Mayo Clin. Proc. *45*:81, 1970.

Grabb, W. C., MacCallum, M. S., and Tan, N. G.: Results from tattooing port-wine hemangiomas. Plast. Reconstr. Surg. *59*:667, 1977.

Greenspan, R. G., Simon, A. L., Ricketts, H. J., et al.: In vitro magnification angiography. Invest. Radiol. *2*:419, 1967.

Griffin, J. M., Vasconez, L. O., and Schatten, W. E.: Congenital arteriovenous malformations of the upper extremity. Plast. Reconstr. Surg. *62*:49, 1978.

Harris, K. E., and Wright, G. P.: A case of haemangiectatic hypertrophy of a limb and observations upon rate of growth in the presence of increased blood supply. Heart *15*:141, 1930.

Holman, E.: Abnormal arteriovenous communications: Great variability of effects with particular reference to delayed development of cardiac failure. Circulation *32*:1001, 1965.

Holman, E.: *Abnormal Arteriovenous Communications*, 2nd ed. Springfield, IL: Charles C Thomas, 1968.

Horton, B. T.: Hemihypertrophy of extremities associated with congenital arteriovenous fistulas. JAMA *98*:373, 1932.

Horton, B. T., and Ghormley, R. K.: Congenital arteriovenous fistulae of the extremities visualized by arteriography. Surg. Gynecol. Obstet. *60*:978, 1935.

Johnson, E. W., Jr., Ghormley, R. K., and Dockerty, M. B.: Hemangiomas of the extremities. Surg. Gynecol. Obstet. *102*:531, 1956.

Klippel, M., and Trenaunay, P.: Du noevus variqueux osteohypertrophique. Arch. Gen Med. *3*:641, 1900.

Leonard, F. C., and Vassos, G. A., Jr.: Congenital arteriovenous fistulation of the lower limb. N. Engl. J. Med. *245*:885, 1951.

Lewis, D. D.: Congenital arteriovenous fistulae. Lancet *2*:621, 1930.

Lewis, T.: The adjustment of blood flow to the affected limb in arteriovenous fistula. Clin. Sci. *4*:277, 1940.

Malan, E., and Puglionisi, A.: Congenital angiodysplasias of the extremities (Note I: Generalities and classifications; venous dysplasias). J. Cardiovasc. Surg. *5*:87, 1964.

Malan, E., and Puglionisi, A.: Congenital angiodysplasias of the extremities (Note II: Arterial, arterial and venous, haemolymphatic dysplasias). J. Cardiovasc. Surg. *6*:255, 1965.

Matas, R.: Congenital arteriovenous angioma of the arm. Metastases eleven years after amputation. Ann. Surg. *111*:1021, 1940.

Matolo, N., Kastagir, B., Stevens, L., et al.: Neurovascular complications of brachial arteriovenous fistula. Am. J. Surg. *121*:716, 1971.

May, J. W., Jr., Athanasoulis, C. A., and Donelan, M. B.: Preoperation magnification angiography of donor and recipient sites for clinical free transfer of flaps or digits. Plast. Reconstr. Surg. *64*:483, 1979.

McNeill, T. W., Chan, G. E., Capek, V., and Ray, R. D.: The value of angiography in the surgical management of deep hemangiomas. Clin. Orthop. *101*:176, 1974.

Miller, S. H., Smith, R. L., and Shochat, S. J.: Compression treatment of hemangiomas. Plast. Reconstr. Surg. *58*:573, 1976.

Miller, T. A.: Surgical management of lymphedema of the extremity. Plast. Reconstr. Surg. *56*:633, 1975.

Moore, A. M.: Pressure in the treatment of giant hemangioma with purpura; case report and observations. Plast. Reconstr. Surg. *34*:606, 1964.

Moore, J. R., and Weiland, A. J.: Embolotherapy in the treatment of congenital arteriovenous malformations of the hand: A case report. J. Hand Surg. *10A*:135, 1985.

Morel-Fatio, D.: Essai de traitement des angiomes plans par poncage colore de la peau congelee. Ann. Chir. Plastique *9*:327, 1964.

Mulliken, J. B.: Cutaneous vascular lesions of children. In Serafin, D., and Georgiade, N. G. (eds.): *Pediatric Plastic Surgery*. St. Louis: C. V. Mosby, 1983, pp. 137–154.

Mulliken, J. B. and Glowacki, J.: Hemangiomas and vascular malformations in infants and children: A classification based on endothelial characteristics. Plast. Reconstr. Surg. *69*:412, 1982a.

Mulliken, J. B., and Glowacki, J.: Classification of pediatric vascular lesions. Plast. Reconstr. Surg. *70*:120, 1982b.

Nevaiser, R. J., and Adams, J. P.: Vascular lesions in the hand: Current management. Clin. Orthop. *100*:111, 1974.

Newmeyer, W. L.: In Green, D. P. (ed.): *Vascular Disorders in Operative Hand Surgery*. London: Churchill-Livingstone, 1984, pp. 1695–1754.

Nicoladoni, C.: Phlebarteriectasie der rechten oberen Extremität. Arch. Klin. Chir. *18*:252, 1875.

Niechajev, I. A., and Karlsson, S.: Vascular tumors of the hand. Scand. J. Plast. Reconstr. Surg. *16*:67, 1982a.

Niechajev, I. A., and Karlsson, S.: Angiomatosis osteohypotrophica. Scand. J. Plast. Reconstr. Surg. *16*:77, 1982b.

Nisbet, N. W.: Congenital arteriovenous fistula in the extremities. Br. J. Surg. *41*:658, 1954.

Noe, J. M., Barsky, S. H., Geere, D. E., and Rosen, S.: Port-wine stains and the response to argon laser therapy: Successful treatment and the predictive role of color, age and biopsy. Plast. Reconstr. Surg. *65*:130, 1980.

Norris, G.: Varicose aneurysm at the bend of the arm: Ligature of the artery above and below the sac; secondary hemorrhages with a return of the aneurysmal thrill on the tenth day; cure. Am. J. Med. Sci. *5*:27, 1843.

Olcott, C., IV, Newton, T. H., Stoney, R. J., and Ehrenfeld, W. K.: Intra-arterial embolization in the management of arteriovenous malformations. Surgery *79*:3, 1976.

Ozeran, R. S., Gral, T., Sokol, A., and Gordon, H. E.: Long-term experience with arteriovenous shunts for hemodialysis. Amer. Surg. *38*:259, 1972.

Parkes Weber, F.: Hemangiectatic hypertrophy of limbs—congenital phlebarteriectasis and so-called congenital varicose veins. Brit. J. Child. Dis. *15*:13, 1918.

Pearse, H. E., and Morton, J. J.: The stimulation of bone growth by venous stasis. J. Bone Joint Surg. *12*:97, 1930.

Pemberton, J., and Saint, J. H.: Congenital arteriovenous communications. Surg. Gynecol. Obstet. *46*:470, 1928.

Pisko-Dubienski, Z. A., Baird, R. J., Wilson, D. R., Bayliss, C. E., Gardiner, J. H., and Sepp, H.: Identification and successful treatment of congenital microfistulas with the aid of directional Doppler. Surgery *78*:564, 1975.

Reid, M. R.: Studies on abnormal arteriovenous communications, acquired and congenital. I. Report of a series of cases. Arch. Surg. *10*:601, 1925a.

Reid, M. R.: Abnormal arteriovenous communications, acquired and congenital. II. The origin and nature of arteriovenous aneurysms, cirsoid aneurysms and simple angiomas. Arch. Surg. *10*:996, 1925b.

Rodriguez-Erdman, F., Burron, L., Murray, J. E., and Moloney, W. L.: Kasabach-Merritt syndrome: Coagulo-analytical observations. Am. J. Med. Sci. *261*:9, 1971.

Sabin, F. R.: Origin and development of the primitive vessels of the chick and of the pig. Contrib. Embryol. *6*:61, 1917.

Seeger, S. J.: Congenital arteriovenous anastomoses. Surgery *3*:264, 1938.

Stephenson, H. E., Jr., and Lichti, E. L.: Application of the Doppler ultrasonic flowmeter in the surgical treatment of arteriovenous fistula. Am. Surg. *37*:537, 1971.

Storey, B. G., George, C. R. P., Stewart, J. H., Tiller, D. J., May, J., and Sheil, A. G. R.: Embolic and ischemic complications after anastomosis of radial artery to cephalic vein. Surgery *66*:325, 1969.

Stout, A. P.: *Tumors of the Soft Tissues.* In Armed Forces Institute of Pathology Atlas of Tumor Pathology, Washington, D.C., 1953.

Szilagyi, D. E., Elliott, J. P., DeRusso, F. J., and Smith, R. F.: Peripheral congenital arteriovenous fistulas. Surgery *57*:61, 1965.

Szilagyi, D. E., Smith, R. F., Elliott, J. P., and Hageman, J. H.: Congenital arteriovenous anomalies of the limbs. Arch. Surg. *111*:423, 1976.

Upton, J., Mulliken, J. B., and Murray, J. E.: Classification and rationale for treatment of vascular anomalies in the upper extremity. J. Hand Surg. *10A*:970, 1985.

Veal, J. R., and McCord, W. M.: Congenital abnormal arteriovenous anastomoses of the extremities with special reference to diagnosis by arteriography and by the oxygen saturation test. Arch. Surg. *33*:848, 1936.

Wakim, K. B., and Janes, J. M.: Influence of arteriovenous fistula on the distal circulation in the involved extremity. Arch. Phys. Med. Rehabil. *39*:431, 1958.

Ward, C. E., and Horton, B. T.: Congenital arteriovenous fistulas in children. J. Pediatr. *16*:746, 1940.

Watson, W. L., and McCarthy, W. D.: Blood and lymph vessel tumors: A report of 1,056 cases. Surg. Gynecol. Obstet. *71*:569, 1940.

Weinberg, M., Jr., Steiger, Z., and Fell, E. H.: Unusual congenital anomalies of the arteriovenous system. Surg. Clin. North Am. *40*:67, 1960.

Woollard, H. H.: The development of the principal arterial stems in the forelimb of the pig. Contrib. Embryol. Carnegie Inst. *14*:139, 1922.

Yao, S. T., Needham, T. N., Lewis, J. B., and Hobbs, J. T.: Limb blood flow in congenital arteriovenous fistula. Surgery *73*:80, 1973.

Young, A. E.: Congenital mixed vascular deformities of the limbs and their associated lesions. *Birth Defects: Original Article Series 14*:289, 1978.

CHAPTER EIGHTEEN

Intra-abdominal and Pelvic Vascular Malformations

A. E. Young

with a contribution by

A. Senapati

VASCULAR MALFORMATIONS IN THE GASTROINTESTINAL TRACT

Classification

Cutaneous vascular malformations are usually recognized early in life, often at birth. By contrast, abdominal vascular malformations, since they are not readily visible, usually present only when complications develop. Their prevalence is thus difficult to determine. In addition, these lesions may shrink before autopsy or may be very small and pass unnoticed.

Current terminology to delineate visceral vascular malformations is misleading. In the literature, the term "hemangioma" is often mistakenly used to describe *malformations*. In this chapter, the following anatomical classification is employed:

1. *Venous malformations*: These are low flow anomalies occurring in many forms, including phlebectasia, bleb-like lesions, polypoid lesions, and diffuse forms involving all layers. These anomalies constitute 2–12% of all vascular malformations of the bowel and 0.05% of all intestinal tumors (Taylor and Torrance, 1974). First described by Gascoyen in 1860, they may be single or multiple and may occur at any site in any organ (Gascoyen, 1860).

2. *Arteriovenous malformations (AVM)*: These have been divided by Moore into three types (Moore et al., 1976).
   a. *Type 1 AVM*: Thought to be acquired and often erroneously called "angiodysplasia" (meaning an abnormality of embryonic vascular development). These anomalies usually present in patients over the age of 55 and are believed to be a vascular degenerative process related to aging.
   b. *Type 2 AVM*: Tend to be large and complex and present before the age of 50 years.
   c. *Type 3 AVM*: Multiple punctate malformations associated with the Rendu-Osler-Weber syndrome (hereditary hemorrhagic telangiectasia). Symptoms usually begin in middle age.

3. *Aneurysms:* These are rarely congenital. They sometimes occur in the Menkes syndrome, in which there is a weakening of the arterial wall as a result of an inherited defect in copper absorption. Copper is an integral part of the enzyme lysyl amine oxidase, essential for the cross-linkage of collagen (Danks, 1977; Smith, 1982).

4. *Lymphatic malformations*: Intra-abdominal lymphatic malformations are usually associated with anomalies of the lymphatic system outside the abdomen. Three types

381

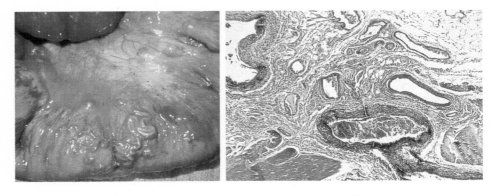

A   B

Figure 18–1. *A,* Intraoperative photograph of small bowel in a teenage girl with intestinal bleeding and Turner's syndrome. Multiple anomalous vessels extend over the serosa to the antimesenteric border. Despite several bowel resections, the patient continues to bleed slowly; over the past 12 years, she has received over 2000 units of washed frozen red blood cell transfusions. (Courtesy of Judah Folkman, M.D.) *B,* Low-power photomicrograph of resected bowel of patient in *A.* Elastic stain demonstrates increased number of arteries and ectatic thickened veins in the intestinal wall. (Courtesy of Judah Folkman, M.D.)

are encountered: *lymph cysts, chylous ascites,* and *intestinal lymphangiectasia.* This last may cause a protein-losing enteropathy (Kinmonth and Eustace, 1975). Lymphatic anomalies of the retroperitoneum, liver, spleen, gastrointestinal tract, and mesentery are also seen combined with venous anomalies—a Klippel-Trenaunay syndrome of the trunk and intra-abdominal viscera (see Figs. 14–27 to 14–29). The multiple intestinal polyps of Peutz-Jeghers syndrome are a cause of chronic gastrointestinal bleeding in the young but are not vascular malformations (Smith, 1982, p. 386).

Presentation

1. Gastrointestinal blood loss: acute severe bleeding, chronic intermittent bleeding, and iron deficiency anemia, all of which may occur if the malformation is in the bowel wall or in communicating structures, such as the liver or pancreas.
2. Obstruction
3. Intussusception
4. Congestive cardiac failure in malformations with a large blood flow (e.g., arteriovenous fistulae or large AVM)
5. As part of other syndromes (Shepherd, 1953). In Rendu-Osler-Weber syndrome, the cutaneous manifestations are always present when there is gastrointestinal involvement.

6. In association with other diseases, e.g. Turner's syndrome (Burge et al., 1981) (Fig. 18–1), Hippel-Lindau syndrome, von Willebrand's disease (Conlon et al., 1978), and the CRST syndrome (calcinosis cutis, Raynaud's phenomenon, sclerodactyly, and telangiectasia) (Winterbauer, 1964).

Diagnosis

Chronic gastrointestinal blood loss in a young patient, for which no cause can readily be found, is often due to vascular malformations. Confirming the diagnosis may, however, be very difficult and may only be by selective mesenteric angiography (Nusbaum and Baum, 1963; Cavett et al., 1977). The Seldinger technique of aortic or selective angiography is used and has a mortality of 0.06% and a morbidity of 0.7% (Land, 1963) and is hence a safe diagnostic procedure.

The radiologic diagnostic features include:
1. Large aberrant vessels
2. Dilated small vessels
3. Rapid venous filling
4. Vascular tufts
5. Pooling of contrast medium during capillary phase

Digital subtraction angiography (DSA) using venous injection of contrast material is not of value in the context of gastrointestinal malformations. Studies with intra-arterial dye injection may be of great value, as the technique allows the detection of the relatively small amounts of contrast that pool in small but significant lesions or are bled into the lumen of the bowel during the examination. The use of isotopes to localize sources of bleeding is discussed in Chapter Eight.

Small Bowel Vascular Malformations

Localized venous malformations compose 2–12% of small intestinal "tumors" and are the most common vascular anomalies in the gastrointestinal tract (Hansen, 1948). River and colleagues, in a review of 127 cases, reported an equal distribution between the jejunum and ileum, with only 3 cases involving the entire gastrointestinal tract (River et al., 1956). The colon was involved only rarely. Taylor and Torrance describe two cases involving the entire small intestine, of which one involved congenital asplenia (Taylor and Torrance, 1974). Their patients were young, and the lesions were presumed to be congenital. The bowel mucosa is usually involved, which accounts for the acute and chronic blood loss. The peritoneum is usually intact. The more distal the lesion, the more likely it is to bleed. Associated cutaneous vascular malformations are common and may be part of a generalized syndrome that assists in the diagnosis (e.g., blue rubber bleb nevus syndrome). The literature has been well reviewed by Hansen (1948) and by River and colleagues (1956).

Diagnosis

These anomalies rarely undergo intussusception but may cause obstruction. Hematological assessment will exclude bleeding disorders and barium studies exclude other lesions, though they rarely show the malformation. In 30% of cases the lesion may be localized at laparotomy by inspection, palpation, and transillumination.

The traditional "string test"—passing a piece of string down the small intestine and looking for blood staining—has now been superceded by angiography. Chromium labelled red cells and technetium sulfur colloid have also been used to localize the bleeding site (Markisz et al., 1982). The former has a higher yield but is anatomically less accurate than the latter.

Treatment

Surgical resection is the best treatment if the lesion can be identified. The biggest problems in operative treatment are localization and the difficulty of resecting some parts of the bowel if they are affected (e.g., the duodenum). "Blind" bowel resection is of little value (Gianfrancisco and Abcarian, 1982), and, in general, bowel should not be resected without extensive preoperative attempts at localizing the site of hemorrhage. Local measures include electrocoagulation at endoscopy, oversewing the lesion, and argon laser photocoagulation. Vasopressin is sometimes used in all types of malformations, and estrogens have been used in the Rendu-Osler-Weber syndrome. Embolization is only a safe procedure in areas of dual blood supply, such as the stomach and rectum.

Proximal Gastrointestinal Vascular Malformations

Until 1967, there were only 36 cases of gastric vascular malformations reported in the world literature (Bongiovi and Duffy, 1967). However, since then, endoscopic examination has led to recognition of these lesions in the esophagus, stomach, and duodenum, the incidence varying between 0 and 4.5% of benign gastric tumors (Farup et al., 1981).

Ninety to 95% of upper gastrointestinal bleeds are due to a well-recognized lesion (ulcers, erosions, carcinoma, etc.) (Sarrasis et al., 1983). The remaining 5% are often undiagnosed, but now more of these are being found to be due to vascular abnormalities. The most common of these is the AVM Type 1, usually referred to as "angiodysplasia." (Many reports describe the lesions as "telangiectasia.") These patients tend to be over 50 years of age, and the lesions are probably *acquired* (Lewis et al., 1981; Roberts et al., 1981). They are usually 5–10 mm in diameter and can be removed with biopsy forceps at endoscopy. They have also been described in association with chronic renal failure (Cunningham, 1981).

Other lesions seen in association with gastric vascular malformations are splenic artery and hepatic artery aneurysms and arteriovenous fistulae (Halpern et al., 1968).

Diagnosis

Contrast radiology rarely demonstrates these lesions. Endoscopy must be performed carefully, the lesions being looked for prior to passage of the endoscope lest they be mistaken for traumatic abrasions.

Treatment

These lesions are rare; hence, evaluation of the relative efficacy of various methods of treatment is difficult (Lewis et al., 1981). Surgical resection, endoscopic coagulation (Weaver et al., 1979), estrogen therapy (to increase the thickness of the gastric mucosa), and laser coagulation have all been tried.

Vascular Malformations of the Colon

Most early reports of vascular abnormalities were of lesions in the rectum or sigmoid colon and have been well reviewed by Shepherd (1953), but since the advent of selective angiography the right colon and cecum have become well recognized sources of bleeding from vascular malformations commonly known as "angiodysplasia" (Boley et al., 1977; Singh et al., 1977; Baum et al., 1977; Editorial, Lancet, 1981). As these lesions generally occur in patients over the age of 60 and are not associated with cutaneous or visceral vascular anomalies, it is assumed that such lesions, involving the right side of the colon, are acquired. These lesions tend to be more common in women. They may present with torrential bleeding, or after a long period of mild blood loss. Cardiac disease, most commonly aortic stenosis, has often been reported in association with this condition (Galloway et al., 1974; Baer and Ryan, 1976), and in one series was associated in 63% of patients (Baum et al., 1977).

Etiology

The most favored etiological theory is that of Boley (Boley et al., 1977) and of Baum (Baum et al., 1973; Baum et al., 1977). They postulate that chronic increase in intra-abdominal pressure obstructs the transmuscular veins that drain the submucosal venous plexus and hence the mucosa. Repeated episodes of raised pressure result in dilatation of the submucosal and mucosal veins. Unlike

the sigmoid colon, in which high pressure peristaltic waves are of short duration, high pressure in the cecum is sustained, so that the veins are obstructed for long periods of time. Other theories include that of Baer, who proposes that mucosal veins dilate as a result of localized obliteration of precapillary tone (Baer and Ryan, 1976). Another theory is that pre-existing mucosal shunts with high blood flow divert blood from the mucosa, rendering it ischemic. Histologic resemblance suggests a common cause with the arteriovenous malformations in Rendu-Osler-Weber syndrome, but the similarity ends there. Cholesterol emboli are sometimes seen in areas adjacent to the abnormality, which suggests that shunting away from the embolized area may occur. Galloway has put forward two other hypotheses (Galloway et al., 1974): first, that atherosclerosis with peripheral ischemia and arteriovenous shunting may occur; and second, that a decreased cardiac output in patients with aortic stenosis may result in mucosal ischemia. A report of a patient at the age of 19 years has led to the speculation that the underlying fault is, indeed, of developmental origin (Allison and Hemingway, 1981). Congenital abnormalities of the bowel microvasculature may predispose to causing this condition in later life.

Diagnosis

Even if these lesions are suspected clinically, their existence may be difficult to confirm and their position hard to localize. At colonoscopy, they may be mistaken for an abrasion and may become invisible as a result of overdistension. Recent advances in selective angiography have improved diagnostic accuracy. *Postmortem* studies have identified these lesions by the injection of gelatin-barium mixtures into the vasculature of resected specimens.

Application of a Doppler ultrasonic flow detector to the segment of colon at laparotomy has been advocated to help localization (Fowler et al., 1979).

Treatment

Torrential bleeding may only be controllable by surgical resection. Often angiography is the only way of localizing these lesions, because they cannot be seen from outside the bowel wall at laparotomy. Lesions that are not bleeding severely, or at all, may be co-agulated by colonoscopy. Where bowel resection is undertaken, angiography of the resected specimen should confirm complete excision (Sheedy et al., 1975).

Rectal Venous Malformations

The rectum may be the primary or sole site of a diffuse venous malformation of the gastrointestinal tract. These were first reviewed in 1924 by Brown, who collected 20 cases; more recently, they have been reviewed by Bell (Bell et al., 1972) and by Coppa (Coppa et al., 1984).

The patients present with episodic bright rectal bleeding in infancy, though there is one instance recorded in which the bleeding did not begin until the patient was 36. The bleeding may be serious enough to cause the death of the patient. Gentry has reported a mortality rate of 45% in 20 untreated patients with diffuse cavernous malformations of the colon and rectum (Gentry et al., 1949).

Hemorrhoids are often associated, and the patient may have a history of unsuccessful hemorrhoidectomy. Additional symptoms described have included constipation, tenesmus, and blood-stained diarrhea. There are no typical proctoscopic findings. The patient may have obvious, even pedunculated, vascular lesions or distended vessels in the rectal wall, or nothing more striking than narrowing of the rectal lumen with congestion of the mucosa. Radiography may show multiple pelvic phleboliths. Bell has reviewed the surgical management of this condition and concludes that because of the difficulties in controlling hemorrhage at operation and delineating the lesion, an aggressive approach employing a combined abdominoperineal resection of the rectum should be employed (Bell et al., 1972). Because the lesions usually involve all coats of the rectal wall, and perirectal tissues, sphincter saving and pull-through operations may fail, though Jeffrey has reported continence after such operations (Jeffrey et al., 1976). Injection sclerotherapy also has minimal effect. Sometimes the lesion may be more generalized and involve other perineal structures and/or urethrovesical mucosa. In the French literature, this latter condition is sometimes referred to as "Esau Bensaude" type, whereas the malformation restricted to the rectum is known

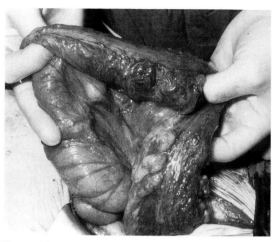

Figure 18–2. Extensive venous malformation of the upper rectum and sigmoid colon shown at operation. This 12 year old with multiple cutaneous and systemic venous and lymphatic malformations of the limbs and trunk presented with hematuria and rectal bleeding.

as the "Barker-Kausch" type (Bensaude and Bensaude, 1932). Multiple cutaneous venous malformations may be associated with similar malformations in the small and/or large bowel (Fig. 18–2). Rectal bleeding may also occur in association with Klippel-Trenaunay syndrome (see later discussion).

VASCULAR MALFORMATIONS OF THE LIVER

In infants, the most common hepatic vascular tumor is the hemangioma, synonymous with "hemangioendothelioma." These tumors present with a liver mass, a bruit, and congestive heart failure, with or without cutaneous hemangiomata. (See Chapter Three for discussion of this entity.) A true arteriovenous malformation of the liver is also a rare cause for cardiac failure in the newborn period. Cardiac failure is usually manifested in the hepatic arteriovenous malformation within a few days of life, whereas circulatory signs usually appear later in hepatic hemangioma cases. Fellows and coworkers believe that it is possible to differentiate these two pathological entities angiographically (Fellows and Mulliken, 1986). Hepatic arteriovenous malformation is a more diffuse lesion and demonstrates (1) an absence of parenchymal or nodular stain; (2) dense filling of vascular spaces; (3) enlarged collateral vessels, particularly inferior phrenic and inter-

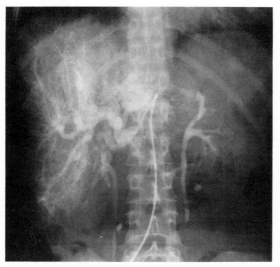

Figure 18–3. Selective hepatic arteriogram of a diffuse hepatic vascular malformation. The hepatic artery and its branches are dilated and supply a diffusely abnormal liver with multiple irregular small vessels, an abnormal hepatogram, and large hepatic veins. Anastomotic channels to the hepatic circulation were noted from the right renal and superior mesenteric arteries. In addition, multiple abnormal vessels were seen supplying the duodenum and proximal jejunal loops.

costal arteries; and (4) impressive extrahepatic arterial supply with prominent arteriovenous shunting.

The majority of vascular lesions in the liver are venous malformations. They are often inappropriately listed as the most common benign liver tumors and are said to account for 0.4% of hepatic neoplasms (Walt, 1977). McLoughlin has shown a 0.35% prevalence in adults at autopsy (McLoughlin, 1971). The lesions are usually asymptomatic and, in life, are most often discovered as incidental findings at laparotomy, ultrasonography, CT scanning, or hepatic scintigraphy. When they are found during ultrasound or scintigraphy, the diagnosis cannot confidently be made without further investigation (Fig. 18–3) unless there is calcification in the lesion (Pantoja, 1968; Jensen and Klinge, 1976) (Fig. 18–3). This change tends only to be seen in older patients. The appearances of CT scanning are of well-defined circular or oval lesions of low density, indistinguishable from metastases and hepatomas until contrast is given, when typical sequential enhancement properties may be seen suggesting, but not confirming, the diagnosis (Barnett et al., 1980; Johnson et al., 1981) (Fig. 18–4). When the CT study is not diagnostic, an hepatic angiogram may be helpful (Fig. 18–5).

Liver function tests and alphafetoprotein assays are normal. Accurate diagnosis in 14 patients was demonstrated using radionuclide scanning with 99m-Tc labelled red blood cells (Front et al., 1981). Preliminary studies using magnetic resonance imaging show that this technique is highly sensitive in detecting venous anomalies of the liver; however, the specificity of this new technology remains in question (Glazer et al., 1985).

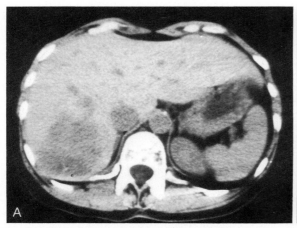
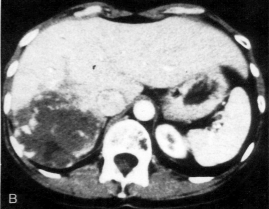

Figure 18–4. *A,* Unenhanced CT scan of this patient's liver shows a diffuse mass posteriorly in the right lobe. *B,* Dynamic infusion of contrast shows peripheral enhancement, and further scanning over the next few minutes showed a gradual increase in the density of the lesion, diagnostic of a venous malformation. (Radiographs courtesy of P. Simons, M.D.)

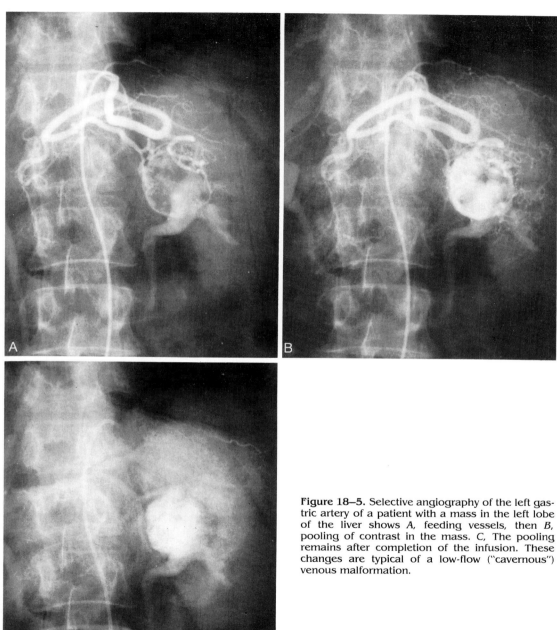

Figure 18–5. Selective angiography of the left gastric artery of a patient with a mass in the left lobe of the liver shows *A*, feeding vessels, then *B*, pooling of contrast in the mass. *C*, The pooling remains after completion of the infusion. These changes are typical of a low-flow (``cavernous'') venous malformation.

Treatment

There is no place for corticosteroids in the treatment of an infant with life-threatening congestive heart failure secondary to a liver arteriovenous malformation. In addition to digitalis and diuretics, embolization has been tried with equivocal success. Whenever possible, resection is the treatment of choice.

Asymptomatic venous malformations need no treatment, though large ones should be monitored. Spontaneous rupture requires surgical intervention and partial hepatic resection (Sewell and Weiss, 1961).

Effect of Oral Contraceptives

Lesions resembling hemangiomas or cavernous venous malformations are sometimes encountered in women taking oral contraceptive agents. This association between vascular hepatic adenomas and the oral contraceptive pill was first made by Baum and colleagues in 1973, with the reporting of seven cases (Baum et al., 1973). Since then, there has been a surge of literature of, usually, isolated cases or reviews (Baek et al., 1976; Editorial, Brit. J. Med., 1977). The relation of these lesions to vascular abnormalities is that the characteristic histologic appearance is that of *peliosis hepatis* (Pliskin, 1975; Sherlock, 1975; Terblanche, 1977), which has been described as showing phlebectasia, blood-filled cystic spaces, focally dilated sinusoids, and thickening of arterial and venous walls. These changes with the contraceptive pill may also occur in the absence of an adenoma (Terblanche, 1977).

VASCULAR MALFORMATIONS OF THE PANCREAS

Vascular malformations of the pancreas are rare but are well recognized. They tend to present at a younger age than other intra-abdominal vascular malformations but have been reported in all age groups (Brinley and Palubinskas, 1977; Mizutani et al., 1981). They are most commonly associated with the Rendu-Osler-Weber syndrome, but in the instances in which they are not there may be a forme fruste of this condition. These anomalies have been reported in association with malformations of the uterus, parametrium,

kidneys, and retroperitoneum (Ishikawa, 1979).

The prevalence in children suggests that they are true congenital abnormalities.

Diagnosis

The abnormal vascular pattern and extent of the anomaly can be readily outlined by angiography (Chuang et al., 1977; Walter et al., 1977). Hemorrhage from the pancreas is more commonly due to pancreatic disease, but in these instances bleeding is usually associated with upper abdominal pain, whereas bleeding from malformations is usually painless.

Treatment

Surgical excision is successful and, indeed, has been recommended as prophylaxis if the lesion is found incidentally; however, excision is not recommended if the anomaly is associated with Rendu-Osler-Weber syndrome, in which the lesions are likely to be widespread.

VASCULAR MALFORMATIONS OF THE SPLEEN

A vascular malformation of the spleen is a very rare condition when it occurs in isolation (Pitlik et al., 1977), though it is said to be the most common benign "tumor" of the spleen, occurring in 0.03–1.4% of autopsies (Husni, 1961). Splenic vascular malformations and hemangiomas may be associated with such lesions in other organs, particularly the liver (Pinkhas et al., 1968). Splenic vascular malformations occurring in isolation are most commonly incidental findings at autopsy, though they may also present as asymptomatic splenomegaly, hypersplenism (Pinkhas et al., 1968), portal hypertension (Pitlik et al., 1977), abdominal pain (Pinkhas et al., 1968), or spontaneous rupture (Husni, 1961; Campbell, 1962; Pitlik et al., 1977; Kaplan and McIntosh, 1987). The hematological complications include anemia, thrombocytopenia, and consumptive coagulopathies (Benjamin et al., 1965; Shanberge et al., 1971). Angiography usually demonstrates the splenic lesions; however, they also can be imaged with computed tomography or ultrasonography (Fig. 18–6). Splenectomy is the treatment of choice. The differential diagnosis between splenic vascular malformations and other causes of isolated splenomegaly may be difficult to establish clinically and can usually only be made with certainty on the basis of histology obtained by splenectomy (Case Records of M.G.H., 1985). The differential

diagnosis includes hemangiosarcoma, hairy cell leukemia, lymphatic malformations, and purpura.

Whitley records a case in which a splenic vascular anomaly may have undergone malignant degeneration with fatal metastatic hemangiosarcoma (Whitley and Winship, 1954). Published histologic details of that case do not, however, afford confirmation that

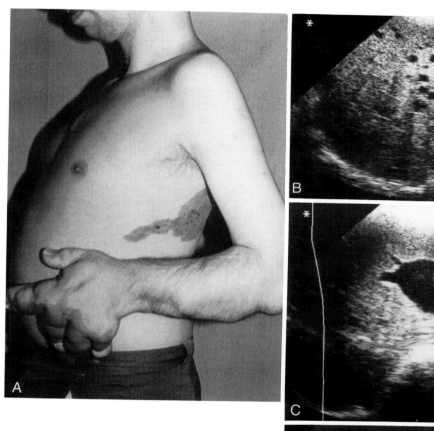

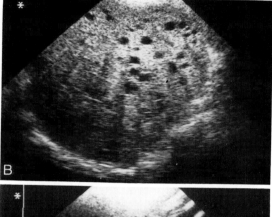

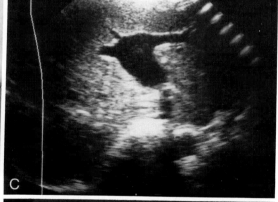

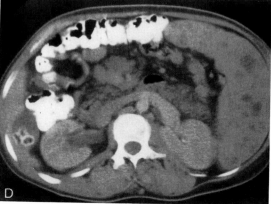

Figure 18–6. *A,* Fifteen year old male with combined vascular anomaly of right lower extremity and buttock, and crossed dissociation with involvement of the left upper extremity, left hypochondrium, and viscera. *B,* Longitudinal ultrasonogram of spleen showing multiple cystic areas. *C,* Transverse ultrasound study demonstrates ectatic portal vein within liver. *D,* Transverse computed tomographic scan with enhancement reveals that the cystic spaces within the enlarged spleen are fluid-filled, i.e., lymphatic and not venous. The mesentery is diffusely involved with lymphaticovenous anomaly (old term, "lymphangiomatosis"). The enlarged portal vein is seen; note meglumine diatrizoate (Gastrografin) within the bowel.

malignant degeneration in fact occurred in a previously benign vascular malformation in the spleen.

RENAL MALFORMATIONS

Vascular malformations of the kidney are rare. The mixed myomatous/angiolipomatous lesions of tuberous sclerosis are not true vascular malformations (Bissada et al., 1975).

Arteriovenous Fistulae

Of 102 renal arteriovenous fistulae recorded by Leary and Utz (1971), 25 were congenital, presenting as congestive cardiac failure (60%), hypertension (50%), flank pain, and/or hematuria. Diagnosis could only be achieved by angiography. Treatment is by nephrectomy or occasionally by branch artery ligation or partial nephrectomy.

The clinical features of *low flow vascular malformations* are more difficult to discern because they are described in the literature as hemangiomas and this appellation tends to include arteriovenous malformations. Papers by Mitchell (Mitchell et al., 1982) and by Rodriguez (Rodriguez and Befaler, 1967) note that symptomatic lesions reveal themselves as hematuria and that this may occur at any age, though most patients are aged less than 40. The malformations have no predilection for side or sex, and 12% are multiple. Most are less than 2 cm in diameter. Diagnosis is only achievable preoperatively by angiography, and even then differentiation from a vascular renal carcinoma may be difficult.

PELVIC VASCULAR MALFORMATIONS

Iliac Vein Compression

The anatomical abnormalities that form the basis of iliac vein compression are described in Chapter Eleven. When symptoms of swelling and heaviness are the sole markers of the condition, conservative management with elastic compression suffices. Cases presenting acutely with venous thrombosis occurring either spontaneously or as a complication of a surgical procedure or preg-

nancy are treated with elevation and anticoagulation. Only in those patients with severe symptoms, particularly of venous claudication, should an operation be considered. Venography should be used to confirm patent distal and femoral veins, and the femoral vein pressure should be measured. Only if the pressure is raised in relation to the opposite femoral vein pressure is a surgical procedure likely to succeed. Direct attack on the abnormal segment of iliac vein, whether by rerouting the iliac artery or by freeing or patching the abnormal segment, has not proved successful. A series treated by transposition of the long saphenous vein from the unaffected limb to the femoral vein of the affected limb (Palma operation) (Palma and Esperon, 1960) produced symptomatic improvement in a majority of patients, but this was not always sustained (Cockett and Young, 1980). In most cases, however, the long saphenous vein is unlikely to improve on the capacity of the naturally occurring rich bypasses afforded by the pelvic cross-collaterals. For a fuller description of this syndrome, see the report by May and DeWeese (1979).

Iliac Vein Atresia/Hypoplasia

Cases of iliac vein atresia with or without hypoplasia are rare, and the indications for surgical intervention are unclear. Peck operated on a 2½ year old girl with apparent iliac vein atresia and found constricting adventitia that could be stripped from the vein, allowing it to re-expand (Peck, 1957). Five year follow-up evaluation showed less pronounced disparity in limb length than before the operation. Kirtley (in the discussion of Peck's paper) recorded that he had bypassed an obstructed iliac vein with an arterial homograft, and although this clotted he reported improvement in limb length disparity similar to Peck. Oda bypassed an atretic iliac vein with prosthetic graft, but, in spite of a substantial pressure gradient across it, the graft clotted 6 months after placement (Oda et al., 1962). Bereston had a similar disappointing result (Bereston and Roberts, 1965). Our patients with atretic iliac veins remain well without exploration (Fig. 18–7). In most instances, there is little virtue in exploring an atretic iliac vein unless there are definite features of distal venous hypertension. Even when this is present, failures are common and largely reflect the general deficiencies of venous reconstructive surgery. The large venous collaterals that are so prominent on the anterior abdominal wall of these patients must not be excised or ligated.

Pelvic Involvement in Klippel-Trenaunay Syndrome

In most cases of Klippel-Trenaunay syndrome, the veins and lymphatics of the whole limb bud, and thus also of the pelvis, are abnormal, and thus the pelvis and its viscera are also involved (Fig. 18–7). This involvement is usually asymptomatic, though in the St. Thomas' Hospital series nine patients (18%) reported rectal bleeding and five of these had also experienced hematuria (Baskerville et al., 1985). Patients may also have hemorrhoids, and, on proctoscopy, engorged submucosal rectal veins can be seen. At colonoscopy, these engorged veins can be seen extending well into the sigmoid colon. We

are not aware of any accounts in the literature showing that any specific difficulties are encountered during pregnancy by patients with Klippel-Trenaunay syndrome. Servelle reports, however, on six children with Klippel-Trenaunay syndrome and associated femoral vein hypoplasias who experienced severe hematuria and rectal bleeding (Servelle et al., 1976). In one case this was fatal, in another rectal resection was required, and in another cystectomy was needed. All patients presented between the ages of 4 and 6. Klein has reported on two similar children (Klein and Kaplan, 1975). The engorgement of the pelvic vasculature in such patients can be attributed to the greatly increased venous flow in the internal iliac veins and their dilated collaterals. This engorgement is secondary to the main venous outflow of the limb, being not through the femoral vessels but via anomalous veins, such as the lateral vein connecting through the gluteal notch into the internal iliac system (Fig. 18–8). This causes not only dilatation of the rectal and

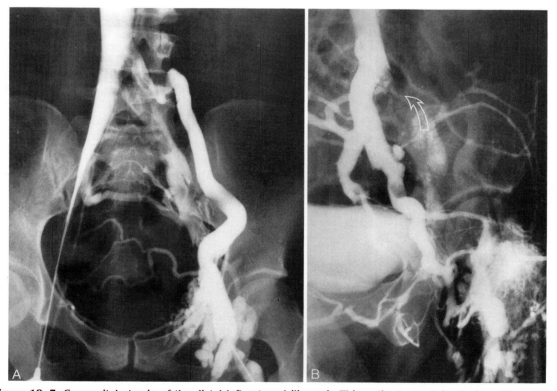

Figure 18–7. Congenital atresia of the distal left external iliac vein. This patient complained of swelling of the left leg. *A,* Left femoral venography together with right iliac venography shows the extensive collateral system. *B,* The pertrochanteric venogram shows the internal iliac to be patent (arrow). Atresia of the vein was confirmed at operation.

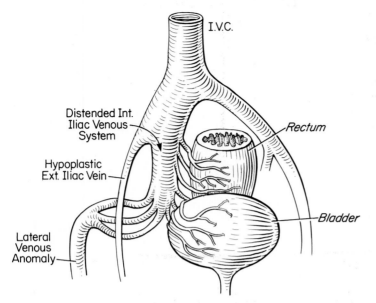

Figure 18–8. This drawing illustrates Servelle's concept of the pathophysiology of rectal bleeding and hematuria in the Klippel-Trenaunay syndrome. Because the bulk of the venous return from the limb enters the internal iliac system rather than the external, the whole internal iliac system including its branches to the rectum and bladder become dilated. Rupture of these vessels leads to hematuria and rectal bleeding. Venographic illustration of this venous enlargement is shown in Figure 9–39.

vesical veins but also dilatation of the upper vaginal veins. Patients with femoral vein underdevelopment may develop large vulval collaterals; one of Servelle's cases, a male, presented with a very large varicocele. We have seen such patients with penile varices (Fig. 18–9). Servelle claims that patients with Klippel-Trenaunay syndrome and symptomatic pelvic venous congestion may be helped by freeing up constrictions of the femoral veins, thus encouraging venous return via the femoral and external iliac veins and reducing excess flow into the internal iliac venous system (Servelle, 1985).

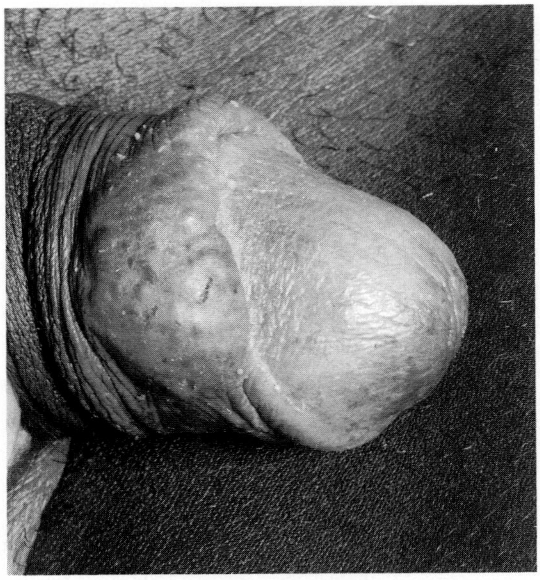

Pelvic Arteriovenous Malformations

Considering the complexity of the pelvic vasculature, one might expect arteriovenous malformations to be common in the pelvis. They are, in fact, extremely rare. In their literature review of 1975, Neifeld and coworkers could only identify 5 males and 11 females who had congenital arteriovenous malformations solely located within the pelvis. Other cases have been reported (Szilagyi et al., 1976; Beggs and Garvin, 1983; Natali et al., 1984). The majority of arteriovenous abnormalities in the pelvis are acquired and follow operative trauma, especially after gynecological procedures and laminectomy (Decker et al., 1968).

In the *female*, the features of arteriovenous malformations are pain in the pelvis, back, and leg, radiating into the perineum; a pulsatile mass on pelvic examination; swelling of the legs; antepartum hemorrhage; postpartum hemorrhage; enlargement of the uterus; and menorrhagia. Most of the malformations come to medical attention in the teens and twenties, and they may be incidental findings. Two of Benson's three patients went through pregnancy (one by cesarean section, two by

Figure 18–9. A venous malformation of the prepuce in a patient with the Klippel-Trenaunay syndrome.

vaginal delivery) without problems, and in one patient in whom it was measured there was no significant increase in cardiac output, nor was there progression of the lesion during pregnancy (Benson et al., 1965). Benson considered that interruption of the pregnancy was not indicated, though Natali (Natali et al., 1984) agreed with Mortensen (Mortensen and Ellsworth, 1965) that pregnancy may activate symptomatically latent arteriovenous malformations.

In the *male*, cases have presented with urinary tract symptoms such as dysuria, frequency (Beggs and Garvin, 1983), impotence (Neifeld et al., 1975), loin pain, and hematuria (Flye et al., 1983). Lower bowel symptoms of tenesmus and constipation have also been noted.

Surgical extirpation of pelvis arteriovenous malformations is both difficult and dangerous and should never be undertaken unless the clinical indications are substantial. Difficulties are encountered because the flow

through a symptomatic arteriovenous malformation is usually so great, and the feeding vessels so multitudinous, that good angiographic delineation of the lesion is difficult to obtain and the operation is thus, to some extent, "blind." It is also difficult to assess the degree of involvement of the rectum, bladder, and pelvic organs. Computerized tomographic scans with contrast enhancement may help as, in the future, may digital vascular imaging techniques. Hemorrhage during resection is difficult to control; Natali cites an average blood loss of 3.4 liters (Natali et al., 1984). He advises the use of autotransfusion apparatus where this is available.

Malformations supplied from the anterior branches of the internal iliac artery are frequently inoperable, in the sense of surgical ablation, though preoperative embolization may make some angiographically localized lesions resectable. Nonetheless, the few cases of direct surgical attack reported in the literature show that the prospect of cure is

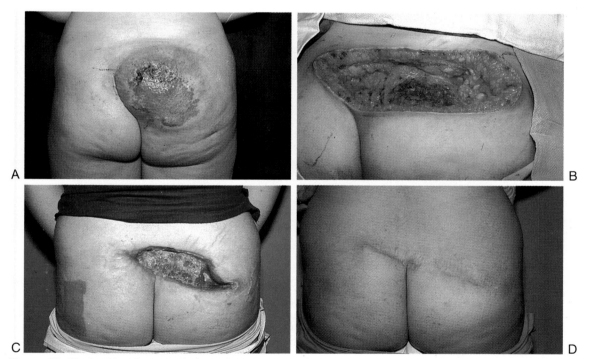

Figure 18–10. A, This 13 year old girl had an apparently innocent port-wine stain over the left upper buttock, present since birth. With onset of puberty, the area began to enlarge and eventually the skin ulcerated. B, Computed tomographic and angiographic studies confirmed that the anomaly was arteriovenous with microshunting. Wide excision was performed. C, Following delayed primary closure with split-thickness skin grafting. D, Four years following excision of the grafted area, there is no evidence of persistent vascular malformation. (Procedure by J. B. Mulliken, M.D.)

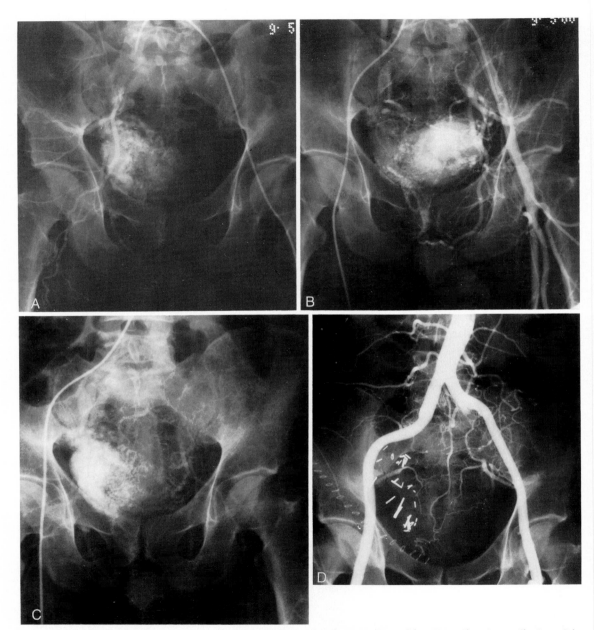

Figure 18–11. Serial angiograms indicating the difficulty that is encountered in attempting to eradicate pelvic arteriovenous malformations. The selective arteriograms are of a 49 year old man who presented wth flank and perineal pain associated with hematuria. *A*, Initial angiography showed a large pelvic arteriovenous malformation. This was treated by embolization and shortly afterwards by right internal iliac artery ligation. The symptoms were not improved. *B*, After ligation of the internal iliac artery, angiography demonstrated that the malformation was continuing to fill through collaterals. The left internal iliac artery and its branches and the inferior mesenteric artery were therefore ligated and a portion of the malformation excised. *C*, Postoperative angiography again showed persistence of the malformation, and at a third operation the right internal iliac artery, its branches, circumflex branches from the external iliac and common femoral arteries, and the arteriovenous malformation itself were excised. *D*, The final postoperative arteriogram no longer shows the arteriovenous malformation, and the patient has remained well. (From Flye, M. W., et al.: Surgery *94*:740, 1983.)

poor. Szilagyi reported two cases made worse by the complications of operative intervention (Szilagyi et al., 1976). In both patients, the lesion was not eradicated. Malan and Puglionisi (1965), Decker and colleagues (1968), and Natali and coworkers (1984) have also noted poor results from operation.

Arteriovenous malformations in the territory of the posterior branch of the internal iliac artery are relatively more common, usually presenting as arteriovenous malformations of the buttock (Fig. 18–10). Constantini and coworkers commented that radiotherapy caused some diminution of a pelvic arteriovenous malformation (Constantini et al., 1943). Azzolini and Tardito described a three-stage repair starting with internal iliac artery occlusion followed by en bloc excision and subsequent reconstruction with bipedicled gluteal flap transposed medially (Azzolini and Tardito, 1974).

Embolization is now preferred to iliac artery ligation, as it has been shown that ligation of one or both internal iliac arteries alone does little or nothing to control pelvic arteriovenous malformations (Adams, 1951; Natali et al., 1984). In the normal patient, such ligations (for instance, as may occur after bilateral renal transplantation) do not devascularize the pelvic organs, nor do they halt hemorrhage from pelvic trauma. Constantini described a case in which revascularization of an arteriovenous malformation occurred within a few days of internal iliac artery ligation (Constantini et al., 1943). In addition

to its failure to control the lesion, iliac artery ligation alone makes subsequent operation very difficult, because the collaterals are tortuous, thin-walled, and friable. However, the major reason for deprecating iliac artery ligation is that by performing the procedure subsequent access for embolization is lost, though if the iliac arteries have been ligated it may be possible to embolize the malformation through collaterals. Natali has described such cases, though there was only limited success from the embolization (Natali et al., 1984). Olcott and colleagues reported a patient with a painful adnexal malformation treated initially by internal iliac-hypogastric artery ligation (Olcott et al., 1976). This led to 3 weeks' relief from the pain. Angiography showed revascularization through lumbar, inferior mesenteric, and external iliac arteries. These were embolized, with relief of symptoms persisting to the end of the reported 9 month follow-up period. Flye reports a case of a 49 year old man with an extensive pelvic arteriovenous malformation who was treated initially with embolization and internal iliac artery ligation without benefit (Flye et al., 1983) (Fig. 18–11A and B). Subsequently, the left internal iliac artery, its branches, the inferior mesenteric artery, and part of the malformation were excised, with benefit (Fig. 18–11C). At a third operation, the right internal iliac artery and its branches and collaterals from the external iliac artery and the femoral artery were excised, together with the malformation. The patient has re-

Figure 18–12. Genital vascular anomalies. A, Coronal venous malformation in a teen-ager. B, Capillary-venous malformation of the scrotum; this 18 year old young man had trouble with large external hemorrhoids.

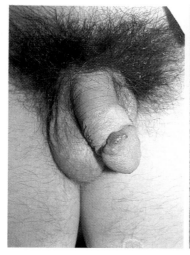

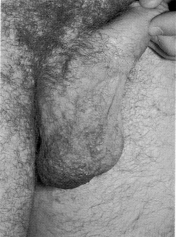

A   B

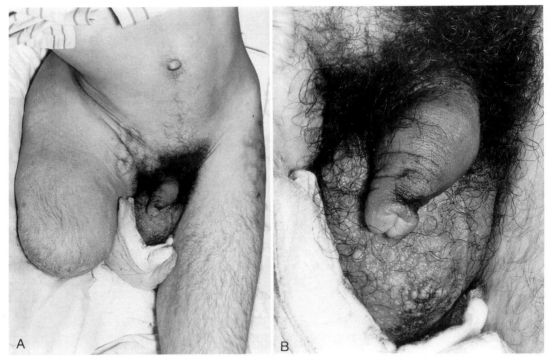

Figure 18–13. A, Chylous reflux into the scrotum of a young man with multiple arteriovenous fistulae of the right lower limb requiring amputation because of pain, ulceration, and contractures. B, Multiple chyle filled vesicles on the scrotum continually leaked.

mained symptom-free at 2 years (Fig. 18–11D). Theoretically, a ligated internal iliac artery can be reconstructed to allow access for embolization. Natali attempted this in two patients, but the procedure failed because of blood loss (Natali et al., 1984).

Genital Vascular Malformations

Penile vascular malformations are rare. Azzolini and Tardito reviewed the literature and found only 12 malformations of the glans and 5 of the shaft of the penis (Azzolini, 1967; Azzolini and Tardito, 1974). Only one of these was an arteriovenous malformation; the others were venous anomalies (Fig. 18–12).

Pelvic Lymphatic Malformations

Genital lymphedema may occur in association with lower limb lymphedema or may present in the absence of clinical disease in the limbs. If the underlying lymphatic abnor-

mality is hypoplasia, edema is the most common clinical manifestation; however, two thirds of these patients will, in addition, suffer discharge from lymphatic vesicles, and this may be complicated by secondary infection. When the underlying lymphatic abnormality is hyperplasia—occurring either alone or in association with multiple arteriovenous fistulae—reflux of chyle may become the major problem. Chyle may be discharged through the scrotal or vulval skin, or into the uterus (chylometrorrhea), vagina, or bladder (Fig. 18–13).

The management of these difficult problems has been described in detail by Kinmonth (Kinmonth, 1976, 1982).

References

Adams, H. D.: Congenital arteriovenous and cirsoid aneurysms. Surg. Gynec. Obst. 92:693, 1951.
Allison, D. J., and Hemingway, A. P.: Angiodysplasias: Does old age begin at nineteen? Lancet 2:979, 1981.
Azzolini, A.: Le lesioni angiodisplasiche del pene: Un caso di angioma artero-venoso. Min. Chir. 22:974, 1967.

Azzolini, A., and Tardito, E.: Non visceral localisations of vascular malformations. In Malan, E.: *Vascular Malformations*. Milan: Carlo Erba, 1974, p. 199.

Baek, S. M., Sloane, C. E., and Futterman, S. C.: Benign liver cell adenoma associated with use of oral contraceptive agents. Ann. Surg. *183*:239, 1976.

Baer, J. W., and Ryan, S.: Analysis of cecal vasculature in the search for vascular malformations. Am. J. Roent. *126*:394, 1976.

Barnett, P. H., Zerhouni, E. A., White, R. I., and Siegelman, S. S.: Computed tomography in the diagnosis of cavernous hemangioma of the liver. Am. J. Roent. *134*:439, 1980.

Baskerville, P. A., Ackroyd, J., Lea Thomas, M., and Browse, N. L.: The Klippel-Trenaunay syndrome. Brit. J. Surg. *72*:232, 1985.

Baum, S., Athanasoulis, C. A., Waltman, A. C., and Ring, E.J.: Angiographic diagnosis and control. Advances in Surgery 7:149, 1973.

Baum, S., Athanasoulis, C. A., Waltman, A. C., et al.: Angiodysplasia of the right colon: A cause of gastrointestinal bleeding. Am. J. Roentgenol. *129*:789, 1977.

Baum, J. K., Holtz, F., Bookstein, J. J., and Klein, E. W.: Possible association between benign hepatomas and oral contraceptives. Lancet 2:926, 1973.

Beggs, I., and Garvin, D. D.: Pelvic arteriovenous malformation in a man. Brit. J. Clin. Pract. *37*:186, 1983.

Bell, G. A., McKenzie, A. D., and Emmons, H.: Diffuse cavernous hemangioma of the rectum. Report of a case and review of the literature. Dis. Colon Rectum *15*:377, 1972.

Benjamin, B. I., Mohler, D. N., and Sandusky, W. R.: Hemangioma of the spleen. Arch. Intern. Med. *115*:280, 1965.

Bensaude, R., and Bensaude, A.: D'angiome caverneux du rectum. Presse Méd. No. *93*:1739, 1932.

Benson, R. C., Dotter, C. T., Peterson, C. G., et al.: Congenital arteriovenous fistula and pregnancy. Am. J. Obstet. Gynec. 92:672, 1965.

Bereston, E. S., and Roberts, D.: Congenital hypertrophy of the extremities. Southern Med. J. *58*:302, 1965.

Bissada, N. B., Smith, P. L., White, H. J., et al.: Tuberous sclerosis complex and renal angiomyolipoma. Collective review. Urology 6:105, 1975.

Boley, S. J., Sammartano, R., Adams, A., et al.: On the nature and etiology of vascular ectasias of the colon (degenerative lesions of aging). Gastroenterology *72*:650, 1977.

Boley, S. J., Sprayregen, S., Sammartano, R. J., et al.: The pathophysiologic basis for the angiographic signs of vascular ectasias of the colon. Radiology *125*:615, 1977.

Bongiovi, J. J., Jr., and Duffy, J. L.: Gastric hemangioma associated with upper gastrointestinal bleeding. Arch. Surg. 95:93, 1967.

Brinley, J. L., and Palubinskas, A. J.: Congenital arteriovenous malformation of the pancreas. Brit. J. Radiol. *50*:219, 1977.

Burge, D., Middleton, A., Kameth, R., and Fasher, B.: Intestinal haemorrhage in Turner's syndrome. Arch. Dis. Child. *56*:557, 1981.

Campbell, W. S.: Rupture of haemangioma of the spleen in pregnancy. J. Obst. Gynaec. Brit. Comm. *69*:665, 1962.

Case Records of the Massachusetts General Hospital (Case 48-1985). New Engl. J. Med. *313*:1405, 1985.

Cavett, C. M., Selby, J. H., Jr., Hamilton, J. L., and

Williamson, J. W.: Arteriovenous malformation in chronic gastrointestinal bleeding. Ann. Surg. *185*:116, 1977.

Chuang, V. P., Pulmano, C. M., Walter, J. F., and Cho, K. J.: Angiography of pancreatic arteriovenous malformation. Am. J. Roent. *129*:1015, 1977.

Cockett, F. B., and Young, A. E.: Results of the Palma operation for iliac vein compression. Paper read before Vascular Society of Great Britain and Ireland, London, 1980.

Conlon, C. L., Weinger, R. S., Cimo, P. L., et al.: Telangiectasia and von Willebrand's disease in two families. Ann. Int. Med. 89:921, 1978.

Constantini, Fabriani, Raynal, and Torreilles: Les angiomies cavernaux cirsoïdes de la fesse. J. de Chir. *59*:11, 1943.

Coppa, G. F., Eng, K., and Localio, S. A.: Surgical management of diffuse cavernous hemangioma of the colon, rectum and anus. Surg. Gynec. Obstet. *159*:17, 1984.

Cunningham, J. T.: Gastric telangiectasis in chronic haemodialysis patients: A report of six cases. Gastroenterology *81*:1131, 1981.

Danks, D. M.: Copper transport and utilization in Menkes' syndrome and in mottled mice. Inorganic Perspectives in Biology and Medicine *1*:73, 1977.

Decker, D. G., Fish, C. R., and Juergens, J. L.: Arteriovenous fistula of the female pelvis. Obstet. Gynec. *31*:799, 1968.

Editorial: Liver tumours and the pill. Brit. Med. J. 2:345, 1977.

Editorial: Angiodysplasia. Lancet 2:1086, 1981.

Farup, P. G., Rosseland, A. R., Stray, N., et al.: Localized telangiopathy of the stomach and duodenum diagnosed and treated endoscopically. Endoscopy *13*:1, 1981.

Fellows, K. E., and Mulliken, J. B.: Angiographic differentiation between hemangioma and arteriovenous malformation of the liver in infancy. Presented at the 6th International Workshop for the Study of Vascular Anomalies, Boston, 1986.

Flye, M. W., Jordan, B. P., and Schwartz, M. Z.: Management of congenital arteriovenous malformations. Surgery 94:740, 1983.

Fowler, D. L., Fortin, D., Wood, W. G., et al.: Intestinal vascular malformations. Surgery 86:377, 1979.

Front, D., Royal, H. D., Israel, O., et al.: Scintigraphy of hepatic hemangiomas: The value of Tc-99m–labelled red blood cells. J. Nuc. Med. *22*:684, 1981.

Galloway, S. J., Casarella, W. J., and Shimkin, P. M.: Vascular malformations of the right colon as a cause of bleeding in patients with aortic stenosis. Radiology *113*:11, 1974.

Gascoyen: Case of a naevus involving the parotid gland, and causing death from suffocation. Naevi of the viscera. Transactions of the Pathological Society of London *11*:267, 1860.

Gentry, R. W., Dockery, M. B., and Clagett, O. T.: Vascular malformations and vascular tumors of the gastrointestinal tract. Int. Abstr. Surg. 88:281, 1949.

Gianfrancisco, J. A., and Abcarian, H.: Pitfalls in the treatment of massive lower gastrointestinal bleeding with "blind" subtotal colectomy. Dis. Colon Rectum 25:441, 1982.

Glazer, G. M., Aisen, A. M., Francis, I. R., et al.: Hepatic cavernous hemangioma: Magnetic resonance imaging. Radiology *155*:417, 1985.

Halpern, M., Turner, A. F., and Citron, B. P.: Hereditary hemorrhagic telangiectasia. Radiology *90*:1143, 1968.

Hansen, P. S.: Hemangioma of the small intestine. Am. J. Clin. Path. *18*:14, 1948.

Husni, E. A.: The clinical course of splenic hemangioma with emphasis on spontaneous rupture. Arch. Surg. *83*:681, 1961.

Ishikawa, T.: Congenital arteriovenous malformations involving the pelvis and retroperitoneum: A case report. Angiology *30*:70, 1979.

Jeffrey, P. J., Hawley, P. R., and Parks, A. G.: Colo-anal sleeve anastomosis in the treatment of diffuse cavernous haemangioma involving the rectum. Brit. J. Surg. *63*:678, 1976.

Jensen, J. T., and Klinge, T.: Hemangioma of the liver. Report of two cases. Acta Radiologica Diag. *17*:61, 1976.

Johnson, C. M., Sheedy, P. F., Stanson, A. E., et al.: Computed tomography and angiography of cavernous hemangiomas of the liver. Radiology *138*:115, 1981.

Kaplan, J., and McIntosh, G. S.: Spontaneous rupture of a splenic vascular malformation. Report of 3 cases and a review of the literature. Journal of the Royal College of Surgeons of Edinburgh *32*(6), 1987.

Kinmonth, J. B.: Disorders of the circulation of chyle. J. Cardiovasc. Surg. *17*:329, 1976.

Kinmonth, J. B.: *The Lymphatics*, 2nd ed. London: Edward Arnold, 1982.

Kinmonth, J. B., and Eustace, P. W.: Gut protein loss in lymphoedema. Proc. Roy. Soc. Med. *68*:673, 1975.

Klein, T. W., and Kaplan, G. W.: Klippel-Trenaunay syndrome associated with urinary tract hemangiomas. J. Urol. *114*:596, 1975.

Lang, E. K.: A survey of the complications of percutaneous retrograde arteriography. Radiology *81*:257, 1963.

Leary, F. J., and Utz, D. C.: Miscellaneous vascular lesions affecting the urinary tract. In Emmet, J. L., and Willen, D. M. (eds.): *Clinical Urography.* Philadelphia: W. B. Saunders Co., 1971, Vol. 3, p. 1637.

Lewis, J. W., Mason, E. E., and Jochimsen, P. R.: Vascular malformations of the stomach and duodenum. Surg. Gynec. Obst. *153*:225, 1981.

Malan, E., and Puglionisi, A.: Congenital angiodysplasias of the extremities (Note II: arterial, arterial and venous, and haemolymphatic dysplasias). J. Cardiovasc. Surg. *6*:255, 1965.

Markisz, J. A., Front, D., Royal, H. D., et al.: An evaluation of 99mTc labelled red blood cell scintigraphy for the detection and localisation of gastrointestinal bleeding sites. Gastroenterology *83*:394, 1982.

May, R., and DeWeese, J. A.: Surgery of the pelvic veins. In May, R. (ed.): *Surgery of the Veins of the Leg and Pelvis.* Stuttgart: George Thieme, 1979, p. 158.

McLoughlin, M. J.: Angiography in cavernous hemangioma of the liver. Am. J. Roent. *113*:50, 1971.

Mitchell, A., Fellows, G. J., and Smith, J. C.: Partial nephrectomy for renal haemangioma. J. Roy. Soc. Med. *75*:766, 1982.

Mizutani, N., Masudo, U., Naito, N., et al.: Pancreatic arteriovenous malformation in a patient with gastrointestinal hemorrhage. Am. J. Gastroenterol. *76*:141, 1981.

Moore, J. D., Thompson, N. W., Appelman, H. D., and Foley, D.: Arteriovenous malformations of the gastrointestinal tract. Arch. Surg. *111*:381, 1976.

Mortensen, J. D., and Ellsworth, H. S.: Internal iliac

arteriovenous fistula developing postpartum. Amer. J. Cardiol. *16*:292, 1965.

Natali, J., Jue-Denis, P., Kieffer, E., et al.: Arteriovenous fistulae of the internal iliac vessels. J. Cardiovasc. Surg. *25*:165, 1984.

Neifeld, J. P., Doppman, J. L., and Chretien, P. B.: Congenital pelvic arteriovenous fistulas: Report of a case and review of the literature. J. Urol. *114*:648, 1975.

Nusbaum, M., and Baum, S.: Radiographic demonstration of unknown sites of gastrointestinal bleeding. Surg. Forum *14*:374, 1963.

Oda, F. T., McLaughlin, J. S., Yeager, G. H., et al.: Vascular anomalies of the extremity associated with abnormal growth. Am. Surgeon *28*:775, 1962.

Olcott, C., Newton, T. H., Stoney, R. J., and Ehrenfeld, W. K.: Intra-arterial embolization in the management of arteriovenous malformations. Surgery *79*:3, 1976.

Palma, E. C., Esperon, R.: Vein transplants and grafts in the surgical treatment of the postphlebitic syndrome. J. Cardiovasc. Surg. *1*:94, 1960.

Pantoja, E.: Angiography in liver hemangioma. Am. J. Roent. *104*:874, 1968.

Peck, M. E.: Obstructive anomalies of iliac vein associated with growth shortening in the ipsilateral extremity. Ann. Surg. *146*:619, 1957.

Pinkhas, J., Djaldetti, M., DeVries, A., et al.: Diffuse angiomatosis with hypersplenism: Splenectomy followed by polycythemia. Am. J. Med. *45*:795, 1968.

Pitlik, S., Cohen, L., Hadar, H., et al.: Portal hypertension and esophageal varices in hemangiomatosis of the spleen. Gastroenterology *72*:937, 1977.

Pliskin, M.: Peliosis hepatis. Radiology *114*:29, 1975.

River, L., Silverstein, J., and Tope, J. W.: Benign neoplasms of the small intestine. Int. Abstracts Surg. *102*:1, 1956.

Roberts, L. K., Gold, R. E., and Routt, W. E.: Gastric angiodysplasia. Radiology *139*:355, 1981.

Rodriguez, S., and Befeler, D.: Renal angiomas. Amer. J. Surg. *113*:574, 1967.

Sarrasis, M., Pang, G., and Hunter, F.: Telangiectasias of the upper gastrointestinal tract. Report of six cases and review. Endoscopy *15*:85, 1983.

Servelle, M.: Klippel and Trenaunay's syndrome. Ann. Surg. *201*:365, 1985.

Servelle, M., Bastin, R., Loygue, J., et al.: Hematuria and rectal bleeding in the child with Klippel and Trenaunay syndrome. Ann. Surg. *183*:418, 1976.

Sewell, J. H., and Weiss, K.: Spontaneous rupture of hemangioma of the liver. Arch. Surg. *83*:729, 1961.

Shanberge, J. N., Tanaka, K., and Gruhl, M. C.: Chronic consumption coagulopathy due to hemangiomatous transformation of the spleen. Am. J. Clin. Pathol. *56*:723, 1971.

Sheedy, P. F., Fulton, R. E., and Atwell, D. T.: Angiographic evaluation of patients with chronic gastrointestinal bleeding. Am. J. Roent. *123*:338, 1975.

Shepherd, J. A.: Angiomatous conditions of the gastrointestinal tract. Brit. J. Surg. *40*:409, 1953.

Sherlock, S.: Hepatic adenomas and oral contraceptives. Gut *16*:753, 1975.

Singh, A., Shenoy, S., Kaur, A., et al.: Arteriovenous malformation of the cecum. Dis. Colon Rectum *20*:334, 1977.

Smith, D. W.: Menke's syndrome. In Smith, D. W.: *Recognizable Patterns of Human Malformations*, 3rd ed. Philadelphia: W. B. Saunders Co., 1982, p. 150.

Smith, D. W.: Peutz-Jeghers syndrome. In Smith, D. W.:

Recognizable Patterns of Human Malformations, 3rd ed. Philadelphia: W. B. Saunders Co., 1982, p. 386.

Szilagyi, D. E., Smith, R. F., Elliott, J. P., and Hageman, J. H.: Congenital arteriovenous anomalies of the limbs. Arch. Surg. *111*:423, 1976.

Taylor, T. V., and Torrance, H. B.: Haemangiomas of the gastrointestinal tract. Brit. J. Surg. *61*:236, 1974.

Terblanche, J.: Liver tumours. Brit. J. Hosp. Med. *19*:103, 1977.

Walt, A. J.: Cysts and benign tumours of the liver. Surg. Clin. North Am. *57*:449, 1977.

Walter, J. F., Chuang, V. P., Bookstein, J. J., et al.: Angiography of massive hemorrhage secondary to pancreatic disease. Radiology *124*:337, 1977.

Weaver, G. A., Alpern, H. D., David, J. S., et al.: Gastrointestinal angiodysplasia associated with aortic valve disease: Part of a spectrum of angiodysplasia of the gut. Gastroenterology *77*:1, 1979.

Whitley, R. D., and Winship, T.: Splenic hemangioma with fatal hemangiosarcoma. Surgery *35*:787, 1954.

Winterbauer, R. H.: Multiple telangiectasia, Raynaud's phenomenon, sclerodactyly and subcutaneous calcinosis: A syndrome mimicking hereditary hemorrhagic telangiectasia. Bull. Johns Hopkins Hosp. *114*:361, 1964.

Vascular Malformations of the Lower Limb

A. E. Young

with contributions by

P. Baskerville
M. Smith
G. Stewart

INTRODUCTION

The lower limb is a common site for all forms of vascular malformations. Many of these will be asymptomatic, but at the time of presentation a clinical attempt at diagnosis should be made. If the patient is a young child, invasive and in-hospital investigation should be avoided unless the condition is progressing and not clinically diagnosable, or unless the symptoms dictate that surgical intervention is necessary.

The details of diagnosis and investigation of the patients are outlined in Chapter Eight. If diffuse arteriovenous malformations are suspected, limb blood flow should be assessed by whatever method is locally available. Arteriography need only be undertaken if there is clinical evidence of localized fistulae. Where there is clearly a venous anomaly, the state of the deep veins must be assessed, ideally by phlebography. If there is edema, lymphography may also be needed to elucidate the exact cause. When the malformation is situated at the root of the limb, care is taken to assess the degree of concomitant intra-abdominal malformation. This may require sigmoidoscopy and cystoscopy, ultrasound, or computed tomographic scanning of the pelvis in addition to normal clinical examination.

In extensive lesions, a prognosis should only be given after investigations are complete and, even then, it should not be dogmatic. We have observed frequently that even after full investigation the future behavior of the limb is difficult to predict.

Treatment should normally be conservative and should wait upon the development of symptoms, except in situations in which prophylaxis against complications or progression is feasible. Such prophylaxis includes:

1. Elastic support for venous hypertension
2. Prophylactic orthopedic procedures to control overgrowth in length
3. Excision of small, well-localized arteriovenous malformations
4. Excision of surface lesions that cause bleeding or ulceration

This expectant policy may be difficult for parents and patient to accept unless it is carefully explained.

MANAGEMENT PROBLEMS

The following specific problems may be encountered:
1. The cutaneous vascular malformation
2. Abnormal veins
3. The large leg
4. Skeletal abnormalities
5. Ulcers
6. Venous thrombosis and thromboembolism

The Cutaneous Vascular Malformation

Capillary vascular malformations are rarely a cause of symptoms, and their extent is such

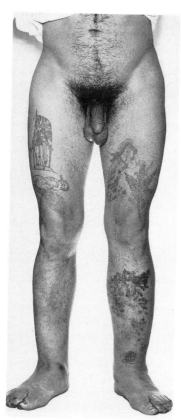

Figure 19–1. Diffuse combined cutaneous malformation of the left lower leg. This patient's lesions were largely asymptomatic. The patient's solution to the cosmetic problem was to distract the eye!

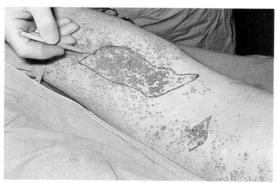

Figure 19–2. This young man's leg had an extensive lymphatic vesicle with a circumscribed area causing troublesome leakage. It was possible to excise this area and obtain linear closure without need for an extensive operation.

that any attempt at treatment for purely cosmetic reasons is unlikely to be worthwhile (Fig. 19–1). Complex lesions, particularly those with friable venules or lymphatic vesicles in them, and those adjacent to arteriovenous malformations, may be a source of repeated trouble from bleeding, sepsis, ulceration, lymphatic leakage, pain, and contracture. These may be difficult to treat. A small lesion can be excised *in toto* with linear closure or grafting. Larger lesions require staged excisions or grafts (Fig. 19–2), though difficulties may be encountered because such areas heal badly, with a tendency to hypertrophic scarring. Furthermore, an apparently superficial lesion is often only the tip of a deep-seated lesion, and excision may be impossible. Free grafts placed on this abnormal deep tissue may "take" badly and may be lifted off by oozing blood or lymph. Mesh grafts are sometimes useful. Free tissue transfers with microvascular anastomosis allow more extensive excision and predictable skin cover of problematic areas. Coexistent venous hypertension, whether from arteriovenous malformations or from venous anomalies, may need to be separately treated, either surgically or by elastic compression before excision of a cutaneous malformation is attempted. Persisting sepsis as cellulitis is often a problem where there is an ulceration and/or lymphatic leakage from a surface malformation and is particularly common where there is coexistent lymphedema. In such cases, long-term prophylactic antibiotics are required and simple antistreptococcal drugs, such as the broad spectrum penicillins, usually suffice.

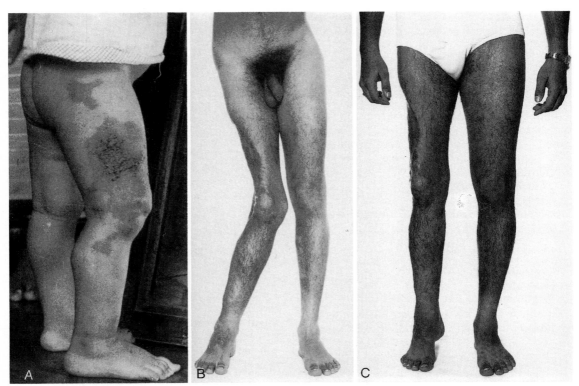

Figure 19–3. The damaging effects of radiotherapy used inappropriately to treat a cutaneous vascular malformation. *A,* As a child, this patient was noted to have Klippel-Trenaunay syndrome and there was a cosmetically unsatisfactory surface malformation on the lateral side of the thigh over the lateral venous anomaly. It was treated initially with radiotherapy and subsequently with excision and grafting. *B,* Radiotherapy damage to the epiphysis at the knee caused a gross varus deformity as the boy grew. *C,* The deformity was corrected by a femoral osteotomy, but radiation damage to the epiphysis reduced the growth in the limb, which is now shorter than its fellow (procedure by F. W. Heatley, FRCS).

There have been many older reports of the use of radiotherapy for the treatment of cutaneous malformations, but current opinion is that it is of no value and, indeed, may worsen the situation (Fig. 19–3). Cryotherapy and local steroid therapy are similarly unhelpful. Persisting sepsis, lymph leakage, pain, and disability from contractures in superficial lesions in the face of repeated, failed attempts at extirpative cure are, in our experience, best treated by amputation.

Management of Cystic Lymphatic Malformations

In the past, the treatment of these so-called "lymphangiomas" has included carbon dioxide snow, liquid nitrogen, excisional surgery, electrocautery, x-rays, thorium-X, and radium. Little or no benefit has previously been reported, unless the involved area was small. In addition, recurrences are common whatever form of treatment is used. The lesions seem to be totally resistant to radiation therapy, which is contraindicated because of the risk of growth disturbance and late malignancies (Saijo et al., 1975). Occasionally, these lesions are best left alone and treatment with compression dressings are used to control the skin vesicles and underlying cysts. However, the troublesome leakage and cosmetic disfigurement commonly encountered with these lesions suggest that active treatment of some form is desirable in most cases.

On the basis of Whimster's hypothesis (Whimster, 1976), our unit considers that the treatment of these lesions would be more successful, and the cosmetic results better, if the principal part of the operation was the excision of the subcutaneous cisterns, leaving as much skin intact as possible. This allows better skin closure with or without skin grafting but, occasionally, leaves some skin vesicles that might eventually collapse. Using the same theoretical concept, some surgeons have attempted to destroy the deep component with injections of boiling water or, more recently, with hypertonic saline or bleomycin (Ikeda et al., 1977). Used alone, these latter methods have proved ineffective, though they may be useful as an adjunct during excisional surgery. Browse and his colleagues have reviewed the results of procedures based on the operative principle of excising the deep cisterns with preservation of as much skin as possible (Browse et al., 1986). Twenty-nine patients were reviewed 2 to 8 years after operation. It was shown that, for management purposes, there are two categories of cystic lymphatic anomalies: (1) small lesions (less than 7 cm in diameter) in favorable sites of the body that are potentially curable, and (2) large lesions (greater than 7 cm in diameter) with an even larger area of subcutaneous cysts in which complete excision of all the skin vesicles requires skin grafting. Eight patients had small lesions, and none of these have had recurrence following excision of the lesion. Nineteen patients had large but resectable lesions. Progression was controlled and the cosmetic appearance improved in 16 patients by radical excision of as much of the cyst-bearing subcutaneous tissue as possible, leaving enough skin to allow linear closure, even though skin vesicles were left. These results show that although only small lesions can be cured, the natural history of steady progression of the larger lesions can be controlled, and sometimes reversed, by wide excisional surgery, with a high degree of acceptance by the patient. The subsequent disappearance of many of the residual skin vesicles supports Whimster's hypothesis that the skin vesicles are secondary to the rhythmic contractions and pressure pulses in the deep cysts.

Abnormal Veins

The predominant cause of symptoms in venous ectasias, Klippel-Trenaunay syndrome, and Parkes Weber syndrome is venous hypertension. This hypertension is a composite of back-flow down large, valveless veins (Baskerville and coworkers (1985) have shown that the volumes involved may be as high as 500 ml), obstruction of deep veins, and arteriovenous fistulae. The simplest, safest, and most effective way to counteract the

venous hypertension is elastic support. This should be of the graduated compression type, in the range of 30–40 mmHg. The stockings must be individually fitted and regularly replaced, as the elastic gradually perishes. Such support will frequently alleviate the patient's symptoms. Only 30% of patients with Klippel-Trenaunay syndrome in the Mayo Clinic series needed operation (Gloviczki et al., 1983). Veins that are cosmetically unacceptable or in which gross reflux is manifested may require excision, but only if the deep veins are phlebographically normal. Particular care must be taken to ensure that the phlebographic assessment of the deep veins is accurate. Lea Thomas has discussed venographic artifacts in his book *Phlebography of the Lower Limb* (1982), but there are particular additional pitfalls in relation to congenital venous anomalies. Most authors report instances in which deep veins of the leg are present but, on initial phlebography, are erroneously believed to be absent or hypoplastic. This may be due to dilution of contrast material or to diversion of the contrast into large superficial trunks. Malan and Puglionisi recommend elastic bandaging of the whole leg prior to venography so as to empty the superficial system (Malan and Puglionisi, 1964). They also note that direct injection into the deep system (e.g., the popliteal vein) may be necessary to demonstrate it. It has also been suggested that retrograde venography from the groin may be necessary to verify a patent femoral system that has not filled because of a band constriction in the popliteal fossa. Müller and Schmidt recorded two cases in which the deep veins were only seen during the venous phase of an arteriogram (Müller and Schmidt, 1969).

Lindenauer demonstrated that in the presence of deep vein atresia or obstruction, ligation and/or stripping of superficial veins precipitates edema or worsens pre-existing edema (Lindenauer, 1965). Thirteen of his 14 patients were made worse by operation, and the varices rapidly recurred. Nonetheless, deTakats (1932), Homans (1946), and Myers and Janes (1955) have advocated the excision of unsightly superficial varices, and this has also been our policy in carefully selected cases in which deep veins have been shown to be normal and symptoms problematic. Not only have we found the results of excision, in such cases, to be cosmetically satisfactory; in addition, excision has also reduced symptoms, particularly in patients with large valveless lateral venous anomalies that contribute to venous reflux into the lower leg.

Although traditional vein strippers can be used to remove ectatic leg veins, major branches and perforating veins must be exposed and ligated or divided under direct vision before the vein is stripped. Abnormal veins do not always lie free in loose connective tissue and fat, as do adult "banal" varicose veins. This is particularly so below the knee, where the palpable abnormal vein may be merely a central channel amidst a meshwork of vascular spaces. For this reason, many surgeons prefer direct excision through long incisions placed over the veins. Direct exposure of all types may precipitate extensive thrombosis in remaining veins and pulmonary embolism. The risk of this is increased if tourniquet hemostasis is used at operation.

Injection sclerotherapy with chemical or physical irritants such as sodium tetradecyl sulfate or hyperosmolar saline is only of value if the injected anomalous veins can be compressed after injection and if the anatomy of the abnormal area is sufficiently well-documented to be sure that there is no risk of the sclerotherapy agent leaking into deep veins. Sclerotherapy also may be of value when it is combined with surgical excision.

Deep vein abnormalities have been discussed and attention drawn to the difficulty that may be experienced in identifying the nature and extent of the abnormality. If careful phlebography, both antegrade and, if necessary, retrograde, confirm an atretic or hypoplastic segment, a direct surgical approach may be of benefit, though the number of recorded cases of benefit is extremely limited (with the exception of those that Servelle has operated upon) (Servelle, 1985). Servelle claims that the deep "hypoplasias" of femoral and popliteal veins may be due to fibrous bands ("brides fibreuses localisées") obstructing them, and advocates exposure and division of the constricting band together with lysis of congenital fibrous constrictions that are encountered around the deep veins ("fendre la gaine de la veine"). He notes that this procedure allows the vein to return to normal diameter and function and among many other cases records a case of Klippel-Trenaunay syndrome operated upon in 1943 for relief of a band reducing the lumen to 1–2 mm. When the leg was re-explored in 1957, the vein at that point was 5 mm in diameter (Servelle, 1965).

Belov claims that by "functional hemodynamic studies" he was able to discover arteriovenous shunts in all four Klippel-Trenaunay syndrome patients that he had seen who had deep vein aplasia and reports that on angiography "numerous direct arteriovenous anastomoses were found in all four patients" (Belov, 1972). Belov treated one patient by exposing the anomalous lateral vein and dividing the arteriovenous anastomoses to it ("skeletonization"), with apparent relief of symptoms. Unfortunately, we are not aware of any publications that offer a full clinical follow-up analysis with objective data from which to assess the purported benefits of exploring and operating upon the deep veins in Klippel-Trenaunay syndrome. However, it is clear that patients with Klippel-Trenaunay syndrome, including those with deep vein abnormalities, do *not* suffer gross symptoms, and milder symptoms can be controlled with elastic support. Therefore, we cannot recommend the routine surgical exploration of deep veins found on venography to be abnormal.

The Large Leg

The large leg is frequently a composite of different abnormalities:

1. Overgrowth of all the tissues (gigantism)
2. Enlargement by the bulk of the vascular malformation
3. Edema secondary to the venous hypertension encountered in venous and arteriovenous malformations
4. Edema secondary to concomitant abnormalities of the lymphatic system
5. Edema secondary to high output cardiac failure in patients with large arteriovenous malformations
6. Edema secondary to hypoproteinemia, which may occur when lymphangiectasia of the bowel is present causing a protein-losing enteropathy

These last two contributors to the large leg are very rare.

Swelling and Lymphatic Problems in the Limb

The multiple causes of thickening and swelling of a limb involved by a vascular malformation have been enumerated. Several of these causes may be present in any patient. The participation of the lymphatic system in the swelling is often substantial and is frequently overlooked, though from the time of the earliest case reports descriptions are found of vascular malformations associated with signs that clearly indicate disorders of the lymphatic system.

Beck, reporting a case of combined vascular deformity of the arm in 1837, described the hypertrophy as being accompanied by "une densité et d'un épaissement de tissu cellulaire souscutane . . . cette augmentation de volume paraissait dependre moins d'une hypertrophie des muscle que d'une épaississement de la couche celluleuse et de la distension de la peau," suggesting that this was lymphedema (Beck, 1837). The cutaneous lesions of Friedberg's case were described as chronic pemphigus but were probably lymphatic vesicles (Friedberg, 1867). The patient of Monod that stimulated the Trélat and Monod review of 1869 was described as suffering from "une infiltration graisseuse et oedémateuse des tissus" (Trélat and Monod, 1869). The grossness of the edema in this case again suggests that it was lymphedema, but Trélat and Monod attributed the edema to venous disease. Indeed, they went so far as to say "on n'a remarque ni trouble, ni changement, ni anomalie dans l'appareil de la circulation lymphatique."

Klippel and Trenaunay barely mention any abnormalities that could be attributable to the lymphatic system, apart from remarking that the skin may occasionally be "elephatiasque, écailleuse, irrégulière et oedémateuse" (Klippel and Trenaunay, 1900). They only mention the lymphatic system to discard the theory of Bull and of Pollosson, that the cutaneous nevus may be the result of an "altération du système lymphatique."

Parkes Weber notes only that the cutaneous alteration may be "lymphangiomatous" but never suggests that there could be a more general lymphatic abnormality (Parkes Weber, 1918).

The involvement of the lymphatic system in patients with definite arteriovenous fistulae went unremarked upon until Robertson's review in 1956 (Robertson, 1956). He observed that a "degree of lymphoedema is not infrequently present," but included this as a regional effect of the arteriovenous fistulae. In three patients with diffuse arteriovenous fistulae he recorded huge lymphatics in the groin and commented that "The co-existence

of two lesions is not surprising when one remembers that lymphatics have a close development relation to veins."

In 1957, Servelle described two patients in whom there was lymphedema that was secondary to obstruction of the lymphatic pathways by compressing bands, one in the popliteal fossa and the other in Hunter's canal (Servelle et al., 1957). The distal lymphatics were dilated in both these cases, and the edema was "improved" by release of the constriction. In this paper, Servelle also recorded two cases of chylous reflux and one of chylothorax occurring in patients who he describes as suffering from Klippel-Trenaunay syndrome. In his book *Oedémes Chroniques des Membres*, published in 1962, Servelle recorded eight further cases of Klippel-Trenaunay syndrome associated with "elephantiasis" (Servelle, 1962). He specifically stated that he had never encountered elephantiasis in association with multiple congenital arteriovenous fistulae.

Specific studies of the lymphatic system in vascular malformations have been performed by Pokrovosky (19 patients) (Pokrovosky et al., 1971) and by Biasi (12 patients) (Biasi et al., 1973); a study by Young is reported (Young, 1978) in which he examined 33 patients with Klippel-Trenaunay syndrome or Parkes Weber syndrome involving the lower limbs. A third of these patients had no stigmata of lymphatic disease, yet this analysis clearly showed several features:

1. Limbs that have no clinical evidence of lymphatic disease will often have an asymptomatic lymphatic abnormality. This abnormality may involve both limbs, even though only one is the site of the blood vascular malformations.

2. In Klippel-Trenaunay syndrome, there is usually an associated lymphatic hypoplasia with less lymph trunks and less nodes than normal. These changes seem to be primary, and not the secondary result of sepsis. The incidence of these changes in Klippel-Trenaunay syndrome is not known, though in Kinmonth and Young's series half of the patients without clinical evidence of lymphatic disease had, in fact, bilateral lymphographic changes (Kinmonth et al., 1976). Servelle has noted megalymphatics in Klippel-Trenaunay syndrome (Servelle, 1985).

3. In patients with multiple diffuse arteriovenous fistulae, two lymphographic patterns are seen:

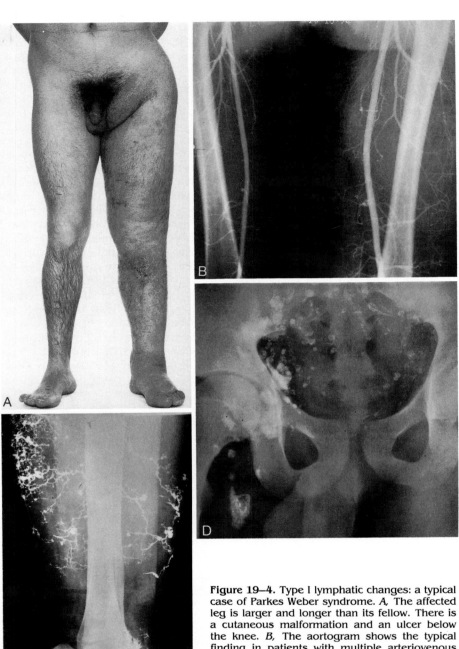

Figure 19–4. Type I lymphatic changes: a typical case of Parkes Weber syndrome. *A*, The affected leg is larger and longer than its fellow. There is a cutaneous malformation and an ulcer below the knee. *B*, The aortogram shows the typical finding in patients with multiple arteriovenous malformations: a larger artery in the affected leg with a greater number of branches. The femur is also noted to be denser than the normal one. *C*, There are dilated varicose dermal lymphatics. *D*, The lymphadenogram shows multiple small scattered lymph nodes in the pelvis on both the affected and clinically unaffected sides.

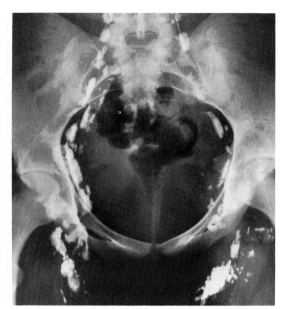

Figure 19–5. Type II lymphatic changes in an arteriovenous malformation. The lymphadenogram shows a normal number of lymph nodes, but these are enlarged.

a. *Type I*: Dilated varicose lymph trunks; filling of dermal lymphatics; multiple small spotty lymph nodes; proximal malformations, importantly including thoracic duct obstructions; prolonged transit time of the contrast material from the foot to the thoracic duct; occasional cutaneous lymphatic vesi-

cles; and occasional chylous reflux. These are essentially the changes seen in some patients with primary hyperplastic lymphedema and may be taken to be a primary failure of proper development of the lymphatic system (Fig. 19–4).

b. *Type II*: Distended lymph trunks, normal in number; enlarged lymph nodes in the groins and pelvis, but normal in position and number; and normal thoracic duct (Fig. 19–5). These Type II changes can be mimicked by fashioning an arteriovenous fistula in the hind limb of the dog (Sokolowski, 1971) (Fig. 19–6), but similar results are not seen following femoral arteriovenous fistulae made in children to encourage limb growth (Kinmonth and Negus, 1974). It is assumed that these Type II changes are due to distension of a normal lymphatic system by increased flow. All these changes may be associated with lymphedema.

The clinical problems produced by lymphatic abnormalities in association with vascular malformations are as follows:

1. Grossly lymphedematous legs (Fig. 19–7)

2. Lymphatic vesicles that may leak chyle or clear lymph

3. Associated chylous ascites or chylothorax

4. Localized cystic lymphatic malformations

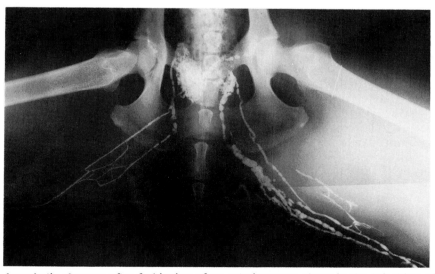

Figure 19–6. Lymphatic changes after fashioning of an arteriovenous shunt in the left thigh of a dog. The lymphatics on the side of the shunt are noted to be enlarged and varicose.

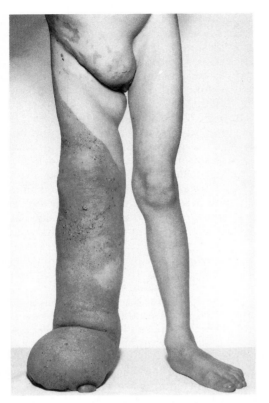

Figure 19–7. A gross example of a combined malformation in the right leg of a 7 year old. There are ectatic veins and cutaneous and subcutaneous vascular malformations, with vesicles and lymphedema. The limb is short.

Gross Lymphedema

Obsessional conservative treatment may prevent progression. This treatment involves compulsive elastic support (Fig. 19–8); careful attention to skin hygiene to prevent cracking, sepsis, and fungal infections; together sometimes with regular use of an automatic massage/compression boot. Surgical excision is not recommended unless the leg is so large as to impair mobility or if the patient finds it cosmetically *very* unacceptable. If the skin is in good condition, an ablative procedure with preservation of local flaps (Homans or Sistrunk's operation) can achieve good results in the hands of an experienced surgical team (Fig. 19–9). Where the overlying skin has become verrucous or is involved by a dermal vascular malformation and cannot be preserved, excision of lymphedematous tissue and split-thickness skin cover may be occasionally necessary (Charles procedure), though this is generally an unsatisfactory option.

"Physiological" operations to establish a new lymphatic drainage from the leg are only applicable in the rare patient who has obstructed or absent iliac nodes, but has well preserved lymph vessels in the leg and groin and a normal lymph system higher. The details of these procedures for managing lymphedema are described in *The Lymphatics,* by J.B. Kinmonth (1982), and in Hurst and coworkers (1985).

Lymphatic Vesicles

If lymphatic vesicles leak only lymph and are well localized, excision should be undertaken and the wound grafted, if necessary. Where there is chylous discharge from the groin or genitalia, local excision of the leaking points does not resolve the problem and a more extensive procedure to ligate the congenital megalymphatics on the posterior abdominal wall is required. Ligation of the abnormal lymphatics at the groin has proved less successful. The importance of accurate lymphography followed by an abdominal operation has been stressed by Kinmonth, who recorded patients in whom even amputation failed to resolve chylous leak (Kinmonth, 1982).

Other Chylous Diseases

Chylous ascites, chylothorax, and exudative enteropathy are all encountered rarely, either alone or in association with lymphedema of the periphery, and sometimes where there is a cutaneous capillary malformation. For further discussion of this subject, the reader is referred to the work of Kinmonth (1982).

Skeletal Abnormalities

The Long Leg/Gigantism

The majority of children with major vascular malformations of the lower limbs have a disparity in limb length if the malformation is unilateral. Trélat and Monod were the first to notice the association, and Klippel and Trenaunay and Parkes Weber embodied it as a feature of the syndromes that bear their names (Trélat and Monod, 1869; Klippel and Trenaunay, 1900; Parkes Weber, 1918). The first case of a combined vascular malformation ever illustrated, Friedberg's case, shows

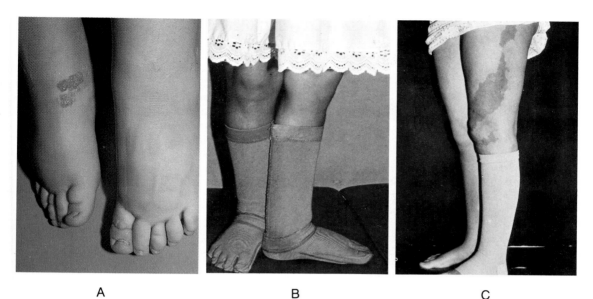

A   B   C

Figure 19–8. Elastic support is the mainstay of conservative therapy for combined vascular anomalies of the lower extremities. *A,* This little girl has bilateral lymphedema as a result of lymphatic anomalies. The edema is most pronounced in the forefoot and toes. Note vesicles on dorsum of right foot. *B,* The elastic stockings of the girl shown in A are custom made to enclose the toes, and she wears them even during her ballet practice (third position shown). *C,* Elastic support can be less tight, but is still necessary, for combined vascular malformations that are predominantly venous. The toes need not be included.

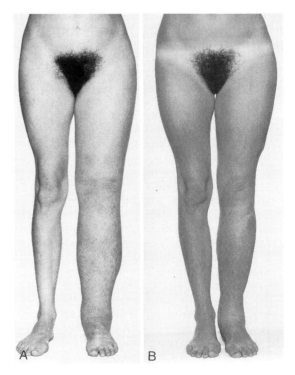

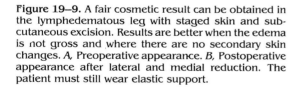

Figure 19–9. A fair cosmetic result can be obtained in the lymphedematous leg with staged skin and subcutaneous excision. Results are better when the edema is not gross and where there are no secondary skin changes. *A,* Preoperative appearance. *B,* Postoperative appearance after lateral and medial reduction. The patient must still wear elastic support.

a dramatic overgrowth of the affected leg (Friedberg, 1867). In adults, this is a fixed discrepancy; in children, owing to growth, the leg length difference often increases and, in addition, may be aggravated by the development of an associated deformity, such as the following:

1. Proportional hypertrophy (proportional gigantism)
2. Disproportionate gigantism
3. Shortening

Proportional hypertrophy exists when the leg is uniformly enlarged, the skeletal enlargement occurring *pari passu* with soft tissue enlargement and without distortion of the normal proportions of the leg. This form is the most common and can occur with any extensive vascular malformation, but it is particularly seen in patients with diffuse microfistulous arteriovenous malformations (see Fig. 19–4A). The Mayo Clinic series showed it in 53 of 69 patients (Gloviczki et al., 1983), and the author's own review found it in 22 of 24 patients (Young, 1978).

Disproportionate gigantism is the gross enlargement of parts of a limb out of proportion to the remainder. It is seen particularly with multiple lymphatic-venous anomalies and in some patients with Klippel-Trenaunay syndrome.

Shortening is seen with intraosseous and venous or lymphatic malformations and, more rarely, with deep vein atresias or hypoplasias. All these congenital anomalies of size may be encountered without any clinical evidence of a vascular lesion. Not all leg length discrepancies are consequent upon a true difference in bone length. Alterations in the pattern of growth secondary to vascular malformation may cause an angular deformity as a result of asymmetrical growth at the epiphyseal plate giving rise to varus, valgus, or flexion deformities. Occasionally a deformity is seen in which the epiphysis itself is affected, and the most common consequence of this is a fixed flexion deformity. Where there is a vascular malformation in the soft tissues immediately adjacent to a joint, this can give rise to deformity also. Care must be taken, therefore, to measure true leg lengths, and where a deformity is present it is important to establish the precise cause and to determine whether or not it is of bone or soft tissue origin.

Leg length discrepancy can be caused by other pathological conditions. Coexistent neurologic disease involving disuse can produce quite severe shortening and may be encountered in those patients with paretic limbs secondary to spinal vascular malformations. Other causes associated with, but unrelated to, the primary vascular malformation may also occur, and these include congenital dislocation of the hip; Perthes disease of the hip; or fractures of the long bones, which may occur in these patients, who can have an osteoporotic bone in association with the vascular malformation.

Finally, it should be noted that a leg length disparity of a centimeter or so can be considered as within the normal range.

Etiology

The literature is replete with investigations and arguments about the nature of the association between vascular malformations and skeletal abnormality. From the clinical point of view, this is a sterile activity, having minimal bearing on treatment. The arguments center on two imponderables. The *first* is whether the hypertrophy is caused by hemodynamic changes or whether the two are separate endpoints derived from a common genetic failure of developmental control. The *second* argument involves speculation about how altered hemodynamics might affect bone growth.

Arguments in favor of abnormal hemodynamics directly causing hypertrophy or hypotrophy can be summarized as follows:

1. Arteriovenous malformations are more likely to cause limb hypertrophy when they are near an epiphysis.
2. Experimental and therapeutic arteriovenous fistulae can produce changes in limb length, though not always in a predictable way. Janes and Musgrove made iliac arteriovenous fistulae in puppies and produced overgrowth of femurs and tibias (Janes and Musgrove, 1950); however, when Janes and Jennings formed fistulae to treat 33 children with short legs, they produced corrective extra growth in the majority but in 28% the length discrepancy worsened (Janes and Jennings, 1961).
3. When difference in blood flow is assessed between a hypertrophic leg and its normal fellow, disparity in blood flow is found to be proportional to the inequality in length. Malan says that this is not so, but he does not appear to have made blood flow

measurements in all his patients (Malan and Puglionisi, 1965).

4. Proximal venous obstruction by ligature or tourniquet stimulates growth in animals and in humans (Schüller, 1889, Kishikawa, 1936; Hutchison and Burdeaux, 1954), though the contrasting finding is that of Bloom and colleagues, who found that acquired femoral artery obstruction following catheterization in children produced shortening of the limb (Bloom et al., 1974).

5. Hyperemia induced at an epiphysis by infection, heating, and trauma encourages overgrowth.

The mechanism by which changed hemodynamics alter the growth is not known, nor how the possible factors interact. These include venous hypertension itself, changes in capillary oxygen, blood pH, ischemia as a result of shunting, and the opening of Sucquet-Hoyer channels in the face of venous obstruction.

6. The vascular pattern in the developing embryonic limb bud is considered to have an important influence on skeletal and muscular development, controlling this through the medium of shifting concentrations of essential low molecular weight compounds such as nicotinamide and oxygen (Caplan and Koutroupas, 1973).

The arguments for hemodynamic abnormalities *not* being causally connected with skeletal abnormalities center on the following observations:

1. Skeletal overgrowth and undergrowth can occur in the absence of any demonstrable vascular abnormality.

2. Hypertrophy and vascular malformations can occur in the same patient but in different limbs, a state Klippel and Trenaunay refer to as "crossed dissociation" (Klippel and Trenaunay, 1900). Oda illustrates an interesting case of Klippel-Trenaunay syndrome in which a leg is shorter than its fellow, but in which the patient also has a small arm not involved by the vascular malformation (Oda et al., 1962).

3. Bizarre and gross skeletal malformations may coexist with vascular malformations in the limb that are not anatomically juxtaposed.

4. The coexistence of other skeletal malformations with vascular malformations is common. We have noted vertebral segmentation defects, rudimentary ribs, fibrous dysplasias, melorheostosis, Perthes disease, coxa vara, congenital dislocation of the hip, failed fusion of obturator foramen, talipes calcaneovarus and equinovarus, syndactyly, accessory phalanges, absent phalanges, Köhler's disease of the tarsal scaphoid, and other anomalies (Fig. 19–10) (see Table 14–3). There is also the specific coexistence of enchondromas with vascular malformations (Maffucci's syndrome), and van der Molen (1976) has noted osteomas. Kessler has noticed sclerosing bone disease (melorheostosis, osteopoikilosis, and osteopathia striata).

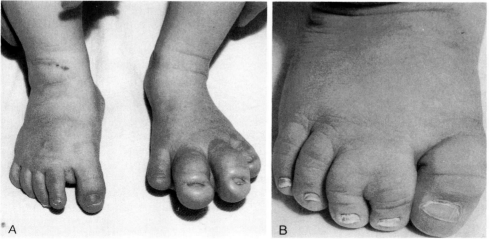

Figure 19–10. Skeletal abnormalities in association with vascular malformations frequently occur in the foot. *A,* Giant toes. *B,* Syndactyly.

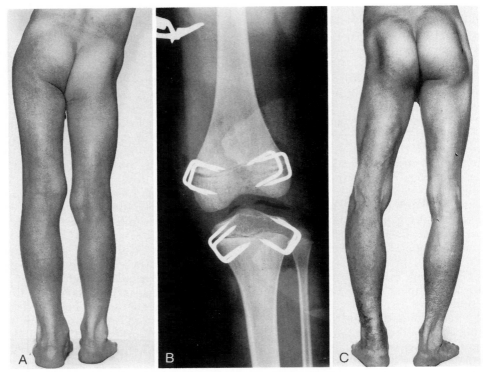

Figure 19–11. Correction of overgrowth in a patient with multiple arteriovenous fistulae. *A* shows the discrepancy (age 12). *B* shows the staples placed for epiphyseal arrest. *C* shows that the discrepancy has been corrected but that a valgus deformity has produced slight shortening (12 years after operation).

The Management of Leg Length Inequality

A discrepancy of 3 cm or more in limb length can, and often does, result in a marked compromise of function of the lower limb and impairment of body form. There may be an abnormal posture with compensatory scoliosis, unphysiological gait, and an abnormal stress on both the joints of the lower back and of the lower limb (Fig. 19–11). In addition, such asymmetry of limb length and posture can have a psychological effect on boys and, principally, girls. Significant discrepancy in leg length, therefore, should be corrected. A discrepancy of 3 cm of less can often be compensated for. A discrepancy of more than 3 cm that requires treatment can be managed by non-operative or operative means. It should be emphasized that no matter which method is adopted, full cooperation of the patient and parents is essential if these deformities are to be overcome successfully.

Non-operative methods include shoe raise, shoe insert, and surgical appliances incorporating a raise. These are simple and easy to adjust and are reversible, but they have two principal disadvantages. The first is that the raise can be very bulky; second, the raise can only be applied to the shoe and therefore may be far from the site of the deformity. This may, for example, lead to a difference in the levels of the knees.

Despite reports early in this century (Codovilla, 1905) proposing leg lengthening, owing to the complexity of the surgery and the high incidence of complications, most orthopedic surgeons, with few exceptions (notable among those being Anderson [1952]), concentrated on correction of a leg length discrepancy either by fitting prosthesis or by shortening the long limb. In the last decade or two, the expectations of patients and their families, allied to improved surgical techniques and external fixation devices (Cauchoix and Morel, 1978), have resulted in more patients undergoing operative correction of their lower limb discrepancies. Although such operations may involve either the longer or the shorter limb, increasingly surgeons have been concentrating on the leg lengthening procedures. There is still a significant complication rate, ranging from 20% (Kawamura et al., 1981) to 80% (Coleman and Noonan, 1967). These complications include infection, non-consolidation of the elongated segment, angulation of the fragments, fracture, soft tissue contracture, neurologic deficit, and arterial insufficiency. Despite this formidable list, provided there is close cooperation between the surgeon and the patient and meticulous attention to detail, leg lengthening remains a viable procedure.

Purely venous malformations almost never produce leg length disparity serious enough to warrant intervention, but between 10% and 20% of those patients with diffuse arteriovenous malformations may need active treatment for disparity in length between limbs.

The same principles that apply to the surgical management of leg lengthening apply to lengthening of bones in the upper limbs. Indications for this are few and far between, and experience recently has been confined to congenital dysplasias, notable among these being the achondroplastics and pseudoachondroplastics.

Assessment of Leg Length Discrepancy

Where asymmetry of the lower limb has been clinically established, and while there is still potential for growth, the patient should be assessed and measured both clinically and radiologically. This should include scannograms, in order to measure accurately both the leg length and any discrepancy that may exist, and radiographs of the hand, to establish the bone age precisely. These should then be repeated at regular intervals.

From the family history, the heights of the parents and siblings will have given an idea of the final height of the patient. This, along with any discrepancy between the limbs, can be accurately measured from the serial scannograms. In addition, not only can this difference be identified but also any change, and the rate of that change, can be monitored. Having properly defined the problem, one is then in a position to advise on treatment. It should be stressed that in patients with a leg length discrepancy secondary to a vascular malformation, the deformity may not be confined to the bone. This is particularly important when surgical correction is being considered, as, for example, any significant joint deformity in the hip, knee, or ankle is a contraindication to femoral or tibial lengthening.

The following operative procedures may be considered:
1. Surgery to the longer limb
   a. Epiphyseal arrest
   b. Femoral shortening
   c. Tibial shortening
2. Surgery to the shorter limb
   a. Single stage elongation of
      (1) Femur
      (2) Tibia
   b. Lengthening by continuous distraction of
      (1) Femur
      (2) Tibia

When the limb bearing the vascular malformation is elongated, operations to lengthen the normal opposite limb are not recommended. These operations are technically difficult and may be complicated by nerve damage and impairment of bone and muscle function; these are risks that are particularly unacceptable when the operated limb, although short in comparison, is otherwise normal. It is better to detect a leg length disparity early in growth so that operation to elongate the short leg can, it is hoped, be avoided, possibly by procedures on the epiphyses on the longer side immediately prior to the end of growth. When a disparity in leg length exceeds 4 cm by the age of 10 years, it is likely that some form of orthopedic intervention will be required. Disparity in the length of the arms, by contrast, is rarely noticed by the patient and seldom requires correction. We cannot support the proposal of Servelle (1985) that the popliteal vein of the short (normal) leg be ligated to help achieve equality of leg length, because popliteal vein ligation carries a serious risk of later complications. Other vascular operations, such as arteriovenous fistula formation, have been tried but have not produced the anticipated increase in growth in the shorter leg in the growing child.

Operations on the Longer Limb

During growth, all patients with a leg length discrepancy should be seen at regular intervals, as described previously, and monitored. In this way, not only can the difference in leg length be measured accurately, but also any rate of change can be noted. By applying these measurements to various growth graphs, the two most reliable being those of Green and Anderson (1951) (Fig. 19–12) and of Moseley (1977), one can predict the final

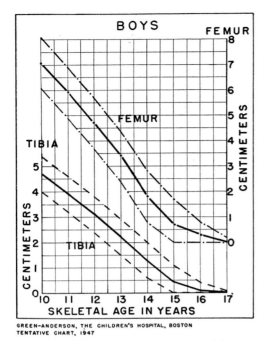
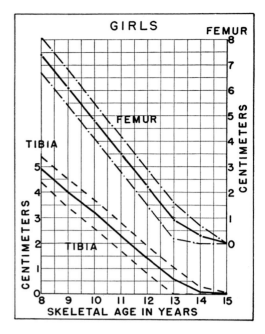

GREEN-ANDERSON, THE CHILDREN'S HOSPITAL, BOSTON
TENTATIVE CHART, 1947

Figure 19–12. Charts showing centimeters of limb length correction that may be achieved from arrest of distal femur or proximal tibia. The central line represents the average correction, the secondary lines the useful range. Results are very variable, and extremes are not shown on these charts from Green and Anderson. (Reproduced with permission from Green, W. T., Anderson, M.: Journal of Bone and Joint Surgery 29A:659, 1947.)

height and also the final disparity in leg length at full maturity. The orthopedic surgeon is then in a position to plan the timing of an arrest of epiphyseal growth.

Epiphyseal Arrest. There are two principal methods of arresting epiphyseal growth: stapling and epiphysiodesis. Stapling, as described by Blount in 1952, can be performed earlier and is theoretically not permanent, because if the staples are removed within 3 years and provided there is still growth potential, growth may resume. Unfortunately, stapling is unreliable and there is a high incidence of complication, with loosening or breaking of staples and asymmetrical arrest of epiphyseal growth leading to both angular and rotational deformity (see Fig. 19–11C). It is therefore not recommended. A more reliable but permanent solution is epiphysiodesis as described originally by Phemister. As it is permanent, this requires an accurate prediction of the required correction, which can be made by use of the regular measurements described previously. By inserting a bone block across both sides of the epiphyseal plate of either the distal femoral epiphysis or the proximal tibial epiphysis, a reliable and symmetrical cessation of growth can be achieved. It must be remembered that if the

proximal tibial epiphysis is arrested, the proximal fibular epiphysis should also be arrested to avoid complication.

Femoral Shortening. A shortening osteotomy of the femur in the longer limb is the simplest and most effective method of correcting a limited leg length discrepancy. It can be performed at either the distal or, more commonly, the proximal metaphysis, or in the diaphysis. At all three sites, soft tissue dissection is kept to a minimum and care must be taken to maintain correct alignment. Metaphyseal correction has the added advantage of being able to correct any associated axial deformity at the same time as the shortening osteotomy. The osteotomy is held by rigid internal fixation by means of a plate or angled plate with compression. The diaphyseal osteotomy can be held by an intramedullary rod; rotation is controlled by performing a step osteotomy. All these methods have the advantage that early mobilization is possible. The maximum correction obtainable by this method, depending on the overall height of the patient, is approximately 6 cm.

Tibial Shortening. Shortening osteotomy of the tibia and fibula has precise indications; a unilateral elongation secondary to vascular disease is amenable to this form of surgery.

The fibula is resected by the required amount in the middle third of its length. The tibia then undergoes a shortening osteotomy at either metaphysis in the diaphysis. The osteotomy is held by a plate or angled plate in compression, as with the femoral osteotomies. A diaphyseal shortening osteotomy can be performed, and as with the femur a stepcut osteotomy will help to control rotation. Fixation at this site can be by medullary nail, which has the particular advantage of permitting earlier weight bearing.

Operations on the Shorter Limb

Before one considers a procedure to elongate either the femur or the tibia, both the back, the joints of the affected leg, and the soft tissues must be carefully examined to establish no other coexisting deformity or contracture that might be aggravated by any lengthening procedure. The examination of the joint should include radiography, as asymptomatic dysplastic joints can be adversely affected by lengthening procedures. Coexisting deformities of bone should also be identified, as they may either be a contraindication to surgery or may be amenable to correction at the same time.

Single Stage Elongation of the Femur. This is best performed in the diaphysis. This can be by means of either a transverse osteotomy or a step-cut osteotomy followed by internal fixation by a plate and screws. The bone gap so created should be packed with autologous cancellous bone graft. An intramedullary nail has no part to play in such procedures. If there is an associated deformity such as a valgus deformity distally, a supracondylar osteotomy with opening is the preferred operation. This again requires autologous bone grafting to fill the gap following the opening wedge corrective osteotomy. This is established by an angled plate with screws, which permits early postoperative rehabilitation. A maximum of 4 cm. in length can be obtained in one operation.

Single Stage Elongation of the Tibia. This is contraindicated, owing to the high complication rate with soft tissue complications and joint deformity. Therefore, for practical purposes, single stage elongation should be confined to the femur.

Lengthening by Continuous Distraction. The principle of this method is that following a transverse osteotomy of the diaphysis of the shaft of the long bone, lengthening takes place by a process of slow and continuous distraction. This is accomplished by means of an external fixator, which is attached to the proximal and distal metaphyses by percutaneous pins. The external fixator may be in the form of a fixed frame (Anderson, 1952) or a smaller portable device (Wagner, 1971, 1977). By means of the fixator, the fragments can be stabilized and precise and accurate distraction can take place. This is usually carried out at the maximum rate of approximately one mm a day. The maximum lengthening achievable is approximately 10 cm in the femur and 5 cm in the tibia. As has already been mentioned, the discrepancy in length, although the more obvious presenting symptom, may not be the only problem in the affected limb. Joints and soft tissues may also be involved. Care must therefore be taken in the management of those patients in whom leg lengthening procedures are undertaken. Prophylactic soft tissue lengthening to prevent contracture, commonly Achilles tendon lengthening and hamstring lengthening, may be performed at the outset. During the distraction process, these same soft tissues must be carefully watched and if there is any evidence of neurologic or vascular compromise, the process must be stopped immediately and if necessary reversed. All these details emphasize the need for meticulous surgical management. Therefore, it is recommended that these procedures be undertaken in a specialist unit.

Further advances, both in surgical technique and in instrumentation, have resulted in different techniques in leg lengthening to try and further minimize complications, the time involved, and the number of surgical procedures. For example, the Wagner method can involve up to three or more major operative procedures (Wagner, 1977). Ilizarov (1971) described a method of lengthening of the tibial and femoral shafts with a correction of up to 40%, ranging from 4 to 11.5 cm. This method involved a corticotomy of either the proximal tibial metaphysis or distal femoral metaphysis with preservation of the periosteum and the incorporation of the operated bone in a special cylindrical frame. At the same time, he advocated soft tissue lengthening procedures. This method has been modified by De Bastiani and his coworkers (1986). He advocates osteotomy of the proximal femoral diaphysis and the proximal tibial diaphysis and describes lengthening of the proximal humerus just distal to the insertion of the deltoid. Like Ilizarov, De Bastiani advocates a corticotomy, carefully preserving the periosteum and where possible the medulla, by completing the osteotomy by circumferential drilling. The fragments are held in place by an external fixator that had been applied prior to completing the osteotomy. There is then a delay of up to 2 weeks to allow early callus formation. Limb lengthening then takes place by callus distraction or callotasis. In this way, soft tissue complications are minimized, and the need for any further fixation following completion of the lengthening is avoided.

Chondrodiastasis or controlled symmetrical distraction of the epiphyseal plate has also been described by De Bastiani and his co-workers (1986). Most of the patients included in this trial were achondroplastic, although up to a third were non-achondroplastic. This method involves distraction of the distal femoral and/or distal tibial epiphyseal plates. There are two methods, either a large force with rapid distraction or a smaller force with slow distraction of the growth plate. Chondrodiastasis that involves slow distraction, thereby avoiding rupture or fracture, hopes

to preserve future potential epiphyseal growth. The increase in leg length is achieved by temporary acceleration. At present, however, this method tends to be used in those patients who are within a year of closure of the growth plate. Lengthening of up to 5 cm can be achieved by this means, but again great care must be taken in the management of the soft tissues.

Other Orthopedic Problems/ Amputation

Localized gigantism is particularly a problem when the toes are involved and the difficulties in finding appropriate footwear for infants may lead to early amputation of the malformed digits. If the width of the foot is normal, simple amputation will suffice, but if the foot is broad or if there are supernumerary digits, a ray amputation is preferable. The grossly abnormal foot may require transmetatarsal amputation (Fig. 19–13A and B). Grotesque involvement, as seen in a few instances of Klippel-Trenaunay syndrome, may necessitate a more proximal amputation in order to reduce tissue bulk and permit am-

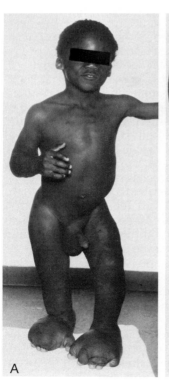 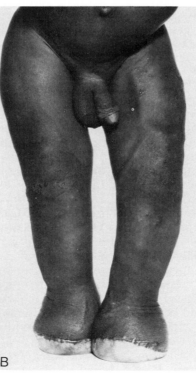

A   B

Figure 19–13. A, Gross deformity of the forefeet in association with a venous malformation of the lower limbs. B, Treated by bilateral transmetatarsal amputation. Although the surgical result appears ungainly, mobility is excellent.

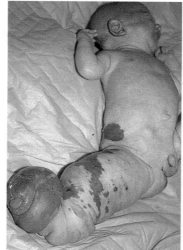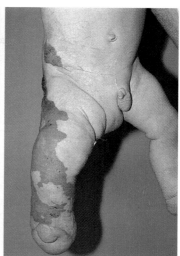

Figure 19–14. *A,* Infant with grotesque Klippel-Trenaunay type of right lower limb malformation. *B,* Following Syme's amputation of the useless foot. Walking will be feasible.

A   B

bulation, e.g., Syme's amputation or disarticulation at the knee, or even hip disarticulation (Ravitch, 1951; Herrington, 1953) (Figs. 19–14 to 19–16).

Other skeletal problems are produced by involvement of the soft tissues around the joint. This, together with bleeding into the joints, may necessitate tenotomies or capsulotomies. Vascular malformations involving the joint may need to be treated by synovectomy (Doig and Lea Thomas, 1972). Bergoin records a patient with multiple cystic venous

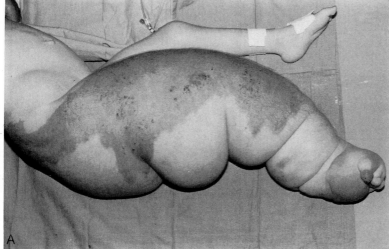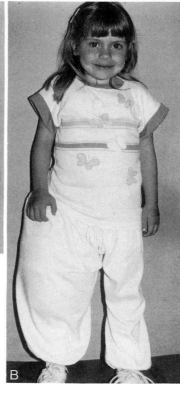

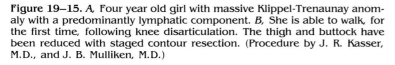

Figure 19–15. *A,* Four year old girl with massive Klippel-Trenaunay anomaly with a predominantly lymphatic component. *B,* She is able to walk, for the first time, following knee disarticulation. The thigh and buttock have been reduced with staged contour resection. (Procedure by J. R. Kasser, M.D., and J. B. Mulliken, M.D.)

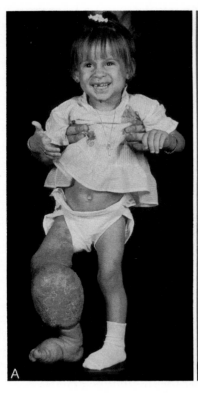
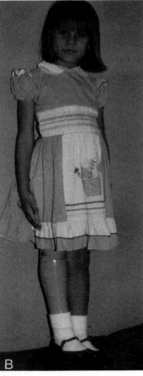

Figure 19–16. *A,* Little girl with complex vascular anomaly of the right lower limb. *B,* Four years following mid-thigh amputation. The distal portion of the femur, with its epiphysis, was reattached to the proximal stump in an effort to maximize subsequent growth. (Procedure by J. B. Emmons, M.D., and J. B. Mulliken, M.D.)

lesions and phlebectasia who suffered progressive destruction of knee and hip joints in infancy requiring arthrodesis of the knee and total hip replacement (with good results) (Bergoin et al., 1976).

In some cases, orthopedic surgery may be required to correct the effects of previously ineffective treatment. For example, Figure 19–3 shows a child whose surface malformation had been treated with radiotherapy, leading to lateral epiphyseal arrest and gross valgus deformity at the knee requiring osteotomy.

In a few instances, painful contractures at joints, together with a widespread vascular malformation, may make *amputation* unavoidable. In the author's series of 46 vascular malformations of the lower limbs, 5 have required limb amputation. In the upper limb, amputations are usually for ischemia. In the lower limb, however, the indications are for mixtures of ischemia, sepsis, hemorrhage, lymph leakage, scarring, joint contractures, and, in one case, paresis secondary to a spinal vascular malformation. Very rarely, a functionally "normal" limb must be amputated because of the cardiac effects of multiple arteriovenous fistulae in it.

Normal techniques of amputation have to be modified when applied to patients with vascular malformation, particularly when diffuse malformations are present. Because malformations may involve the whole territory of the limb bud, even high amputation may not eradicate them. It is often necessary, therefore, to cut unconventional flaps in order that there be healthy skin covering those parts of the stump on which pressure of friction from a prosthesis will be experienced. Figure 19–17 shows an example of this problem. The patient's malformation is so extensive that several further operations were required to excise involved skin traumatized by the prosthesis.

Ulcers

In vascular malformations, ulcers are not uncommon. Their etiology may be multifactorial, and a clear elucidation of the underlying cause is thus essential for effective management. Possible causes include:

1. Direct trauma to the friable skin over or involved by a malformation

2. Primary or secondary infection of a mal-

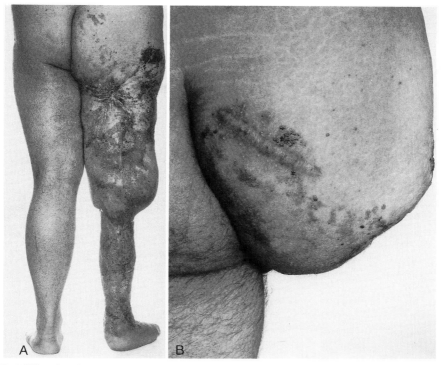

Figure 19–17. Difficulties following amputation. *A,* This extensive combined malformation eventually was associated with contractures, hemorrhage and recurring sepsis. Disarticulation amputation was necessary. *B,* Residual malformations on the stump bled when traumatized by the prosthesis, and further resections of these lesions were necessary.

formed area or skin already broken—exacerbated in some instances by inadequate lymphatic drainage

3. Venous hypertension
4. Ischemia
5. Ill-advised treatment of a vascular malformation by radiotherapy, caustics, sclerosant injections, etc.

Any or all of these may coexist.

The important combination is that of venous hypertension and ischemia seen in high flow arteriovenous malformations. The mechanism by which this combination produces ulceration is discussed in Chapter Thirteen. Often venous hypertension is the prime agent by which an arteriovenous malforma-

Figure 19–18. Ulcers in association with arteriovenous malformations may occur on the forefoot, and in such instances they may still nonetheless be due to venous hypertension rather than to forefoot ischemia.

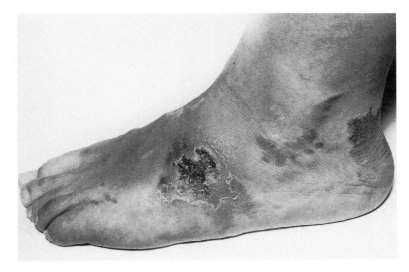

tion causes ulceration, and the ulcers may then closely mimic those seen in banal venous disease, sometimes known as "stasis" or "gravitational" ulcers (Fig. 19–18). The presence of severe or persistent pain in such ulcers should, however, warn of superadded arterial ischemia.

Management

Malformations that break down when traumatized may be protected by regular bandaging and elastic stockings with padding beneath. Simple elastic stockings may themselves suffice. Footwear may need to be specially made or altered if it contributes to the trauma.

Secondary infection restricted to the ulcer itself is best treated by regular cleaning with mild antiseptics and rebandaging. The presence of surrounding cellulitis requires systemic antibiotics. The organism usually responds to penicillin or erythromycin. The bacteria cultured from the floor of the ulcer is not necessarily the organism causing the cellulitis. Where coexistent lymphatic insufficiency encourages repeated infection with ulceration, long-term prophylactic antibiotics may be indicated. Topical applications of antibiotics are of minimal value and may cause sensitization of the skin with eczema and may occasionally lead to extension of the ulcer.

In ulcers in which venous hypertension is suspected as the prime cause, conservative measures are indicated first, namely:

1. Treatment of infection
2. Control of the venous hypertension by elevation and/or elastic or compression bandaging or support stockings.

Even in the presence of high flow arteriovenous malformations with some ischemia, it may be possible to achieve and maintain healing by these simple expedients. If not, angiography should be performed to indicate whether there are particularly troublesome local arteriovenous connections that can be ligated, excised, or embolized. It is unusual to demonstrate such local lesions. In the absence of a specific causative lesion inviting treatment, an indolent ulcer can itself be widely and deeply excised together with underlying perforating veins. Skin cover can be achieved with split-thickness skin grafts. The healing thus achieved must be maintained with firm, consistently applied elastic bandaging (Fig. 19–19).

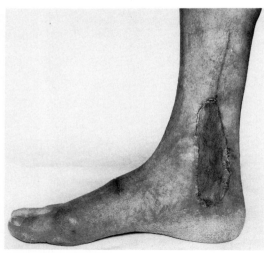

Figure 19–19. An ulcer at the ankle secondary to multiple arteriovenous fistulae around the ankle. The lesion was successfully treated by excision of the ulcer and the underlying tissues, ligation of perforating veins deep to the fascia, and split-thickness skin grafting. Healing was maintained by continued elastic support.

Persisting painful ulcerations, particularly when associated with extensive anomalies, recurrent bleeding and infection, lymphatic weeping, or contractures, may be better treated by an early well-planned amputation than by a demoralizing and painful series of unsuccessful attempts at local excision and grafting (Fig. 19–20).

Venous Thrombosis and Thromboembolism

Patients with the Klippel-Trenaunay type of congenital venous dysplasia have an increased likelihood of developing a deep venous thrombosis or pulmonary embolus spontaneously. In the St. Thomas' Hospital series of 49 patients, 11 had episodes of thromboembolism, occasionally multiple (Baskerville et al., 1985). These were all confirmed radiologically or by ventilation-perfusion scanning, and one of these patients required a pulmonary embolectomy. This incidence of 22.4% is much greater than the published incidence of thromboembolic episodes of 0.0055% (Dupont, 1975).

Predisposing Factors

Anatomical Factors. Abnormalities in the venous architecture are likely to be one of

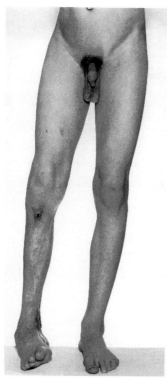

Figure 19–20. Chronic ankle ulceration secondary to multiple arteriovenous fistulae causing a contracture and secondary talipes equinovarus. Amputation was eventually necessary.

the most important factors predisposing to thrombosis in the veins of the affected limb. As discussed elsewhere, these deep venous abnormalities can be divided into two types: one type being constriction or atresia of the main stem veins and the other being dilatation or reduplication of these veins. In the St. Thomas Hospital series, 40% of patients had these abnormalities on phlebography. Because arterial inflow in the affected limbs lies within normal limits, blood velocity within these numerous ectatic venous channels will be reduced, which may encourage thrombus formation. The excessive number of pelvic phleboliths in such a young group of patients tends to support this view. Furthermore, a more detailed analysis of the distribution of venous thromboembolism among the patients reveals that it is precisely within the group of patients who have dilated and multiple stem veins that most of these episodes occur.

Hematological Factors. It has been known for some time that some congenital vascular abnormalities are associated with coagulation abnormalities. The most common abnormality arising in malformations is a consumptive coagulopathy, as in the thrombocytopenia that accompanies some forms of large and/ or diffuse venous anomalies and which, in extreme cases, may precipitate purpura (Dube et al., 1975). Even extensive malformations are almost never associated with Kasabach-Merritt syndrome (a term that should be strictly associated with true hemangioma), in which platelet survival may be reduced from the normal half-life of 45 days to just a few hours. There may, however, be increased consumption of clotting factors as indicated by raised levels of fibrin split products. However, such hematological abnormalities will work against the development of major thrombosis and embolism.

Therefore, it would appear that the most likely predisposing factor in the development of deep vein thrombosis in these patients is the abnormality of venous anatomy, though a defect in vein wall fibrinolytic ability cannot be excluded. This possibility is at present being explored. Immunohistochemical studies indicate that vein wall plasminogen activators are concentrated within smooth muscle. Varicose veins have been shown to have reduced plasminogen activator activity, and this may correlate with the deficiency in smooth muscle of such veins (Layer et al., 1986).

Three of the St. Thomas' Hospital patients had deep venous thromboses after minor vein operations, two of whom also had pulmonary emboli. This postoperative incidence of thrombosis is considerably higher than that recorded following either general surgical or varicose vein operations (Kinmonth, 1955).

Prophylaxis

In view of these findings, we strongly suggest that no patient with extensive venous or combined malformations receive estrogen for contraceptive or other purposes. Because of the venous congestion and the increased skin blood flow, the use of prophylactic anticoagulation will make an operation more difficult; however, on balance, we would recommend that all patients should also be offered antithrombotic prophylaxis prior to any form of surgical intervention.

References

Anderson, W. V.: Leg lengthening. J. Bone Joint Surg. *34*:150, 1952.

Baskerville, P. A., Ackroyd, J. S., Lea Thomas, M., and Browse, N. L.: The Klippel-Trenaunay syndrome. Brit. J. Surg. *72*:232, 1985.

Beck, G.: Hypertrophie congéniale d'un membre. Archiv. Gén. Méd. Tome *1*:99, 1837.

Belov, S.: Congenital agenesia of the deep veins of the lower extremities. J. Cardiovasc. Surg. *13*:594, 1972.

Bergoin, M., Carcassonne, M., Legre, G., and Huguet, J. F.: Dysplasie veineuse congénitale du membre inférieur droit associée à un syndrome de Kasabach-Merritt chez une enfant de 14 ans. Chirurgie *102*:68, 1976.

Biasi, B., Sala, A., and Bigloli, R.: La linfografia nelle angiodisplasie degli arti. Angiologia: Minerva Chir. *28*:918, 1973.

Bloom, J. D., Mozersky, D. J., Buckley, C. J., and Hagood, C. O.: Defective limb growth as a complication of catheterization of the femoral artery. Surg. Gynec. Obstet. *138*:524, 1974.

Blount, W. P., and Zeier, F.: Control of bone length. JAMA *148*:451, 1952.

Browse, N. L., Whimster, I., Stewart, G., et al.: The surgical management of lymphangioma circumscriptum. Brit. J. Surg. *73*:585, 1986.

Caplan, A. I., and Koutroupas, S.: The control of muscle and cartilage development in the chick limb. The role of differential vascularization. J. Embryol. Exp. Morph. *29*:571, 1973.

Cauchoix, J., and Morel, G.: One stage femoral lengthening. Clin. Orthop. *136*:66, 1978.

Codovilla, A.: On the means of lengthening the lower limbs, the muscles and tissues which are shortened through deformity. Am. J. Orthop. Surg. *3*:353–369, 1905.

Coleman, S. S., and Noonan, T. D.: Anderson's method of tibial lengthening by percutaneous osteotomy and gradual distraction. J. Bone Joint Surg. *49*:263, 1967.

De Bastiani, A., and Briviol, A. R.: Allungamento diafisario del' arto inferiore (studio di 78 casi). Chir. Organi. Mov. *70*:111, 1985.

De Bastiani, A., Briviol, A. R., and Trivella, G.: Chondrodiastasis—controlled symmetrical distraction of the epiphyseal plate. J. Bone Joint Surg. *68B*:550, 1986.

deTakats, G.: Vascular anomalies of the extremities. Surg. Gynec. Obstet. *55*:227, 1932.

Doig, R. L., and Lea Thomas, M.: Haemangioma of the knee joint. J. Cardiovasc. Surg. *13*:620, 1972.

Dube, B., Pillai, P. N., Singhal, G. D., and Khanna, N. N.: Blood coagulation studies in children with surface hemangiomas. Internat. Surg. *60*:524, 1975.

Dupont, P. A.: In Nicolaides, A. N. (ed.): *Thromboembolism*. Lancaster, England: Med. and Tech. Publ., 1975, p. 1.

Friedberg, H.: Riesenwuchs des rechten Beines. Virchow's Archiv f. Path. Anat. *40*:353, 1867.

Gloviczki, P., Hillier, L. G., Telander, R. L., et al.: Surgical implications of Klippel-Trenaunay syndrome. Ann. Surg. *197*:353, 1983.

Green, W. T., and Anderson, M.: Experiences with epiphyseal arrest in correcting discrepancies in length of the lower extremities in infantile paralysis. J. Bone Joint Surg. *29A*:659, 1947.

Green, W. T., and Anderson, M.: AAOS Instructional course lectures. *VIII*:294, 1951.

Herrington, J. L.: Congenital angiomatous malformation involving the entire lower extremity. Report of hemipelvectomy in a 25-day-old infant. Surgery *34*:759, 1953.

Homans, J.: Surgery of the veins. In Bancroft, F. W., and Humphreys, G. H.: *Surgical Treatment of the Soft Tissues*. Philadelphia: J. B. Lippincott Co., 1946, p. 427.

Hurst, P. A. E., Stewart, G., Kinmonth, J. B., and Browse, N. L.: Long-term results of the entermesenteric bridge operation in the treatment of primary lymphedema. Brit. J. Surg. *72*:272, 1985.

Hutchison, W. J., and Burdeaux, B. D.: The influence of stasis on bone growth. Surg. Gynec. Obstet. *99*:413, 1954.

Ikeda, K., Suita, S., Hayashida, Y., and Yakabe, S.: Massive infiltrating cystic hygroma of the neck in infancy with special reference to bleomycin therapy. Zeit. Kinderchir. *20*:227, 1977.

Ilizarov, G. A.: Basic principles of trans-osseous compression and distraction osteosynthesis (Russian). Ortop. Traumatol. Protez. *32*(11):7, 1971.

Janes, J. M., and Jennings, W. K.: Effects of induced arteriovenous fistula on leg length. Mayo Clinic Proc. *36*:1, 1961.

Janes, J. M., and Musgrove, J. E.: Effect of arteriovenous fistula on growth of bone: An experimental study. Surg. Clin. North Am. *30*:1191, 1950.

Kawamura Hosono S., and Takahashi, T.: The principle and techniques of limb lengthening. Int. Orthop. *5*:69, 1981.

Kessler, H. B., Recht, M. P., and Dalinka, M. K.: Vascular anomalies in association with osteodystrophies—a spectrum. Skeletal Radiol. *10*:95, 1983.

Kinmonth, J. B.: Experience of the stripping operation for varicose veins. Proc. Roy. Soc. Med. *48*:442, 1955.

Kinmonth, J. B.: *The Lymphatics*, 2nd ed. London: Edward Arnold, 1982.

Kinmonth, J. B., and Negus, D.: Arteriovenous fistulae in the management of lower limb discrepancy. J. Cardiovasc. Surg. *15*:447, 1974.

Kinmonth, J. B., Young, A. E., Edwards, J. M., et al.: Mixed vascular deformities of the lower limbs, with particular reference to lymphography and surgical treatment. Brit. J. Surg. *63*:899, 1976.

Kishikawa, E.: Studien über einige lokale Reize, welche das Längenwachstum des Langröhren knockens steigern. Fukuoka Acta Med. *29*:4, 1936.

Klippel, M., and Trenaunay, P.: Du noevus variqueux ostéohypertrophique. Arch. Gén. Méd. Tome *III*:641, 1900.

Layer, G., Pattison, M., Evans, B., et al.: Tissue fibrinolytic activity is reduced in varicose veins. Proc. of First United Kingdom Meeting, Union Internationale de Phlebologie, Negus, D., ed. London: John Libbey, 1986.

Lea Thomas, M.: *Phlebography of the Lower Limb*. Edinburgh: Churchill Livingstone, 1982.

Lindenauer, S. M.: Klippel-Trenaunay syndrome: Varicosity, hypertrophy and hemangioma with no arteriovenous fistula. Ann. Surg. *162*:303, 1965.

Malan, E., and Puglionisi, A.: Congenital angiodysplasias of the extremities (Note I: venous dysplasias). J. Cardiovasc. Surg. *5*:87, 1964.

Malan, E., and Puglionisi, A.: Congenital angiodysplasias of the extremities (Note II: arterial, arterial and venous, and haemolymphatic dysplasias). J. Cardiovasc. Surg. *6*:255, 1965.

Moseley, C. F.: A straight-line graph for leg-length discrepancies. J. Bone Joint Surg. *59A*:174, 1977.

Müller, J. H. A., and Schmidt, K. H.: Angiographische befunde beim Klippel-Trenaunay-Weber syndrom. Fortschr Roentgenstr. *110*:540, 1969.

Myers, T. T., and Janes, J. M.: Comprehensive surgical management of cavernous hemangioma of the lower extremity with special reference to stripping. Surgery *37*:184, 1955.

Oda, F. T., McLaughlin, J. S., Yeager, G. H., et al.: Vascular anomalies of the extremity associated with abnormal growth. Am. Surgeon *28*:775, 1962.

Parkes, Weber, F.: Haemangiectatic hypertrophy of the limbs—congenital phlebarteriectasis and so-called congenital varicose veins. Brit. J. Child Dis. *15*:13, 1918.

Phemister, D. B.: Operative arrestment of longitudinal growth of bones in the treatment of deformities. J. Bone Joint Surg. *15A*:1, 1933.

Pokrovosky, A. V., Moskalenko, J. D., and Tkhor, S. N.: The state of the lymph system in congenital arterial and venous diseases of the extremities. Vestn. Khir. *107*(9):74, 1971.

Ravitch, M. M.: Radical treatment of massive mixed angiomas (hemolymphangiomas) in infants and children. Ann. Surg. *134*:228, 1951.

Robertson, D. J.: Congenital arteriovenous fistulae of the extremities. Ann. Roy. Coll. Surg. Engl. *18*:73, 1956.

Saijo, M., Munro, I. R., and Mancer, K.: Lymphangioma: A long-term follow-up study. Plast. Reconstr. Surg. *56*:642, 1975.

Schüller, M.: Mittheilung über die künstliche Steigerung des Knochenwachsthums beim Menschem. Berl. Klin. Wschr. *26*:21, 1889.

Servelle, M.: Agénésie d'une des veines principales du membre inférieur. Coeur et Med. Int. *4*:53, 1965.

Servelle, M.: *Oedemes Chroniques Des Membres*. Paris: Masson, 1962.

Servelle, M.: Klippel and Trenaunay's syndrome. Ann. Surg. *201*:365, 1985.

Servelle, M., Albeaux-Fernet, M., Laborde, M., Chabot, J., and Rougeulle, J.: Lésions des vaisseaux lymphatiques dans les malformations congénitales des veines profondes. Presse Méd. *65*:531, 1957.

Sokolowski, J.: Lymph circulation within the extremity with arteriovenous fistulae. Pol. Przegl. Chir. *43*:1243, 1971.

Trélat, U., and Monod, A.: De l'hypertrophie partielle ou totale du corps. Arch. Gén. de Méd. *13*:636, 676, 1869.

van der Molen, H. R.: Association d'angiome et d'anomalies osseuses en dehors du la maladie Klippel-Trenaunay. Phlébologie *29*:25, 1976.

Wagner, H.: Operative beinverlängerung. Der Chirurg. *42*:260, 1971.

Wagner, H.: Surgical lengthening and shortening of femur and tibia: Technique and indications. Hungerford, D. S. (ed.): In *Progress in Orthopaedic Surgery*. Berlin: Springer-Verlag, 1977.

Whimster, I. W.: The pathology of lymphangioma circumscriptum. Brit. J. Derm. *94*:473, 1976.

Young, A. E.: Congenital mixed vascular deformities of the limbs and their associated defects. Birth Defects; Original Article Series *14*:289, 1978.

CHAPTER TWENTY

Laser Therapy of Port-Wine Stains

Joel M. Noe

INTRODUCTION

To understand lasers, one must first understand light. Light is a form of energy. In 1666, Newton observed that when sunlight passes through a prism, it is broken up into many different wavelengths. Our eyes perceive a band of wavelength as a specific color; hence, white light is seen by us, after it passes through a prism, as composed of many different colors. Light is part of the electromagnetic spectrum, which has a visible and nonvisible component. The visible light is in the central part of the electromagnetic spectrum. Argon lasers utilize the blue-green wavelength, whereas ruby lasers and helium neon lasers consist of red light. The far red, invisible infrared section is used for CO_2 lasers (Fig. 20–1).

The word laser is an acronym that signifies "*Light Amplification by Stimulated Emission of Radiation.*" The laser is essentially a machine that produces light. However, laser light is distinguished from common bulb illumination by four characteristics. First, it is monochromatic, whereas light from a bulb has many wavelengths. Second, laser light is collimated, that is, all the beams are in phase; therefore, laser light can be focused. The third characteristic is coherence, that is, laser light is in phase both temporally and spatially. The fourth attribute of laser light is its intense brightness.

A laser has three components: (1) a power supply, (2) a medium (either gas, liquid, or solid), and (3) a set of mirrors. The nature of the medium defines the type of laser. Examples of gas lasers are argon and krypton. A CO_2 laser is in a liquid medium; the ruby laser is in a solid state. The power supply (e.g., electricity) induces electrons in an atom to "lase," that is, to pass from a higher energy level to a lower energy level (Fig. 20–2). This orbital shift of electrons gives off a "quantum," or packet of energy, in the form of light. This packet of energy, or photon, then bounces back and forth between parallel mirrors, being amplified in the process, until a high enough energy level is reached, whereupon the laser light comes out through an opening in one of the mirrors.

HISTORY

The conceptual basis for modern lasers can be traced to Albert Einstein's postulation (1905) that all radiant energy must be absorbed or emitted by a body in quanta whose magnitude depends on the frequency (Einstein, 1917; Maiman, 1960). Thus, Einstein's generalization of the quantum theory of light led to our understanding of stimulated emission, stimulated absorption, and spontaneous emission. In 1964, Basov and Prokharov received the Nobel Prize in physics for microwave application. Townes and Webber, in the United States, furthered these concepts and extended lasers into the optical frequency range, as suggested by Schawlow and Townes in 1958. On July 7, 1960, Theodore H. Maiman, of Hughes Aircraft Research Laboratory, built the first working laser, a 4 inch cylinder containing the ruby red rod encircled by a flash tube. It emitted a brilliant coherent red light at 694.4 nm. New lasers developed rapidly based on this prototype. The argon laser was invented in 1964, also at Hughes Aircraft Research Laboratory, by William B. Bridges.

The first medical application of lasers was the treatment of retinal detachment. Two

centers in the United States were initially involved in the clinical use of lasers to treat conditions of the skin. One center was the Palo Alto Medical Clinic, where Zwang, an ophthalmologist, used the argon laser to treat diseases of retinal vessels (Zwang and Flocks, 1965). Stimulated by his work, Lash and Maser, plastic surgeons in Palo Alto, began to use an argon laser to treat cutaneous vascular lesions. They initially treated a patient with a small "strawberry" hemangioma and thereafter, a patient with a port-wine stain (Lash and Maser, 1972). At about the

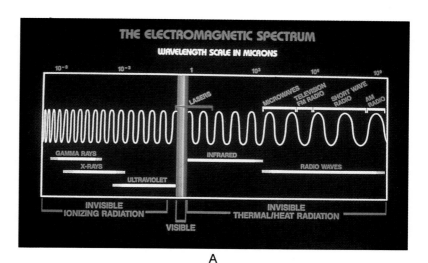

A

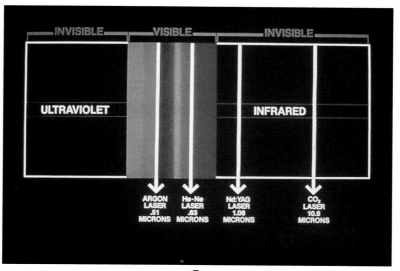

B

Figure 20–1. *A*, The electromagnetic spectrum. *B*, Lasers exist in both the visible and the non-visible spectra. (Reproduced with permission of Xanar, Inc.)

ENERGY LEVEL DIAGRAM FOR ARGON ION

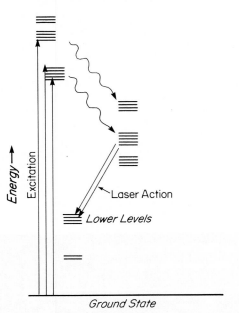

Figure 20–2. The argon ion "lases": a photon of light is emitted as electrons pass from a high energy orbit to a lower level.

same time, Goldman, a dermatologist, was working independently at the Medical Laser Laboratory at the Children's Hospital Research Foundation in Cincinnati. By 1967, he had treated 45 patients with port-wine stains, using the ruby, neodymium-YAG and argon lasers (Goldman and Rockwell, 1972). He found blanching of the treated stains, which remained unchanged during 3 years of observation. In the 1970s, inspired and instructed by Lash and Maser, other investigators began to refine the application of the argon laser for treating port-wine stains: Cosman in New York, Noe in Boston, and Apfelberg in Palo Alto (Noe et al., 1980; Cosman, 1980; Apfelberg et al., 1976).

ARGON LASER INTERACTION WITH PORT-WINE STAINS

Since the port-wine stain is composed of an increased number of ectatic vessels in the superficial reticular and papillary dermis, it is well within the range of the argon laser, which only penetrates 1.0–1.5 mm beneath the epidermis. The argon laser emits light that is preferentially absorbed by colored

materials such as red hemoglobin and brown melanin. The light energy changes to heat, and thrombosis ensues, causing a decreased blood flow and a subsequent collapse of the blood vessels. With less red hemoglobin flowing through these dermal channels, the color of the skin lightens. The surface flattens as a result of diminished vessel size in combination with dermal scarring and contraction.

The mechanism just described is overly simplistic. The argon laser emits light, not just in two wavelengths but in multiple wavelengths. Although there are two major bands (488 nm and 514 nm), there are also eight minor bands. Therefore, the light is not only absorbed by hemoglobin; it is also absorbed by the other dermal components, including collagen, as well as by the overlying epidermis, including melanin. Thus, the released heat can also damage surrounding dermal collagen. Unlike a conventional thermal burn injury, the adnexal structures usually survive argon laser absorption. The skin appendages show resistance to the laser, specifically the hair follicles. Sweat glands are generally spared. Skin histologic examination following present-day argon laser treatments demonstrates a superficial necrosis of the overlying epidermis and the superficial dermis (Apfelberg et al., 1979; Finley et al., 1981). With time, dermal scarring is seen. It is unknown what might be the relative contribution to lightening because of selective absorption of heat energy by the vessels and direct vascular damage, and what might be caused by relatively non-specific absorption of light energy by the surrounding tissues with secondary compression of vessels. Suffice to say, argon laser therapy results in a controlled dermal scar with smaller vessels that have fewer red blood cells. Subsequently, lightening and smoothening of the involved skin also result.

Predictive Role of Color, Age, and Biopsy in Response of Port-wine Stains to Argon Laser Therapy[*]

Color

The infant's port-wine stain is flat, pink-colored, smooth-surfaced, and most commonly located in the head and neck area. As

---

[*]Noe et al., 1980.

the child ages, the color may darken from pink to red to purple and the smooth skin becomes irregular and possibly a "cobblestone" surface. The darker the skin color, the more hemoglobin is present in the abnormal vascular channels. Thus, there is more chromophore to absorb the laser light, and a better result can be expected. An excellent result is defined as marked skin lightening without scarring, and a poor result is insufficient lightening with or without scarring.

Age

With aging, the stain color darkens, the skin surface becomes more irregular, and the skin thickens. Thus with time and with thickening and deeper color of the skin, the hemoglobin content increases, and hence, better results are expected with the argon laser therapy.

Histology

Light microscopy of skin biopsies of port-wine stains from infants shows an increased number of ectatic vessels in the superficial dermis (Barsky et al., 1980; Apfelberg et al., 1979). This changes with time, that is, there is a progressive ectasia, while the number of

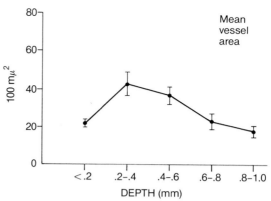

Figure 20–4. The relationship of mean vessel area to increasing subepidermal depth. The mean vessel area is also highest at 0.2–0.4 mm, just as for the vascular area. (From Barsky, S., Rosen, S., Geer, D., Noe, J. M.: The nature and evolution of port wine stains: A computer-assisted study. J. Invest. Dermatol. 74:154–157, 1980. Copyright 1981, The Williams and Wilkins Co.)

vessels stays constant. With this progressive dilatation, the color darkens from pink to red to purple, and the surface changes from smooth to irregular to "cobblestone" pattern (Figs. 20–3 to 20–8).

The therapeutic usefulness of a biopsy was studied by Noe and colleagues in 100 patients aged 7 to 66 with a port-wine stain involving from 2 to 99% of the face (Noe et al., 1980; Finley et al., 1981). A graded color chart was prepared in an attempt to achieve an objec-

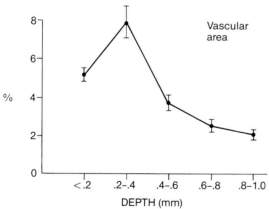

Figure 20–3. The relationship of vascular area to dermal depth in biopsies of port-wine stains. The percentage of dermis occupied by vessels (vascular area) is highest at 0.2–0.4 mm beneath the epidermis. The variation is expressed as standard error of the mean. (From Barsky, S., Rosen, S., Geer, D., Noe, J. M.: The nature and evolution of port wine stains: A computer-assisted study. J. Invest. Dermatol. 74:154–157, 1980. Copyright 1981, The Williams and Wilkins Co.)

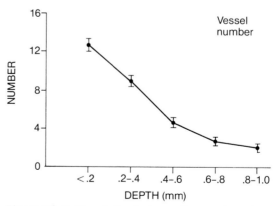

Figure 20–5. Correlation between the number of vessels and dermal depth. In port-wine stains the vessel number is highest just beneath the epidermis and decreases rapidly into the dermis. (From Barsky, S., Rosen, S., Geer, D., Noe, J. M.: The nature and evolution of port wine stains: A computer-assisted study. J. Invest. Dermatol. 74:154–157, 1980. Copyright 1981, The Williams and Wilkins Co.)

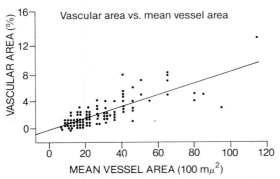

Figure 20–6. Relationship of percentage of dermal area composed of vessels (vascular area) to mean vessel area. As would be expected, there is a strong correlation (Pearson coefficient 0.79) between these two parameters. (From Barsky, S., Rosen, S., Geer, D., Noe, J. M.: The nature and evolution of port wine stains: A computer-assisted study. J. Invest. Dermatol. 74:154–157, 1980. Copyright 1981, The Williams and Wilkins Co.)

tive characterization of port-wine stain color and response to argon laser therapy. This chart encompassed the patient's normal skin color and the port-wine stain range from pink to purple. The port-wine stain was assigned a number—a higher number indicating a darker tone. Prior to argon laser treatment, a 3 mm punch biopsy was obtained from a representative region of the lesion (Fig. 20–9A and B). Lidocaine (Xylocaine) without epinephrine was used for the biopsy and subsequent test patch. The gross features of each lesion and the patient's associated clinical characteristics were noted. A detailed analysis of each biopsy, including both vessel and non-vessel parameters, was made with the assistance of a computer. In comparison with normal skin, the principal abnormalities noted in port-wine stains were an increased vessel number and ectasia. In the port-wine stain biopsies, the vessel number was higher in the immediate subdermal area, and then rapidly diminished (see Fig. 20–5). The mean vessel number was 0.46 ± 0.17 mm. In contrast, in the port-wine stain skin, the mean vessel area showed less variation throughout the dermis (see Fig. 20–4). The product of both factors determines the percentage of dermis occupied by vessels (vascular area), but it is the mean vessel area that is the major determinant of area (see Figs. 20–3 to 20–7). Although age correlated poorly with vessel number, it correlated well with both progressive vessel ectasia and color shift (pink to purple) (see Fig. 20–8A and B). Of the mul-

tiple vessel parameters analyzed (vessel number, vessel area, wall thickness, angulation, and luminal erythrocytes), each exhibited strong layer to layer correlation with the first 0.8 mm of tissue beneath the epidermis, indicating homogeneous vessel characteristics within the lesion (Table 20–1). The size of the lesion and the facial quadrant distribution did not change with age, nor were they related to histologic parameters. This particular study also noted that port-wine stains are found most commonly on the right side and lower quadrants of the face. A distinctive pattern of involvement of both eyelids was present in patients who have glaucoma; mental retardation was noted when a larger percentage of the facial area was stained.

Thus, the best results with laser therapy are achieved in those patients who have the most red blood cells and the most dilated vessels in the superficial dermis. These patients tend to be older and to have darker colored stains with a more irregular skin surface (Table 20–2).

Recommendations

The results of argon laser therapy can be predicted on the basis of the skin color, patient age, and biopsy (Figs. 20–9 and 20–10). It is safe to treat patients with dark

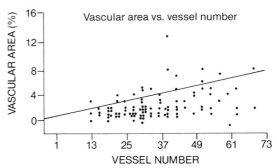

Figure 20–7. Relationship of vascular area and vessel number. The modest relationship between vascular area and vessel number (Pearson correlation coefficient 0.37), in contrast to the strong correlation between mean vessel area and percentage of dermal area composed of vessels (vascular area, Fig. 20–3), indicates that the most significant determinant of vascular area is *mean vessel area* rather than number of vessels. (From Barsky, S., Rosen, S., Geer, D., Noe, J. M.: The nature and evolution of port wine stains: A computer-assisted study. J. Invest. Dermatol. 74:154–157, 1980. Copyright 1981, The Williams and Wilkins Co.)

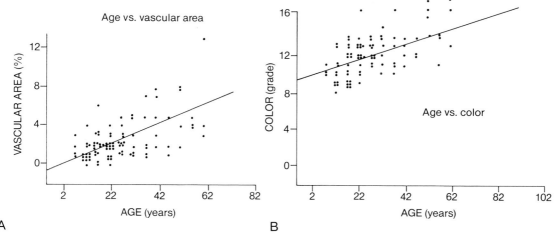

Figure 20–8. Relationship of age to percentage of dermal area composed of vessels (vascular area) *(A)* and color *(B).* As age increases, so does vascular area (Pearson correlation coefficient 0.63). There is an equally good relationship between age and deepening color (Pearson correlation coefficient 0.60). (From Barsky, S., Rosen, S., Geer, D., Noe, J. M.: The nature and evolution of port wine stains: A computer-assisted study. J. Invest. Dermatol. 74:154–157, 1980. Copyright 1981, The Williams and Wilkins Co.)

port-wine stains and irregular surfaces because the benefit, in addition to lightening, will be smoothening of the surface (Fig. 20–11). Dixon reported a 38% incidence of scarring in children treated with laser under the age of 12 (Dixon et al., 1984). Hypertrophic scarring is particularly likely in the lips and perialar regions, just as seen in children following thermal burn injury. At the present time, it is best not to treat children in this age group. Unfortunately, it is the children with port-wine stains who most deserve therapy for obvious social and psychological reasons.

Benefit-Cost Ratio

Argon laser therapy is a procedure, and like any other therapeutic modality, it should be evaluated from a benefit-cost viewpoint to a patient. The benefits (Table 20–3) include lightening, flattening of an irregular or "cobblestone" surface, breaking up a homogeneous port-wine stain into smaller areas that tend to be less visible, and decreased vascularity with less chance of bleeding (see Fig. 20–10). The natural evolution from pink to red to purple and the change from smooth

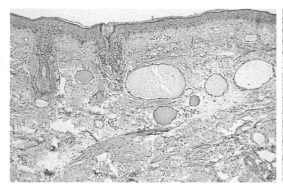

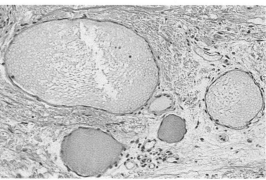

A   **B**

Figure 20–9. *A,* Skin biopsy from a 32 year old male with a facial port-wine stain. Note the thin, dilated vascular channels in the papillary and upper reticular dermis. (Hematoxylin and eosin; the bar is 0.3 mm, reduced from magnification × 50). *B,* Higher power magnification to show the anomalous thin-walled channels, filled with red blood cells.

Table 20–1. CORRELATIONS WITHIN THE PORT-WINE STAIN[a]

Thickness	% Erythrocyte Filled Vessels	Wall Thickness	Vessel Angulation[b]	Vascular Area	Mean Vessel Area	Vessel Number	Eccen-tricity[c]
<.2 vs. < .4 + >.2	.48	.51	.40	.35	.36	.28	.20
<.4 + >.2 vs. < .6 + >.4	.49	.37	.30	.51	.36	.40	.11
<.6 + >.4 vs. < .8 + >.6	.20	.37	.38	.38	.30	.23	.01
<.8 + >.6 vs. <1.0 + >.8	.10	.11	.25	.63	.10	.25	−.05

[a]Pearson product-moment correlation coefficient: >.32 significant, $p = .001$; >.25 significant, $p = .01$; >.19 significant, $p = .05$.
[b]60° and 90° oriented vessels divided by total number of vessels minus those with 45° orientation.
[c]Long divided by short axis.
From Noe, J. M., Barsky, S. H., and Geer, D. E.: Port wine stains and the response to argon laser therapy: Successful treatment and the predictive role in color, age and biopsy. Plast. Reconstr. Surg. 65:130, 1980.

to irregular to "cobblestone" seem to be minimized after laser therapy. There is less need for costly, thick cosmetics, and time is saved. There is also the psychological benefit noted not only from lightening but also from the other changes previously cited (Kalick et al., 1981; Noe, 1983). The untreated patients with port-wine stains who live in northern climates remark that in the winter the stained areas darken during exposure to cold weather, whereas the uninvolved skin is lighter when more time is spent indoors. Hence, they note increased contrast in winter, compared with decreased contrast in the summer. In the warm weather, the port-wine stain is redder and the surrounding, non-involved skin also deepens in color, as a result of time spent in the sun and in outdoor activities. Hence, these patients tend to prefer summer to winter. After laser therapy, this contrast between normal and stained skin is diminished; this is particularly noticeable in the colder months.

The major complication of laser therapy is scarring, both atrophic and hypertrophic. As noted previously, scarring occurs most commonly in children under the age of 12. Scars in all age groups tend to have a propensity for the upper melolabial area (Fig. 20–12). Some of the scars are hypertrophic both in appearance and behavior, and therefore show some improvement with time. One might question why children might have a higher incidence of scarring from an instrument whose mechanism is heat. As a general rule, children produce more scar tissue than adults. Thermal damage to the dermis could account for scar production, as seen in healing of a deep dermal burn. The heat generated by the laser induces fibroblasts to synthesize collagen. The increased incidence of scarring around the mouth may also be related to motion in this area.

An additional cost of laser therapy is the

Table 20–2. ANALYSIS OF FACTORS DETERMINING RESPONSE TO ARGON LASER THERAPY

	Desirable*	Undesirable*	Scarring*
Age (year)			
<17	5	7	3
≥17 <37	24	10	3
≥37	16	0	1
Color (graded units)			
Pink (8–9)	1	8	4
Red (10–13)	20	9	2
Purple (≥14)	24	0	1
Vascular area (%)			
<2	0	8	2
≥2<5	11	6	3
≥5	34	3	2
Mean vessel area (100 μm²)			
<15	4	10	3
≥15<25	11	6	2
≥25	30	1	2
Fullness (%)			
≤3	0	12	6
>3<15	10	5	0
≥15	35	0	1

*Indicates numbers of patients.
From Noe, J. M., Barsky, S. H., and Geer, D. E.: Port wine stains and the response to argon laser therapy: Successful treatment and the predictive role in color, age and biopsy. Plast. Reconstr. Surg. 65:130, 1980.

Table 20–3. BENEFITS OF ARGON LASER THERAPY

Lightens
Smooths
Flattens nodules
Breaks up "mass" effect
Stops evolution, i.e., progressive ectasia
Decreases time and cost of cosmetics
Decreases bleeding
Provides psychological benefits

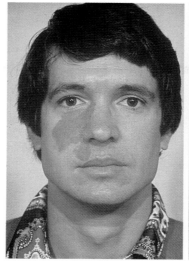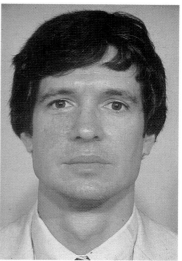

Figure 20–10. *A,* Thirty-five year old male with a homogeneous port-wine stain within the right maxillary area. *B,* Following argon laser therapy: "an excellent result." (Courtesy of the late Bard Cosman, M.D., Columbia University, College of Physicians and Surgeons.)

A   B

time required for multiple treatments. The laser also causes pain from the heat; hence, local anesthesia must be used. The laser wound is much like that of a second degree burn, although, as noted previously, histologically there tends to be more sparing of the adnexal epidermal structures. It usually takes 1–3 weeks for the wound to heal by re-epithelialization and new dermal collagen production. Dressings must be worn during this period, and time may be lost from work or school. Most insurance companies now cover the cost of laser therapy when they agree that it is medically warranted.

Technique

The procedure is performed on an outpatient basis using local anesthesia (2% lidocaine [Xylocaine]) to maximize vessel dilatation. Each treatment session lasts 1½–2

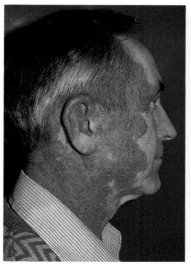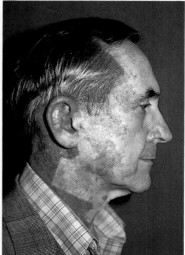

Figure 20–11. *A,* Fifty-eight year old male with a thick, nodular, purple port-wine stain of the right side of the face. *B,* Two years following argon laser therapy: graded a "good" result. Although the stain is lighter and flatter, there is scattered atrophic and some hypertrophic scarring.

A   B

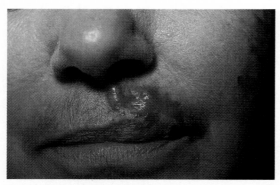

Figure 20–12. An erythematous, pruritic, hypertrophic scar, 4 months following argon laser therapy for a vascular stain of the upper lip in a 33 year old female.

hours, and afterward a dressing is applied. One to three weeks later, the transudation stops, and a scab may or may not form. The skin turns a bright red color, which then begins to fade. After about 4 months, one will have an approximate impression of what the final result will be. Lightening continues to occur for a total of 15–18 months before the final result is noted. The skin is protected during this time from both trauma and ultraviolet light. A sunscreen is recommended during the healing phase, particularly in the summer. Likewise, the patient is asked to protect the skin from ultraviolet light prior to treatment. The fear is that the sunburn or erythema produced would absorb the laser light, increasing the damage to the epidermis and decreasing the damage to the ectatic vessels in the dermis.

A laser test patch should always be performed prior to treatment. This will allow the patient and family, as well as the physician, to evaluate the results before the whole area is treated. It is best to wait at least 4 months after the test patch before assessing the results. At that time, a larger area can be safely treated. After this latter wound is healed, another segment is treated.

There are no data to suggest any advantage to the "stripe" technique (Apfelberg et al., 1983). Theoretically, by leaving untreated areas, the rate of re-epithelialization should be expedited with a decreased incidence of scarring. In practice, however, this decreased rate of scarring has not been realized. A bizarre appearance may result from this "striping" or zebra technique. Likewise, a dilemma is created when an undesirable re-sult is obtained after the first use of the striping technique. If no further treatment is warranted, the patient's partially treated stain has an odd, striped appearance.

CO_2 LASER THERAPY

CO_2 laser emits a light in the non-visible infrared area. To be clinically useful, it must be aligned with a visible light that acts as a guide, for example, the red light of the helium-neon laser. The CO_2 laser is very powerful. It acts by the absorption of infrared light by any cell that retains water, with subsequent destruction and vaporization. When used in a patient with a port-wine stain, this type of laser causes destruction of the epidermis, superficial dermis, and ectatic vessels. Healing proceeds slowly by re-epithelialization from the deep, undamaged adnexal skin structures. Thus, the CO_2 laser causes a more non-specific thermal burn, in comparison with the argon laser. As much damage occurs to the surrounding dermal structures, including collagen, as to the ectatic vessels of the port-wine stains. The CO_2 laser is too non-specific for the commonplace port-wine stain, the exception being the patient with a very thick, nodular, hypertrophic lesion (Balin, 1983; Arndt and Noe, 1982).

FUTURE CONSIDERATIONS

Argon laser treatment of cutaneous vascular lesions has been an accepted procedure for many years. Although this modality yields excellent results in many cases, there remains a definite incidence of scar formation even in the hands of the most skillful practitioner. The laser treatment actually produces a second degree burn with fairly uniform destruction, extending from the stratum corneum to 0.4–0.5 mm below the dermal-epidermal junction. The ideal goal is destruction solely of the abnormal vasculature, with sparing of the surrounding tissue. Unfortunately, this ideal simply has not been demonstrated with conventional argon laser treatment. Therefore, modifications of the present argon technique are currently under investigation. It is possible to protect the overlying epidermis and the surrounding dermal structures from the deleterious effects of this light energy. Gilchrest and coworkers (1982) use cold application to protect overlying epidermis during the passage of light energy and subsequent heat generation.

It is possible to make the ectatic vessels absorb blue-green light more selectively. This is desirable because laser destruction of abnormal dermal vasculature, without extensive tissue damage to adjacent normal tissue, can only be achieved by restricting the absorption of laser energy to the blood vessels alone. This requires selective absorption of the laser energy by blood, and a short irradiation time. Selective absorption is possible only if a wavelength of light can be chosen for which blood is highly absorbent, and if the other tissue is highly transparent. Fortuitously, hemoglobin is a strongly absorbing chromophore that is found only in blood (Fig. 20–13). The absorption band of oxyhemoglobin has several peaks, ranging from the ultraviolet through the near infrared portions of the spectrum. The strongest absorption is in the Soret band near 410 nm, and the double absorption peaks in the 530–580 nm region. The spectrum for reduced hemoglobin is quite similar to that of oxyhemoglobin. The double absorption peaks in the 530–580 nm region are replaced with a single absorption peak, which is nearly centered between the two peaks of oxyhemoglobin. Clinical use of this feature will necessitate laser interaction with both arterial and venous blood; consequently, the design of the laser should take both spectra into account. When lasing occurs through skin, another chromophore, melanin, becomes important. Melanin absorption decreases with approximately the fourth power of wavelength within this range. Therefore, in order to minimize laser absorption of mel-

anin and consequent injury to the epidermis and melanocytes of the basal layer, the laser wavelength should be as long as possible. This favors the absorption peaks in the 530–580 nm region, over the Soret bands at the shorter wavelengths.

A dye laser, tuned to approximately 576 nm, should offer an optimum wavelength match for selective destruction of ectatic vessels. Promising clinical trials resulting with a pulsed dye laser have been reported (Greenwald et al., 1981; Andersen and Parrish, 1981; Tan et al., 1986–1987). The tunable dye laser at 576 nm appears to produce very good results in patients with light port-wine stains, in younger patients, in patients who might scar easily, and in patients who have not responded well either to Argon or to CO_2 laser treatment. At present, it is unclear which wave length and which pulse duration will be best for the tunable dye laser. Also, it is unclear as to how permanent this quite selective vascular damage will be. Because of the selectivity, the tunable dye laser may require more treatment sessions for the same area than the one session per treatment area for the argon laser. Studies are under way to define the optimal wave length and the optimal pulse duration as well as the best treatment technique.

Argon lasers have a multiwavelength emission spectrum; however, most of the energy is contained in two bands, at 488 nm (blue) and 514 nm (green). The blue light can be eliminated with optical techniques, allowing passage of only the green light, which is much closer to the optimum spectral absorption range. Studies are under way to see if only the green light alone will provide more selec-

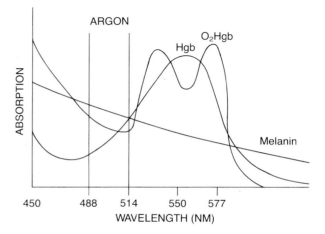

Figure 20–13. The absorption peaks of reduced hemoglobin, oxyhemoglobin, and melanin in relation to argon laser radiation. Although only the two major argon emission bands are shown at 488 nm and 514 nm, there are also eight minor bands.

tive absorption than the present combination of both.

Just as the wavelength of irradiation is important, so is the time constant for irradiation. As the laser energy is absorbed by hemoglobin, it is converted into thermal energy. For the purposes of this discussion, we may consider this transformation to be instantaneous. The released thermal energy diffuses into adjacent tissues. The thermal diffusion length, L, is related to the time during which thermal diffusion occurs, t, by the equation:

$$L^2 = 4Kt$$

K, the thermal diffusivity constant of living tissue, is very nearly the same as that of water, and can be taken as 0.0015 cm²/sec. To destroy abnormal vascular tissue, it is necessary thermally to damage the wall of the blood vessel in order to cause contraction, vessel collapse, and/or thrombosis. The wall can vary, from one cell width for capillaries to many cell thicknesses for larger vessels. Thus, a distance of about 25 microns (corresponding to an exposure time of approximately 1 msec) should be adequate to damage the full thickness of most capillary and venule vessel walls. In commonly available argon cutaneous units, the shortest available laser pulse time is 0.2 seconds. This corresponds to a diffusion length of approximately 0.35 mm. Thus damage from such a laser pulse may extend radially outward from every irradiated, blood-filled vessel for a distance that is about half the thickness of the dermis. This accounts for the extensive, non-specific damage produced with these current units.

The Medical Laser Research and Development Corporation is presently developing a device called the "Dermascan" for treating cutaneous vascular lesions (Tang et al., 1985). The Dermascan is a laser terminator that controls delivery of the laser beam to the skin. It utilizes rapid scanning to control the irradiation time of any given point and limit the effects of thermal diffusion. This device is presently being tested with the argon ion laser, both full spectrum and green only, as well as with a dye laser. Using this device, specific vascular damage can be demonstrated. The Dermascan is designed to destroy abnormal, ectatic blood vessels permanently. When used to irradiate normal skin, it seems to have no effect, and gives only a warm sensation.

Although the skin is a highly vascular organ, most of its rheologic capacity is unused except when the body is placed under severe thermal stress. Therefore, increased blood flow to the skin serves to dispel excess heat. Under conditions of normal room temperature and physical activity, the blood content of the skin is so low that it is a fairly transparent target for the laser beam, even that delivered by the Dermascan.

SUMMARY

The argon laser is now an established method of treating port-wine stains. The blue-green light is selectively absorbed by the red-colored hemoglobin molecules within the ectatic dermal vasculature. Heat-generated thrombosis occurs with resultant lightening of the port-wine stain and flattening of its surface. Thermal damage to the perivascular dermis may also be beneficial by narrowing the dermal vessels. However, heat can also cause unnecessary dermal damage that results in scarring, particularly in children. The age and color of the stain and a preliminary biopsy are all helpful ways to predict the response to treatment with the argon laser.

The tunable dye laser is producing very promising results when treating young children, patients with light port-wine stains, and those whose skin is very sensitive to heat. The optimal wave length and pulse duration are yet to be defined.

Future investigations will be focused on (1) ways to modify the skin blood flow, thus minimizing the heat damage; (2) devising new lasers that will selectively treat only ectatic vessels, sparing the surrounding tissue; and (3) evaluating the different wave lengths, different pulse durations, and different techniques on presently available lasers.

References

Anderson, R. R., and Parrish, J. A.: Microvasculature can be selectively damaged using dye lasers: A basic theory and experimental evidence in human skin. Lasers in Surg. Med. *1*:263, 1981.

Apfelberg, D., Flores, J., Maser, M., and Lash, H.: Analysis of complications of argon laser treatment for port wine hemangiomas with reference to stripe treatment. Lasers in Surg. Med. *2*:357, 1983.

Apfelberg, D., Kosek, J., Maser, M., and Laub, D.: Histology of port wine stains following argon laser treatment. Brit. J. Plast. Surg. *32*:232, 1979.

Apfelberg, D., Maser, M., and Lash, H.: Argon laser management of cutaneous vascular deformities. West. J. Med. *124*:99, 1976.

Arndt, K., and Noe, J.: Lasers in dermatology. Arch. Dermatol. *118*:295, 1982.

Balin, P.: Use of the CO_2 laser for non-PWS cutaneous lesions. In Arndt, K., Noe, J., and Rosen, S. (eds.): *Cutaneous Laser Therapy: Principles and Methods.* New York: John Wiley and Sons, 1983, pp. 187–200.

Barsky, S. H., Rosen, S., and Noe, J. M.: The nature and evolution of port wine stains: A computer-assisted study. J. Invest. Dermatol. *74*:154, 1980.

Cosman, B.: Experience in the argon laser therapy of port wine stains. Plast. Reconstr. Surg. *65*:119, 1980.

Dixon, J., Huether, S., and Rotering, R.: Hypertrophic scarring in argon laser treatment of port wine stains. Plast. Reconstr. Surg. *73*:771, 1984.

Einstein, A.: Zur quantum theori der strahlung. Phys. Z. *18*:121, 1917.

Finley, J., Noe, J. M., Geer, D., et al.: Healing of port wine stains after argon laser therapy. Arch. Dermatol. *117*:486, 1981.

Gilchrest, B., Rosen, S., and Noe, J.: Chilling port wine stain improves the response to argon laser therapy. Plast. Reconstr. Surg. *69*:278, 1982.

Goldman, L., and Rockwell, J. R., Jr.: Lasers reactions in living tissue. In Goldman, L., and Rockwell, J. R., Jr.: *Lasers In Medicine.* New York: Gordon and Breach, 1972, pp. 163–185.

Greenwald, J., Rosen, S., Anderson, R., Noe, J., et al.: Comparative histological studies of the tunable dye (at 577 nm) laser and argon laser: The specific vascular effects of the dye laser. J. Invest. Dermatol. *77*:305, 1981.

Kalick, M., Goldwyn, R., and Noe, J.: Social issues and body image concerns of port wine stained patients undergoing laser therapy. Lasers in Surg. Med. *1*:205, 1981.

Lash, H., and Maser, R.: Presentation, American Society for Plastic and Reconstructive Surgery Meeting, Las Vegas, Nevada, September 19–23, 1972.

Maiman, T.: Stimulated optical radiation in ruby lasers. Nature *187*:493, 1960.

Noe, J.: Laser use in dermatology. In Dixon, J. (ed.): *Plastic Surgery in Surgical Applications of Lasers.* Chicago: Year Book Medical Publishers, Inc., 1983, pp. 125–147.

Noe, J. M., Barsky, S. H., and Geer, D. E.: Port wine stains and the response to argon laser therapy: Successful treatment and the predictive role in color, age and biopsy. Plast. Reconstr. Surg. *65*:130, 1980.

Tan, O. T., Carney, J. M., Margolis, R., Seiki, Y., Boll, J., Anderson, R. R., and Parrish, J. A.: Histologic responses of port-wine stains treated by argon, carbon dioxide, and tunable dye lasers. A preliminary report. Arch. Dermatol. *122*:1016, 1986.

Tang, S., Arndt, K., Gilchrest, B., Itzkan, I., Noe, J., Stern, R., and Bourgelais, D.: Clinical comparison of millisecond versus conventional argon laser treatment of the *in vivo* vascular skin lesions, Boston Laser Group, Tufts and Harvard Medical Schools, Boston, MA. Lasers in Surg. Med. *5*:177, 1985.

Zwang, H. C., and Flocks, M.: Clinical experience with laser photocoagulation. Fed. Proc. *24*:565, 1965.

CHAPTER TWENTY-ONE

Embolization of Vascular Malformations

Marie-Claire Riché and Jean-Jacques Merland

INTRODUCTION

Early attempts at therapeutic embolization were made for intracranial vascular lesions, but the nonselective techniques were empirical and the results were uncertain (Brooks, 1930; Luessenhop and Spence, 1960). Neuroradiologists introduced selective arteriography and then embolization (or endovascular therapy), first in spinal intramedullary malformations (Djindjian et al., 1973), then in the branches of the external carotid artery (Djindjian et al., 1972; Doppman et al., 1968). From the delicate craniofacial vasculature, embolization was then extended to simpler vascular territories that exist in the kidney and the digestive system (Doyon et al., 1975; Kuss et al., 1975).

Embolization was used first to stop bleeding, then to devascularize tumors; application to vascular malformations was the legitimate next step (Haughton, 1975; Cunningham and Paletta, 1970; Bennett and Zook, 1972; Longacre et al., 1972; Olcott et al., 1976). Because these malformations consist of clusters of abnormal blood vessels, it is important that the anomaly be occluded at its center. This is a significant concept. For many years, it was thought that ligation of the main feeding vessels would be sufficient to reduce the vascularity of the lesion. Experience with arterial ligation demonstrates that after a temporary reduction in size, the lesion re-expands as before, and often enlarges further as collaterals open up (Riché et al., 1980).

Our technique depends on radiography to visualize the vascular anomaly. Intravascular catheters are introduced as near as possible to the lesion, and emboli, either particles or fluid, are then released to follow the blood flow into the malformation (Natali and Merland, 1976). Embolization, therefore, differs totally from proximal vascular ligature because blood serves as a vehicle to carry the emboli into the central malformation (Wolpert and Stein, 1979). Embolization may be used alone as a single treatment, or, in some cases, it is performed to devascularize the operative field prior to surgical extirpation.

Embolization should not be considered a solitary treatment modality. Investigators have much to learn about the pathogenesis, natural history, and abnormal physiology of vascular malformations. For this reason, in 1978, we formed our multidisciplinary clinic for the study and management of these lesions. The patients are evaluated by a surgeon, hematologist, cardiologist, therapeutic radiologist, and members of other disciplines. Patients are entered into treatment protocols; therapeutic decisions and outcomes are carefully monitored and analyzed. Only by such an interdisciplinary approach can we learn more about the abnormal rheology and assess the outcome of new treatments for malformations.

Over 700 vascular anomalies have been

embolized in our department since 1973. These include malformations of the vertebral-medullary-cephalic region (N = 190), cervical-cephalic area (N = 380), extremities (N = 97), pelvis (N = 18), thorax (N = 4), and visceral or genital organs (N = 13).

MATERIALS AND METHODS

Our method has evolved considerably over the past 5 years for four main reasons:

1. Improved radiological equipment has become available, including better fluoroscopy, real-time digital subtraction techniques during arteriography, and biplane arteriography for documentation, all of which reduce contrast and radiation dose as well as diminish the duration of the procedure.

2. Marked improvement in catheter technology has occurred with the development of miniaturized flow-guidable and coaxial catheters, which allow for placement of embolic material deep into the lesions.

3. Painless, slightly hyperosmolar contrast dyes reduce the need for general anesthesia, simplify protocols, and facilitate clinical surveillance during treatment.

4. A wide range of embolic material are now available, as seen in Table 21–1. Each product has its advantages, its particular specifications, and its dangers. We have found that, after the choice of solid or liquid material, the most important feature is the absorbability. Biodegradable substances are usually well tolerated but do not always remain in the lesion long enough to impede blood flow permanently. On the other hand, a non-absorbable product permanently obstructs vessels, and little is known about the long term consequences of this persistent foreign material. No single product is ideal; combinations of embolic material are often necessary.

Gelfoam (gelatin sponge, the Upjohn Co., Kalamazoo, MI) is the most commonly used absorbable embolic material. It is cut into 1 × 2 mm strips or made into particles with a hand punch and injected through catheters. Gelfoam is used primarily as a temporary occlusive agent in the presurgical devascularization of lesions. *Polyvinyl alcohol foam* (Ivalon, Unipoint Industries, Inc., High Point, NC) is the most commonly employed nonabsorbable material. Ivalon is made radiopaque with 60% tantalum oxide or 66% barium sulfate and is pre-cut into 0.3–1.0 mm diameter particles with a conventional angiographic hand punch. These particles expand 10–15 times in size several seconds after contact with fluids. Ivalon's tendency to clump in the catheter can be minimized by combining it with Gelfoam particles.

Isobutylcyanoacrylate (IBCA, formerly available from Unipoint Industries, Inc.) is a fast-polymerizing tissue adhesive of low viscosity that can be injected through a flow-guided balloon tipped catheter that has a hole at its end. This allows injection of relatively precise quantities of the mixture deep within the lesion. It is used in the treatment of high flow fistulous vascular malformations (Debrun et al., 1982a). This material's major disadvantage is its tendency to "glue" the catheter to the vessel wall; it is a difficult product to handle. The other compounds, both liquid and solid, are usually administered through catheters that are inserted close to the lesion via a larger coaxial catheter. Chemical analogs of IBCA have been shown to have carcinogenic potential in animals; therefore, application of IBCA is restricted in the U.S. by the Food and Drug Administration.

Table 21–1. EMBOLIZATION MATERIAL

	Resorbable	Permanent Solid Particles	Polymerizing Liquid (Non-resorb.)	Fibrosing Agent (Resorb.)	Thrombosing Agent
Autogenous clot	3 days				
Gelfoam powder	5–10 days				
Occluding balloons		+			
Ivalon		+			
Dura mater		+			
Calibrated microbeads		+			
IBCA			+		
Ethibloc				+	
Ethanol					+
Tetradechol					+

Ethibloc (Ethicon GmbH, Hamburg, West Germany) is a new liquid embolizing compound, developed in Germany, that can be administered directly into a vascular anomaly by percutaneous technique. It is a vegetable protein, predominantly prolamine or corn amino acids. It is mixed with amidotrizoic acid to give it radiopacity; it is dissolved in oleum and then mixed with ethanol. It was developed initially for occlusion of the pancreatic duct, and during the initial studies it was noted that autolysis of the gland occurred after occlusion of the pancreatic duct with this material (Phillip and Schmid, 1977; Rosch et al., 1979). Subsequently, it was used experimentally to occlude the renal arteries in several animal systems, and this demonstrated a similar parenchymal autolytic effect as in the pancreas. Since then, Ethibloc has been used in clinical trials in France and Germany for occlusion of vascular malformations as well as for obliteration of renal arteries (Kuhne and Helmke, 1982). A minor disadvantage is its relatively significant viscosity compared with IBCA, as well as the moderate inflammatory response induced in the early post-injection period. An advantage to Ethibloc is that there is no danger of gluing the catheter to the vessel wall, and the material is biodegradable and is cleared by phagocytosis over an extended period of time.

Detachable *balloons* mounted on the end of catheters have been utilized to occlude arteriovenous fistulae or high flow arteriovenous malformations in which the channels are too dilated for the smaller particulate matter to be used (Debrun et al., 1978; Debrun et al., 1982b). Occasionally, a balloon catheter is employed to occlude a high flow malformation temporarily ("balloon flow arrest") so that one of the other occlusive compounds such as Ethibloc or IBCA can be used. The disadvantages of balloons are that they need a relatively large coaxial system to be introduced intra-arterially, and occasionally they can be difficult to release in the exactly desired location.

Ethanol (95%) has been reintroduced into the angiographer's armamentarium over the last few years. Alcohol injection for thrombosis of cervicofacial vascular malformation is discussed in the textbook by Lasjaunias and Berenstein (1987). Although its viscosity is low and it is easy to inject both percutaneously and via catheters, alcohol is not easy to control within an arteriovenous anomaly and significant amounts pass through into the venous side, creating the risk of thrombosis. In addition, the profound sclerotic reaction and easy passage of the alcohol into normal adjacent vascular territories can produce significant ischemia and necrosis in unwanted areas, such as skin and nerves.

Nevertheless, it is worthwhile to pursue the therapeutic goal of localized thrombosis of low flow vascular anomalies. Intravascular sclerotherapy is now accepted for prophylactic and therapeutic control of esophageal varices (Jensen, 1983; Brooks, 1984). Several of the variceal sclerosing agents are currently undergoing clinical trial for treatment of congenital venous anomalies. *Sodium morrhuate,* a naturally occurring mixture of sodium salts of cod liver oil, is still available but seems to cause more complications than the newer synthetic agents. *Ethanolamine oleate,* derived from oleic acid, has similar properties to sodium morrhuate, and is still used in Great Britain. *Sodium tetradecyl sulfate* (tetradechol, STS, Sotradecol) is a synthetic anionic detergent currently favored for sclerotherapy in the U.S. *Hydroxypolyethoxydodecan* (HPD, polidocanol, Aethoxysklerol) is the preferred variceal sclerosant in West Germany.

COMPLICATIONS AND PITFALLS

Complications

Experience has shown that complications are related to two factors: (1) the ability of the angiographer to position catheters and use the embolization products, and (2) knowledge of malformation angiostructure. Problems are often the result of inexperience, and this is why these procedures should always be performed in specialized centers. The potential for complications also depends on the territory where the embolization is performed; for example, in the central nervous system or spinal region, the slightest problem may result in significant neurologic impairment. A complication in an extremity may have minor consequence but could result in ischemia of a distal part necessitating amputation (Fig. 21–1).

An analysis of our series of 122 embolizations within the extremities (vascular malformations and tumors) revealed 13 complications (10%): 10 were asymptomatic, 2 cases responded to local treatment, and 4 cases required operative correction (2 surgical revascularizations and 2 surgical resections in the territory of the malformation). None of the patients had functional impairment. On the contrary, in the spinal cord area, out of 90 cases, there were 4 complications (4%), but all of these were of the utmost gravity: 1 death, 2 patients with paraplegia, and 1 patient with transient triplegia.

Pitfalls

False diagnosis of the lesion is a potential pitfall. A patient with a vascular lesion referred for embolic therapy should be evaluated as having a potentially malignant tumor. Another pitfall is an incorrect angiographic estimation of the architecture of the anomalous channel, so that a large embolus becomes lodged in a dominant feeding vessel—equivalent to arterial ligation. Also, if the emboli are too small relative to the caliber of the arteriovenous communications, the particles may pass into a draining vein and into the general circulation.

It is difficult to assess the proper indications for embolization. Many quiescent vascular anomalies should be left alone. In our institution, 40% of the patients with head and neck vascular malformations referred and studied were embolized. However, in the extremities, only 20% of the patients were embolized; this was usually in an attempt to improve functional ability.

PRIMARY LESIONS

Low Flow Malformations

The arteries are not dilated in low flow malformations; the site of developmental anomaly is either the capillary bed or the veins. There is considerable stagnation, sometimes increased by the lack of normal venous drainage.

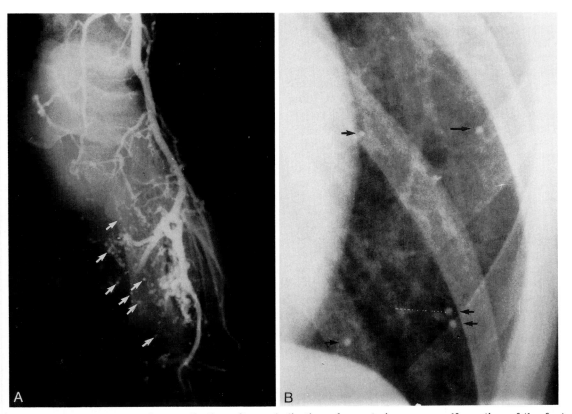

Figure 21–1. A, Asymptomatic complication after embolization of an arteriovenous malformation of the foot with microbeads (arrows). B, Some of the beads are seen in the lung fields (arrows).

Capillary-Venous Malformations

Capillary-venous malformations produce a clinically obvious swelling that is increased by dependent position as a result of increased venous pressure. Venous angiography reveals multiple ectasias (resembling a bunch of grapes). Thrombosis within the anomaly leads to phleboliths, so often seen on plain films. Latent intravascular coagulopathy can be accentuated by embolization. Hematologic evaluation should include measurement of fibrin degradation products in the peripheral blood and, if possible, in a blood sample taken directly from the vascular anomaly. Heparin therapy may be indicated prior to embolization or surgical resection.

The arterial approach for embolization of capillary-venous lesions is often difficult, because the injected material may be swept into normal undilated arteries. Skin necrosis is a real potential hazard. Therefore, perarterial embolization of venous malformations is not recommended.

We have studied another approach to these malformations, the direct injection of a fibrosing material (Ethibloc) (Riché et al., 1983). Caution is necessary not to allow the sclerosant to enter the venous drainage. External compression is used to stagnate Ethibloc within the malformation until it hardens sufficiently (10 minutes). This product causes a mild inflammatory period, after which time tissue remodeling occurs. If necessary, the sclerosed lesions can be surgically excised after 10 days (Fig. 21–2). Progressive fibrosis is expected over 2–3 months. Because the long term results of this product are still unknown, most sclerosed venous malformations should be removed surgically. The use of Ethibloc alone is usually restricted to those areas where excision would be deforming, such as the commissure of the lip, forehead, or masseter area.

We have also tried Ethibloc in a few cases of arteriovenous malformations. It was difficult to handle via the arterial route because of its viscous nature and prolonged time of polymerization. We have discontinued its use in these lesions. We have also had some success in the direct injection of Ethibloc in selected cases of small, localized, cystic lymphatic malformations.

Ethibloc is fully authorized for use in Germany and France. It is undergoing laboratory evaluation and authorized clinical trials in the U.S. and is not as yet approved for clinical use by the Food and Drug Administration.

Localized Venous Malformations

Angiographically, venous anomalies appear as non-partitioned pouches, either attached to major vessels (like the jugular vein) or located within muscle compartments. Isolated jugular and supraclavicular venous lesions can often be easily dealt with by surgical excision. The more diffuse intramuscular anomalies are best managed by sclerotherapy with a fibrosing material, such as Ethibloc.

Diffuse Venous Malformations

Extensive venous dysplasia necessitates a detailed study of the major deep veins, as these are often indistinct or hypoplastic. Superficial dysplasias often reflect deep venous malformation; sometimes the superficial veins must be preserved, as they alone are functional. In cases in which deep venous trunks are normal, the superficial varicosities may be thrombosed by sclerosing agents injected percutaneously.

Venous-Lymphatic Malformations

Venous-lymphatic lesions consist of combined abnormal venous and lymphatic channels. They may be located anywhere, either in the subcutaneous area or in deep muscular regions. One particular location amenable to embolic therapy is the anterior part of the tongue, which is usually enlarged and covered with vesicles. Periodic inflammation leads to intermittent bleeding. In these cases, the arteriogram is normal and shows small arteries. Embolization through the arterial route with small particles is an efficient way to reduce the volume of the tongue and suppress periodic inflammatory episodes (Fig. 21–3).

High Flow Malformations

Arteriovenous Fistula

By definition, an arteriovenous fistula consists of a single arteriovenous communication supplied by one or several arteries leading directly into a vein. Although sometimes definitely post-traumatic, as in the case of ca-

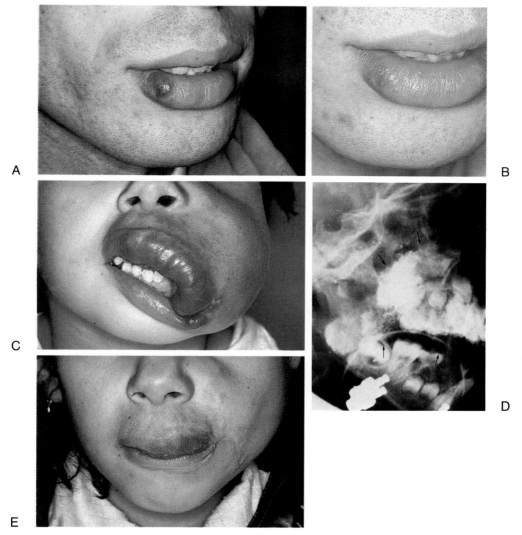

Figure 21–2. Two examples of the use of Ethibloc. *A*, A small venous malformation of the lip before embolization. *B*, Result 3 months later. *C*, Capillary-venous malformation of the lip and temporomasseteric region in a girl of 5 years. *D*, Lipiodol mixed with Ethibloc highlights the intravascular extension of the material within the anomaly (arrows). *E*, Result 6 months after subsequent surgical resection and reconstruction. The malformation on the cheek has not yet been identified. (Courtesy of Dr. E. Hadjean.)

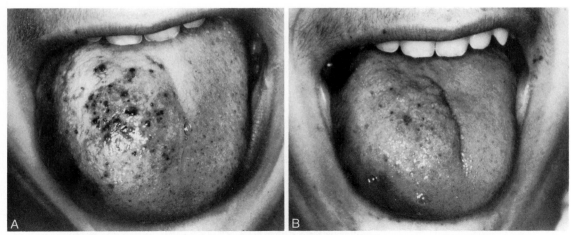

Figure 21–3. Combined venous-lymphatic malformation of the tongue with hemorrhage. *A,* Before embolization. *B,* Six months after embolization of the right lingual artery. Note the decrease in volume and fewer hemorrhagic vesicles.

rotid-cavernous fistulae and some vertebro-vertebral fistulae, many of these are indisputably of developmental origin, for example, an extramedullary fistula supplied by the anterior spinal artery.

When the feeding artery is sufficiently dilated, the ideal treatment of a solitary fistula consists of release of an inflated balloon into the fistula, hence obliterating the abnormal communication while maintaining both arterial and venous flow. In other cases, the afferent supply is by several narrow arteries, and non-absorbable embolic material, either dura mater or IBCA, can be used. Embolization may be performed with venous compression so that the material will lodge in the fistula without entering the vein (Fig. 21–4). Direct puncture into the fistula is used in some cases. Should the arterial route fail, it is theoretically possible to use the vein as access to perform a retrograde occlusion, as in the case of a draining vein with multiple small arterial feeders.

Arteriovenous Malformation

When this high flow lesion is visualized by angiography, a network of abnormal vessels is seen, featuring one or several shunt zones (nidus) that short-circuit the capillary bed. There are usually several dilated afferent arteries and multiple draining veins. The congenital nature of these often quiescent arteriovenous malformations is not always obvious. They sometimes reveal themselves later on in life, or following injury or a change in hormonal status (puberty, pregnancy, or oral contraception). Embolization or surgical removal may be considered equally satisfactory treatment. Incomplete therapy of either type causes collateral formation and further expansion. Embolization must therefore be complete, reaching the shunt zones (nidus), and must neither be limited to distal arterial occlusion nor go beyond the shunt zones into the veins. Experience has taught us that there are several configurations that occur in both large and small shunt arteriovenous malformations and that the number and the size of the shunts cannot be inferred from the caliber of the afferent artery. Our understanding of these shunts has advanced with the use of arteriography with venous compression and microspheres for measuring the size of the arteriovenous connections.

In some cases, the anatomical site of the arteriovenous malformation (for example, the face or pelvic region) makes surgical removal feasible only after embolization. The extent of anatomical resection is not diminished by preoperative embolization. However, the blood loss and decreased likelihood of re-expansion are helped by preoperative embolization. In such cases, preoperative embolization is usually straightforward, using resorbable material such as Gelfoam. Surgical resection should normally be performed as soon after embolization as possible.

SPECIFIC LOCATIONS

Head and Neck

Capillary-Venous Lesions

Capillary-venous anomalies and isolated facial venous ectasias can be managed by embolization techniques followed, in some cases, by surgical excision. An exception is the venous anomaly of the buccal fat pad (boule de Bichat), the clinical diagnosis of which is easy

and a lesion that may be treated surgically without embolization.

Considerations for embolic therapy include the size and site of the malformation and the patient's age. The extent of the lesion is a critical factor, because attempted removal of a large malformation is hazardous and there is always the danger of massive bleeding and the need for extensive resection causing mutilation. Embolization can succeed in progressively reducing the malformation's size and improving the patient's appearance.

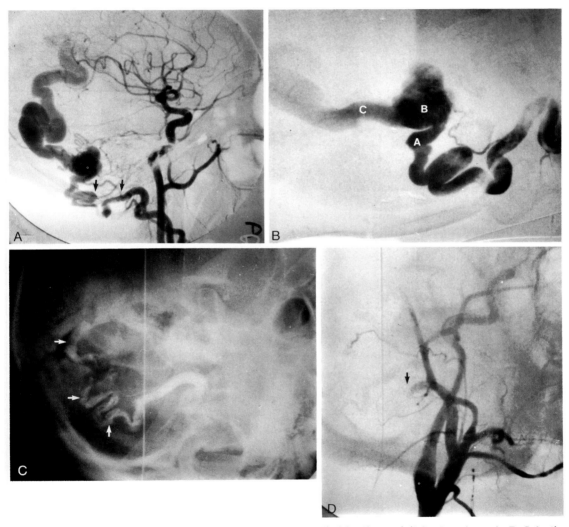

Figure 21–4. *A,* Large arteriovenous fistula of the scalp supplied by the occipital artery (arrow). *B,* Selective arteriography of the occipital artery with compression of external carotid artery demonstrates location of the fistula. A = occipital artery; B = site of the fistula; C = draining vein. *C,* After embolization with IBCA, the terminal occipital artery and the fistula are filled with polymerizing material (arrows); there is no leakage into the draining veins. *D,* Study of the common carotid artery shows the disappearance of the fistula after embolization (arrow).

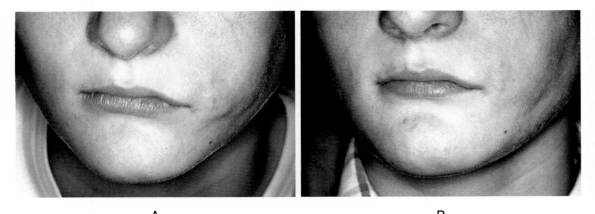

A   B

Figure 21–5. *A,* Small capillary-venous malformation of the left cheek, including the lip commissure. This malformation was treated by two successive direct injections of Ethibloc. *B,* One year after treatment; note that the bulging has disappeared, as has much of the bluish coloration of the skin.

Small malformations are easy to treat by embolization, particularly when they are located in cosmetically sensitive areas (Fig. 21–5).

The location of the lesion also influences management. For example, malformations in the masseter, the lip commissure, the eyelids, and the forehead are best treated by embolization alone because surgical excision in these locations can be mutilating. In other locations, for example, the lips, anterior portion of the tongue, and cervical region, resection may be undertaken 10 days after embolization (Fig. 21–6).

Although vascular malformations are present from birth, the ideal age for commencing treatment is 6 or 7 years, before the malformation expands extensively. In massive malformations, several embolic procedures may be required prior to excision (Fig. 21–7).

Arteriovenous Malformation

Serious hemodynamic and aesthetic consequences of facial arteriovenous malformations justify the continued search for better therapeutic solutions. Embolization has been used in a small series of patients from several centers (Schrudde and Petrovici, 1981; Leikensohn et al., 1981; Berenstein and Kricheff, 1981; Azzolini et al., 1982). When one is treating these lesions, the close relationship between the internal and external carotid vessels and the vertebral arteries must be taken into account. Unfortunately, this is demonstrated by ill-conceived ligature of the external carotid artery to control an expand-

ing arteriovenous malformation. After proximal ligation, the malformation remains unchanged while the internal carotid vessels, the vertebral arteries, and the contralateral external carotid artery branches enlarge and take on the extra circulatory load. In addition, patients in whom ligation of the external carotid artery has been performed usually have substantial arteriovenous malformations and often suffer from postoperative trophic skin changes as a result of obstruction of venous blood flow or diminished nutritive skin flow. Embolization following proximal ligature is extremely difficult; however, it can be achieved by puncture of the external carotid artery beyond the ligature or puncture of the internal maxillary artery, or by surgical exposure of a facial or superficial temporal artery. In some cases, embolization can only be carried out after surgical revascularization, for example, a venous patch at the origin of the external carotid or an interposition vein graft. In other cases, it may be necessary to achieve direct surgical access to the vertebral artery at the level of C1–C2 (Merland et al., 1980).

The guiding concept is that embolization for an arteriovenous malformation must be complete, totally obliterating the central nidus; otherwise, flow will resume via collaterals inaccessible to embolization. As far as possible, the aim should be total eradication of the lesion by the combined use of embolization and surgical ablation (Fig. 21–8).

In some cases, the intricate relationship between internal and external arteries requires complicated therapeutic measures,

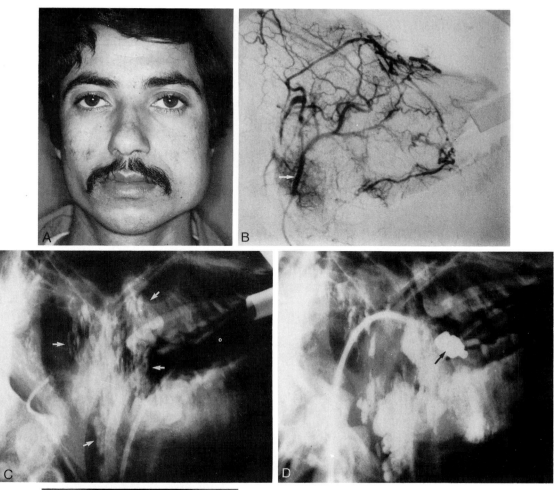

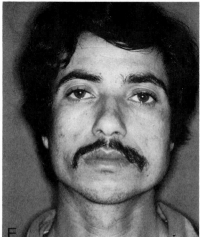

Figure 21–6. Extensive capillary-venous malformation of the left cheek, including the masseter. *A,* Clinical appearance before embolization and operation. *B,* Selective catheterization of the transverse facial artery (arrow) shows normal appearance on early films. *C,* On late films, the typical "bunch of grapes" appearance is seen (arrows); careful perarterial embolization was performed with the dura mater. *D,* Direct puncture into the malformation (arrow) confirmed its pathologic anatomy and allowed filling of the various pouches with Ethibloc. *E,* Excision was performed (preoperative heparin was used to control the intravascular clotting disorder). Result after 6 months is shown. (Courtesy of Dr. E. Hadjean.)

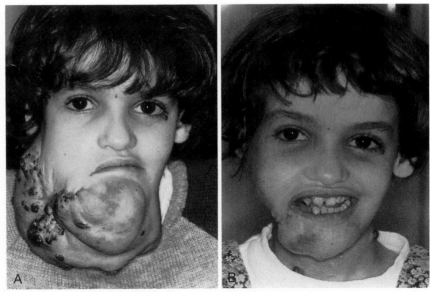

Figure 21–7. Giant capillary-venous malformation. Seven embolization procedures, primarily with IBCA and some Ethibloc, were necessary prior to surgical removal. *A,* At outset. *B,* Postoperatively. (Courtesy of Dr. E. Hadjean.)

even in the absence of arterial ligation (Fig. 21–9).

Extremities

Experience has demonstrated that treatment of malformations in the extremities is invariably difficult. The primary objective, preservation of limb function, takes precedence over aesthetic consideration. At present, embolic therapy of extremity vascular anomalies is recommended only for complicated cases. Among the 500 patients referred to our department for vascular malformations of the extremities, only 97 have been embolized. The majority are managed with supportive measures, particularly elastic stockings.

The following four complications may occur necessitating intervention.

Pain

Pain may be caused by multiple factors: venous congestion in dysplasias or an arteriovenous malformation inducing a sensation of heaviness; thrombosis or deep hematoma; tense hemarthroses in synovial malformations; or bone pain in high flow malformations with bone erosion. Dystrophic skin changes are frequently associated with these malformations, probably secondary to shunting of nutritive flow.

In venous malformations, even very large varicose veins can be sclerosed or surgically ablated, provided that a complete radiological survey has proved the existence of an open, deep venous system. In other cases, pain stems from a localized thrombus as a result of venous stagnation and medical treatment with anti-inflammatory agents may be appropriate.

Embolization may be indicated in an arteriovenous malformation causing persistent pain. It is carried out after superselective catheterization of the main feeding vessels. In large arteriovenous malformations, the technique used is injection of microscopic particles into the bloodstream while exerting compression on the normal major blood vessels. Embolization in these instances must be prudent, aiming not at total eradication of the malformation but at symptomatic relief. In a highly localized arteriovenous malformation, direct puncture of the supplying artery and injection of a small quantity of a liquid material such as IBCA or Ethibloc may suffice.

Ulceration and Hemorrhage

Hematoma and hemorrhage occurring as a result of localized intravascular coagulopathy in vascular malformations are best treated by heparin.

An active arteriovenous malformation can also cause hemorrhagic ulceration. The initial phenomenon, related to hemodynamic stealing, can be complicated by severe hemorrhage as a result of erosion of blood vessels. These chronic ulcers will not heal with conservative wound care. Embolization alone has also had disappointing results. Whichever technique is employed, any reduction in necrosis is, unfortunately, often short-lived. At present, the most satisfactory management appears to be embolization followed immediately by skin grafting or flap coverage. It is important to avoid obstruction of venous drainage and thus minimize venous hypertension, which leads to tissue breakdown (Fig. 21–10). In advanced cases in which amputation is inevitable, preoperative embolization may allow more distal amputation.

Lengthening of Limbs

Both low and high flow malformations can cause early overgrowth of the extremity, which may even reach 3 or 4 cm of extra length. This must be watched from an early age, not only by clinical examination, which tends to be unreliable, but also by periodic radiological measurements. Skeletal length must be compared in the various bone segments. Superselective embolization of the arteries supplying the articular cartilages, using microparticles, stabilizes growth and can be

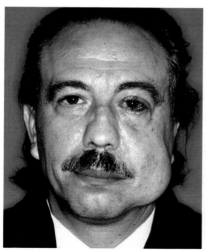
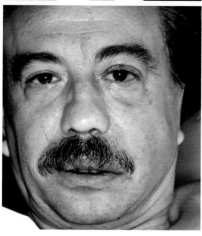
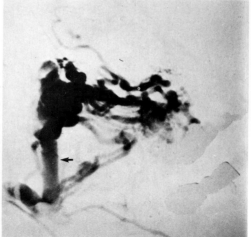

Figure 21–8. *A*, Arteriovenous malformation of the face. *B*, The bulging lower eyelid is caused by compression of venous return. This malformation was supplied mainly by an enlarged internal maxillary artery (arrow). *C*, Embolization was carried out with autogenous clots prior to subtotal excision, which was accomplished with minimal blood loss. (Courtesy of Dr. E. Hadjean.)

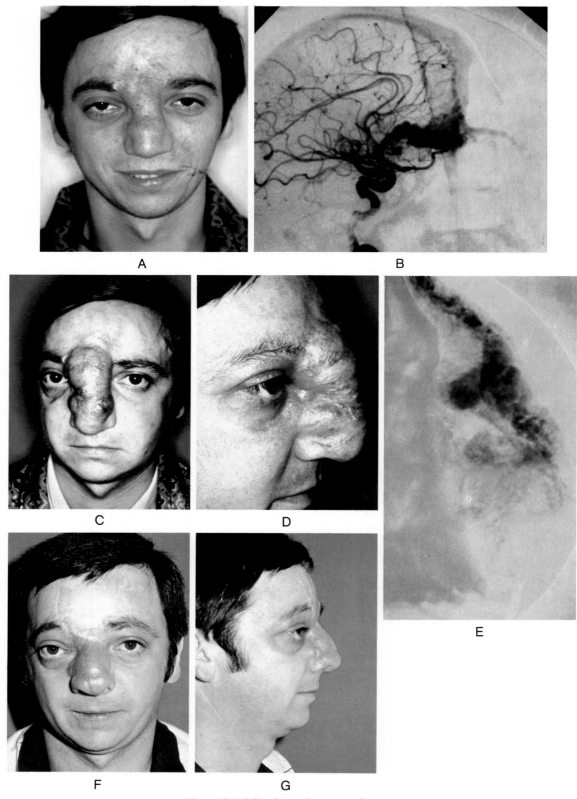

Figure 21–9 *See legend on opposite page*

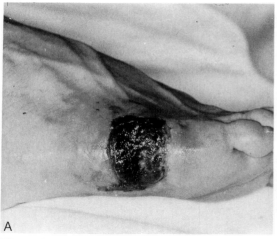 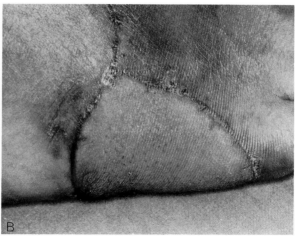

Figure 21–10. *A*, Arteriovenous malformation of the foot with hemorrhage and persistent ulceration. *B*, After embolization, a local flap was rotated to cover the remaining malformation. Lesion is stable after 2 years. (Courtesy of Prof. Servant.)

used even in the absence of hypervascularization. Embolization must be associated with suitable venous tourniquets to retain the emboli at the epiphyses (Fig. 21–11).

Cardiac Failure

Cardiac failure is not rare in a diffuse arteriovenous malformation of the limbs. Cardiac output can be measured by Fick's method at the time of cardiac catheterization. Embolization is indicated when the output is in excess of 10 liters per minute and there is cardiac enlargement or symptoms. An extensive arteriovenous malformation may be surprisingly hemodynamically quiescent; some have only a few large shunts, easily obstructed by large particles; others consist of multiple, small shunts that must carefully be obstructed one by one, usually with IBCA. The stabilization of expansion of the anomaly and control of high cardiac output can be long lasting.

Gastrointestinal Tract and Liver

Gastrointestinal Tract

Pure congenital malformations of the gastrointestinal tract are seldom encountered. Colonic arteriovenous malformations often described in the literature are found in old patients and are probably acquired lesions.

Two congenital lesions may present with intestinal hemorrhage: the blue rubber bleb syndrome (Bean syndrome) and Rendu-Osler-Weber syndrome. Arteriographic findings are usually deceptive in Bean syndrome, and embolization has not been performed in these cases. Rendu-Osler-Weber disease affects the digestive tract, as well as the spleen and liver. Arteriography shows many scattered telangiectatic lesions. The telangiectasias may be helped by laser therapy, but where lesions are not accessible to the laser beam, embolization can be used to stop repeated bleeding. The end-artery configuration of the mesenteric vasculature makes per-

---

Figure 21–9. Bonnet-Dechaume-Blanc syndrome. *A*, This patient was first seen in 1972 for repeated epistaxis secondary to an arteriovenous malformation of the nose. *B*, Angiogram showed enlarged branches of the external carotid artery and an intraorbital and intracerebral arteriovenous malformation supplied by the internal carotid artery. *C* and *D*, Repeated embolization of the internal maxillary and facial arteries controlled epistaxis, but the malformation continued to expand; the ulceration became life threatening. Management involved three phases; first, the large ethmoidal arteries were clipped surgically, thus interrupting the blood supply coming from the internal carotid artery. *E*, Later, preoperative embolization was performed through both external carotid branches, followed by removal of the superficial lesion and reconstruction with a forehead flap. *F* and *G*, Results 4 years later. (Courtesy of Dr. E. Hadjean.)

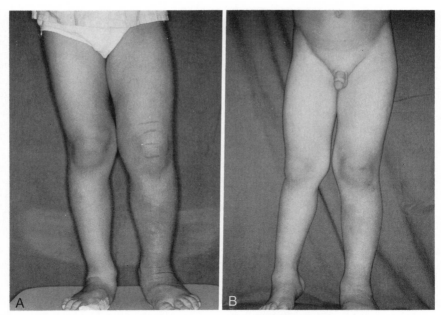

Figure 21–11. Arteriovenous malformations of the limb. *A,* Pain and limited knee movement were associated with a difference in leg length of 3.8 mm in this 6 year old boy. Embolization was performed with microparticles under compression of the adjacent arteries. *B,* One year later, pain completely disappeared, the leg has a more normal appearance, and the overgrowth is now 2.8 mm. The child wears elastic support stockings. (Courtesy of Prof. J. Natali.)

foration of the bowel a feared complication. Therapeutic embolization for hereditary telangiectasia must always be approached with caution; surgical resection should also be considered.

Liver

Hepatic venous anomalies are usually quiescent; these malformations do not bleed but may cause persistent pain. Arteriographically, they appear on late films as a tumor-like scattered blush. They may be multiple, of various size, either on the surface of the liver or deep in the lobes. Embolization with small particles may be used to occlude the feeders selectively, followed by hepatic resection when necessary.

Pelvis

Whereas embolization and resection is seldom used in malformations of the extremities, this combined approach plays an important part in the treatment of arteriovenous anomalies within the pelvis. Preoperative embolization has transformed surgical ther-

apy, enabling near total ablation of these malformations. Because of the multiple vascular branches, embolization is lengthy, sometimes requiring several sessions. Resorbable material can be used, as the embolization is preoperative. Nevertheless, surgical ablation is often accompanied by significant blood loss despite successful embolization, because of the existence of gigantic dilated veins (Fig. 21–12).

Spinal Cord

Arteriovenous Malformation Supplied by the Anterior Spinal Artery

The peculiarities of spinal cord vascular anatomy explain both the difficulties and the dangers of embolization and its extraordinary success. The anterior spinal artery, which vascularizes the anterior two thirds of the spinal cord, is supplied by only a few radicular arteries, and there is little chance for collateral flow. Embolization, therefore, carries the danger of interrupting this anterior vascular axis. Rigorous precautions must be taken to ensure that emboli reach only the malformation (Riché et al., 1982).

Before embolization is undertaken, the existence of a potential alternative vascular supply to the cord must be established, for example, subjacent and overlying radicular arteries or posterior spinal arteries for the conus medullaris. In addition, temporary clamping tests are necessary in some cases. Lastly, the use of rapidly polymerizing liquid material (IBCA) is dangerous and should not be employed; small solid particulate emboli should be used instead. The poor medullary vascularization enables remarkable stability of the cord vascular anomaly after embolization. Medullary vascular malformations seem unable to recruit collaterals from other regions. This is why even partial embolization may provide excellent functional results by reducing vascular flow and preventing recurrent hemorrhage. However, even when a spinal arteriovenous malformation is completely occluded, the patient's recovery also depends on the extent of previous anatomical lesions that are due to hemorrhage or ischemia. In the long run, little is known of the evolution of arteriovenous malformations thrombosed by embolization: cavitation or compression by the thrombosed elements could occur. Nevertheless, it seems that whenever possible, embolization should be preferred to a surgical approach in this region.

Paraspinal Arteriovenous Malformations

Paraspinal arteriovenous malformations are often of gigantic size, covering several thoracic or lumbar levels, and have much in common with arteriovenous malformations of limbs as potential causes of heart failure. In addition, their massive venous blood flow often erodes adjacent vertebrae. Surgical eradication is usually impossible. Embolization is particularly indicated in young patients to reduce cardiac flow and to stabilize the lesion (Merland et al., 1979).

Central Nervous System

The possibilities for vascular collateral flow are multiple; these malformations, when they are dearterialized but not thrombosed, can always be revascularized by neighboring ar-

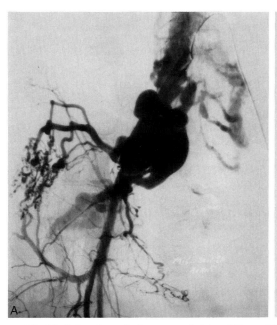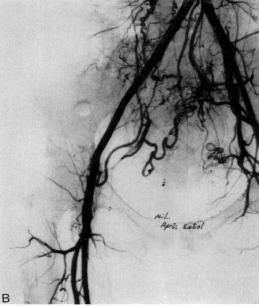

Figure 21–12. Extensive arteriovenous fistula of the pelvis. This arteriovenous malformation was unsuccessfully treated by ligation of the hypogastric artery performed prior to this arteriogram *(A)*. It was possible to embolize the main pedicle of the superior gluteal artery. The after-embolization arteriogram *(B)* is satisfactory, and this malformation could then be extirpated with acceptable blood loss. (Courtesy of Prof. J. Natali.)

teries. This is why it is imperative to reach the core of the lesion. Moreover, the danger of embolization in this region should never be overlooked because there is always a risk that embolizing a functional territory will cause dramatic neurologic impairment. Two approaches are possible:

1. *Directed flow embolization:* A non-releasable balloon is temporarily positioned at the origin of the healthy arteries to be protected; embolization particles of a caliber equal to the diameter of the malformed vessels are then introduced, to be carried preferentially toward the malformation.

2. *Selective embolization by a calibrated leak balloon:* A balloon pierced with a calibrated hole is allowed to approach the malformation via the supplying arteries. Once close to the malformation, this pierced balloon can be used to inject a mixture of IBCA, iophendylate (Pantopaque), and tantalum powder into the nidus.

The same problem hinders both of these techniques, namely, that only total eradication of the malformation guarantees permanent cure. In most cases, the malformation is only 70–80% obliterated and can reappear at any time. In some cases, complementary stereotaxic irradiation may diminish flow to the remaining lesion when it is smaller than 2–3 cm in diameter.

There is increasing evidence that a combined angiographic-surgical treatment may be a useful approach. After surgical exposure, the superficial feeder vessels are catheterized in the operating room by the neurosurgeon and then embolized by the radiologist. The thrombosed arteriovenous malformation is left in place, and subsequent embolization may be used to block the remaining deep vessels.

References

Azzolini, A., Bertani, A., and Riberti, C.: Superselective embolization and immediate surgical treatment: Our present approach to treatment of large vascular hemangiomas of the face. Ann. Plast. Surg. 9:42, 1982.

Bennett, J. E., and Zook, E. G.: Treatment of arteriovenous fistulas in cavernous hemangiomas of face by muscle embolization. Case Report. Plast. Reconstr. Surg. 50:84, 1972.

Berenstein, A., and Kricheff, I. I.: Microembolization techniques of vascular occlusion: Radiology, pathologic, and clinical correlation. Amer. J. Neuroradiol. 2:261, 1981.

Brooks, B.: The treatment of traumatic arteriovenous fistula. South Med. J. 23:100, 1930.

Brooks, W. S., Jr.: Variceal sclerosing agents. Amer. J. Gastroent. 79:424, 1984.

Cunningham, D. D., and Paletta, F. X.: Control of arteriovenous fistulae in massive facial hemangioma by muscle emboli. Plast. Reconstr. Surg. 46:305, 1970.

Debrun, G., Lacour, P., Caron, J. P., Hurth, M., Comoy, J., and Keravel, Y.: Detachable balloon and calibrated-leak balloon techniques in the treatment of cerebral vascular lesions. J. Neurosurg. 49:635, 1978.

Debrun, G., Vinuela, F., Fox, A., and Drake, C. G.: Embolization of cerebral arteriovenous malformations with bucrylate. J. Neurosurg. 56:615, 1982a.

Debrun, G., Vinuela, F., Fox, A., and Kan, S.: Two different calibrated leak balloons: Experimental work and application in humans. AJNR 3:407, 1982b.

Djindjian, R., Cophignon, J., Théron, J., Merland, J. J., and Houdart, R.: L'embolisation en neuro-radiologie vasculaire. Technique et indications à propos de 30 cas. Nouv. Presse Médicale 1:2153, 1972.

Djindjian, R., Cophignon, J., Théron, J., Merland, J. J., and Houdart, R.: Embolization by superselective arteriography from the femoral route in neuroradiology. Review of 60 cases: I. Technique, indications, complications. Neuroradiology 6:20, 1973.

Doppman, M. L., DiChiro, G., and Ommaya, A.: Obliteration of spinal cord arteriovenous malformation by percutaneous embolization. Lancet II:477, 1968.

Doyon, D., Mouzon, A., Vadrot, D., Franco, D., and Bismuth, H.: Embolisation transhépatique des varices oesophagiennes. J. Radiol. Electrol. 56:917, 1975.

Haughton, V. M.: Hemoclip-Gelfoam emboli in the treatment of facial arteriovenous malformations. Neuroradiology 10:69, 1975.

Jensen, D. M.: Sclerosants for injection sclerosis of esophageal varices. Gastrointest. Endoscop. 29:815, 1983.

Kuhne, D., and Helmke, K.: Embolization with 'Ethibloc' of vascular tumors and arteriovenous malformations in the head and neck. Neuroradiology 23:253, 1982.

Kuss, R., LeGuillou, M., Merland, J. J., LePage, T., and Bories, J.: L'embolisation en pathologie urogénitale. Ann. Urol. (Paris) 9:1, 1975.

Lasjaunias, P., and Berenstein, A.: *Surgical Neuroangiography.* Heidelberg: Springer-Verlag, 1987, Volume II, Chapter 9, p. 394.

Leikensohn, J. R., Epstein, L. I., and Vasconez, L. O.: Superselective embolization and surgery of non-involuting hemangiomas and AV malformations. Plast. Reconstr. Surg. 68:143, 1981.

Longacre, J. B., Benton, C., and Unterthiner, R. A.: Treatment of facial hemangioma by intravascular embolization with silicone spheres. Case report. Plast. Reconstr. Surg. 50:618, 1972.

Luessenhop, A. J., and Spence, W. T.: Artificial embolization of cerebral arteries: Report of use in a case of arteriovenous malformation. JAMA 172:1153, 1960.

Merland, J. J., Chiras, J., and Riché, M.D.: Arteriovenous malformations of the posterior wall of the thorax and abdomen. J. Neuroradiol. 6:221, 1979.

Merland, J. J., Tricot, J. F., Hadjean, E., Riché, M. C., and Enjolras, O.: Les malformations vasculaire cervico-céphaliques. Protocole actuel de traitement. A propos de 230 cas. Phlébologie 33:95, 1980.

Natali, J., and Merland, J. J.: Superselective arteriography and therapeutic embolisation for vascular malformations (angiodysplasias). J. Cardiovasc. Surg. *17*:465, 1976.

Olcott, C., Newton, T. H., Stoney, R. J., and Ehrenfeld, W. K.: Intra-arterial embolization in the management of arteriovenous malformations. Surgery *79*:3, 1976.

Phillip, J., and Schmid, A.: Chronishe Pankreatitis—Konservative versus operative Therapie unter prognostischen Aspekten. Fortschr. Med. *95*:1875, 1977.

Riché, M. C., Hadjean, E., Tricot, J. F., Henriquez, C., and Merland, J. J.: Les risques de la ligature de la carotide externe dans le traitement des angiodysplasies cervico-faciales. Ann. Oto-Laryng. (Paris) *97*:1, 3, 1980.

Riché, M. C., Modenesi-Freitas, J., Djindjian, M., and Merland, J. J.: Arteriovenous malformations (AVM) of the spinal cord in children. A review of 38 cases. Neuroradiology *22*:171, 1982.

Riché, M. C., Hadjean, E., Tran-Ba-Huy, P., and Merland, J. J.: The treatment of capillary-venous malformations using a new fibrosing agent. Plast. Reconstr. Surg. *71*:607, 1983.

Rosch, W., Phillip, J., and Gebhardt, C. H.: Endoscopic duct obstruction in chronic pancreatitis. Endoscopy *11*:43, 1979.

Schrudde, J., and Petrovici, V.: Surgical treatment of giant hemangioma of the facial region after arterial embolization. Plast. Reconstr. Surg. *68*:878, 1981.

Wolpert, S. M., and Stein, B. M.: Factors governing the course of emboli in the therapeutic embolization of cerebral arteriovenous malformations. Radiology *131*:125, 1979.

CHAPTER TWENTY-TWO

The Emotional Impact of a Vascular Birthmark

Alexandra M. Harrison

INTRODUCTION

In Hawthorne's *The Birthmark*, Aylmer says to his lovely young wife, "You came so nearly perfect from the hand of Nature that this slightest possible defect, which we hesitate whether to term a defect or a beauty, shocks me, as being the visible mark of earthly imperfection" (Hawthorne, 1846). Such references to cutaneous marks in literature and in legend testify to the impact of these blemishes on the bearer and on the viewer (Shaw, 1981). This discussion explores the ways in which vascular birthmarks affect psychosocial development and self-esteem.

Vascular birthmarks can be separated into two major categories, hemangiomas and malformations, which are distinguishable by clinical examination, natural history, and laboratory studies (Mulliken and Glowacki, 1982). Hemangiomas and vascular malformations have a different time course and prognosis. This temporal difference highlights the developmental framework used as a basis for understanding the emotional consequences of a vascular birthmark on the child and on the family.

GENERAL REMARKS ABOUT BIRTHMARKS

The factors that influence the effect of birthmarks on the patient's emotional life include location, type, size and contour, and parental and societal attitudes.

The location of the birthmark is critical. Facial birthmarks usually have a more devastating effect than blemishes of corresponding size and color on other parts of the body. It is particularly disturbing when there is deviance from an internal image of what a normal human face should look like. Infant observation studies demonstrate that babies have innate preferences for the visual configuration of the human face and develop a schema for what an average face should look like, probably within the first months of life (Stern, 1985). Cross-cultural studies show impressive consistency in the association of particular facial expressions with specific feelings such as happiness, fear, and sadness (Izard, 1971).

The type of vascular birthmark is relevant because of the differences in presentation and in natural history. A hemangioma typically appears after birth, rapidly increases in size, and then slowly involutes. The vascular malformation, on the other hand, is usually noted at birth and remains relatively unchanged, growing commensurately with the child.

The size and contour of the vascular anomaly are also important, not only because of the proportionate impact on physical appearance but also because of the manner in which body defects influence personality development. The more severe the disfigurement,

454

the more vigorous the psychological defenses that form to protect the person from the pain attached to having the defect. Heavy reliance on relatively primitive defenses, such as denial and avoidance, requires significant compromises in all areas of personality growth. Excessive use of denial can also affect satisfaction with treatment by impairing the patient's capacity for realistic assessment of therapeutic goals (Kalick et al., 1981).

The parents' response to their child's birthmark has a critical influence on the child's emotional adjustment to the blemish. The birth of a child with a disfiguring birthmark is a major challenge to the parents' self-esteem and to their capacity to parent. Irrational guilt and the tendency to focus on the child's vulnerabilities may cause the parents to be overprotective and distort their perceptions of the child's true strengths and weaknesses.

Societal attitudes to the blemish are another powerful factor. The social psychology literature on "deviance" emphasizes the deleterious effect on an individual of being singled out as different (Asch, 1951). There are also studies that demonstrate the strong effect physical appearance can have on people's estimation of a person's character. Pleasing physical appearance is associated with positive personality characteristics, whereas unpleasing physical appearance is associated with negative personality traits (Dion et al., 1972).

THE BIRTHMARK AND THE DEVELOPING CHILD

Each stage of personality development, from infancy through toddlerhood and the preschool period, into the school years, adolescence, and adulthood, carries with it a particular set of conflicts. The toddler years are characterized by conflicts surrounding the child's new awareness of himself as an individual and his need to establish himself as separate from his parents. Conflicts resulting from a somatic defect, and feelings about looking different from other people, may become confused with the developmental tasks. When this happens, successful resolution of either set of conflicts may become impossible. Family issues, such as marital conflict or depression in a parent, also influence the child's reaction to a vascular birthmark.

In order to promote effective problem solving, the various intermingled conflicts must be disentangled from one another. Certain aspects of child and family development critically influence how a birthmark affects the child's emotional life.

Infancy

All family members are affected by the birth of a child with a bodily defect. Each member tends to project his or her own feelings of vulnerability and imperfection onto the "defective child." Although these reactions begin in infancy, they will persist throughout the life of the birthmarked child. Parents feel tremendous guilt, as evidenced by their question, "What did I do wrong?" They struggle with this irrational guilt and with the fantasy that they are somehow to blame for their child's deformity (Mintzer et al., 1984). The mother may go through lists of foods eaten or medication taken during pregnancy, or the family tree may be scrutinized, searching for evidence of a similar defect. In folklore, the mother's witnessing a conflagration or the slaughter of animals, especially if she simultaneously touches her face, has been used to explain her child's birthmark. Likewise, the mother's craving for or overeating brightly colored foods such as strawberries has been linked with birthmarks. (See Chapter One for a discussion of "maternal impressions.")

For parents, childbirth carries restorative fantasies of "making good" what they consider "bad" or "wrong" about themselves. These fantasies of restoration are suddenly disappointed by the reality of a newborn with a defect. Solnit and Start (1961) discuss how parents of a deformed child find it difficult to deal with normal ambivalence of anger and disappointment about the loss of their anticipated "perfect child." Vascular malformations are present from birth and are usually obvious. In these cases, the typically happy, restorative birth experience is intruded upon by a visible bodily defect. In contrast, 70% of hemangiomas are not present at birth, whereas 30% may be seen only as a small, red spot (Mulliken and Glowacki, 1982). Parents of children with hemangiomas often describe a joyous birth experience, unaware of a problem. Their fantasy of giving birth to a "perfect" child seems to have come true, and their self-esteem is enhanced. However, as the hemangioma suddenly appears in the baby's skin, the parents feel as if their gift, the idealized "perfect child," has been taken away; they now have a fantasy of being punished. As the hemangioma grows daily during the first few months, the parents focus on the birthmark, which now has an out-of-control quality. Parents are particularly fearful when the hemangioma proliferates to involve the eyes, lips, or nose, or obstructs the upper airway. Necrosis and ulceration of a hemangioma cause further alarm. This anxiety is underscored by the folklore and superstition linking birthmarks with blood and violence.

During the first few months at home, a baby is usually introduced to the community. Display of normal offspring, in a sense, increases the self-esteem of family members. A vascular birthmark may interfere with this healthy exhibitionism. Parents describe their pain at being deprived of the pleasure of "showing off" their child, their distress at being unable to dress their baby in pretty clothes and take her for a walk without the fear of negative reactions from strangers. Here again, the normal developmental process of parenting is complicated by the presence of a vascular anomaly.

Toddlerhood

In the first 12–18 months of life, a child does not make the same discriminating observations about himself as he does in the period following. Age 18–24 months is the critical stage in the cognitive development of self-awareness. In this period, children first recognize a rouge spot placed on their nose when they look at themselves in a mirror (Lewis and Rosenblum, 1978). Also at this age, language develops, allowing the child to label objects. Now the child may first appear to notice the birthmark and may ask the parents about it, or begin to refer to the birthmark by a name. A child may indicate an awareness of looking different from the parents or from other children, begin to finger or manipulate the birthmark, or appear self-conscious in front of strangers. One mother of an unusually articulate preschool child reported that when her daughter was about 2 years old, she seemed to become aware of her facial hemangioma for the first

time. She touched her cheek and then touched her mother's cheek and asked, "Where's yours? Where's *your* oomangiu?" Another child at this same age suddenly became preoccupied with looking at her birthmark in the mirror and touching it, much to her parents' concern.

In addition to these important cognitive changes, 1½ to 2 year old children are attempting to move out into the world and explore their potential as autonomous beings. Because their capacity for independence is still precarious, they tend to be very sensitive to separation from parents and often become oppositional or clinging at bedtime, when leaving home, or when confronted with strangers.

If parents do not understand the developmental changes taking place, they may interpret the child's sudden attention to a birthmark as a function of the birthmark alone, and not see it in the context of increasing self-awareness. For example, a child's sudden shyness with strangers or fussiness about leaving home is a normal behavior and not a reaction to a birthmark. Distinguishing developmental conflicts from concerns about the birthmark allows parents to manage their child's behavior in a relaxed manner. It is a mistake to assume that the birthmark is "the problem" and that it must be quickly removed.

Preschool Period

In the preschool period, developmental conflicts about competition (girls with their mothers and boys with their fathers) eventually lead to an identification with the parent of the same gender. Before this resolution is achieved, the child struggles with feelings of inadequacy and inferiority in relation to his or her adult competitor. For example, the little girl feels like a "have-not" in comparison with her mother, who has many things she desires but cannot yet have, such as a husband, baby, or career. All bodily defects, including vascular birthmarks, seem to share the general feature of becoming a focus for feelings of badness and inferiority. When, for example, the little girl focuses on her birthmark as the reason she feels inferior to her mother, she may act sad or regress to babyish behavior. The same sorting of the two sets of conflicts, as described previously, can facilitate parental decisions about child rearing and about the birthmark and can also free the child to continue her developmental course (Harrison, 1983). This situation is illustrated by the following example:

Susan, a charming 4 year old girl, began sucking her thumb and pulling at her facial hemangioma shortly after making the transition from a small play group to a large nursery school. This behavior was unusual for Susan, who was a precocious child. In spite of her hemangioma, which presented a significant disfigurement during her toddler years, her parents had taken pains to fill her life with rich experiences in an extended community of neighborhood, church, and school. They were gratified to recognize signs of healthy self-esteem in their daughter. A brother was born when she was 3, and Susan seemed to accommodate herself well to her new rival. Her brother, however, became more mobile and more a real competitor after his first birthday. Several weeks after Susan started nursery school, the family took a trip to visit extended family in a distant state. During the visit, she said to her father, "Daddy, I don't think this hemangioma looks pretty on my face." Then, after seeing a dramatization of the Nativity, she said, "Could I be Mary? No, I think I couldn't be . . . because of this (indicating her hemangioma), and also because I'm so young." Her parents noted that the thumb sucking seemed to coincide with Susan's negative remarks about her hemangioma and her entrance into nursery school. Thus, they became concerned that the involuting hemangioma had suddenly become a focal problem for Susan. They asked her if she wanted to see the surgeon about having it removed. Susan said to the surgeon, "I want it off." Five minutes later, she said, "Well, maybe we should wait." Her confused parents consulted a child psychiatrist to help them make a decision about surgical excision.

In a play interview with Susan, the child psychiatrist noted several themes. First, there were conflicts about competition with people she loved and depended upon, especially her mother and brother. Second, she had fantasies that there was something bad or wrong with her. Finally, there were feelings of positive attachment to her hemangioma. The psychiatrist made sense of the play material and the parents' history in the following way.

Susan was struggling with developmental conflicts characteristic of girls her age. Competitive feelings toward her brother for her parents' love and toward her mother for her father's love came into conflict with her love for her mother and brother and caused her to feel like a bad girl. Conflicts about her hemangioma emerged from her positive feelings for it along with her realization that a beautiful Madonna does not have a facial blemish. Susan had confused the two sets of conflicts; she suspected that her birthmark, which distinguished her from the other child in the family and from her "Madonna" mother, was evidence of some badness or inferiority that made her the loser in both competitions. Temporarily overwhelmed by these intermingled conflicts, she regressed into a more infantile position and developed the symptoms of thumb sucking and separation anxiety. Because Susan had strong psychological defenses and was basically a healthy child, the interviewer suggested to the parents that they put off the issue of an operation and wait to see what happened. The evaluator also recommended postponing the excision because of Susan's fear that she might be punished for having angry wishes, and because of the tendency for children to imagine that the procedure might be a punishment for their sins.

The School-Aged Child

The school-aged child attempts to put some distance between himself and his family and concentrates on building competence at school and with friends. Stage-specific developmental conflicts focus on competence issues, such as separating from home and going to school and performing at academic and athletic tasks, and making and getting along with friends. Feelings about a birthmark may become mixed up with these developmental conflicts. For example, a child may believe that the birthmark is the reason he cannot make friends, or the reason he cannot do well at school. Sometimes it is difficult to sort out how much of the problem is related to the birthmark, and how much is a function of the child's lack of competence in peer relationships, particularly when a child complains that other children make fun of him because of his birthmark.

The Adolescent

The adolescent struggles with adult sexuality and with the need to separate from home and family in order to become independent. Mrs. R, a woman with a venous malformation on her face, described the distressing first emergence of her venous anomaly at age 12, when she entered puberty. The appearance of the vascular stain, compounded by a number of misdiagnoses and upsetting treatment encounters, presented a significant complication to her early experience of herself as a woman. Mrs. R recalled associating this time with a memory of a sign on the wall of the pediatric ward: "Handicapped Children are God's Special Children." Her remembrance of the sign reflects two characteristic defenses used to cope with the pain of the appearance of the vascular anomaly. One is regression from the adolescent position backward into childhood, as she made an identification with handicapped "children." The second is her taking in the association the sign connoted between "handicapped" and "special" as a means of turning something bad into something good. This gave the adolescent task of identity formation an unwelcome feature—the identity of "handicapped." In the same way, Mrs. R talked about the response of other people to her: "People look at the birthmark, not at you as a person." Another woman described the childhood experience of watching the eyes of the people she was talking to travel from her eyes to her facial birthmark, and sensing their loss of contact with her as a whole person.

Mrs. R talked of the complications introduced by her venous malformation when she attempted to master the adolescent task of separating from her parents and finding a peer group. She described her confused and angry rejection of her parents; she thought her parents were "ashamed" of her because of the vascular deformity. She said that the birthmark "affects your eye contact . . . makes you inhibited when you talk to people. . . . It makes you do obnoxious things when you're different. I said the stupidest things (to boys her age). It may be just due to being an adolescent, but you think it's because of your face. . . . If you go to a party dressed inappropriately, you're not going to have a good time at the party (but you think you had a bad time because your face made you different)."

The Young Adult

Mrs. R also spoke eloquently about how her vascular malformation influenced her adult development. "People would come up on the street and ask, 'What happened to your face?' You got numb. It's not something you can talk about very well unless you bring it up yourself. First you have to deal with other people's feelings, help other people with their feelings, before you can get any support yourself." Her skill at helping other people with their feelings contributed to her choice of nursing as a profession. Also, as she said, "People accept you as a nurse because you're nice to them, no matter what you look like." She also concluded that her choice of a passive, dependent man as a husband was influenced by her skill at taking care of others and her difficulty in asserting herself on behalf of her own needs.

Unhappily, when Mrs. R became pregnant with her first child, her vascular malformation began to enlarge secondary to the hormonal changes. "It's insulting to think that your body would pop up with this. You're supposed to enjoy becoming a woman and having a child. If something like this happens . . . it interferes with the pleasure." Tragically, Mrs. R had a stillbirth. Although the doctors told her there was no evidence that her facial anomaly caused this event, she remained feeling confused and responsible. "You feel real guilty about something like this. I felt I caused it. I was different and I must have done something bad." Although these words described feelings about her birthmark, it seemed that on an unconscious level the birthmark had become a metaphor for a more general sense of badness or defectiveness.

Another example of the impact of a vascular birthmark on the unconscious mind is the following case of a young woman with a port-wine stain type of malformation. Mrs. S joined a religious group whose special mission isolated members of the group from the outside world. She married within this community. She and her husband were identified strongly with the religious teachings of the group, for example, "Beauty is on the inside; it's what's inside that counts." This adjustment, successful in many ways, still required her to deny some of her own thoughts and feelings, and left her vulnerable to life challenges that might confront the hidden part of her mental life.

THE ASSOCIATION OF BIRTHMARKS WITH BADNESS AND FRIGHTENING FANTASIES

The symbolic power of a somatic defect derives, in part, from its association with wickedness or unacceptable feelings and fantasies. At a primitive cognitive level, an equation is made between good and beautiful versus bad and ugly. Literature is full of references to physical defects as symbols of evil (Shakespeare, *Richard III*; *Midrash*, 1939; Robbins, 1959). In Hawthorne's story *The Birthmark*, Georgiana's perfect beauty is marred for her husband by a vascular stain on her cheek in the shape of a tiny hand. As the story unfolds, it becomes clear that one of the "imperfections" the mark represents is the "animal instinct," that is, sexuality, which distinguishes mortals from heavenly beings. The theme of animality also appears in the biblical story of Cain, and in a Kipling story, "The Mark of the Beast," in which the desecration of a holy figure is associated with animality and guilt (*Midrash*, 1939; Kipling, 1918).

Thus, legend and fiction provide clues to our understanding of the fantasies people have about vascular birthmarks. The mother of a child with such a birthmark imagines having caused the defect by eating strawberries ("forbidden fruit") or by viewing a forbidden sight. Parents report stories of strangers in stores accusing them of beating their children. These brutal accusations demonstrate a lack of social judgment by the accusers. However, they probably also reveal primitive fantasies such as of uncontrolled aggression, which are closer to the consciousness of seriously disturbed people but which form part of everyone's psychological repertoire.

RECOMMENDATIONS TO PHYSICIANS

A physician confronts several dilemmas when consulted about a vascular birthmark. The primary question is: How does the birthmark itself affect the child's emotional growth? If the physician decides that the birthmark is indeed interfering with the child's healthy development, what should he recommend be done about the situation? Should he advise surgical intervention? Should he suggest a wait-and-see attitude?

Should he refer the family to another specialist? How can he take into account the parents' attitude toward the birthmark?

The physician should focus on one important question in the initial assessment: Does the presentation of the problem made by the patient and his family conform to the degree of objective deformity caused by the birthmark? If the vascular mark is minor but the patient expresses great concern, this discordance may be a clue that there are significant underlying emotional issues. What is the next step in sorting out the effect of the birthmark itself on the child's emotional state? In order to address these complicated questions, I have organized the symptoms that might reflect the emotional impact of a vascular birthmark on a child into a symptom hierarchy (Table 22–1). This scheme lists the symptoms of children with vascular birthmarks in terms of the relative likelihood that the symptom could be successfully managed by treating the birthmark per se.

Category I in the hierarchy includes the symptoms with the highest likelihood of improving with successful treatment of the birthmark. It includes those rare children who have a functional impairment caused by a vascular malformation, and the larger group of well adjusted children who have specific symptoms related to their birthmarks. In the first, "functional" set, a severe vascular anomaly may interfere with a baby's eating, sleeping, breathing, or vision. In adolescence, a severely disfiguring birthmark may make it very difficult for a child to make an adequate sexual adjustment. In these cases, appropriate treatment should focus on removing or diminishing the birthmark, to promote healthy psychological development. The second set, the group of otherwise healthy children who persist in complaining about a disfiguring birthmark, also belong in Category I. Self-consciousness or shame about a disfiguring birthmark interferes with the child's attempts to master developmentally appropriate tasks, such as becoming part of a peer group in the school-aged child and becoming attractive to the opposite sex in the adolescent. These symptoms are relatively specific to the effect of the birthmark and may be expected to ameliorate as the birthmark improves.

Category II symptoms include those that are more clearly multifactorial and not as easily related to the birthmark as those in Category I. They usually indicate greater

Table 22–1. SYMPTOM HIERARCHY FOR CHILDREN WITH VASCULAR BIRTHMARKS

Importance of Birthmark in Successful Treatment of Symptoms	Symptoms	Recommendation
Category I Handicapped child: Birthmark causes functional interference with basic needs *or* Healthy child: *Specific* problems with self-esteem related to objectively disfiguring birthmark	1. Infancy: Problems with eating, sleeping, breathing, vision, or activity 2. Toddler: Problems with talking, walking 3. School age: Problems with school attendance socialization, learning 4. Adolescence: Problems with sexual behavior, independence; fear of rejection by opposite sex because of birthmark 5. Child persistently complains about birthmark in words or actions (hiding, hitting birthmark) 6. Afraid to try new situations because of birthmark	Focus on treatment of birthmark
Category II Poorly adjusted child: *Non-specific* problems related to birthmark	1. Fears: shy, clinging behavior 2. Excessive struggles 3. Overly shy or overly aggressive 4. Learning problems 5. Testing limits 6. Adolescent problems with sex, drugs, alcohol 7. Sleeping disorder 8. Eating disorder 9. Elimination problems (enuresis, encopresis, etc.) 10. Depression 11. Inconsistent complaints about birthmark	Psychiatric evaluation, then focus on treatment of *either* birthmark *or* emotional problems
Category III Severely disturbed child	1. Extreme fears 2. Severe learning problems 3. School refusal, truancy (chronic) 4. Delinquent behavior 5. Deviant sexual behavior 6. Serious depression 7. Psychosis	Focus on treatment of emotional disorder

emotional disturbance that probably would not go away, even if the birthmark disappeared. In this category, I have placed inconsistent complaints about the birthmark, under the assumption that ambivalent feelings about it indicate something different from dislike. These symptoms and inconsistent complaints do not suggest greater emotional disturbance in the child.

Category III is made up of symptoms of pervasive developmental disturbance, which may or may not be related to the birthmark but which would definitely not be expected to improve significantly if the birthmark were to disappear.

The complexity of the issues involved in

the decision of whether or not to attempt a surgical excision of a vascular birthmark lends itself to a "best case–worst case" approach rather than to a set of specific directives. In general, however, the "best case" will be that in which the symptoms are in Category I, and the "worst case" includes all those symptoms in Category III.

Example 1: "Best Case." An adolescent, who is a successful student and is well liked by her peers, consistently complains that boys will not give her a chance because of the disfiguring vascular birthmark on her face. She says she knows that if a boy would make an effort to look beyond her birthmark and get to know her as a person, he would find the effort worthwhile. She is anxious about going out on dates and having sexual relationships, and says she is "retarded" compared with her girl friends. Her parents admit they are a little overprotective of their daughter because they don't want her to get hurt. They acknowledge the degree of her deformity, but say that she is a beautiful person. Both child and parents are in agreement about desiring surgical excision if it is possible.

Example 2: "Worst Case." A preschool child is brought to the surgeon by her parents, who request excision of a large facial vascular birthmark. The parents explain that the child has been anxious and fearful since infancy because of the negative reactions of people to the birthmark. When the child was a few months old, the parents were told by their pediatrician that the birthmark could be removed before she went to school. Now they are reluctant to let her attend nursery school because they fear it would be traumatic to her. In fact, they rarely take her out at all because they cannot bear to see her unhappy, and because she has had to bear so much pain already.

It is clear that most cases will fall somewhere between these two examples. However, the general principles of specific conflict about the birthmark in the midst of an otherwise reasonably healthy development, contrasted with a troubled development complicated by the birthmark, may be applied to intermediate cases. This is not to say that a patient with generally disturbed development might not benefit from amelioration of the birthmark, but only that symptomatic improvement cannot be assured in these cases and that postoperative courses in these patients can be expected to be rocky and unpredictable. In these complicated cases, the physician may wish to recommend psychiatric consultation in order to clarify the emotional impact of the birthmark. With any patient for whom surgical intervention is being considered, a psychiatric consultation may provide valuable data to the physician making the recommendation.

SUMMARY

Vascular birthmarks can cause serious emotional problems in the developing child and adult. A birthmark is a life stress, having a stage-specific influence on the child and his or her family. In this context, the concept of an association between bad and ugly is pertinent to understanding the psychology of birthmarks. There are special characteristics for the various types of vascular birthmarks. Central to the issue is the basic concept of imperfection in relation to the parent-child relationship. In a sense, parents of children with a visible birthmark are challenged to a degree beyond the universal challenge of parenthood: They must love a child who has a defect. In Hawthorne's story, Alymer could not tolerate Georgiana's imperfection, and in his attempt to eradicate her birthmark he "rejected the best the earth could offer" and killed his wife with the same magic potion that erased the birthmark. Parents of children with vascular birthmarks will sometimes make a comment such as, "I forget about the birthmark until I see a stranger's reaction to it. To me, she is just my Nancy, and she is beautiful." In making such a comment, the parent is not denying the birthmark, but he has clearly taken back projections of his own feelings of defectiveness and is able to see his child as a complicated person in her own right, and to love her. In struggling successfully with this challenge, parents of children with birthmarks provide an inspiration to all of us.

References

Asch, S. E.: Effects of group pressure upon the modification and distortion of judgment. In Guetzkow, H. (ed.): *Groups, Leadership, and Men.* Pittsburgh: Carnegie Institute Press, 1951.

Dion, K. K., Berscheid, E. L., and Walster, E.: What is beautiful is good. J. Pers. Soc. Psychol. 24:285, 1972.

Harrison, A. M.: Body image and self esteem. In Ablon, S. L., and Mack, J. E. *The Development and Sustaining of Self-Esteem in Childhood.* New York: International Universities Press, Inc., 1983, p. 90.

Hawthorne, N.: The Birthmark. In *Mosses from an Old Manse.* New York: Wiley and Putnam, 1846, p. 32.

Izard, C. E.: *The Face of Emotion.* New York: Appleton-Century-Crofts, 1971.

Kalick, S. M., Goldwyn, R. M., and Noe, J. M.: Social issues and body image concerns of port wine stain patients undergoing laser therapy. Lasers in Surgery and Medicine 1:205, 1981.

Kipling, R.: *The Mark of the Beast and the Head of the District.* Girard, KS: Haldeman-Julius Co., in Collected Stories. New York: Little Leather Library Corp., 1918.

Lewis, M., and Rosenblum, L. A. (ed.): *The Development of Affect.* New York: Plenum Press, 1978, p. 220.

Midrash, ibid., on the story of the curse of Cain. *Midrash,* vol. Genesis, on the story of the mark of Cain. London: Soncino Press, 1939.

Mintzer, D., Als, H., Tronick, E. Z., and Brazelton, T. B.: Parenting an infant with a birth defect: The regulation of self esteem. Psychoan. Stud. Child. *39*:561, 1984.

Mulliken, J. B., and Glowacki, J.: Hemangiomas and vascular malformations in infants and children: A classification based on endothelial characteristics. Plast. Reconstr. Surg. *69*:412, 1982.

Robbins, R. H.: *The Encyclopedia of Witchcraft and Demonology.* New York: Crown Pub., 1959.

Shakespeare, W.: *Richard III.*

Shaw, W. C.: Folklore surrounding facial deformity and the origins of facial prejudice. Brit. J. Plast. Surg. *34*:237, 1981.

Solnit, A. J., and Start, M. H.: Mourning and the birth of a defective child. Psychoanal. Stud. Child. *16*:523, 1961.

Stern, D.: *The Interpersonal World of the Infant.* New York: Basic Books, Inc., 1985.

Glossary

Herein is a brief lexicon of vascular anomalies. Some of the terms are incorrect, outmoded, or uncommon; yet all words deserve consideration even if some should be discarded on the basis of present knowledge. This section also offers a translation of old terms and eponyms into current nomenclature.

Anastomotic Aneurysm: Circumscribed arteriovenous malformation with visible, prominent vessels. *Syn*. Aneurysm by anastomosis (Bell), arteriovenous aneurysm.

Anderson-Fabry Disease: *Syn*. Fabry disease.

Aneurysmal Varix (Varix Aneurysmaticus): Circumscribed venous ectasia with dilatation. *Syn*. Varicose wen of Petit, "phlebangioma."

Aneurysm Racemosum: Circumscribed arteriovenous malformation. *Syn*. Cirsoid aneurysm, angioma racemosum of Virchow.

Angel's Kiss: *Syn*. *Naevus flammeus nuchae*, "stork bite," salmon patch.

Angiectoid Nevus: A cutaneous vascular malformation of unspecified type.

Angiodysontogenesia: Term used by Malan to indicate a vascular malformation consisting primarily of anomalous vessels rather than a solid mass of tissue.

Angiodysplasia: Any congenital vascular abnormality. Used by Malan to specify a malformation retaining the capacity for growth by cellular proliferation.

Angioendothelioma: Acquired vascular tumor of intermediate malignancy.

Angiokeratoma Circumscriptum: Hyperkeratotic vascular lesions, appearing over trunk and lower extremities. Confusing term, referring to localized form of Fabry disease or capillary-lymphatic vascular malformation.

Angiokeratoma Corporis Diffusum (Universale): *Syn*. Fabry disease, *vide infra*.

Angiokeratoma of Fordyce: Degenerative ectatic vascular lesion of the adult scrotal skin.

Angiokeratoma of Mibelli: Telangiectasias progressing to hemorrhagic papules over hands and feet of adolescent females. *Syn. Naevus a pernione*.

Angiolymphoid Hyperplasia: A vascular tumor, with eosinophilia, of adults sometimes known as "epithelioid hemangioma" or Kimura disease.

Angioma: Loosely used term to indicate any circumscribed vascular lesion. Should be restricted to those with a potential for growth by cellular multiplication.

Angioma Cavernosum (of Virchow): Circumscribed arteriovenous or venous malformation with large channels. Outdated histopathological term.

Angioma Racemosum (of Virchow): Vascular malformation consisting of markedly dilated interconnecting vessels. Outdated pathologically based term. Includes arteriovenous malformations.

Angioma Serpiginosum (of Hutchinson): Acquired extensive punctate telangiectasias in gyrate or serpiginous pattern in abnormally pink skin. *Syn*. Generalized essential telangiectasia.

Angioma Simplex (of Virchow): Vascular lesion consisting predominantly of capillaries usually applied to hemangioma of infancy. Outdated pathologically based term.

Angiomatosis Osteohypotrophica: Multiple circumscribed vascular malformations associated with underdevelopment of bone.

Angio-Osteohypertrophy Syndrome: Association of congenital vascular malformation(s) with limb hypertrophy and a cutaneous capillary nevus. Unhelpful composite term embracing Klippel-Trenaunay and Parkes Weber syndromes.

Angiosarcoma Multiplex: *Syn*. Kaposi's sarcoma.

Arterial Angioma: Circumscribed arteriovenous malformation.

Arterial Cavernous Angioma: Circumscribed arteriovenous malformation.

Arterial Racemose Angioma: Circumscribed arteriovenous malformation.

Arteriovenous Aneurysm: Circumscribed arteriovenous malformation with visible, enlarged vessels.

Arteriovenous Angioma: Inexact term usually meaning a well-localized arteriovenous malformation.

Arteriovenous Fistula: Identifiable, single abnormal communication between an artery and a vein bypassing the capillary bed. Congenital or acquired.

Arteriovenous Malformation: Any vascular maldevelopment characterized by the presence of abnormal channels joining the arterial circulation to the venous without the interposition of a normal capillary bed. Usually characterized by high flow.

Arteriovenous Shunt: Any communication between the arterial and venous systems bypassing the capillary bed. Includes anatomically normal structures such as Sucquet-Hoyer channels.

Ataxia Telangiectasia: Autosomal recessive inherited telangiectasias of the face, conjunctivae, and sometimes the extremities associated with ataxia (CNS degeneration) and immunoparesis. *Syn.* Louis-Bar syndrome.

Bannayan Syndrome: Macrocephaly with subcutaneous lipomas and vascular malformations. Partly subsumed by the term "Proteus syndrome."

Barker-Kausch Syndrome: Diffuse venous malformation confined to the rectum and perirectal tissues.

Bean Syndrome: *Syn.* Blue rubber bleb nevus syndrome.

Beckwith-Wiedemann Syndrome: Transient midfacial dermal stain associated with macroglossia, umbilical defects, and cellular abnormalities of pancreas, liver, and kidneys.

Bell's Anastomotic Aneurysm: *Syn.* Arteriovenous malformation.

Berenbruch-Cushing-Cobb Syndrome: *Syn.* Cobb syndrome, *vide infra.*

Bloom Syndrome: Cutaneous photosensitivity, telangiectases, malar hypoplasia, and stunted growth.

Blue Angioma (of Broca): Circumscribed venous malformation.

Blue Rubber Bleb Nevus Syndrome: Multiple circumscribed venous malformations of skin and viscera. Associated with gastrointestinal bleeding. May be familial.

Boder-Sedgwick Syndrome: *Syn.* Ataxia telangiectasia, Louis-Bar syndrome.

Bonnet-Dechaume-Blanc Syndrome: Telangiectatic facial nevus associated with a retinal and intracranial vascular malformation, especially around the mesencephalon. *Syn.* Wyburn-Mason syndrome in the British medical literature.

Brushfield-Wyatt Syndrome: Cutaneous capillary malformation in the "trigeminal" area associated with a calcified cerebral cortex and vascular malformations.

Capillary Angioma: Inexact term. Has been used synonymously with "strawberry" hemangioma, "port-wine" capillary malformation, and *naevus flammeus.*

Capillary-Cavernous Hemangioma: Confusing term embracing true hemangioma of infancy involving upper and deep dermis and subcutaneous tissues. In other patients, applied to venous malformation.

Cavernous Hemangioma: Confusing term sometimes referring to non-involuting, bulky venous malformation; sometimes referring to deep, involuting, true hemangioma.

Caviare Tongue: Venous or lymphatic malformation of the tongue or buccal mucosa in the form of multiple small blebs.

Chylous Reflux: Pathological condition: reflux of chyle into incompetent distal lymphatics, usually of pelvis, genitalia, or limbs.

Cirsoid Aneurysm (Tumor Circoideus) (Aneurysma Circoideus): Circumscribed arteriovenous malformation with visible prominent vessels.

Cobb Syndrome: Association of verrucous or port-wine capillary malformations of skin (sometimes with café au lait patches and ipsilateral hypertrophy) with a vascular malformation of the spinal cord adjacent to the cutaneous malformation. *Syn.* "Cutaneomeningospinal angiomatosis."

Cockett Syndrome: *Syn.* Iliac compression syndrome.

Congenital Avalvulosis: Rare condition. Absence of most or all venous valves.

Congenital Livedo: *Syn.* Cutis marmorata.

Congenital Varicose Veins: Unhelpful term used loosely to include all varicose veins presenting in infancy and childhood. Includes embryological venous remnants and varices developing as a result of obstruction or malfunction or secondary to arteriovenous malformation.

Cutaneomeningospinal Angiomatosis: *Syn.* Cobb syndrome, *vide supra.*

Cutis Marmorata Telangiectatica Congenita: Literally means "marbled skin." Widespread diffuse ectasia of cutaneous venules and capillaries. *Syn.* Van Lohuizen syndrome.

Cystic Hygroma: A predominantly cystic lymphatic malformation occurring at the root of the neck.

Disappearing Bone Disease: *Syn.* Gorham syndrome, *vide infra.*

Divry–Van Bogaert Syndrome: Association of cutis marmorata, cerebral vascular malformations in absence of intracranial calcification, mental retardation, and spasticity.

Dysplastic Venopathy: *Syn.* Venous dysplasia. Unhelpful term encompassing all congenital maldevelopments of veins, including primary varicosis, ectasias, hypoplasias, and atresias.

Ectasia: Congenital dilatation of a vessel, e.g., arteriectasia, phlebectasia, lymphangiectasia.

Elephantiasis Congenita Angiomatosa: Co-existence of lymphedema and diffuse vascular malformation in a limb.

Elephantiasis Telangiectodes: Gross enlargement of a limb by a vascular malformation, with or without lymphedema.

Encephalotrigeminal Angiomatosis: *Syn.* Sturge-Weber syndrome.

Epithelioid Hemangioma: Angiolymphoid hyperplasia with eosinophilia. *Syn.* Histiocytoid hemangioma, Kimura disease.

Esau-Bensaude Malformation: Diffuse cavernous venous malformation of rectum and perineum, sometimes also involving the ureterovesical mucosa.

Fabry Disease: *Syn.* Angiokeratoma corporis diffusum universale, Anderson-Fabry syndrome, a sex-linked recessive disorder of sphingolipid metabolism presenting with hemorrhagic skin vesicles.

Foix-Alajouanine Syndrome: Intra- and extramedullary vascular malformations in spinal cord with enlargement in caliber and thickness of the vessels and varicose postspinal vein. Often leads to paraplegia.

Fungus Hematodes: Old descriptive term for a cutaneous vascular malformation of venous or arteriovenous type.

Giant Limb: Abnormally large limb, the enlargement involving all tissues. Used in the sense of congenital macrosomia, not hypertrophy. Can be proportionate or disproportionate.

Giant Limb of Robertson: Giant limb associated with diffuse arteriovenous malformation. Almost synonymous with Parkes Weber syndrome.

Gigantism (Local): Gross or malproportioned overgrowth of part of the body, most commonly a digit or digits.

Gorham Syndrome (Gorham-Stout Syndrome): Multiple areas of osteolysis that are probably due to intraosseous vascular anomalies (usually venous). *Syn.* Disappearing bone disease, phantom bone disease, Trinquoste syndrome, or (when involving the arm) "hemangiomatosis braquial osteolytica of Martorell." See also *Haferkamp Syndrome.*

Haferkamp Syndrome: Severe and generalized form of Gorham syndrome. It is additionally characterized by malignant vascular proliferation, lipid dysmetabolism, fatty degeneration, atherosclerosis, and anemia.

Hamartia: Malformed tissue (from Greek *hamartīa*, to sin, to err).

Hamartoma (of Albrecht): A lesion of developmental origin with the capacity for benign cellular proliferation. Requires the presence of two or more tissue types.

Hamartoma Angiomateux Sudoripor Secretant (of Vilanova): *Syn.* Sudiparous angioma (*vide infra*).

Hemangiectasia Hypertrophicans: *Syn.* Klippel-Trenaunay syndrome and Parkes Weber syndrome.

Hemangiectatic Hemihypertrophy: Term used by Parkes Weber to describe his syndrome. Subsequently misused to include other conditions with association of a vascular malformation and over-growth.

Hemangioendothelioblastoma: Malignant acquired vascular tumor.

Hemangioendothelioma: An acquired vascular tumor, the term "benign hemangioendothelioma" has been used synonymously for the common hemangioma of infancy; both cutaneous and visceral locations.

Hemangioma: Generic term used to describe a wide variety of vascular lesions both congenital and acquired and of different etiologies and natural history.

Hemangiomatosis: Generalized, miliary, or multiple cutaneous and visceral hemangiomas of infancy. Unfortunately, has often been applied to extensive vascular malformations. Does *not* indicate presence or potential malignant change or metastasis.

Hemangiomatosis of Jaffe: *Syn.* Blue rubber bleb nevus syndrome.

Hemangiopericytoma: Acquired tumor of vascular pericytes. Benign or malignant.

Hematoncus: Localized vascular birthmark. Antique term used by Alibert, subdivided into *Haematoncus fongoïdes* (mushroom-like), *Haematoncus framboesia* (raspberry-like), and *Haematoncus tuberosus* (potato-like).

Hemolymphangioma: Congenital cutaneous or deep vascular malformation containing combined lymphatic and blood vascular elements. *Syn.* "Elephantiasis congenita angiomatosa," if extensive.

Hemorrhagic Sarcoma: *Syn.* Kaposi's sarcoma.

Hereditary Hemorrhagic Telangiectasia: Telangiectases of skin and mucous membranes associated with recurrent bleeding. Familial. *Syn.* Rendu-Osler-Weber syndrome, Babington syndrome, and Goldstein syndrome.

Hypertrophic Angioma: Old term, unfortunately used synonymously for angiokeratoma and sometimes for the entirely different common hemangioma of infancy.

Hypertrophic Naevus Flammeus: Hypertrophic form of congenital capillary-lymphatic malformation. *Syn.* "Verrucous hemangioma."

Iliac Vein Compression Syndrome: Congenital obstruction of common iliac vein (usually left) by superimposed iliac artery, leading to swelling of leg and venous claudication. *Syn.* Cockett syndrome.

Infantile Angioectatic Hypertrophy Syndrome: Association of congenital vascular malformation(s) with limb overgrowth and a cutaneous capillary nevus. An unhelpful composite term. Includes Klippel-Trenaunay syndrome and Parkes Weber syndrome.

Jahnkhe Syndrome: Sturge-Weber syndrome without ocular involvement.

Juvenile Angioma: *Syn.* "Strawberry" hemangioma.

Kaijser Syndrome: Generalized intestinal involvement by venous-lymphatic malformations.

Kasabach-Merritt Syndrome: Association of thrombocytopenic purpura with large or extensive hemangiomas.

Kast Syndrome: *Syn.* Maffucci syndrome.

Klippel-Trenaunay Syndrome: Association of congenital varicose veins with a cutaneous capillary malformation and limb hypertrophy. *Syn.* Hemangiectasia hypertrophicans, osteohypertrophic naevus flammeus, naevus verrucosus hypertrophicans (see *Klippel-Trenaunay-Weber syndrome*).

Klippel-Trenaunay-Weber Syndrome: Mixing together of Klippel-Trenaunay syndrome and Parkes Weber syndrome to form an unhelpful composite term indicating the association of congenital vascular malformation(s) with limb hypertrophy and a cutaneous capillary nevus but failing to consider the presence or absence of clinically important arteriovenous fistulae. Synonymous with angioosteohypertrophy syndrome and infantile angioectatic hypertrophy.

Klippel-Trenaunay-Weber-Rubashov Syndrome: *Syn.* Klippel-Trenaunay-Weber syndrome (in Russian literature).

Lateral Venous Anomaly: Persistent postaxial embryonic vein in lower limb. Usually seen as part of Klippel-Trenaunay syndrome. Sometimes known as vein of Servelle.

Lawford Syndrome: Facial capillary malformation with glaucoma but without enlargement of the globe.

Lithogenic Phlebangiomatosis: *Syn.* Gorham syndrome, *vide supra*.

Livedo Reticularis: Adult equivalent of infantile cutis marmorata. Accentuated pattern of dermal venules.

Louis-Bar Syndrome: Telangiectasias of face, head, conjunctivae, and sometimes extremities associated with degeneration of parts of the central and peripheral nervous system leading to ataxia. There may be associated immunologic deficiency. Neoplasms such as gliomas may develop. *Syn.* Ataxia telangiectasia Type I, Boder-Sedgwick syndrome.

Lymphangiectasis: Dilatation of a lymph vessel.

Lymphangiohemangioma: *Syn.* "Hemolymphangioma." Outdated term for a combined venous and lymphatic vascular malformation.

Lymphangioma: Inaccurate term for a lymphatic malformation. May be diffuse or localized. Finds most common usage in term "lymphangioma circumscriptum."

Lymphangioma Circumscriptum: Apparently localized area of micromulticystic lymphatic malformation. Because the lesion may be more widespread than it appears, it has been referred to as a "lymphangioma diffusum" by Kinmonth.

Lymphangioma Simplex: Cutaneous lymphatic blebs; distinct from "lymphangioma cavernosum," which is a deep cystic lymphatic anomaly.

Lymphatic Hyperplasia: Lymphatic vessels and/or lymph nodes that are larger and/or more numerous than normal.

Lymphatic Hypoplasia: Lymphatic vessels and/or lymph nodes that are smaller and /or less numerous than normal.

Lymphatic Vesicle: Intradermal lymph cyst or blister.

Macula Materna, Macula Matricis: Old terms for a vascular birthmark.

Maffucci Syndrome: Dyschondroplasia of a limb or limbs, with enchondromas, associated with a vascular malformation (usually venous and venous-lymphatic). *Syn.* Maffucci-Kast syndrome, Kast syndrome, Ollier-Klippel syndrome.

Martorell-Servelle Syndrome: Anomalous, ectatic, superficial veins associated with obstructed, plastic, or atretic deep veins. Partly encompassed by Klippel-Trenaunay syndrome.

Miliary Hemangiomata of the Newborn: Multiple hemangiomas in various tissues, present at birth. *Syn.* Generalized hemangiomatosis and, erroneously, "disseminated hemangiomatosis."

Milles Syndrome: Sturge-Weber syndrome with choroidal involvement but no glaucoma.

Mixed Vascular Malformation: Congenital vascular malformation involving two or more elements of the vascular system: capillaries, arteries, veins, and lymphatics. *Syn.* Mixed vascular deformity, "Hemolymphatic angiodysplasia."

Naevus a Pernione: *Syn.* Angiokeratoma of Mibelli.

Naevus Anaemicus: Congenital anomaly of cutaneous capillaries, blotchy areas of pallor being interspersed in pink skin.

Naevus Angiomatodes: Extensive subcutaneous vascular malformation.

Naevus Arachnoideus: "Spider" nevus. Rarely seen during infancy; usually develops between ages 6 and 10.

Naevus Araneus: *Syn.* "Spider nevus."

Naevus Flammeus: *Syn.* Port-wine stain.

Naevus Flammeus Nuchae: Self-limiting dermal vascular ectasia involving nape of neck. Same lesion as is commonly seen on eyelids and glabella in neonates.

Naevus Maternus: Any vascular birthmark, but usually refers to "strawberry" hemangioma in old medical literature.

Naevus Sanguineus: Synonym for hemangioma.

Naevus Vascularis Reticularis: *Syn.* Cutis marmorata.

Naevus Vasculosus Osteohypertrophicus: *Syn.* Klippel-Trenaunay syndrome.

Naevus Venosus: Circumscribed, superficial, venous malformation.

Naevus Verrucosus Hypertrophicans: *Syn.* Klippel-Trenaunay syndrome.

Nape Nevus: Capillary malformation on nape of neck. *Syn.* "Stork" mark.

Nevus (British and Latin—Naevus): Any birthmark. Often used synonymously for a capillary vascular malformation.

Osteohypertrophic Naevus Flammeus: *Syn.* Klippel-Trenaunay syndrome.

Osteovascular Dysplasia: *Syn.* Gorham syndrome.

Paine-Efron Syndrome: Ataxia and telangiectasia developing in late childhood. *Syn.* Ataxia telangiectasia Type II.

Parkes Weber Syndrome: Concurrence of

multiple congenital arteriovenous fistulae and an enlarged limb.

Perithelioma Multiplex: *Syn.* Kaposi's sarcoma.

Phacomatosis: Term introduced by Van der Hoeve in 1932 to describe combined neuroectodermal malformations, including Sturge-Weber syndrome, tuberous sclerosis, and von Recklinghausen's neurofibromatosis.

Phantom Bone Disease: *Syn.* Gorham syndrome.

Phlebangiectasia: Venous ectasia.

Phlebangioma: Circumscribed venous malformation. *Syn.* Varicose hemangioma, varicose aneurysm, varicose angiocavernoma, venous racemose angioma, blue angioma of Broca.

Phlebarteriectasis (of Bockenheimer): Congenital ectasia of arteries and veins without the presence of arteriovenous fistulae.

Poikiloderma Congenitale: *Syn.* Rothmund-Thomson syndrome, *vide infra.*

Proteus Syndrome: Partial gigantism of hands or feet (usually bilateral and asymmetrical); macrocephaly, skull exostoses, lipomas, hemihypertrophy, and vascular malformations (typically diffuse patchy dermal staining). Probably subsumes Riley-Smith and Bannayan syndrome.

Pseudo-Kaposi's Sarcoma: Angiodermatitis associated with arteriovenous malformation clinically and histologically mimicking Kaposi's sarcoma.

Pulsatile Fungus Hematodes: Old term for localized arteriovenous malformation.

Pulsating Angioma: Circumscribed arteriovenous malformation.

Purpura Hemorrhagica Nodularis: *Syn.* Kaposi's sarcoma.

Racemose Angioma (of Virchow): Circumscribed arteriovenous malformation.

Rankenangioma: Synonym of cirsoid aneurysm. (From German *ranken*, to grow with tendrils.)

Red Angioma (of Broca): Circumscribed arteriovenous malformation.

Rendu-Osler-Weber Syndrome: Hereditary hemorrhagic telangiectasia.

Riley-Smith Syndrome: Capillary and/or venous malformations associated with lymphatic anomalies, chylous cysts, macrodactyly macrocephaly, and pseudopapilledema. Probably part of Proteus syndrome.

Roberts Syndrome: Midfacial capillary stain associated with low birth weight, microbrachycephaly, hypertelorbitism, exorbitism, thin nares, cleft palate, malformed ears, micrognathia, sparse blonde hair, hypomelia, cryptorchidism, and mental deficiency. Autosomal recessive. *Syn.* Appelt-Gerken-Lenz syndrome, pseudothalidomide or SC syndrome, hypomelia-hypotrichosis-facial "hemangioma" syndrome.

Rothmund-Thomson Syndrome: Diffuse, red reticulation of skin associated with short stature, cataracts, sparse or absent eyebrows and lashes, photosensitivity, etc. Recessive inheritance. *Syn.* "Poikiloderma congenitale."

Rubinstein-Taybi Syndrome: Capillary stain of forehead associated with broad thumbs and great toes and with mental retardation. Typical facies.

Salmon Patch: Pink cutaneous capillary mark that predictably fades during infancy.

Sarcoma Nodulosum Cavernosum: *Syn.* Kaposi's sarcoma.

Schirmer Syndrome: Facial capillary malformation with early glaucoma and buphthalmos. Synonymous with Sturge-Weber syndrome.

Sclerosing Hemangioma: *Syn.* Dermatofibroma and fibrous histiocytoma. An acquired skin tumor.

Serpentine Aneurysm: Arteriovenous malformation.

Servelle Aneurysm: *Syn.* Martorell-Servelle syndrome.

Servelle Vein: *Syn.* Lateral venous anomaly in lower limb.

Simple Angioma: *Syn.* "Strawberry" hemangioma.

Stellate Nevus: *Syn.* Spider nevus.

Stigma Metrocelis: Old term for vascular birthmark.

Storino-Engel Syndrome: "Capillary hemangiomatosis," *vide supra.*

Stork Mark: Self-limiting dermal vascular ectasia involving nape of neck.

Strawberry Nevus: Superficial hemangioma with fruit-like appearance.

Sturge-Weber Syndrome: Facial capillary malformation in first or second trigeminal nerve territory associated with ipsilateral vascular malformations over cerebral cortex and ocular vascular anomalies. Sometimes known as Sturge-

Weber-Krabbe, Kalischer, Cushing, or Dimitri syndrome; also known as Jahnke, Lawford, or Schirmer syndrome.

Sudoriparous Angioma: Blue vascular malformation that sweats profusely when touched.

Telangiectatica Congenita: *Syn.* Cutis marmorata.

Trinquoste Syndrome: *Syn.* Gorham syndrome.

Troncular: Adjective used in publications by Italian authors, meaning "related to main vessels," i.e., fistulae from or dysplasias of; translates into English as "truncal."

True Diffuse Phlebectasia (of Bockenheimer): Generalized venous dilatation not secondary to arteriovenous malformation.

Ullmann's Universal Angiomatosis: Catch-all term for systematized vascular malformations. Not in general use.

Unna's Nevus: Capillary stain on nape of neck. Persistent form of *naevus flammeus nuchae*. *Syn.* Erythema nuchae.

Van Lohuizen Syndrome: *Syn.* Cutis marmorata telangiectatica congenita.

Varicose Aneurysm: Circumscribed arteriovenous malformation.

Varicose Dysplasia: Term used by Schobinger to indicate condition of early appearing "banal" varicose veins associated with a vascular birthmark on the affected limb.

Varicose Hemangioma: Circumscribed venous malformation.

Varicosis Praecox: Idiopathic, "adult" type varicose veins appearing in childhood.

Vascular Neurocutaneous Syndromes: Congenital lesions of central nervous system associated with vascular anomalies in the skin.

Venous Angiocavernoma: Circumscribed venous malformation.

Venous Cavernous Angiectasia: Diffuse ectatic venous malformation.

Venous Dysplasia: Includes all congenital malformation of veins, such as hyperplasias, ectasias, hypoplasias, and atresias. *Syn.* Dysplastic venopathy.

Venous Racemose Angioma: Circumscribed venous malformation.

Venous Spur (of May and Thurner): Congenital anomaly partly obstructing left common iliac vein; part of iliac compression syndrome.

Verrucous Hemangioma: Congenital form of hypertrophic vascular staining; a cutaneous, capillary-lymphatic malformation. *Syn.* Hypertrophic naevus flammeus.

von Hippel–Lindau Syndrome: Benign cerebellar tumor and cyst; about 20 per cent of cases also have retinal lesions, also associated cysts of pancreas and vascular tumors of liver and kidney.

Wyburn-Mason Syndrome: *Syn.* Bonnet-Dechaume-Blanc syndrome.

Index

Note: Page numbers in *italics* indicate illustrations; page numbers followed by t indicate tables.

471